MEL

Diagnostic Imaging

Softcover Edition

Editors:
A. L. Baert, Leuven
K. Sartor, Heidelberg

Springer
Berlin
Heidelberg
New York
Barcelona
Hong Kong
London
Milan
Paris
Tokyo

H. Carty (Ed.)

Emergency Pediatric Radiology

With Contributions by

L. J. Abernethy · R. E. Appleton · A. W. Duncan · D. Grier · K. E. Halliday
A. S. Hollman · S. J. King · S. Macdonald · C. W. Majury · W. Ramsden · P. Rao
J. M. Somers · L. E. Sweeney · N. B. Wright · R. E. R. Wright

Foreword by
A. L. Baert

With 477 Figures in 710 Separate Illustrations and 74 Tables

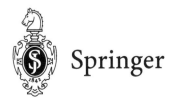

Springer

HELEN CARTY, MB
Professor of Paediatric Radiology
Alder Hey Children's Hospital
Eaton Road
Liverpool L 12 2AP
United Kingdom

MEDICAL RADIOLOGY · Diagnostic Imaging and Radiation Oncology

Continuation of
Handbuch der medizinischen Radiologie
Encyclopedia of Medical Radiology

ISBN 3-540-42292-7 Springer-Verlag Berlin Heidelberg New York

Library of Congress Cataloging-in-Publication Data. Emergency pediatric radiology / ed., H. Carty; with contributions by L. Abernethy ... [et al.]; foreword by A. L. Baert. p. cm. -- (Medical radiology) Includes bibliographical references and index. ISBN 3-540-63882-2 (hard cover; alk. paper) ISBN 3-540-42292-7 (soft cover; alk. paper). 1. Pediatric radiology. 2. Pediatric emergencies--Diagnosis. 3. Pediatric diagnostic imag-ing. I. Carty, Helen. II. Abernethy, L. (Laurence) III. Series.   RJ51.R3 E44 1999   618.92'00757--dc 21   98-40967   CIP

Springer-Verlag Berlin Heidelberg New York
a part of Springer Science+Business Media

http://www.springer.de

© Springer-Verlag Berlin Heidelberg 1999, 2002
Printed in Germany

Cover Design: Verlagsservice Teichmann, Mauer
Typesetting: Best-set Typesetter Ltd. Hong Kong

Foreword

Radiological imaging plays a crucial role in the rapid and appropriate management of medical and surgical emergencies in children. Adequate handling of these conditions in children requires from the radiologist compassion and understanding because she or he is confronted not only with the physical problem of the patient but frequently also with much anguish on the part of the child and/or the parents.

High-level radiological expertise and knowledge are essential for selecting, conducting and interpreting those radiological examinations that may be best suited to solve the acute clinical problem and for counselling the pediatrician or surgeon on the best course of action to be followed in each individual situation.

Rapid development of the new cross-sectional radiological imaging methods as well as new insights and recent technical changes in the field of traditional roentgenology have created a need for a volume dealing specifically with pediatric emergencies.

I am highly pleased that Dr. Helen Carty accepted our invitation to prepare a volume on this topic. Indeed, Dr. Helen Carty, who is Professor of Radiology and head of the department of radiology at the Alder Hey pediatric hospital in Liverpool, is known worldwide for her numerous contributions in the field of pediatric radiology, more particularly in the area of musculoskeletal and acute conditions in infancy and childhood. Moreover she is the editor of a very successful textbook on pediatric radiology and a much appreciated lecturer on this topic not only in the United Kingdom but also throughout Europe and, indeed, worldwide. Dr. Helen Carty has been able to engage an impressive group of distinguished pediatric radiologists from the United Kingdom, each of them outstanding experts in their particular field of interest, as collaborators in this book project. Due to their high-level contributions as well as the attentive and expert editorial coordination by Dr. Helen Carty, both overlapping of topics and lacunas have been successfully avoided in this book. The result is an outstanding and up-to-date comprehensive work that covers adequately all aspects of radiologic emergency care for children.

I have no doubt that many radiologists but also pediatricians and surgeons all over the world will find this excellent volume to be a great tool in their daily practice and a welcome addition to their professional library.

I would appreciate any constructive criticism that might be offered.

Leuven   ALBERT L. BAERT

Preface

The presentation of illness in children is frequently sudden and compelling. The child may present as an acute emergency within hours or days of birth or subsequently, at any time during childhood. Emergency presentation may relate to an acute isolated illness, be the first presentation of what becomes a lifelong problem, or be due to an acute exacerbation or a complication of a known condition. Broadly speaking emergencies fall into three categories: trauma, medical and surgical conditions. Sometimes the problem is obvious, such as an acute asthmatic attack, and the choice of radiological imaging is straightforward. Frequently, the child presents with a symptom, for example vomiting, which has a large number of causes, and imaging and its interpretation are more complex. The radiograph may have a particular pattern, such as a unilateral hyperinflated lung, the interpretation of which is often difficult, particularly as initial interpretation is by a doctor other than a trained pediatric radiologist. It is hoped that *Emergency Pediatric Radiology* will offer the necessary help for radiologists, paediatricians and A&E staff and provide a more detailed description of the radiology of pediatric emergencies than in other texts.

All the chapters are written by pediatric radiologists practising in the U. K. Most describe the A&E radiology of the organ systems. There is a separate chapter on child abuse. Three chapters are based on presenting symptoms. Inevitably, there is a little overlap, as the child presenting with a limp or back pain often shares a common aetiology, but for ease of use, where this exists, the two descriptions have been left in.

No book can be produced without the help of willing authors and secretaries. I would like to record my thanks to my contributors, their partners and secretaries. We all hope that this volume in the series *Medical Radiology* will be of practical help to colleagues when looking after children.

Liverpool   HELEN CARTY

Contents

1 Head and Neck Emergency Radiology

L.E. Sweeney

CONTENTS

1.1 Introduction

Plain film radiography remains the mainstay of imaging of acute head and neck lesions, particularly in infants and children. The role of ultrasound (US) and computed tomography (CT) has increased in recent years. Major technical advances have reduced the scan times, enabling CT examinations more often to be performed without sedation or general anaesthesia. Magnetic resonance imaging (MRI) is also being increasingly used, usually in the follow-up of acute conditions rather than in the emergency situation.

1.2 Head Trauma

Head injury is common in childhood. Most injuries are minor and do not present with or have neurological sequelae. Major trauma is self-evident and when accidental should have an appropriate history. It is important to determine whether there is evidence of intracranial injury. The main clinical issue is exclusion of associated intracranial injury. In most instances this can be assessed clinically and no imaging is required. There is considerable doubt about the value of routine radiographs in head injuries. A fracture of the skull will be shown on radiographic examination in only about 2.7% of children with head injury (LLOYD et al. 1997). In major injury the presence of the fracture does not influence management. A closed head injury cannot be predicted from a skull x-ray. Only 48% of children with extradural and 15% with subdural haematomas have a fracture, so significant treatable intracranial injury in the absence of a fracture is not uncommon. Intracranial injuries are best demonstrated by CT, which must be done if such injuries are suspected. The mechanism of injury is relevant in assessing the likelihood of a significant head injury. This risk is high in road traffic accidents or when a large amount of force is concentrated over a small area, e.g. when a child is hit with a golf club, as well as in the presence of potentially penetrating injuries. Many of these fractures are depressed (LORONI et al. 1996).

L.E. Sweeney, MD, Consultant Radiologist, X-Ray Department, Royal Belfast Hospital for Sick Children, 180 Falls Road, Belfast, BT12 6BE, UK

Table 1.1. Indications for skull radiographs

History of loss of consciousness or amnesia
Scalp bruise, swelling or laceration down to bone
Child under 2 years old; suspected non-accidental injury
Type of injury warrants skull x-ray, e.g. blow by golf club or
    fall from height onto a hard surface

Table 1.2. Indications for CT

Suspected foreign body or penetrating injury to skull
Disorientation or depressed consciousness
Focal neurological symptoms or signs
Cerebrospinal fluid (CSF) from nose or CSF/blood from ear
Tense fontanelle or sutural diastasis
Post-fracture headache (late presentation)

1.2.1
Imaging After Head Injury

In head injury skull x-rays in general are not indicated except (a) in children under the age of 2 years because of concern over missing a fracture in non-accidental injury and (b) when depressed fractures are suspected. In recent years the number of children having skull radiographs has decreased but there is still much debate about their role in the management of children with head trauma (Table 1.1) (BEATTIE 1997; WALLACE et al. 1994; JOHNSTONE et al. 1996; MOREEA et al. 1997). The minimum number of radiographs of a high standard should be obtained and the examination performed by an experienced radiographer. The skull views should include a postero-anterior (PA) and a lateral view. There is usually a good correlation between the site of a fracture and the site of injury; the examination can therefore be tailored accordingly. A single lateral projection is usually sufficient in the severely injured child. This should be done as a decubitus film so that if a fluid level is present within the sphenoid air sinus it may be detected. Additional views such as a Townes if there is injury to the occipital region, a tangential view to show a depressed fracture or the other lateral view may be necessary in some cases to fully demonstrate a suspected fracture.

Computed tomography is the preferred modality for evaluation of both depressed fractures and intracranial injury (Table 1.2) (READ et al. 1995; TEASDALE et al. 1990; MURSHID 1994; DAVIS et al. 1994). It is better at demonstrating fresh blood and most skull fractures than MRI. If there are multiple injuries, other parts of the body can also be scanned by CT. MRI is helpful in selected cases in the follow-

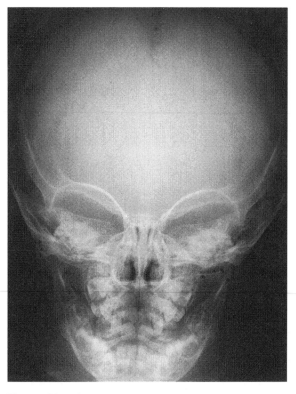

Fig. 1.1. Metopic suture

up of children with intracranial injury to assess prognosis, or where non-accidental injury is suggested. In the latter MRI may show evidence of both recent and old injuries. US has a limited role in trauma as there is poor visualisation of the peripheral cortex and posterior fossa. In infants with an open anterior fontanelle, high-resolution cranial US can be helpful in demonstrating cerebral lacerations and contusions due to non-accidental injury and subdural haematomas. Cerebral perfusion can be monitored by colour Doppler US.

1.2.2
Normal Anatomy

It is important to be familiar with the normal sutures, fissures and vascular grooves in order to distinguish them from fractures (KEATS 1996). Vascular grooves have sharp sclerotic edges while fractures have sharp non-sclerotic edges. The metopic suture is usually closed at birth. A persistently open metopic suture can be misinterpreted as a fracture in the midline of the frontal bone or occipital bone on a Townes view (Fig. 1.1). The mendosal suture may also persist in the neonate. In the base of the skull the most common

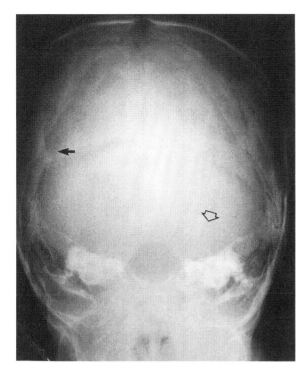

Fig. 1.2. Intrasutural bone (*solid arrow*). Synchrondrosis between the exoccipital and supra-occipital bones (*open arrow*)

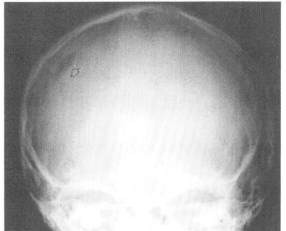

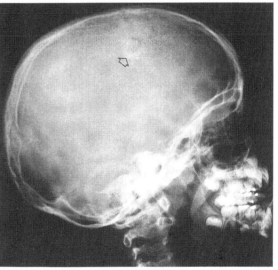

Fig. 1.3 a,b. Depressed skull fracture. a Radiolucent diastatic part of fracture (*arrow*). b Area of sclerosis at periphery due to overlapping fragment of bone (*arrow*)

synchondroses are frontosphenoid, intersphenoid and spheno-occipital. The intersphenoid synchondrosis disappears by the age of 2 years while the spheno-occipital synchondroses can remain open into the late teens. Intrasutural (wormian) bones are also a normal finding, most commonly in the lamboid and posterior sagittal sutures (Fig. 1.2). They later unite with the adjacent skull bones.

1.2.3
Types of Skull Fracture

The most common type of skull fracture is a linear, often hairline fracture. If there is no displacement of bone, no treatment is required. Healing of skull fractures is variable but usually takes less than 6 months in infants, 6–12 months in older children and 2–3 years in adults. Associated intracranial complications, though rare, can occur. If the fracture extends into a paranasal sinus or the mastoid air cells, meningitis can be a complication or, if it crosses a vascular structure, haemorrhage can result. Dural or meningeal tears can be caused by a widely diastatic fracture. Diastatic sutural fractures can occur in isolation or in association with a linear fracture.

Depressed fractures are usually caused by a high-velocity blow. Tangential views show the degree of displacement of these fractures, although CT is indicated for more accurate assessment of the degree of depression of the depressed fragment and damage to the underlying brain (Figs. 1.3–1.5). Penetrating intracranial injuries are caused by high-velocity bullets or, if fired at close range, airgun pellets. They may also occur following accidents with arrows, darts or "sword fighting" with a variety of implements. Apart from contamination associated with the injury, severe brain damage may result. CT is always indicated in the assessment of such injuries.

Basal skull fractures are the most difficult to detect on skull radiographs. If there is clinical evidence of a basal skull fracture, high-resolution CT is indi-

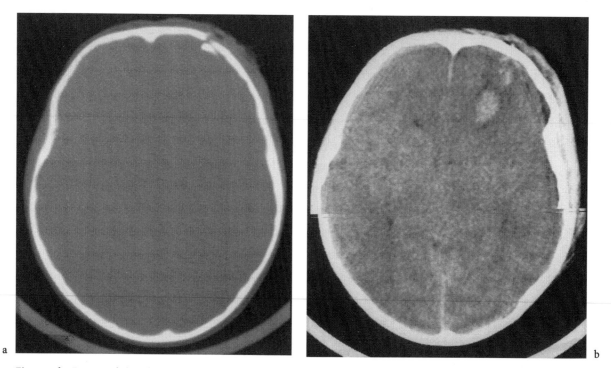

a   b

Fig. 1.4 a,b. Depressed skull fracture. Axial CT scan bone and soft tissue windows. **a** Depressed fragment of left frontal bone. **b** Haemorrhage and contusion of brain

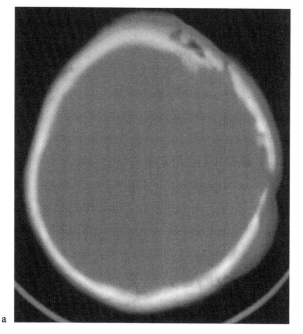
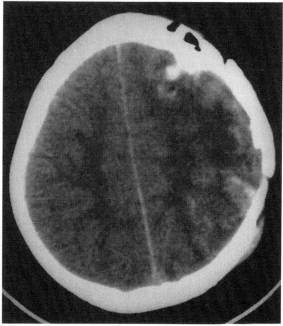

a   b

Fig. 1.5 a,b Depressed skull fracture. **a** Bone window. Depressed fracture of left frontal and parietal bone. **b** Soft tissue window showing the depressed fragment. Laceration of the overlying scalp is present, with air in the soft tissue. There are left frontal and parietal haematomas of high density with low density in the surrounding brain substance due to contusion

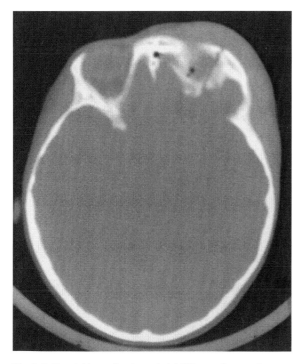

Fig. 1.6. Frontal bone fracture. Axial CT scan shows a fracture involving the roof of the left orbit. Also note orbital emphysema, pneumocephalus and soft tissue swelling

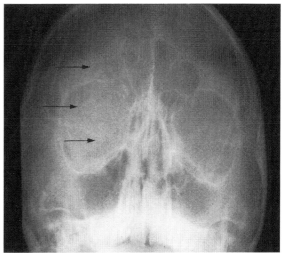

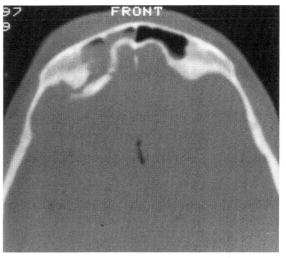

Fig. 1.7 a,b. Frontal bone fracture. **a** Radiograph showing fracture extending from the right frontal bone into the superior and posterior walls of the orbit. Note increased opacity over the right orbit due to soft tissue swelling. **b** Axial CT showing fracture, pneumocephalus and air-fluid levels in the right frontal sinus

cated (ASSANO et al. 1995). Basal skull fractures are suspected clinically when there is bleeding from the ear, discharge of CSF from the ear or nose, cranial nerve dysfunction or conductive deafness. Fractures through the anterior fossa often involve the orbital roof (Figs. 1.6, 1.7). Fractures through the floor of the middle fossa may disrupt the sella or cause an air-fluid level in the sphenoid sinus (Fig. 1.8). The fluid represents blood and will be visible on the cross-table lateral view of the skull. Fractures of the posterior fossa floor usually involve the temporal bone or the posterior part of the occipital bone. A rare form of fracture is a saucer-shaped depression following a forceps delivery or compression of the skull by a round object. It is sometimes known as a "ping pong" fracture (Fig. 1.9).

1.2.4
Intracranial Haemorrhage

1.2.4.1
Acute Epidural Haematoma

Acute epidural haematoma is uncommon in childhood, and is usually due to tearing of dural or

meningeal veins. The most common site is over the temporal or temporoparietal convexity. On CT it has a high-density elliptical shape (Fig. 1.10). This is an acute neurosurgical emergency. Rapidly deteriorating consciousness is the clinical presentation.

1.2.4.2
Subdural Haematomas

Subdural haematomas are caused by a shearing force which tears the veins bridging the subdural space and are relatively common in infants and young chil-

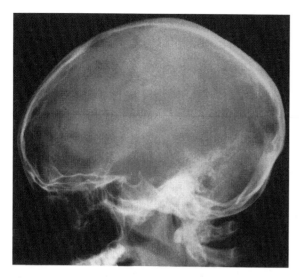

Fig. 1.8. Fracture of base of skull. Lateral radiograph with horizontal x-ray beam shows air-fluid level in the sphenoid sinus

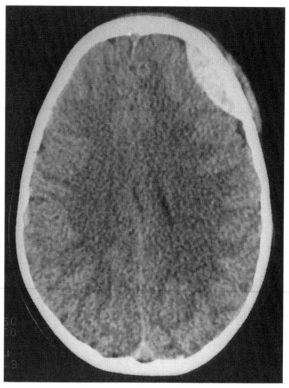

Fig. 1.10. Epidural haematoma. CT scan shows a high-density haematoma with a convex medial edge and small lateral ventricles due to cerebral swelling

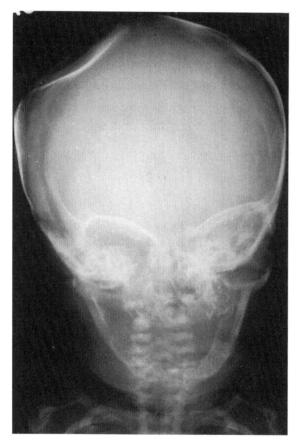

Fig. 1.9. Newborn infant with a "ping pong" or pond fracture of the right parietal bone

dren following non-accidental shaking or strong impact injuries. These infants usually present with seizures, vomiting or irritability. In the acute phase the haematoma will be of high density on CT, but as the blood clot becomes denatured it may appear isodense with the brain. They are more frequently seen over the cerebral convexities and are usually bilateral and conform to the shape of the brain (Fig. 1.11); they are recognised because of displacement of midline structures or ipsilateral ventricular compression. They may extend into the interhemispheric fissure in NAI. Isodense subdural haematomas can also occur in anaemic patients. Intravenous contrast medium can show the displaced cortical vessels and the inner membrane of the subdural haematoma will enhance (HAYMAN et al. 1979). After 2–3 weeks the density of the subdural haematoma will be lower than that of brain and nearer to CSF density.

Subdural haematoma due to accidental trauma usually occurs with major injury such as is seen in road traffic accidents but is very uncommon following simple accidental trauma (LLOYD et al. 1997). When a subdural haematoma occurs following accidental trauma it is most frequently unilateral.

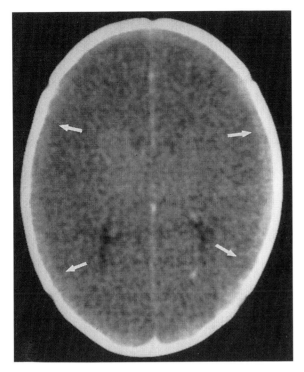

Fig. 1.11. Subdural haematoma in the posterior interhemispheric fissure and over lateral convexities on axial CT scan. Subdural haematomas can be difficult to see when close to the skull vault. Note also intraventricular haemorrhage

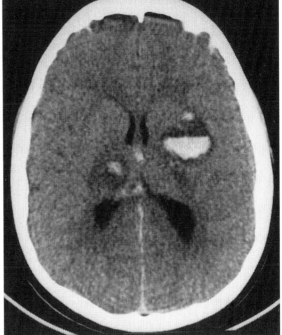

Fig. 1.12. Cerebral and intraventricular haemorrhage. Axial CT scan shows a haematoma in the right thalamus, a fluid level in an organising haematoma in the left parietal lobe and intraventricular haemorrhage and thick irregular linear density in the posterior interhemispheric fissure due to subarachnoid blood

1.2.4.3
Subarachnoid Haemorrhage

Subarachnoid haemorrhage in infants often occurs in non-accidental injury and may be associated with intracerebral haemorrhage. Increased density on CT occurs along the falx and tentorium in subarachnoid haemorrhage. The falx in children can have a high attenuation but should be thin and regular in contour. In the presence of subarachnoid haemorrhage the falx will appear thickened and irregular and there may be extension of haemorrhage into the cortical sulci.

1.2.4.4
Intracerebral Injuries

Intracerebral haemorrhage, which may be associated with cerebral laceration, cerebral contusion or shearing injuries, can be detected by CT (Fig. 1.12). Localised cerebral contusions can result from deceleration, when the brain comes into contact with the skull, a depressed fracture or penetrating injury. Shearing stress injuries due to rapid rotatory deceleration cause tears at the grey-white matter interface and small foci of increased density on CT. These tears can result from violent shaking and when seen are highly suspicious of non-accidental injury.

1.2.4.4.1
CEREBRAL OEDEMA

Generalised brain swelling is common in children after major trauma or asphyxia. CT and MRI show loss of differentiation between grey and white matter, and a diffuse low density of the supratentorial portion of the brain, sometimes referred to as the acute reversal sign, will be seen on CT. The swelling of the brain causes raised intracranial pressure. Obliteration of the basal cisterns is the earliest sign of cerebral oedema. There is compression of the cerebral sulci and the lateral ventricles become slit like (Fig. 1.13).

1.2.4.4.2
TRAUMATIC PNEUMOCEPHALUS

Traumatic pneumocephalus can be shown occasionally on plain skull radiographs but is more clearly defined by CT.

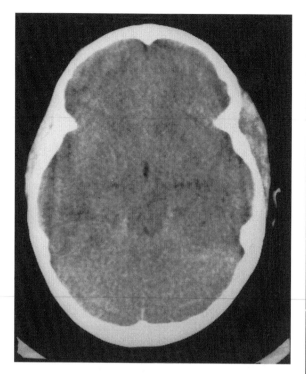

Fig. 1.13. Cerebral swelling. Axial CT scan. There is generalised cerebral swelling with obliteration of the sulci and basal cisterns. The lateral and third ventricles are small. The supratentorial brain substance is of low density compared with the cerebellum: the acute reversal sign

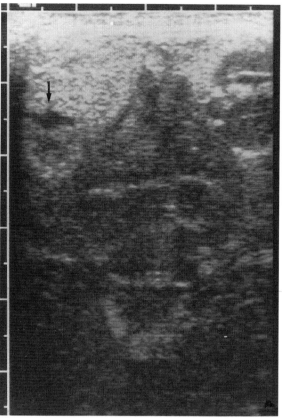

Fig. 1.14. Non-accidental injury. Cranial US scan of a 5-week-old infant showing cerebral contusion as areas of increased echogenicity and a cerebral laceration as a sonolucent area

1.2.4.4.3
NON-ACCIDENTAL INJURY

Non-accidental injury (NAI) should be suspected when the cause of trauma is not evident or easily explained. NAIs are caused by direct trauma to the skull and by shaking (WILKINS 1997). Vigorous shaking causes shearing injuries to the brain. The skull is fractured in approximately 13% of cases of NAI, and 80% of NAIs occur in infants less than 1 year old. Most skull fractures are linear in NAI and are similar to those in accidental trauma, but there is no or an inappropriate history; depressed, diastatic, stellate or multiple bilateral fractures, and fractures which cross sutures, are all suggestive of NAI. Acute intracranial injuries due to NAI are best demonstrated by CT and include subdural and subarachnoid haemorrhage and acute cerebral contusions, foci of parenchymal haemorrhage and shearing injuries of the grey-white matter junction (COHEN 1996). MRI is useful in demonstrating subdural and intraparenchymal haematomas of differing ages and shearing injuries of the white matter (SATO et al. 1989). High-resolution cranial

US can also demonstrate cerebral contusional tears in young infants (Fig. 1.14; JASPAN et al. 1992).

1.2.5
Complications of Head Trauma

Meningitis or intracranial abscess can result from fracture of the sinuses, mastoids and middle ear if there is a persistent communication between the fracture and the intracranial contents, causing a potential route for infection. Most of these complications can be demonstrated by CT or MRI. They usually arise in the immediate post-traumatic period.

Post-traumatic Headache. Most children with head injury recover rapidly within hours of the injury and have no sequelae clinically. Occasionally a child, usually 5 years plus, presents with persistent headache

Table 1.3. Causes of localised swelling or lump on the head

Cephalhaematoma
Subgaleal haematoma
Leptomeningeal cyst
Osteomyelitis
Histiocytosis
Haemangioma – soft tissue or osseous
Bone tumour
Encephalocoele

or vomiting or simply feels "funny" following minor trauma. Skull x-rays are not helpful in the group. A CT scan should be done; it will almost invariably be normal but this is the only way to exclude intracranial pathology.

1.3
Localised Swelling or Lump on the Head

A localised swelling or lump on the head can be caused by a variety of conditions, some of which are listed in Table 1.3. It is most frequently seen following trauma either acutely, as in cephalhaematoma or subgaleal hygroma, or subsequently due to a complication of trauma, as in leptomeningeal cyst. The simplest form of imaging is usually with plain radiographs; if required, further evaluation of the lump with CT or MRI can be carried out.

1.3.1
Cephalhaematoma

Cephalhaematoma occurs in approximately 1% of live births. It is a traumatic subperiosteal haemorrhage, the blood lying beneath the outer layer of periosteum. Cephalhaematoma does not extend beyond a single bone. Cephalhaematomas usually increase in size after birth and present as a firm tense mass. They resolve spontaneously in a few weeks or months. A small number may calcify, a rim of periosteal new bone being laid down around the outer margin of the haematoma (Fig. 1.15). Occasionally they heal with permanent localised thickening of the skull vault. Imaging is not required except possibly during the healing phase, when cephalhaematoma can be clinically misinterpreted as a depressed skull fracture because the edge of the calcified haematoma feels like the edge of a depressed fracture. Plain radiographs of the skull will enable the correct diagnosis to be made.

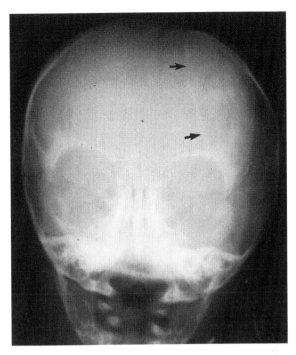

Fig. 1.15. Cephalhaematoma. Radiograph shows calcification over the posterior half of the left parietal bone

1.3.2
Subgaleal Hygroma

Subgaleal hygroma is usually due to trauma from obstetric forceps and is often associated with an underlying skull fracture. Cerebrospinal fluid leaks through tears of arachnoid and dura and passes into the subgaleal space to form a subgaleal hygroma. Subgaleal hygroma can extend across sutures, which distinguishes it from a cephalhaematoma.

1.3.3
Leptomeningeal Cyst

Linear skull fractures which are widely diastatic are often associated with tearing of the underlying dura. The arachnoid membrane herniates through the tear and impinges upon the margins of the fracture. The transmitted intracranial pulse will then erode the skull, causing the fracture to become wider. The enlarging defect in the skull is called a growing fracture; it is usually oval in shape and has scalloped margins (Fig. 1.16). A pulsatile swelling will be clinically palpable in the skull defect. There is usually associated brain damage which can be demonstrated on CT. Surgical repair of the dura may be required to prevent further increase in size of the skull defect.

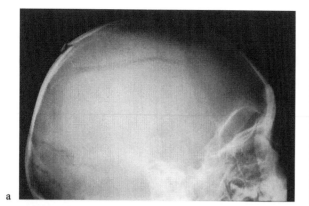

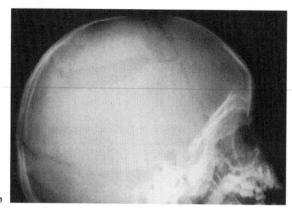

Fig. 1.16. a Diastatic fracture. **b** Growing fracture in same patient. Radiograph taken several months later shows a wide defect with scalloped sclerotic margins

1.3.4
Osteomyelitis

Abscesses of soft tissues of the scalp and osteomyelitis of the skull and facial bones are uncommon. In the past osteomyelitis occurred as a complication of mastoiditis and ear infections. It can occur by haematogenous spread and occasionally it is seen as a complication of a scalp laceration, a compound skull fracture or sinusitis (Fig. 1.17).

1.3.5
Miscellaneous

Some bone tumours are associated with soft tissue swelling, e.g. histiocytosis, and this may be the clinical presentation (Fig. 1.18). Others can cause localised expansion or thickening of the skull vault, e.g. haemangioma and meningoma, but most such tumours are uncommon. Fibrous dysplasia can also cause localised thickening, but is in general a radio-

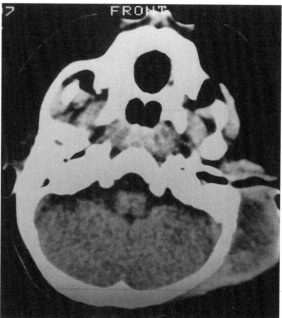

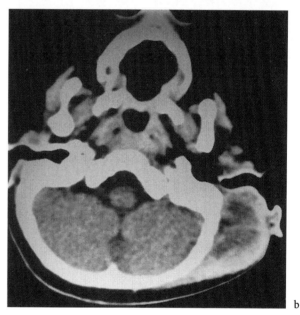

Fig. 1.17 a,b. Pre-auricular abscess. Axial CT **a** pre **b** post contrast shows soft tissue abscess with enhancement of the wall and low attenuation centre

graphic finding rather than a clinical finding Encephalocoeles tend to occur in the midline, usually in the occipital region but sometimes in the frontal area (Fig. 1.19). Any child with such swellings should undergo plain skull radiography, which is often diagnostic. Subsequent views may be required.

Soft tissue tumours involving the scalp are uncommon. US will differentiate a cystic from a solid

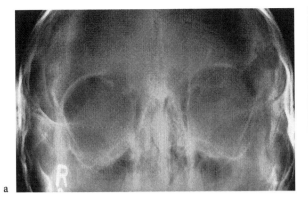

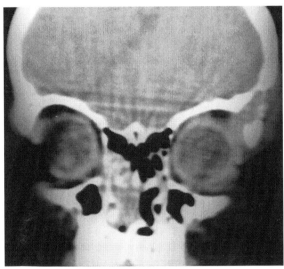

Fig. 1.18 a,b. Langerhans cell histiocytosis. a Radiograph shows osteolytic lesion of the left frontal bone involving the supero-lateral margin of the orbit. b coronal CT shows extension of the soft tissue component into the orbit

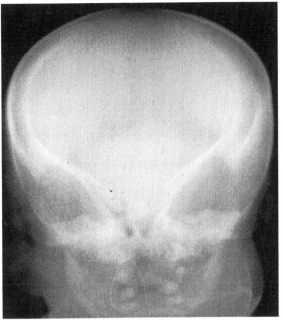

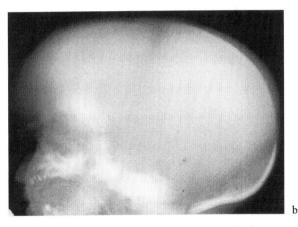

Fig. 1.19 a,b. Encephalocoele. a Frontal radiograph showing separation and depression of the orbits. b Lateral radiograph showing frontal soft tissue mass

lesion and colour Doppler can demonstrate blood flow. Further evaluation by CT and/or MRI is usually required, particularly when surgery is being considered.

1.4
Facial Trauma

1.4.1
Introduction

Facial fractures are not as common in infants and young children as in adults. The reported incidence in children under 12 years varies from 1.5% to 8% of all facial fractures (KABAN 1993). The mid face is the most protected area in children under 2 years be-

cause of its retrusive position relative to the skull vault (HOLLMAN 1994). Mandibular fractures are the most frequently reported fractures of the face, although fractures of the teeth and alveolus are probably more common. The most common aetiology of facial fractures is road traffic accidents, which usually cause multiple injuries.

1.4.2
Imaging of Facial Trauma

High-resolution CT with thin sections (3 mm) is the method of choice for imaging maxillofacial injuries.

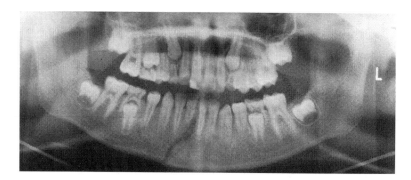

Fig. 1.20. OPG of a 12-year-old boy who fell off a wall, showing an undisplaced fracture of the body of mandible on the right side and fractures of the mandibular condyles. Condylar fractures can sometimes be difficult to see on an OPG

Most facial fractures in children are the result of severe trauma and are associated with multiple injuries. CT has the advantage of being able to image other injuries (Laine et al. 1993; Rehm and Ross 1995) and 3D CT can also be of value prior to surgery. Conventional radiography is infrequently used for evaluation of maxillofacial injuries. Plain radiographs are still occasionally used when the clinical suspicion is low or when CT is not readily available. The 30° occipitomental view is the most useful radiographic projection of the facial bones.

1.4.3
Mandibular Fractures

Fractures of the mandible are often bilateral because of the ring-like configuration at the mandible; however, single fractures also occur. Most can be shown on an orthopantomogram (OPG) (Fig. 1.20) or a PA mandible view although central fractures in the region of the chin will be missed on an OPG. If the child is old enough an OPG may be all that is required if the fracture is demonstrated. A PA mandible and both lateral oblique views may be required to supplement this if the OPG is negative and there is strong suspicion of a fracture or if the injury point is on the chin. Fractures of the mandidular condyles are often greenstick. CT will also readily demonstrate mandibular fractures. Extension of the fracture into a tooth socket constitutes a compound fracture.

1.4.4
Nasal Fractures

Radiographs of the nasal bone are unnecessary if there is clinical evidence of an undisplaced nasal fracture as the treatment is conservative. If there is clinical evidence of a displaced nasal septum or de-pressed nasal fracture then a lateral radiograph of the nasal bones and an occipitomental view may be required prior to surgery.

1.4.5
Zygomatic/Maxillary Fractures

The types of fracture of the facial bones include solitary zygomatic arch fractures, tripod fractures of the zygomatic and maxillary bone complex, isolated maxillary fractures and LeFort fractures of the face. These fractures are usually the result of a direct blow to the face.

The tripod fracture consists of a fracture at the fronto-zygomatic suture, a fracture of the floor of the orbit, a fracture of the lateral wall of the maxillary sinus and fracture of the zygomatic arch. The fracture fragment is usually displaced downwards and outwards (Figs. 1.21, 1.22).

LeFort (middle third) fractures are classified into three types. LeFort 1 is a transverse submaxillary fracture which is above the level of the teeth and separates the upper face from the maxillary alveolus. LeFort 2 is a transverse fracture extending across the maxillary bone and nose. It may extend into the floor of the orbit. LeFort 3 is a complete detachment of the facial bones from the cranium. The fracture line runs through the nasal bones and the medial and lateral walls of the orbits (Fig. 1.23). If there is posterior displacement of the facial bones, occlusion of the airway can occur (Figs. 1.24, 1.25). When a facial fracture is suspected on plain radiographs, further delineation with CT is required (Fig. 1.26).

Computed tomography should be done primarily without plain radiography if there is good clinical suspicion of a fracture. Soft tissue swelling over the cheek causing antral opacity should not be misinterpreted as bleeding into the antrum on plain radiography. Facial soft tissue swelling usually projects above the orbital floor over the eye.

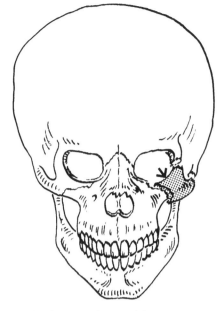

Fig. 1.21. Line diagram of a tripod fracture

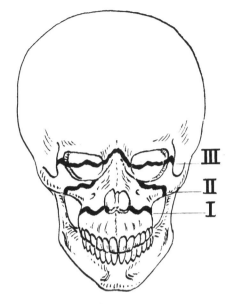

Fig. 1.23. Line diagram of Le Fort fractures

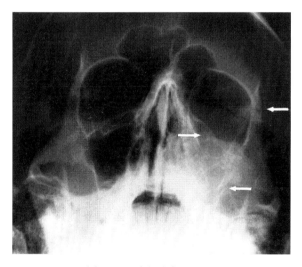

Fig. 1.22. Tripod fracture of the left zygoma. Occipitomental radiograph. The fractures shown include the frontozygomatic suture, the lateral wall of the maxillary sinus and the floor of the orbit

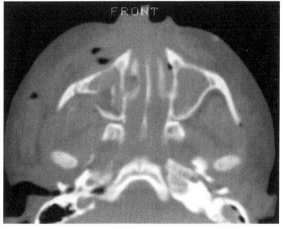

Fig. 1.24. Maxillary fractures. Axial CT scan. There is marked facial soft tissue swelling and air in the soft tissue due to a laceration. There are fractures of the medial and lateral walls of the right maxillary sinus with medial displacement of a fragment of the lateral wall and an undisplaced fracture of the right zygomatic arch

1.4.6
Orbital Trauma

The orbit is frequently involved in complex facial fractures and with extension of frontal bone or basal skull fractures. The optic canal may be damaged if an orbital roof fracture extends posteriorly. Orbital emphysema may occur if a fracture involves the frontal or ethmoid sinuses. Blunt trauma to the orbit causes a blow-out fracture through the floor of the orbit. It usually occurs in isolation but can be associated with other facial fractures. The increased pressure in the globe results in herniation of orbital contents through the fracture site, leading to diplopia. Most blow-out fractures occur in the floor of the orbit; however, sometimes they occur through the medial wall of the orbit or lamina papyracea, which is thin, and extend into the ethmoid sinuses. CT is the best method for evaluation of the orbits, preferably in the coronal plane (Fig. 1.27). The presence of herniation

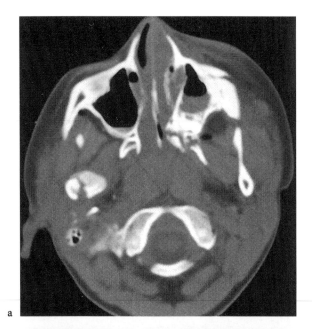

a

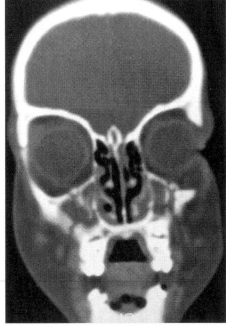

Fig. 1.26. Five-year-old girl hit by car wing mirror. Coronal CT shows bilateral fractures of the lateral wall of the maxillary sinus and orbital floor

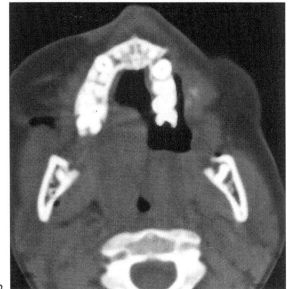

b

Fig. 1.25 a,b. Maxillary fractures. **a** Axial CT scan showing fractures of the anterior and medial walls of the left maxillary sinus, fractures of the left medial and lateral pterygoid plates and a fracture of the right mandibular condyle. Note also the air-fluid level of the left maxillary sinus. **b** Axial CT scan (same patient as in **a**) showing fractures of the left maxilla involving the alveolus

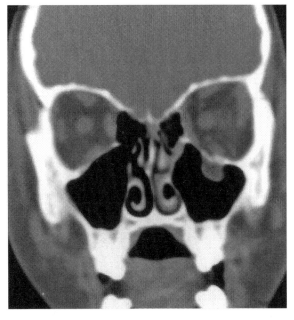

Fig. 1.27. Orbital fracture. Coronal CT scan showing a blow-out fracture of the floor of the left orbit with herniation of orbital fat into the antrum

and trapping of the inferior rectus muscle can be distinguished from herniation of orbital fat. On plain radiographs the trapped content projects herniated material into the antral roof but fat and muscle cannot be distinguished. In acute trauma this may not be visible if there is extensive intrasinus bleeding.

1.5
The Eye

1.5.1
Role of Imaging

Ocular emergencies are common in children. Usually imaging is not required for diagnosis or management as the problem can be identified clinically. When adequate clinical examination of the eye is prevented by opacification of the media by haemorrhage following trauma, the eye can be evaluated by US, provided rupture of the globe has been excluded clinically. Imaging is also required for intra-ocular foreign body localisation and evaluation of the child presenting with proptosis or sudden loss of vision. CT and MRI can demonstrate the retrobulbar and intracranial extension of orbital masses (HOPPER 1992; LATACK et al. 1987; KINGSLEY et al. 1986). The primary imaging approach to suspected orbital tumours should be performance of urgent MRI if this is available. If it is not, CT should be done. CT may also be needed to supplement MRI to establish the extent of bone destruction.

1.5.2
Orbital Ultrasound

Orbital trauma is common in children. US of the eye may be considered whenever opacification of the media prevents adequate clinical examination and rupture of the globe has been excluded clinically (KWONG et al. 1992; ENRIQUEZ et al. 1995; RAMJI et al. 1996). The examination is performed with the patient supine. A small amount of US gel is applied to the closed upper eye lid and the scan is performed with a 7- to 10-MHz linear array transducer. Scanning is done in the transverse and sagittal planes. Care is taken not to apply pressure to the globe.

Ultrasound will demonstrate haemorrhage in the anterior chamber or vitreous humour as increased echogenity (Fig. 1.28). The position and appearance of the lens can be evaluated and retinal detachment can be demonstrated (Fig. 1.29).

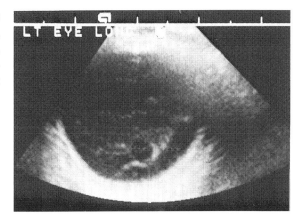

Fig. 1.28. Vitreous haemorrhage shown on orbital US as low-level echoes

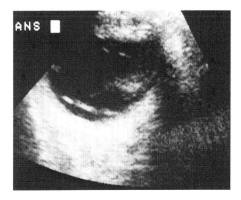

Fig. 1.29. Vitreous haemorrhage and retinal detachment. The curvilinear detached fragment of the retina is shown

Ultrasound is useful in the demonstration of foreign bodies which will appear echogenic and cause reverberation artefact if they are metal. Colour Doppler US can be used to assess the retinal vessels. Air in the eye may prevent visualisation of an ocular lesion.

1.5.3
Intra-ocular Foreign Body

Plain radiographs will reveal foreign bodies of adequate radiopacity depending on the nature and size of the foreign body and the density of surrounding structures. Occipitofrontal and occipitomental 35° views and a lateral view centred on the orbit with the eyes in the primary position are the radiographic views required. US is now the preferred method for localisation of foreign bodies and demonstrates the precise relationship of a foreign body to the globe. It

Table 1.4. Causes of sudden loss of vision

Trauma
Retinal detachment
Optic nerve compression
Papilloedema
Takayasu's arteritis

will show non-radiopaque and small foreign bodies not visible on plain radiographs. CT has a role in foreign body localisation when plain radiography and US are inadequate, such as when the foreign body lies within the orbit but outside the globe, or there is doubt about the nature or location of the foreign body or whether there are multiple fragments (Fig. 1.30).

1.5.4
Sudden Loss of Vision

1.5.4.1
Introduction

Sudden loss of vision is uncommon in childhood. When it does occur there may be little obvious evidence of ocular disease. In the early stages loss of vision may not be noticed, especially in a young child, and chronic or congenital disease may present as sudden loss of vision (Table 1.4). US is useful in demonstrating several of the conditions listed in Table 1.4, but CT or MRI is required for more detailed assessment of tumours prior to treatment.

1.5.4.2
Retinal Detachment

Retinal detachment may occur apparently spontaneously as a result of congenital or old inflammatory defects in the retina. Blunt trauma to the head or any trauma to the eye may lead to retinal detachment after an interval of days, weeks or months. Retinal detachment can be demonstrated by US.

1.5.4.3
Vitreous Haemorrhage

Vitreous haemorrhage is a common finding in severe ocular trauma. The sonographic appearance of vitreous haemorrhage varies from homogeneous

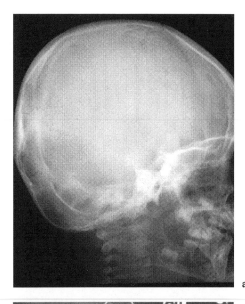

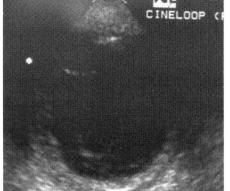

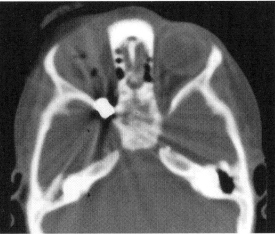

Fig. 1.30 a–c. Appearance following an airgun pellet wound to the eye. **a** Lateral skull radiograph shows a pellet that appears posterior to the orbit. **b** Orbital US shows vitreous haemorrhage as low-level echoes. **c** Axial CT scan shows the pellet posteriorly in the orbit and projecting intracranially as well as orbital emphysema

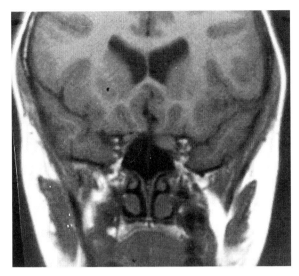

Fig. 1.31. MRI of optic nerve glioma in a child who presented with sudden loss of vision. T1-weighted image showing enlargement of the left optic nerve

1.5.4.4
Optic Nerve Compression

Tumours compressing the anterior visual system can cause unilateral or bilateral visual loss. While US can show intra-ocular tumours such as retinoblastoma, CT or MRI is required for evaluation of retrobulbar and intracranial extension (Fig. 1.31).

1.5.5
Papilloedema

During the early stages, papilloedema can lead to transient episodes of blurring or vision. Occasionally optic disc drusen can be confused with papilloedema on fundoscopy. This is a benign condition which can cause visual impairment and is usually found on US of the eye for an unrelated reason (Fig. 1.32). Drusen consists of deposits of hyaline calcific material within the head of the optic nerve. The use of orbital US in demonstrating dilatation of the optic nerve sheath in the diagnosis of raised intracranial pressure has been described by HELMKE and HANSON (1996). The discovery of papilloedema should lead to urgent referral for MRI or CT to identify the cause.

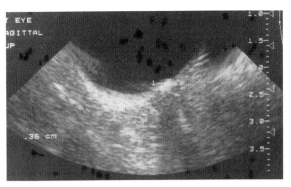

Fig. 1.32. Orbital US showing calcification of the optic nerve (drusen). Drusen can raise the optic disc and clinically simulate papilloedema

Table 1.5. Causes of proptosis

Orbital complications of sinusitis
   Orbital cellulitis
   Subperiosteal abscess
   Orbital abscess
Mucocoele
Intra-orbital tumours
   Retinoblastoma
   Dermoid
   Haemangioma
   Rhabdomyosarcoma
   Optic nerve glioma
   Neuroblastoma
Bone tumours involving the orbit
Hyperthyroidism

1.5.6
Proptosis

The most common causes of proptosis are listed in Table 1.5. They include benign and malignant tumours, vascular malformations and complications of sinus infection. The role of imaging is to assess the retrobulbar and intracranial extent of orbital masses and the presence or absence of bony involvement.

1.5.6.1
Orbital Infection

The majority of orbital infections are a complication of sinusitis. Other causes include trauma, foreign bodies, spread from facial infection and septicaemia. Infection usually spreads from the ethmoid sinuses through the thin lamina papyracea which form the medial wall of the orbit. Infection spreads to the orbit from the sinuses more easily in children than in

---

to heterogeneous depending on the age of the haemorrhage.

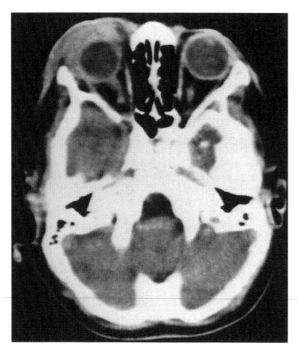

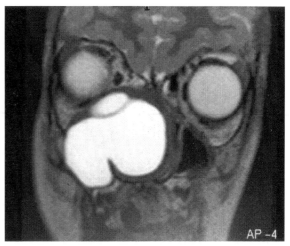

Fig. 1.34. Mucocoele of maxillary sinus. Coronal T2-weighted fast spin-echo image shows high signal intensity of the right maxillary sinus with expansion and thinning of the medial wall

Fig. 1.33. Peri-orbital cellulitis. Axial CT post contrast showing swelling of the right eyelid

adults because of the thin sinus walls, especially the lamina papyracea, and larger communicating veins.

Orbital cellulitis and orbital and subperiosteal abscesses may present with fever, proptosis and eyelid tenderness. It is important to differentiate between these types of infection as treatment varies. Orbital cellulitis is treated with antibiotics whereas orbital and subperiosteal abscesses require surgical drainage (Fig. 1.33). Contrast-enhanced CT is the imaging method of choice. On CT there is increased density or stranding of retrobulbar fat. An orbital abscess consists of a collection of fluid within the orbit and a subperiosteal abscess is characterised by a mass of fluid density usually at the medial side of the orbit, causing lateral displacement of the medial rectus muscle. A complication of orbital infection is cavernous sinus thrombosis. CT scans should be carefully scrutinised for evidence of this; if doubt exists, one should proceed to MRI.

1.5.6.2
Mucocoeles

Mucocoeles are caused by obstruction of the sinus ostia. Clinical presentation is characterised by pain, proptosis or facial swelling. Predisposing conditions include cystic fibrosis, immotile cilia syndrome or an

obstructing mass, although in most affected children these conditions are not encountered. The clinical findings depend on the size and location of the mucocoele. The frontal sinus is the most common site and extension into the orbit may cause proptosis. The secretions become trapped within the sinus and the bony walls of the sinus expand due to the increased pressure. There is a risk of brain abscess or cavernous sinus thrombus due to intracranial extension of a frontal or sphenoid sinus mucocoele. CT with intravenous contrast enhancement will delineate the extent of a mucocoele and has the advantage of demonstration of bone detail. Mucocoeles are low-attenuation or soft tissue density masses arising within a sinus. Areas of high attenuation indicate desiccated secretions or fungal colonisation. On MRI, mucocoeles with high water content are hypointense on T1-weighted images and hyperintense on T2-weighted images (Fig. 1.34). If the protein content of the mucocoele is increased, its signal intensity on T1-weighted images is increased and it has low intensity signal on T2-weighted images.

If the sinus walls are not expanded it is not possible to differentiate a mucocoele from a retention cyst or polyp or tumour.

1.5.6.3
Orbital Tumours

Orbital tumours can be classified into intra- and extra-ocular (SHIELDS et al. 1986). Retinoblastoma is

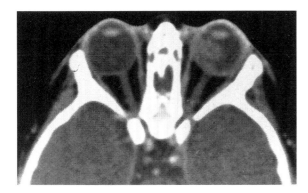

Fig. 1.35. Retinoblastoma. Axial CT shows the soft tissue intra-ocular mass

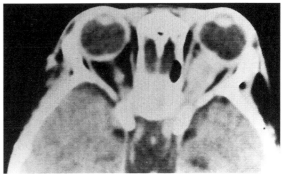

Fig. 1.37. Optic nerve glioma. Axial CT shows enlargement of the optic nerve and proptosis

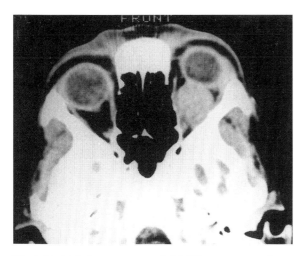

Fig. 1.36. Rhabdomyosarcoma. Axial CT post contrast showing tumour in the right orbit, causing proptosis

the most common intra-ocular tumour in childhood. It is usually unilateral but may be bilateral. Leukokoria (white pupillary reflux) is the most frequent presenting signs and is caused by replacement of vitreous humour by a white or pink mass. There is reduced visual acuity, eye pain, strabismus and proptosis. The tumour may extend outside the globe. Calcification occurs in 95%. These tumours enhance with intravenous contrast on CT (Fig. 1.35). US is a quick method of examining the vitreous, which normally is completely transonic. In retinoblastoma the vitreous is solid and irregular.

Rhabdomyosarcoma is the most common extra-ocular malignant neoplasm in childhood, generally being seen in older children (SOHAIB et al. 1998) (Fig. 1.36). It is much less common than retinoblastoma; in those cases that present to an accident and emergency department, pain or proptosis is usually the reason.

Optic nerve gliomas can occur in children, usually in those with neurofibromatosis type I. Clinical presentation as an emergency is usually with diplopia or failing vision; alternatively the child may present with fits due to the phakomatosis, the tumour then being discovered incidentally (Fig. 1.37).

Benign tumours are more common than malignant orbital tumours. A dermoid tumour is the most frequently seen orbital tumour in children. Orbital dermoids account for 1%–2% of all orbital masses. Sixty percent arise from the upper outer quadrant of the orbit, from sequestration of ectoderm. Most orbital dermoids present in childhood as subcutaneous nodules adjacent to the orbital rim and may be fixed to the underlying periosteum. In young children dermoids are not usually associated with proptosis. Plain radiography of the orbit may show bony changes with a defect in the orbital rim that has a smooth or scalloped sclerotic margin. In adults and older children dermoids are deeper and presentation may be with unilateral proptosis. Imaging with CT or MRI is then indicated. On CT the dermoid will have a low attenuation centre, may contain fat and may show a fluid-fat level (Fig. 1.38). There may also be a thick enhancing rim which can be calcified. Dermoids can also occur in the midline and present as a nasal mass. In more than 50% of nasal dermoids there is communication with the brain, predisposing to infection. CT will show the defect in bone.

Cavernous haemangiomas may bleed, the enlargement leading to clinical presentation with pain and proptosis. Cavernous haemangiomas do not always show contrast enhancement on CT. Haemangiomas are also fairly common in the orbit in children.

Other tumours are rare, e.g. metastatic disease from neuroblastoma or Ewing's sarcoma, teratomas, histiocystosis and lymphoma.

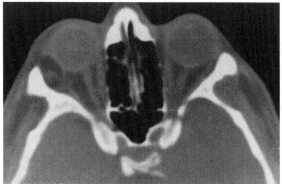

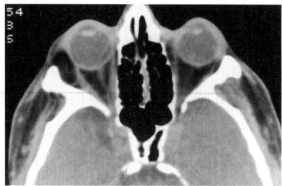

a

b

Fig. 1.38. Dermoid. Axial CT shows a fat containing lesion in the upper outer quadrant of the right orbit. There is mild scalloping of the adjacent bone of the orbital wall

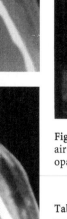

Fig. 1.39. Acute sinusitis. Occipitomental radiograph showing air-fluid levels in the frontal and left maxillary sinuses and opacification of the right maxillary sinus

Table 1.6. Indications for imaging of sinusitis

Chronic sinusitis
Recurrent acute sinusitis
Suspected complications of sinusitis
    Orbital cellulitis
    Osteomyelitis
    Orbital abscess
    Brain abscess
    Cavernous sinus thrombosis
    Mucocoele

1.6
Sinuses and Mastoids

1.6.1
Sinusitis

Acute bacterial sinusitis is a frequent complication of common colds. The ostia of the sinuses become obstructed by congested mucosa, leading to impaired drainage and then superimposed bacterial infection. The diagnosis of sinusitis depends on the history and clinical examination. Clinical findings include headaches, pain or tenderness over the affected sinus, nasal obstruction, mucopurulent nasal discharge, fever, lethargy and malaise. Causative organisms include *Haemophilus influenzae* and *Moraxella catarrhalis*. Imaging is not usually required to make a diagnosis of acute sinusitis.

The main purpose of imaging is to estimate the extent of mucosal thickening and to diagnose complications (Fig. 1.39). Indications for imaging in sinusitis are given in Table 1.6. Plain radiographs of the paranasal sinuses are of limited value in acute

sinus disease as bacterial viral and allergic changes appear similar (ARRUDA et al. 1989).

Interpretation of radiographs is difficult in infants because of their small size. Although the maxillary and ethmoid sinuses are present from birth, they initially measure only a few millimetres. The maxillary sinuses usually mature to adult size by the age of 12 years. The sphenoid sinus is present at 2 years of age and the frontal sinuses are usually not present until 7–10 years of age and reach adult size around puberty. There is also poor correlation of signs and symptoms of paranasal disease with imaging findings.

Opacification of the sinuses is not always pathological. Imaging of the paranasal sinuses is generally not recommended in children under 5 years of age because of the poor development. CT in the coronal plane is the method of choice in the full assessment of sinus disease (MCALISTER et al. 1989; KRONEMER and MCALISTER 1997). It provides excellent anatomical detail, differentiates between bone and soft tissue and is superior to plain radiography. MRI also clearly demonstrates mucosal thickening and fluid within the sinuses but lacks bone detail. Mucosal thickening on MRI is a very common incidental finding in children and must not be over-interpreted.

1.6.2
Acute Mastoiditis

Acute mastoiditis is an acute bacterial infection of the mastoid air cells. It most commonly occurs as a complication of acute otitis media and can also occur with chronic otitis media and cholesteatoma. Clinical presentation is with fever, pain and swelling over the affected mastoid process. Common causative organisms include group A β-*haemolytic streptococci*, *staphylococci* and *Proteus mirabilis*. Treatment is with antibiotics. Surgery may be required if antibiotic treatment fails or there are complications such as brain or subperiosteal abscess. Acute mastoiditis results in oedema or exudate which causes decreased aeration or opacification of the air cells. CT is the imaging modality of choice. The main role is to exclude intracerebral extension or associated subdural empyema. CT should be done if there is suspicion of such disease.

1.7
Neck

Clinical examination of the neck in a young child or infant presenting with an acute swelling in the neck or upper airway obstruction can be difficult. Diagnosis of neck abnormalities in children depends on their precise delineation and a knowledge of the physiology and structure of the neck (ADAMS and CINNAMOND 1997).

1.7.1
Imaging of the Neck

A plain lateral soft tissue radiograph with the neck partially extended can often provide detailed information about the anatomy of the airway. Air within the upper respiratory tract will outline anatomical structures. The retropharyngeal tissues vary in thickness with normal respiration. During expiration there is normal anterior buckling of the trachea, which is exaggerated further if the head is flexed. This causes apparent thickening of the retropharyngeal tissue, mimicking a retropharyngeal abscess

displacing the trachea anteriorly. Therefore, in the infant it is important to obtain the lateral radiograph of the neck in inspiration. The technique of light anterior compression of the larynx can be used to exclude a retropharyngeal mass. The radiologist wears a lead glove and with the index finger applies pressure on the cricothyroid membrane during the radiographic exposure. The compression is gentle and very brief so as not to compromise the airway (POZNANSKI 1976) Alternatively, fluoroscopic observation in difficult cases will show that the "mass" is spurious. In infants the posterior pharyngeal wall can lie more anteriorly than in older children. The prevertebral soft tissue space is no greater than three-quarters of the anteroposterior diameter of the adjacent vertebral body, provided the radiograph is with the neck extended and in inspiration.

High-resolution US with a linear array 7.5-mHz transducer is used as the initial screening procedure for investigation of neck masses, CT and MRI subsequently being used when required. Both CT and MRI provide detailed information about the structures of the soft tissue of the neck, show the extent of a mass and its effect on adjacent structures, and aid in guiding aspiration and/or biopsy.

1.7.2
Lump or Swelling in the Neck

Neck masses in children are common and frequently present acutely at the accident and emergency department. The most common cause of a neck mass in a child is inflammatory lymphadenopathy which will resolve with appropriate treatment. However, there are numerous causes of neck masses in childhood, the more common ones being listed in Table 1.7. Clinical examination is often difficult and imaging with high-resolution US and colour Doppler is the initial method of choice as no sedation is required, no radiation is involved and it is non-invasive (EL-SILIMY and CORNEY 1993; FRIEDMAN et al. 1983; GLASIER et al. 1987; SHERMAN et al. 1985). CT and MRI can be used if further evaluation of the mass is required.

1.7.2.1
Cystic Hygroma

Cystic hygromas or lymphangiomas are congenital malformations of lymphatic channels which frequently present at birth or in the first few weeks of

Table 1.7. Causes of neck masses in childhood

Abscess
Lymphadenitis
Parotitis
Osteomyelitis of mandible
Retropharyngeal abscess
Infection of cystic lesion
Haematoma
Cystic hygroma
Branchial cyst
Thyroglossal duct cyst
Vascular malformation
Leukaemia
Lymphoma
Neuroblastoma
Rhabdomyosarcoma
Histiocytosis
Thyroid abnormality
   Goitre
   Adenoma
   Carcinoma
   Lymphoma

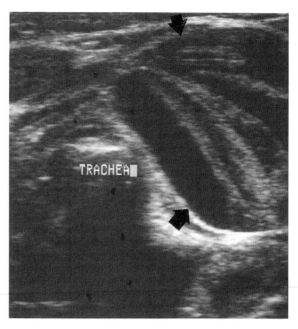

Fig. 1.40. Two-month-old girl with an infected cystic hygroma causing acute respiratory obstruction. Transverse US scan of the neck shows a multiloculated cyst which impinges upon the trachea. There are low-level echoes in some of the loculi

life as a painless soft tissue mass posterior to the sternomastoid muscle. If large, they may cause airway and soft tissue compression in the neck or extend into the mediastinum. Most are slow growing but sudden enlargement can occur due to haemorrhage, inflammation or trauma. US will demonstrate a thin-walled multiloculated cystic mass that may contain septa of various thicknesses (Fig. 1.40; SHETH et al. 1987). The contents of the cyst may be echogenic if there has been recent haemorrhage. Tissues adjacent to the lesion are often indistinct as cystic hygromas tend to infiltrate adjacent structures. A cystic hygroma may rarely consist of a solitary cyst. Full mapping of the lesion requires MRI in axial and coronal planes.

1.7.2.2
Branchial Cysts

Branchial cysts arise from persistence of the branchial clefts. The embryo has five branchial clefts separated by six branchial arches. Second branchial clefts account for 90% of branchial cleft abnormalities, first branchial clefts 8% and third branchial clefts 2%. Branchial cysts occur mainly in the upper neck anterior to the sternomastoid muscle but can occur anywhere from the tonsillar fossa to the supraclavicular area. (BUCKINGHAM and LYNN 1975). On US a branchial cyst is usually a well-defined, thin-walled, cystic mass anterior to the sternocleidomastoid muscle and lateral to the common carotid artery and jugular vein (Fig. 1.41). If there is

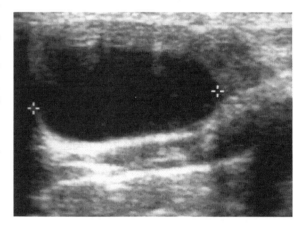

Fig. 1.41. Branchial cyst in a 3-month-old girl who presented with stridor. US of the neck shows a cystic mass

superimposed infection, the wall of the cyst is thickened and the echogenicity of the fluid may increase. Sudden enlargement due to haemorrhage or infection can cause compression of the airway.

1.7.2.3
Haemangiomas

Haemangiomas are developmental vascular anomalies usually found in infants under 6 months of age.

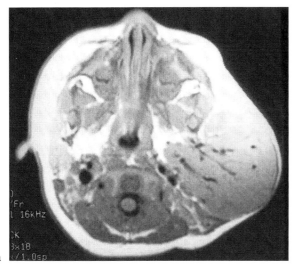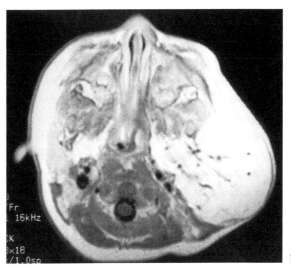

a　　　　　　　　　　　　　　　　　　　　　　　　　　　　　　　　　b

Fig. 1.42 a,b. Haemangioma of parotid gland. **a** Axial T1-weighted MR image shows a homogeneous mass of intermediate intensity. **b** Axial T1-weighted image after gadolinium administration shows marked enhancement of the mass and enlarged feeding and draining vessels

They are usually asymptomatic, but if in the neck they can increase in size to cause compression of the airway and may present as an emergency. They are absent at birth and appear and grow rapidly in the neonatal period. Between the 6th and the 10th month of life haemangiomas usually stop enlarging, and complete regression occurs in more than 70% of cases by the age of 8 years. Plain radiographs may show a soft tissue mass with calcification and phleboliths. There are two major types of haemangiomas, capillary and cavernous, both of which can be localised to the skin or involve deeper soft tissues. On US haemangiomas will have hypoechoic areas with echogenic septations which on colour Doppler will be shown to be vascular. Haemangiomas can appear echogenic because they contain numerous interfaces, proteinaceous material or thrombus. CT and MRI provide excellent tissue differentiation and can define the extent of the haemangioma and its major feeding vessels (Fig. 1.42).

1.7.2.4
Cervical Lymphadenitis

Cervical lymphadenitis usually results from infection of the tonsils, pharynx and teeth or soft tissues of the face. Infections of the oral cavity frequently involve the submandibular and deep cervical lymph nodes. Although viral infections are more common, bacterial infections, particularly with staphylococcus

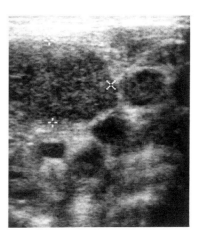

Fig. 1.43. Neck abscess and cervical adenitis in a 2-year-old girl who presented with a painful mass in the left side of the neck. Longitudinal sonogram shows a mass which represents an abscess surrounded by large lymph nodes

or streptococcus, tend to have a more rapid onset and more often progress to suppurative lymphadenopathy. US can identify purulent lymphadenopathy which requires drainage. Inflammatory lymphadenopathy will appear on US as enlarged tender echo-poor oval masses, which, though numerous, are discrete. Suppurating lymph nodes will have a sonolucent centre (Fig. 1.43). Colour flow imaging shows increased vascularity if the nodes are due to inflammation. Tuberculous nodal disease may present in the neck but is usually found in an at-risk patient. It is rare in the native Caucasian population.

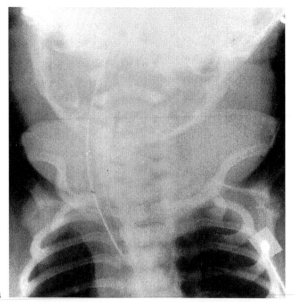

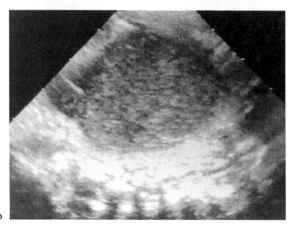

Fig. 1.44 a,b. Neck abscess causing acute respiratory obstruction. **a** Radiograph showing displacement of the trachea to the right by a soft tissue mass. **b** Longitudinal sonogram of the neck in the midline, showing abscess anterior to the cervical spine

Atypical mycobacterial infection is more common. All children with nodal neck disease should have a chest x-ray to exclude both TB and mediastinal nodal disease due to lymphoma.

1.7.2.5
Neck Abscesses

Neck abscesses can be demonstrated by US as a partially or totally fluid-filled mass with a thick wall (Fig. 1.44). Gas bubbles are occasionally seen as areas of echogenicity in the centre of the abscess.

1.7.2.6
Lymphoma

Clinical presentation of lymphoma may follow recognition of the presence of nodes by the child or parent. Ultrasonically lymphomatous masses are often large, and the nodes are no longer discrete. Necrosis may mimic suppuration. In suspected lymphoma the liver, spleen and kidneys should also be examined ultrasonically for lesions. A chest x-ray is mandatory.

1.7.2.7
Acute Suppurative Sialadenitis

Acute suppurative sialadenitis affects the parotid gland more than other salivary glands and tends to occur in dehydrated and/or debilitated patients. It may originate from a septic focus in the oral cavity or dental infection which may depress salivary secretion. Bacterial parotitis is usually unilateral and the commonest pathogen is *Staphylococcus aureus*. The onset is rapid, with swelling and tenderness of the affected gland and pyrexia. US is helpful in identifying the presence of infection by showing enlargement of the gland and the extent of abscess formation (SEIBERT and SEIBERT 1988a, b; GARCIA et al. 1998).

1.7.2.8
Juvenile Recurrent Parotitis

Recurrent parotitis in children is rare. It is characterised by periodic acute or subacute swelling of the parotid gland and/or pain and is usually unilateral. It is often accompanied by fever and malaise. There is non-obstructive cystic dilation of the intraglandular ducts or sialectasis. The aetiology is unknown and it usually resolves spontaneously after puberty. Duct dilation can be demonstrated by US as hypoechoic areas (CHITRE and PREMCHANDRA 1997). If duct dilation is present on US a sialogram can be performed to exclude duct stenosis or obstruction (Fig. 1.45). MRI can also demonstrate sialectasis.

1.7.2.9
Sialolithiasis

The majority of salivary calculi occur in the submandibular gland and in children over 10 years of age

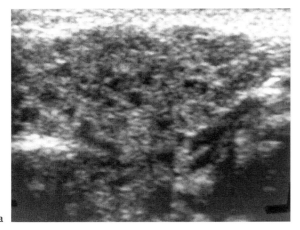

a

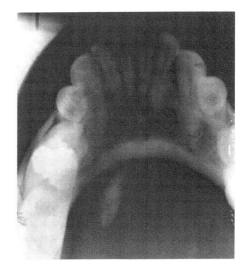

Fig. 1.46. Submandibular calculus. Intra-oral radiograph

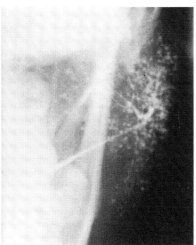

b

Fig. 1.45 a,b. Sialectasis. a US demonstrates multiple hypoechoic areas representing dilated ducts. b Sialogram shows beaded appearance of ectatic ducts

Table 1.8. Causes of acute stridor

Croup
Acute epiglottitis
Foreign body in airway
Neck mass compressing airway, e.g. retropharyngeal abscess
Foreign body aspiration
Angioedema

and they are usually opaque. In children under 10 years of age the submandibular gland is located intra-orally, but in those over 10 years of age the gland is both intra- and extra-oral. Occlusal radiographs will show a stone in the submandibular gland or ducts (Fig. 1.46), US may be helpful in showing a stone which is not visible on plain radiographs because it is superimposed on bone. Sialography may be required to show a radiolucent stone and will also demonstrate sialectasis, which may occur secondary to obstruction of the duct by a stone.

1.7.2.10
Periodontal Abscess and Osteomyelitis

Dental caries which involves the pulp cavity leads to necrosis of the pulp tissue. Infection then ascends to the root tip and involves tissues around the tooth.

This results in widening of the periodontal membrane space and then loss of the lamina dura. If untreated this will be followed by resorption of the surrounding bone.

In older children infection of the tooth socket leading to osteomyelitis can follow dental extraction. The socket fails to heal and there is destruction of the adjacent bone. Clinical presentation is with pain and swelling over the mandible. US will demonstrate bone destruction and periosteal reaction before evidence of osteomyelitis is present on the plain radiograph (KAISER and ROSENBORG 1997; Fig. 1.47).

1.7.3
Acute Upper Airway Obstruction

Obstruction of the airway in the infant and child may occur acutely with rapid onset of signs and symptoms because of the relatively narrow diameter of the airway in early life. Management depends upon rapid assessment of the appropriate level of the obstruction and diagnosis of the obstructing lesion. All forms of acute airway obstruction tend to present with stridor (Table 1.8). When imaging is required

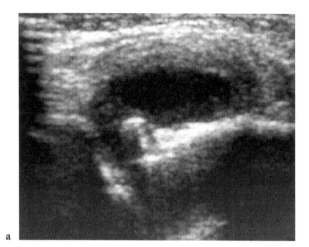

a

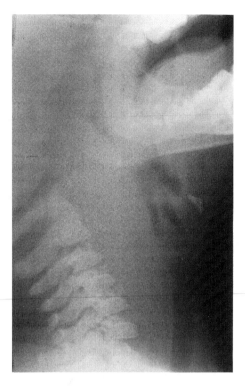

Fig. 1.48. Retropharyngeal abscess. Lateral radiograph showing anterior displacement of the larynx and trachea by a retropharyngeal abscess

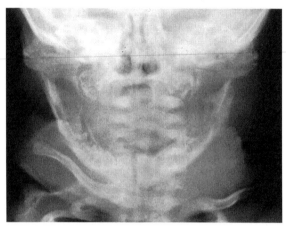

b

Fig. 1.47 a,b. Osteomyelitis of mandible. Five-week-old female infant with facial swelling. **a** US scan shows a periosteal reaction over the left side of mandible and a sonolucent soft tissue abscess. **b** AP view of the mandible shows osteolytic area in the body of mandible

but less common causes of retropharyngeal abscess. Presenting symptoms include stridor, drooling and dysphagia. A soft tissue lateral radiograph of the neck may show an increase in width of the prevertebral soft tissue with anterior displacement of the trachea. If air is present in the abscess the diagnosis of retropharyngeal abscess can be made confidently. If no air is present, US, CT or MRI is required to show the nature of the mass (Fig. 1.48).

plain radiography and fluoroscopy with attention to technique are the mainstays of evaluation of stridor in children (CAPITANO and KIRKPATRICK 1968; DUNBAR 1970; JOHN and SWISCHUK 1992; SWISCHUK 1994).

1.7.3.2
Acute Epiglottitis

Acute epiglottitis is a potentially fatal condition if not recognised and treated promptly. Peak incidence is between 3 and 4 years. Haemophilus influenza type B is the causative organism in the majority of cases. The typical clinical presentation is of pain on swallowing, stridor and drooling. The child will be sitting up and leaning forward because lying back may cause suffocation due to occlusion of the laryngeal inlet by the epiglottis. Radiographs are not indicated if the condition is suspected because of the potential danger of the child becoming acutely obstructed at

1.7.3.1
Acute Retropharyngeal Abscess

Acute retropharyngeal abscess is most common in infancy and young children, in whom it may cause airway obstruction and is potentially very serious. It is usually due to a suppurating retropharyngeal lymph node. Perforation of the pharynx by an unsuspected foreign body or extension of osteomyelitis of the cervical spine into the soft tissue are important

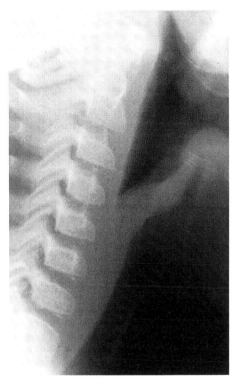

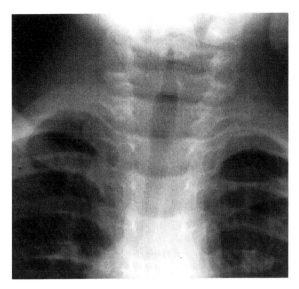

Fig. 1.50. Croup. Radiograph shows narrowing of the subglottic region of trachea and loss of normal shoulder-like lateral convexity

Fig. 1.49. Acute epiglottitis. Lateral radiograph of neck showing thickened epiglottis and aryepiglottic folds

any-time (DAVIS et al. 1981). If radiographs are done inadvertently the entire epiglottis is seen outlined by air in the pharynx (Fig. 1.49).

1.7.3.3
Laryngotracheobronchitis or Croup

Croup is the most frequent cause of upper respiratory tract obstruction in children and is usually caused by viral infection. In most cases croup is mild and imaging is not required (GOEL 1984). Those cases which are severe enough to require radiographic examination have marked dyspnoea, inspiratory stridor and a croupy cough. The typical age group is 11 month–3 years. A chest radiograph which includes the neck will show a narrow subglottis with loss of the shoulder-like lateral convexity and may show ballooning of the hypopharynx. The chest radiograph may show collapsed lobes or overinflation of the lungs. The lateral neck radiograph will also show subglottic narrowing with increased density of the tracheal lumen and is a reliable means of excluding a retropharyngeal abscess or opaque foreign body (Fig. 1.50).

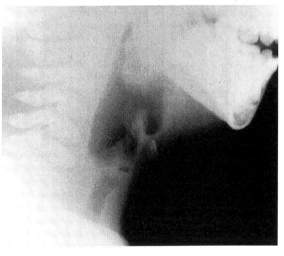

Fig. 1.51. Tonsilitis in a child who presented with difficulty in breathing. Lateral radiograph shows enlarged tonsils

1.7.3.4
Tonsilitis

Occasionally enlarged tonsils can cause a degree of airway obstruction (Fig. 1.51). Imaging is not usually required to diagnose tonsilitis. Enlarged tonsils compressing the airway can be shown on a lateral radiograph of the neck and may be detected incidentally. Similarly enlargement of the adenoids is a common finding in children both with and without symptoms.

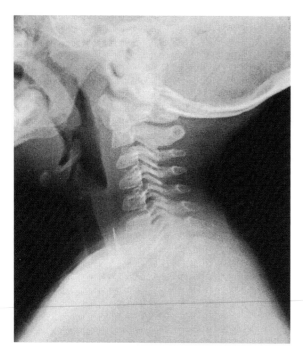

Fig. 1.52. Foreign body in oesophagus. Lateral radiograph shows a fragment of eggshell in the oesophagus

1.7.4
Airway and Oesophageal Foreign Bodies

Airway and oesophageal foreign bodies constitute an acute emergency. Foreign bodies in the pharynx are uncommon: approximately 4% of foreign bodies impact in the pharynx, this eventuality occurring if they are too large to pass through, if they are irregular in shape, or if the edges are sharp and catch on the pharyngeal mucosa. The most common pharyngeal foreign bodies are eggshell fragments, plastic or glass (Fig. 1.52). Fish bones and aluminium ring pulls are also sometimes found.

The majority of ingested foreign bodies pass uneventfully through the gastrointestinal tract. Oesophageal foreign bodies may become embedded in the oesophageal wall, causing oedema and compression of the trachea. Perforation of the pharynx or oesophagus is rare (Fig. 1.53). A retropharyngeal or mediastinal abscess may result. The most common site of hold-up in the oesophagus is at the level of the cricopharyngeus (80%). There is usually a history of choking, coughing, excessive salivation, dysphagia or vomiting. In infants dysphagia may go unnoticed and presentation is with stridor and airway obstruction. A lateral radiograph of the neck and a PA chest film which includes the neck will usually confirm the diagnosis of a radio-opaque foreign body. If the type of foreign body ingested or

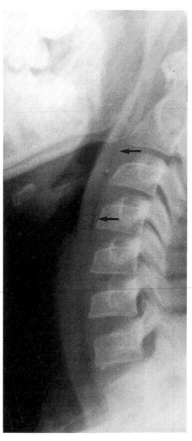

Fig. 1.53. Perforation of oesophagus. This child complained of pain in her throat after eating fish. Lateral radiograph of the neck shows air in retropharyngeal soft tissue (*arrows*) but no evidence of a fish bone

aspirated is known then it can be helpful to x-ray the object to assess its density. In the pharynx a radiolucent foreign body will usually be outlined by air on the lateral neck radiograph (Figs. 1.54, 1.55). A barium swallow may be required to delineate a non-radiopaque foreign body lodged in the oesophagus.

Not all metal is radiopaque. Aluminium objects such as ring pulls from drinks and some coins can be easily ingested. If it is not recognised that aluminium is poorly opaque and difficult to detect on plain radiographs and that a barium swallow is required to make the diagnosis, the diagnosis of ingested foreign body will be delayed with an increased risk of oesophageal perforation (EGGLI et al. 1986).

1.7.5
Thyroid Lumps or Swelling

Thyroid disease is an unusual cause of diffuse swelling or lump in the neck in childhood. The differential

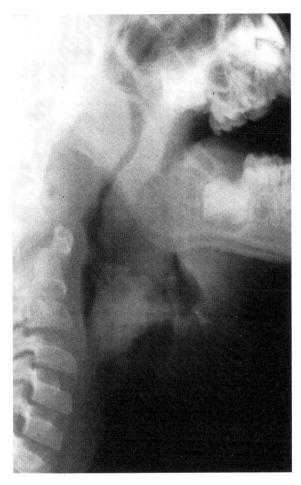

Fig. 1.54. Foreign body in oesophagus. Lateral radiograph of the neck shows a lump of meat lodged in the oesophagus

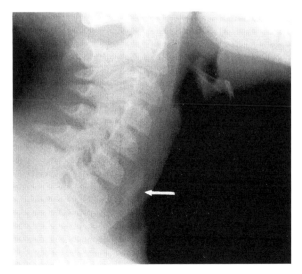

Fig. 1.55. Foreign body in oesophagus. Lateral radiograph of the neck shows an opacity in the pre-vertebral soft tissue (*arrow*) which represents a sweet lodged in the oesophagus

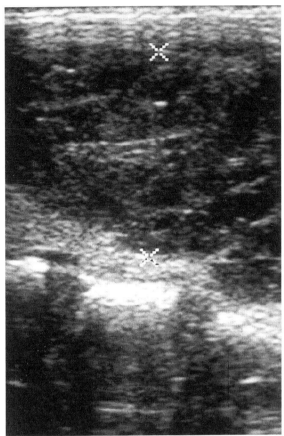

a

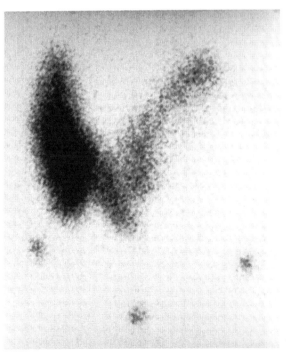

b

Fig. 1.56 a,b. Lymphoma of thyroid. **a** US shows a hypoechoeic mass. A thin rim of normal thyroid is noted posteriorly. **b** Technetium-99 m pertechnetate scan shows a large "cold" mass in the left lobe of the thyroid

diagnosis is narrowed by the clinical information, history, presentation and laboratory data, e.g. thyroid function. US is the primary imaging technique in evaluation of the thyroid. It can distinguish single from multiple nodules and show whether a lesion is solid, cystic or mixed (BACHRACH et al. 1983). Scintigraphy is sometimes useful for further functional assessment.

Simple cysts of the thyroid are uncommon. A midline cyst is most likely to be a thyroglossal duct cyst. The majority occur at or below the hyoid bone. Infection of the cyst can occur. Haemorrhagic cysts can occur as a result of trauma to the thyroid. Sometimes they are due to haemorrhage into an adenoma. Thyroid abscesses are unusual and are associated with fever, pain, tenderness and dysphagia. Recurrent thyroid abscesses are likely to be secondary to a pyriform sinus fistula (AHUJA et al. 1998). A barium swallow will show the sinus tract extending from the pyriform sinus.

Solid masses can be due to thyroid adenomas, lymphoma or carcinoma (Fig. 1.56). The sonographic appearance can be similar and biopsy is required to differentiate between them. Hashimoto's thyroiditis is the result of an immune disorder and is best diagnosed by serology; US is non-specific. Most thyroid lumps are not painful. The child may present as an emergency because the lump has been noticed and causes alarm. Pain in relation to thyroid masses is found with an infected thyroglossal cyst or thyroiditis. Dysphagia is an uncommon presentation but may ensue once the child is aware of the mass. Hoarseness implies involvement of laryngeal nerves and, though rare, indicates either hypothyroidism or malignant infiltration.

References

Adams DA, Cinnamond MJ (1997) Paediatric otolaryngology. In: Kerr AG (ed) Scott Brown's otolaryngology, 6th edn, vol 6. Butterworth - Heinemann, Oxford

Ahuja AT, Griffiths JF, Roebuck DJ, Loftus WK, Lau KY, Yeung CK, Metrewelli C (1998) The role of ultrasound and oesophagography in the management of acute suppurative thyroiditis in children associated with congenital pyriform sinus. Clin Radiol 53:209–211

Arruda LK, Mimica IM, Sole D, Weckx LLM, Schoettler J, Heiner DC, Naspitz CK (1989) Abnormal maxillary sinus radiographs in children: Do they represent bacterial infection? Pediatrics 85:553–558

Assano T, Ohno K, Takada Y, Suzuki R, Hirakawa K, Monma S (1995) Fractures of the floor of the anterior cranial fossa. J Pediatr 39:4:702–706

Bachrach LK, Daneman D, Daneman A, Martin DJ (1983) Use of ultrasound in childhood thyroid disorders. J Pediatr 103:547–552

Beattie TF (1997) Minor head injury. Arch Dis Child 77:82–85

Buckingham JM, Lynn HB (1975) Branchial cleft cysts and sinuses in children. Mayo Clinic Proc 49:172–175

Capitanio MA, Kirkpatrick JA (1968) Upper respiratory tract obstruction in infants and children. Radiol Clin North Am VI:265–277

Chitre VV, Premchandra DJ (1997) Recurrent parotitis. Arch Dis Child 77:359–363

Cohen RA, Kaufman RA, Myero DA, Towbin RB (1986) Cranial computed tomography in the abused child with head injury. Am J Roentgenol 146:97–102

Davis RL, Mullen N, Makela M, Taylor JA, Cohen W, Rwara FP (1994) Cranial computed tomography scans in children after minimal head injury with loss of consciousness. Ann Emerg Med 24:4:640–645

Davis HW, Gartner JC, Galvis AG, Michaelo RH, Mestad PH (1981) Acute upper airway obstruction: croup and epiglottitis. Pediatr Clin North Am 28:859–880

Dunbar JS (1970) Upper respiratory tract obstruction in infants and children. Am J Roentgenol 109:227–246

Eggli KD, Potter BM, Garcia V, Altman RP, Breckbill DL (1986) Delayed diagnosis of oesophageal perforation by aluminium foreign bodies. Pediatr Radiol 16:511–573

El-Silimy O, Corney C (1993) The value of sonography in the management of cystic neck lesions. J Laryngol Otol 107:245–251

Enriques G, Gil-Gibernau JJ, Garriga V, Ribes L, Lucaya J (1995) Sonography of the eye in children: imaging findings. Am J Roentgenol 165:935–939

Friedman AP, Haller JO, Goodman JD, Nagar H (1983) Sonographic evaluation of non-inflammatory neck masses in children. Radiology 147:693–697

Garcia CJ, Flores PA, Arce JD, Chuaqui B, Schwartz DS (1998) Ultrasonography in the study of salivary gland lesions in children. Pediatr Radiol 28:418–425

Glasier CM, Seibert JJ, Williamson SL, Seibert RW, Corbitt SL, Rodgers AB, Lange TA (1987) High resolution ultrasound characterization of soft tissue masses in children. Pediatr Radiol 17:233–237

Goel KM (1984) Are neck radiographs necessary in the management of croup syndrome. Arch Dis Child 59:980

Hayman LA, Evans RA, Hinck VC (1979) Rapid high-dose contrast computed tomography of isodense subdural haematoma and cerebral swelling. Radiology 131:381–383

Helmke K, Hansen HC (1996) Fundamentals of transorbital sonography evaluation of optic nerve sheath expansion under intracranial hypertension. II. Patient study. Pediatr Radiol 26:706–710

Hollman AS (1994) Facial trauma. In: Carty H, Shaw D, Brunelle F, Kendall B (eds) Imaging children. Churchill Livingstone, Edinburgh, pp 1744–1753

Hopper KD, Sherman JL, Boal DK, Eggli KD (1992) CT and MR imaging of the pediatric orbit. Radiographics 12:485–503

Jaspan T, Narborough G, Punt JAG, Lowe J (1992) Cerebral contusional tears as a marker of child abuse - detection by cranial sonography. Pediatr Radiol 22:4:237–245

John SD, Swischuk LE (1992) Stridor and upper airway obstruction in infants and children. Radiographics 12:625–643

Johnstone AJ, Zuberi SH, Scobie WG (1996) Skull fractures in children a population study. J Accident Emerg Med 13:386–389

Kaban CB (1993) Diagnosis and treatment of fractures of facial bones in children 1943-1993. J Oral Maxillofac Surg 51:722–729

Kaiser S, Rosenberg M (1997) Early detection of subperiosteal abscess by ultrasonography. A means for further successful treatment in pediatric osteomyelitis. Pediatr Radiol 24:336–339

Keats TE (1996) Atlas of normal variants that may simulated disease, 6th edn. Mosby, St Louis

Kingsley DPG, Lloyd GAS, Kendal BE (1986) Radiology of orbital masses in children. Acta Radiol 369:354–657

Kronemer KA, McAlister WH (1997) Sinusitis and its imaging in the pediatric population. Pediatr Radiol 27:11:837–846

Kwong JS, Munk PL, Lin DTC, Vellet AD, Levin M, Buckley AR (1992) Real time sonography in ocular trauma. Am J Roentgenol 158:179–182

Laine FJ, Conway WF, Laskin DM (1993) Radiology of maxillo-facial trauma. Curr Prob Diagn Radiol 22:145–188

Latack JT, Hutchinson RJ, Heyn RM (1987) Imaging of rhabdomyosacroma of the head and neck. Am J Roentgenol 8:353–359

Lloyd DA, Carty H, Patterson M, Butcher CK, Roe D (1997) Predictive value of skull radiography for intracranial injury in children with blunt head injury. Lancet 349:821–824

Loroni L, Ciucei G, Piccinini G, Cuseini M, Sorza P, Piola C, Servadei F (1996) Approach to head trauma in childhood in a district general hospital. Eur J Emerg Med 3:141–148

McAlister WH, Lusk R, Muntz HR (1989) Comparison of plain radiographs and coronal C.T. scans in infants and children with recurrent sinusitis. Am J Roentgenol 153:1259–1264

Moreea S, Jones S, Zoltie N (1997) Radiography for head trauma in children. What guidelines should we use? J Accident Emerg Med 14:12–15

Murshid WR (1994) Role of skull radiology in the initial evaluation of minor head injury. Acta Neurochir 129:11–14

Poznanski AK (1976) Practical approaches to pediatric radiology, Year Book Medical Publishers, Chicago, pp 249–251

Ramji FG, Slovis TL, Baker JD (1996) Orbital sonography in children. Pediatr Radiol 26:245–258

Read HS, Johnstone AJ, Scobic WG (1995) Skull fracture in children: altered conscious level is the indication for urgent CT scanning. Injury 26:333–334

Rehm CG, Ross SE (1995) Diagnosis of unsuspected facial fractures on routine head CT scans. J Oral Maxillofac Surg 53:522–524

Sato Y, Yuh WTC, Smith WL, Alexander RC, Kao SCS, Ellerbroek CS (1989) Head injury in child abuse; evaluation with MR imaging. Radiology 173:653–657

Seibert RW, Seibert JJ (1988a) High resolution ultrasonography of the parotid gland in children. Paediatric Radiology 16:374–379

Seibert RW, Seibert JJ (1988b) High resolution ultrasonography of the parotid gland in children. Part II. Paediatr Radiol 19:13–15

Sheth S, Nussbaum AR, Hutchins GM, Sanders RC (1987) Cystic hygromas in children: sonographic-pathologic correlation. Radiology 162:821–824

Sherman NH, Rosenberg HK, Heyman S, Templeton J (1985) Ultrasound evaluation of neck masses in children. J Ultrasound Med 4:127–134

Shields JA, Backawell B, Augsburger JJ, Donoso LA, Benardino V (1986) Space-occupying orbital masses in children. A review of 250 consecutive biopies. Ophthalmology 93:3:379–383

Sohaib SA, Moseley J, Wright JE (1998) Orbital rhabdomyosarcoma – the radiological characteristics. Clin Radiol 53:357–362

Swischuk LE (1994) Upper airway disease. In: Emergency imaging of the acutely ill or injured child, 3rd edn. Williams and Wilkins, Baltimore

Teasdale GL, Murray G, Anderson G, Mendelow AD, MacMillan R, Jennett B, Brookes M (1990) Risks of acute intracranial haematoma in children and adults: implications for managing head injuries. BMJ 300:363–370

Wallace SA, Bennett J, Perez-Avila C, Gullan RW (1994) Head injuries in the accident and emergency department are we using resources effectively? J Accident Emerg Med 11:25–31

Wilkins B (1997) Head injury abuse or accident? Arch Dis Child 76:393–397

2 Emergency Chest Radiology in Children

A.W. Duncan

2.1
Radiographic Assessment of the Chest

Children present to the Accident and Emergency Department with a variety of clinical symptoms in addition to those due to trauma. These presenting symptoms include cough, breathlessness, chest pain and occasionally haemoptysis. Chest pain alone is rarely of sinister significance and is most often musculoskeletal in origin, e.g. effort syndrome, muscle strain or rib injuries. Tietze's syndrome or costochondral chondritis probably of viral origin

A.W. Duncan, MD, FRCR, FRCPCH, DMRD, Consultant Paediatric Radiologist, Department of Radiology, Bristol Royal Hospital for Sick Children, St. Michael's Hill, Bristol BS2 8BJ, UK

may occasionally account for chest pains. Unlike in the adult population, chest pain is rarely due to a cardiac disorder. It may occasionally occur in aortic stenosis. Pain associated with respiratory distress may be due to a pneumothorax, spontaneous or secondary to an underlying pre-existing respiratory disorder such as asthma or cystic fibrosis, or occasionally be secondary to trauma. Lung tissue itself is insensitive to pain and chest pain is usually the result of damage to surrounding structures. Pulmonary consolidation may be entirely painless unless there is pleurisy. Pain may occasionally be the result of ingested or inhaled oesophageal or tracheal foreign bodies. Reflux oesophagitis with or without hiatus hernia, spasm or achalasia, and very rarely with rupture of the oesophagus, may be responsible for chest pain. Pleural irritation may present as pain in the abdomen. Similarly, some abdominal conditions may result in chest pain. This particularly occurs with diaphragmatic irritation since the central portion of the abdomen is innervated from the phrenic nerve. Pain may be the presenting symptom of subphrenic abscesses.

Cough is a more specific symptom of respiratory disease and is usually a reflex stimulated by material in the air passages. In addition to infective causes it may be the result of foreign body. Very rarely in children is it due to compression of the bronchi by vascular structures and mass lesions.

Chronic cough is most commonly due to asthma. Other causes include whooping cough, lower respiratory tract infection compounded by social conditions such as parental smoking, habit cough, foreign body, aspiration, cystic fibrosis, tuberculosis, immunodeficient states and chronic gastro-oesophageal reflux.

Dyspnoea is a frequent presentation of many respiratory diseases. It is due to compromise of the airway either by extramural causes such as tumours and mediastinal glands or compression of the lung due to effusions, pneumothorax or occasionally large hiatal hernias. The two major mural lesions are oedema and paralysis of the larynx. Intramural lesions such as foreign bodies or mucous plugs are seen in asthma and bronchiolitis. Involvement of the lung itself is usually due to infective causes such as pneumonia and pleurisy. Cardiovascular disease may present with dyspnoea due to cardiac failure or pericarditis. Occasionally an abdominal cause with marked distension of the abdomen leads to elevation and splinting of the diaphragm. Rarely psychogenic causes are responsible.

Haemoptysis is a rare presenting feature in children. It may originate in the trachea from tracheitis or more rarely haemangioma. Bronchial causes of haemoptysis include adenoma, bronchitis, bronchiectasis, foreign bodies and newly perforated intrathoracic gastroenteric cysts secondary to ulceration within them. Pulmonary causes include trauma, pneumonia, infarction, tuberculosis, abscesses and pulmonary haemosiderosis.

2.1.1
Interpretation

Any of these symptoms in addition to physical signs elicited in relationship to the chest would prompt in the first instance a request for a chest radiograph. The abnormality itself may be apparent immediately. If it is not, then a systematic approach analysing the chest radiograph may be required to identify an abnormality which at first sight is elusive to the eye. This should begin with scrutiny of the soft tissues of the neck and extend into the mediastinum. Radiopaque foreign bodies may be seen. Duplication cysts and collapsed segments of the lung in or adjacent to the mediastinum can be difficult to see unless actively sought. The outline of the trachea and main bronchi should be searched for narrowing or intraluminal soft tissue opacity. Focal lesions within the lung are usually fairly apparent. However, with collapse/consolidation adjacent to the diaphragm or heart border the only sign may be loss of part of the outline of these structures. Fine interstitial changes, because they are generalised, may be overlooked. Examples are pulmonary haemosiderosis, which may produce small miliary-like nodules, and diffuse peribronchial thickening as seen in infective or allergic states. Visualisation of the right horizontal fissure in the young child is always abnormal beyond the immediate post-natal period after the foetal fluid has resorbed, and is an early indication of interstitial pulmonary oedema or pleural reaction secondary to infection. The costophrenic angle should be checked for blunting, which may indicate pleural fluid, and

the apices for lucencies that may imply a small apical pneumothorax. Mass lesions can easily be overlooked if the clavicle and ribs are projected closely together in this region, obscuring a small soft tissue opacity. The thoracic wall should be searched for rib fractures, congenital anomalies which may indicate a syndrome, notching in coarctation of the aorta and soft tissue swelling or interstitial air. Lucencies may be seen in the mediastinum. Linear ones are due to interstitial air. More focally rounded lucencies are seen in cavities or hiatal hernia.

Vertebral anomalies, widening of the foramina and paravertebral masses may be missed on an under-penetrated film. The ideal exposure for a child's chest x-ray is one in which the vertebrae are seen but the bony detail of the vertebrae is not. The diaphragm height should be checked. Its elevation may imply pathology beneath the diaphragm, paralysis or subpulmonary fluid.

The stomach air bubble should be identified to confirm abdominal situs, which is important in congenital heart disease. This should be differentiated from the bubble, which may indicate free air due to a pneumoperitoneum or subphrenic abscesses. The absence of an air bubble itself may well be fortuitous but occasionally it may imply achalasia, in which case examination of the mediastinum may show an air-fluid level in the dilated oesophagus.

From these initial observations in most instances the diagnosis can be made on the plain radiograph. If on the frontal projection a lesion is seen, a lateral view may be of value for localisation of, for example, a mass in the anterior, middle or posterior mediastinum or a foreign body in the trachea or oesophagus. If there are large areas of opacity such as pleural effusion, ultrasound is indicated to identify any underlying collapsed lung or masses and to aid diagnostic or therapeutic drainage. Further studies in the more difficult cases will require fluoroscopy, contrast studies, computed tomography (CT) or magnetic resonance imaging (MRI), and occasionally the use of radio-isotopes. These further investigations must never be done until the chest x-ray has been carried out. One would consider the appearances of this and the differential diagnosis, with further examinations to elicit the definitive diagnosis.

2.1.2
Pitfalls

There are anatomical differences in children's chest x-rays compared with those of adults that could lead to misinterpretation. The thymus is prominent especially in the first year of life and can mimic masses and pneumonias. The degree of ventilation of the lungs has a greater impact on the degree of pulmonary opacification and mediastinal size compared with adults. The same is true of rotation of the patient, which can lead to increased transradiancy of the side away from the cassette.

2.1.2.1
The Thymus

In the normal chest in the neonate the thymus is prominent and often obscures the true heart size, which is better assessed on a lateral film. In early life the thymus gland consists of two unequally sized pyramidal lobes. Each is surrounded by a fibrous capsule with septa that divide the lobes into small irregular lobules 1–2 mm in diameter. This bilobed appearance with its finely nodular surface gave rise to its name, given by Rufus of Ephesus in the first century. Thymus in Greek means "a warty excrescence like a thyme bud" and in ancient Greek was the name for the herb thyme, itself so named because it was thought to give courage – which is translated from the Greek "*thymon*". The origin if its name is as intriguing as its appearance and function.

The cardiothoracic ratio in the PA projection in older children and adults is normally 50% but is difficult to assess in children under 6 months old since the cardiothymic silhouette is often entirely produced by the thymus. Also the AP projection is usual in this age group, because the film is taken supine, the erect position being difficult. This will magnify the cardiothymic silhouette.

The thymus is a soft structure and its anterolateral border abuts the costochondral junction of the anterior ribs and the bulge between these produces the "thymic ripple" (Fig. 2.1). The trachea normally deviates to the right side because of the left-sided aorta. The thymus may bulge more focally (Fig. 2.2) and even extend to the diaphragm, and to the unwary may mimic a focal mass. A normal thymus, however, does not displace or compress the trachea and its typical anterior sail appearance on the lateral projection usually gives reassurance.

The thymus varies in size and correlates with the body weight in the first year of life (HASSELBATCH

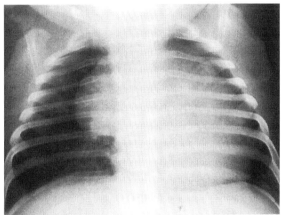

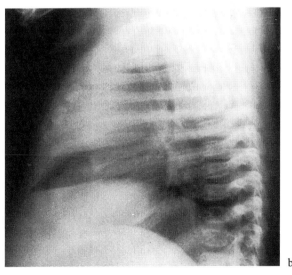

Fig. 2.2. a On this variation the thymus shows a localised bulge at the right-hand border. **b** The lateral view shows a very clear-cut inferior straight margin with the trachea clearly not compressed or displaced, indicating that this is a normal thymus

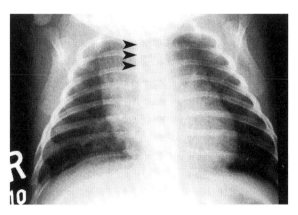

Fig. 2.1. The normal chest: normal thymic silhouette with the ripple shadow clearly seen along the left mediastinal border. The trachea deviates as it extends caudally to the right (*arrowheads*)

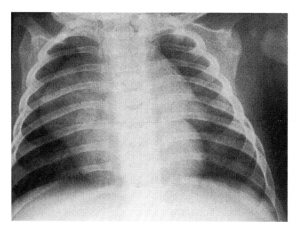

Fig. 2.3. Normal thymus. This radiograph shows a large thymus, a "sail" shape on the left and a more focal bulge on the right

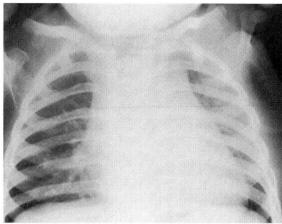

a

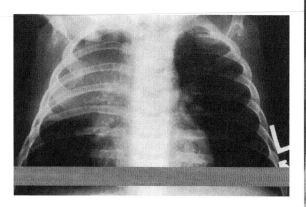

Fig. 2.4. Normal thymus. Rotated film. The thymic silhouette on the right side abuts the right thoracic wall and mimics a pneumonia in the right upper lobe with the clear inferior border appearing as the horizontal fissure. This has been produced by rotation of the patient, causing the normal aerated lateral portion of the lung to lie more posteriorly and not outline the lateral border of the thymus

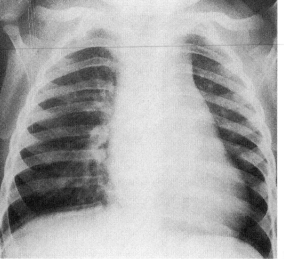

b

Fig. 2.5. a An expiratory film shows widening of the mediastinum and cardiac silhouette, with increased pulmonary vascularity. **b** An inspiratory film in the same child shows normal appearances

et al. 1997). The right lobe is more prominent than the left. Persistence of the large thymic shadow on a chest radiograph beyond 2 years should raise a question about its normality. Occasionally in prepubertal children the thymus may appear as a right superior mediastinal mass. The prominence in early life is largely due to its comparatively large size in relationship to the mediastinum (Fig. 2.3). Its apparent diminution in size after 1 year is due to growth of the child with the thymus remaining almost unchanged in size (ADAMS and IGNOTUS 1993) until puberty. Thereafter thymic remnants may be seen into adulthood.

There are numerous normal thymic variants seen on infants' chests which may cause confusion. A fre-

quent normal appearance is the "sail shadow", which on a rotated film may mimic a pneumonia (Fig. 2.4; OERMANN and MOORE 1996). Other technical factors can contribute to misinterpretation. The expiratory phase, particularly in the neonate, can dramatically increase the cardiothymic silhouette and pulmonary vascularity, mimicking heart failure or right to left shunt. Mediastinal widening in the expiratory film in the older child (Fig. 2.5) can give rise for concern, especially in trauma cases. The thymus may at times mimic a tumour (Fig. 2.6a). A straight film or in difficult cases fluoroscopy will clarify the situation. The thymus is a soft structure and does not displace or compress the trachea. On fluoroscopy it can be seen to change in contour readily with respiration and on rotation of the patient the lateral aspect can

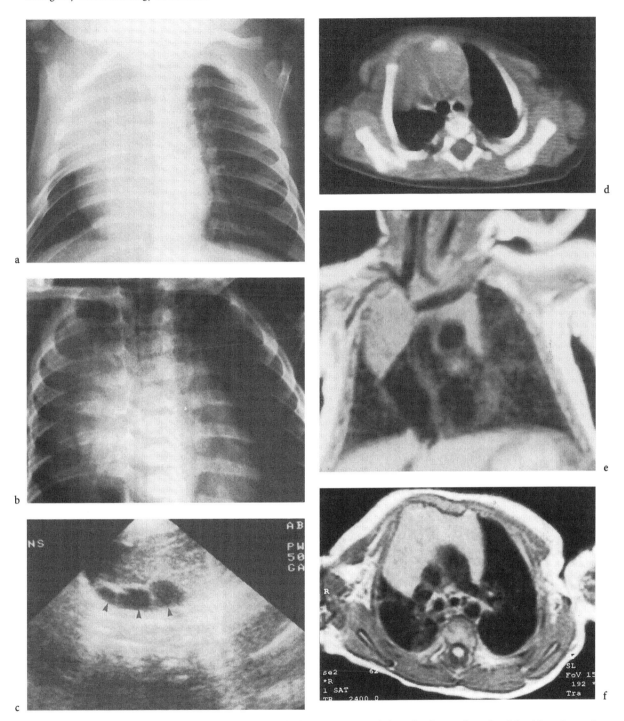

Fig. 2.6. a There is an opacity in the right upper zone, which could be a mass, collapsed upper lobe or the thymus. The film is rotated and renders the interpretation difficult. **b** A straight film shows that this is the thymus and shows its lateral extent. **c** Ultrasound shows the typical echogenic appearance of the thymus lying above the hypoechoic vessels (*arrowheads*). Note that these are not compressed. **d** CT scan. This shows a normal thymus which is more prominent on the right side. Owing to a partial volume effect, it appears that there is exten-sion anteriorly into the chest wall on the right side. **e** Coronal T1-weighted MR image shows the normal angular configuration of the thymus, which is not displacing structures or compressing veins. It has a homogeneous signal, with no focal areas of altered signal. The signal is slightly greater than that of muscle. **f** Axial T2-weighted MR image shows the smooth angular configuration with the signal being higher than that of muscle, but lower than that of fat

be evaluated with regard to differentiating it from mass or pneumonia (Fig. 2.6b). The next imaging investigation should be ultrasound, which may be able to resolve the problem (CARTY 1990), the thymus being of uniform echogenicity, similar to the liver, and having a characteristic shape (ADAMS and IGNOTUS 1993) (Fig. 2.6c). If there is still doubt MRI or, if this is not available, CT will usually resolve the issue. The thymus is angular, being quadrilateral in children up to 5 years, and then more triangular (ST. AMOUR et al. 1987). On both CT and MRI (Fig. 2.6d) the thymus is homogeneous with smooth margins and does not displace structures. On MRI its signal on T1-weighted images (Fig. 2.6e) is slightly greater than that of muscle; on T2-weighted images (Fig. 2.6f) it appears much brighter than muscle, with a signal close to that of fat (SIEGEL et al. 1989b). Posterior extension or ectopic location of the thymus may simulate a posterior mediastinal mass on the chest radiograph but MRI and ultrasound should resolve the problem (VAN MOSSEVELDE et al. 1993).

The thymus is important for the development of immunity; hence its comparatively large size in early life. The absence of the thymus gland such as in di George syndrome will render the child vulnerable to infection. Any child in the first year of life who has recurrent infections and is seen on the radiograph to have persistent absence of the thymus should be considered to be in this category. However, interpretation may be difficult since infections and stress cause rapid involution of the thymus gland within 24h; therefore on a single radiograph in a child of 6 months of age or younger with infection the apparent absence may be due to this rapid involution. The absence of the thymus gland, although suspected on plain films, must be confirmed by MRI, or if this is not available, CT.

Similarly, lack of normal adenoidal tissue in the post-nasal space in children over 6 months should alert one to possible immunological compromise. Conversely, tissue in the post-nasal space in the newborn should raise the possibility of a mass. Although it is rarely pathological, this possibility must be excluded.

The trachea normally deviates to the right due to the normal position of the left-sided aorta. On an expiratory film the trachea kinks contralateral to the site of the descending aorta on the AP projection (Fig. 2.7) and buckles forward on the lateral film. On the lateral film variation with breathing in the width of the soft tissues in the prevertebral region is much greater than that in the older child, where one verte-

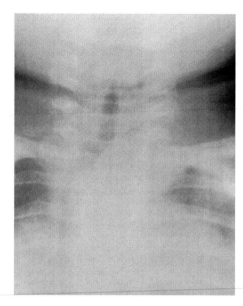

Fig. 2.7. Frontal projection showing normal kinking of the trachea which should not be mistaken for displacement by a mass. If in doubt one should perform a lateral film or repeat AP with the neck extended and full inspiration

bral width is considered the upper limit of normal. This increase in soft tissue space associated with buckling of the trachea may mimic a prevertebral cervical mass such as an abscess or tumour. Fluoroscopy with the head extended will clarify the issue as in this position the "pseudo" mass disappears, but if fluoroscopy is not available a supine lateral film in inspiration with the child's neck extended and gentle pressure of a lead-gloved finger on the larynx will compress the soft tissues and indicate whether the lesion is real or a technical artefact (Fig. 2.8).

Skin folds, especially in the neonatal period, may mimic a pneumothorax (Fig. 2.9). Similarly, a lucency overlying the heart may be due to a hole in the incubator.

2.1.2.2
Sternal Deformity

A depressed sternum will also cause apparent cardiac enlargement (Fig. 2.10). The clinician examining the child can identify the deformity but rarely puts the information on an x-ray request form. In children with pectus cavinatum or excavatum, the ribs have an abnormal angle on the x-ray.

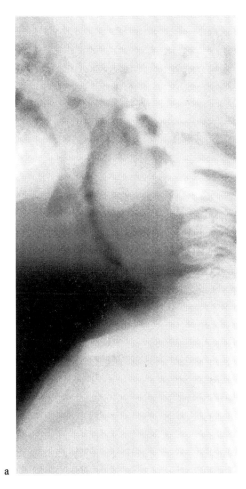

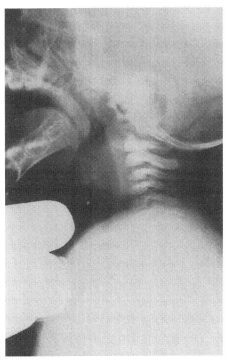

Fig. 2.8. a The lateral projection taken in the expiratory phase with the head slightly flexed gives the impression of a prevertebral mass. b Film taken in the inspiratory phase with the neck in a neutral position. The leaded gloved hand (*white area*) applies gentle pressure and eliminates the artefactual appearance of the prevertebral mass

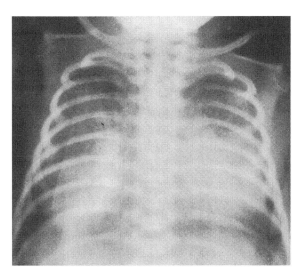

Fig. 2.9. The thin lucent line seen on both sides, but more prominently on the right side, is due to a skin fold and not a pneumothorax

2.1.2.3
The Diaphragm

The right hemidiaphragm is usually one half intercostal space higher than the left but equal height or a higher left hemidiaphragm occurs in the minority of normal individuals. The position of the left hemidiaphragm is due to depression by the cardiac apex. The abdominal situs does not influence the height of the hemidiaphragm. The most common cause of an elevated left hemidiaphragm in infants is gastric distension caused by the ingestion of air during crying. Abnormal elevation may be due to supradiaphragmatic causes, e.g. atelectasis, hypoplasia or overinflated contralateral lung. A subpulmonary effusion, although not strictly causing an elevated hemidiaphragm, gives the same appearance. Diaphragmatic causes such as phrenic nerve palsy and eventration and subdiaphragmatic causes such as subphrenic abscesses, hepatic or splenic en-

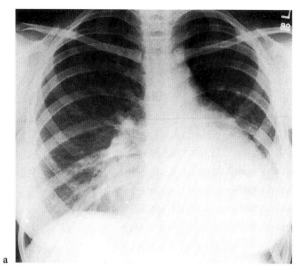

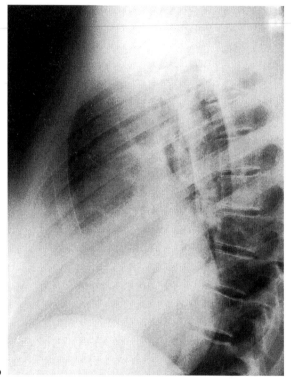

Fig. 2.10. a Depressed sternum in a 16-year-old girl. The posterior portion of the ribs are more horizontal and the anterior portion of the ribs point down more than is normal. There is displacement of the cardiac silhouette to the left. The heart appears enlarged, particularly as the right border is not seen, and is partially obscured by the soft tissue opacity produced by the medial anterior thoracic wall being displaced posteriorly by the depressed sternum. **b** Depressed sternum, lateral projection. This view shows the displacement of the posterior border of the heart. This is not due to cardiac enlargement, but displacement by the sternum, which can be seen as a curvilinear white line overlying the anterior mediastinum

largement and abdominal mass may cause real elevation (Oh et al. 1988). Bilateral elevation is due to abdominal distension by gas or fluid-filled loops of bowel, or abdominal masses. This can impair normal ventilation and decrease oxygen saturation as well as causing basal collapse.

Normal movements of the diaphragm can be assessed by fluoroscopy. The movements are always in the same direction although the excursions may not be symmetrical. If fluoroscopy is not possible because of the patient's condition, e.g. on intensive care, it can be evaluated by ultrasound. Paradoxical movements, i.e. upward movements of the affected hemidiaphragm on inspiration, occur in phrenic nerve palsy due most commonly to thoracic surgery or birth trauma, and are seen in eventrations. Poor or no movements occur in these conditions but are more commonly seen in juxtadiaphragmatic disorders such as subphrenic abscess, pneumothorax, emphysema or atelectasis. The movements should be assessed with deep inspiration as well as sniffing since in a few individuals paradoxical movements occur with sniffing. Severe eventration may be difficult to distinguish from a true diaphragmatic hernia on the plain film. Ultrasound or, if necessary, CT or MRI may distinguish this.

Interposition of bowel between the liver and the right diaphragm is a frequent finding on chest radiographs and is of no clinical relevance but may be mistaken for localised pneumoperitoneum. This is known as Chilaiditi's syndrome and is often a transient phenomenon.

2.2
Respiratory Distress

Chest radiographs are usually performed for respiratory symptoms of dyspnoea, wheeze, cyanosis or sometimes pyrexia. The appearance on the film may correlate with the clinical picture. However, some features may reflect pre-existing disease and it is important to differentiate the appearances that are contributing to rather than incidental to the presenting features. Some incidental features may be pathological and need investigation. Therefore, faced with a radiograph of a child with respiratory symptoms, analysis is of paramount importance to direct one to the definitive diagnosis. In the analysis of the film it is helpful to study the prominent overall appearance. The following categories will be studied:

2.2.1 The large mediastinum
2.2.2 The bubbly chest
2.2.3 Predominantly hyperlucent hemithorax
2.2.4 Mediastinal lucencies
2.2.5 Predominantly opaque hemithorax
2.2.6 Focal lesions
2.2.7 Interstitial disease

Since the pathology varies with age, interpretation will be best considered in two main categories: the young child, including neonates and infants up to the age of about 2 years, and the older child. Some of the conditions discussed are seen mainly in the immediate newborn period and are therefore seen as emergencies in special care baby units or departments of neonatal surgery. Delayed presentation of conditions such as congenital diaphragmatic hernia or lobar emphysema after the child has been well at home can lead to confusion and are discussed in this section as they may present as emergencies.

2.2.1
The Large Mediastinum

Common causes of the large mediastinum are shown in Table 2.1, and a flow chart illustrating the diagnostic pathway is provided in Fig. 2.11.

2.2.1.1
Neonate

2.2.1.1.1
LARGE THYMUS
Most prominent thymic silhouettes are non-pathological; however, true massive thymic hyperplasia that is symptomatic has been described (OBARO 1996; PEDROZA MELENDEZ and LARENAS-LINNEMANN 1997) and may compress and displace structures, unlike normal enlarged thymus (MEZA et al. 1993). Some such cases are associated with other disorders (BEES et al. 1997). Rebound enlargement after chemotherapy may also simulate tumour (BODE and SCHEIDT 1988) but is rarely symptomatic. If it presents a diagnostic problem, MRI will differentiate the two conditions. Gallium-67 scans are of little value as the hyperplastic thymus may accumulate the

Table 2.1. Common causes of the large mediastinum

Neonate/infant	Older child
Normal	Lymphoma
Teratoma	Cardiomegaly
Cardiomegaly	Lymphangioma
Lymphangioma	Malignant germ cell tumour
	Langerhans cell histiocytosis

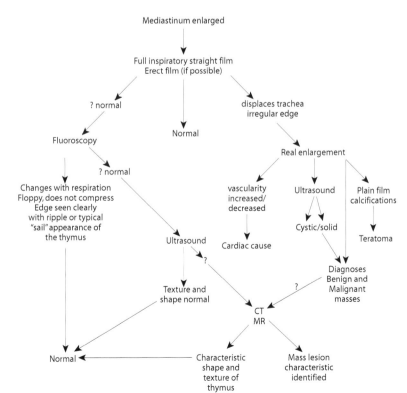

Fig. 2.11. Flow chart illustrating appropriate pathway for investigation of the large mediastinum

isotope. Thallium and the newer radiopharmaceuticals, especially fluorine-18 fluoro-2-deoxy-D-glucose (FDG) and technetium-99m methoxyisobutylisonitrite (MIBI), may have a role in difficult cases in differentiating tumour from rebound thymus with fibrosis. Thymomas and thymic cysts are rare causes of mediastinal enlargement, both being very rare in children. In human immunodeficiency virus, thymic enlargement has been described due to multilocular thymic cyst formation which can be confirmed by CT or MRI (LEONIDAS 1998).

2.2.1.1.2
THYMIC TERATOMA

Thymic teratoma, a germ cell tumour, is usually benign and is the second most common cause of mediastinal widening after a normal large thymus. It accounts for 10% of all childhood mediastinal masses (KING et al. 1982). Most occur in young children below 2 years of age. They are often asymptomatic, but occasionally will cause tracheal compression resulting in dyspnoea and possibly stridor (Fig. 2.12). Haemoptysis may be a rare presentation. The widening of the mediastinum is frequently more prominent on the left side and indistinguishable in most cases from the thymus from which such teratomas may occasionally arise.

Thymic teratomas are formed from totipotential tissue and therefore give rise to a variety of cell types. They may contain calcification, fat or cystic areas. Occasionally the fat will form fluid levels in the cystic areas. These appearances are best identified on CT or MRI. Tissue characterisation is obviously better on MRI and although it will not image calcification directly, if large enough it will appear as an area of signal void. If all these features are present the lesion is usually benign although because of the multipotential nature of the cells, malignancy cannot be excluded in other areas of the mass. Rapid increase in size is not an indication of malignancy and may well be due to haemorrhage into the mass. If there are signs of local invasion this is a sign of malignancy (LEVITT et al. 1984).

Very rarely the teratoma may lie within the pericardium, causing cardiac silhouette enlargement and often presenting with cardiac failure. Ultrasound, CT and MRI will aid in the diagnosis (STY et al. 1992).

2.2.1.1.3
LARGE HEART

The neonate and infant mediastinum can be prominent due to the thymus and may make assessment of the heart size difficult or impossible on the AP pro-

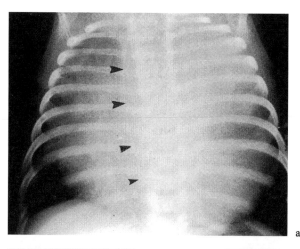

a

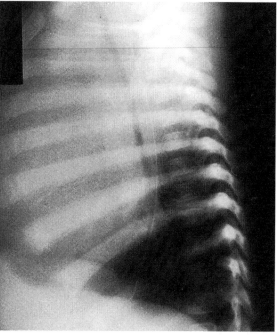

b

Fig. 2.12 a,b. Teratoma. **a** There is marked enlargement of the cardiothymic silhouette. The tracheal displacement is not seen well on this film. The nasogastric tube (*arrowheads*) shows that there is displacement of the oesophagus, indicating a pathological mass. **b** The lateral projection shows posterior displacement of the trachea, as well as compression, which causes respiratory distress. The retrosternal space is obliterated without the horizontal inferior margin of the normal thymus gland being seen

jection. The lateral projection is more helpful but echocardiography is far more accurate in assessing cardiac pathology and should be undertaken in all suspected cases. However, in an emergency situation much information can be obtained from the plain radiographs. Normal vascularity on the AP projection with increase in the transverse diameter of the

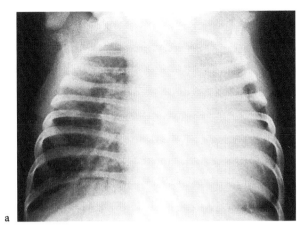

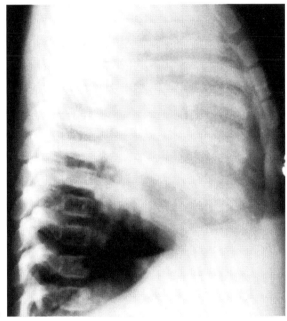

Fig. 2.13 a,b. Left to right shunt. a There is cardiac enlargement, increased vascularity and hyperinflation of the lungs, consistent with a left to right shunt with some indistintness of the vessels, suggesting cardiac failure. In this case it was due to a patent ductus arteriosus. b The lateral projection confirms the cardiac enlargement, with a lateral cardiothoracic ratio greater than 50%. The trachea is displaced posteriorly due to cardiac enlargement but is not compressed

mediastinum should alert one to possible non-cardiac causes. Careful assessment of the lateral projection should be carried out to exclude a mediastinal mass rather than cardiac enlargement. Evenly distributed increased vascularity in a non-cyanosed infant is usually due to a left to right shunt, usually a patent ductus arteriosus or ventricular septal defect (Fig. 2.13). The supine film and the smaller distances from the apex to the base of the lung in an infant do

not produce the same hydrostatic pressure changes seen in the erect older child.

Pulmonary vascularity is more difficult to assess and often is seen more peripherally in children than adults. The assessment of pulmonary vasculature is heavily dependent on the quality of the radiograph. If over-exposed, the pulmonary vasculature cannot be seen. Cardiac failure is usually manifest by indistinctness of the vessels in the neonate without the typical septal line seen in the adult although visualisation of the minor fissure on the right always indicates interstitial oedema. Associated pleural effusions because of the supine position are seen as a diffuse haze over the whole lung due to general peripheral distribution of fluid, with fluid seen in the fissures. Increase in the pulmonary vascular markings may not necessarily indicate a cardiac cause since the tachycardia will make the vascular markings more prominent, as will extracardiac conditions such as arteriovenous malformation and coarctation of the aorta with cardiac failure. Acute or chronic upper airway obstruction such as adenoidal enlargement, especially if associated with skeletal problems such as achondroplasia, may precipitate cardiac failure and should prompt appropriate lateral skull radiographs. The rarer conditions of enlarged heart with pulmonary plethora and cyanosis are usually due to a complex heart lesion, most commonly transposition of the great vessels, truncus arteriosus or non-obstructive pulmonary venous return, and are markedly more frequent in children with chromosomal abnormalities.

Normal pulmonary vascularity with a large cardiothymic silhouette may have a cardiac cause such as cardiomyopathy (Fig. 2.14), pericardial effusion, conduction anomalies or right outflow tract obstructions depending on myocardial compromise. Pericardial effusion (Fig. 2.15) produces globular enlargement of the heart silhouette and widening of the superior mediastinum with obscuration of the aortic knuckle and pulmonary artery, and may have a crisp outline to the heart due to dampening of the myocardial movements. Myocarditis also produces cardiac silhouette enlargement but the superior mediastinum is not enlarged and pulmonary congestion is invariably present, which helps to differentiate this from pericardial effusions.

Oligaemic lungs indicate right heart failure or outflow obstruction (Fig. 2.16). The cardiac silhouette may occasionally provide a definitive diagnosis such as "egg on the side", as seen in transposition of the great vessels. Extracardiac features on a plain film may aid the diagnosis. A right aortic arch iden-

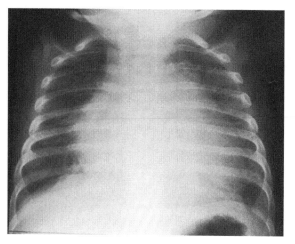

Fig. 2.14. Cardiomyopathy. The heart is enlarged and the pulmonary vascularity is not as prominent as one sees in a left to right shunt, although this is not always the case as it depends on the myocardial function

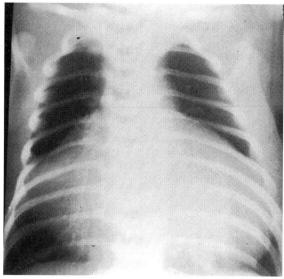

Fig. 2.16. Ebstein's anomaly. Large heart with decrease in the pulmonary vascular markings

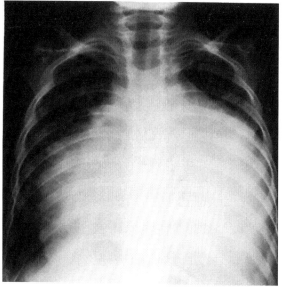

Fig. 2.15. Pericardial effusion. Massive cardiac silhouette enlargement due to a pericardial effusion. This can be confirmed by ultrasound. Note the loss of the aortic knuckle. The pulmonary vascularity depends on the compromise of myocardial function and failure

tified by the trachea deviating to the left on the AP radiograph is seen in Fallot's tetralogy (25%), pseudotruncus arteriosus (50%), truncus arteriosus (25%), double outlet right ventricle (25%), and single ventricle (12.5%) (CONDON 1990), but may occur as an isolated anomaly.

The typical features and appearances of congenital heart disease illustrated in older textbooks are now seldom seen due to earlier diagnosis and treatment.

The bronchial anatomy seen in the mediastinum may indicate complex heart disease with asplenia associated with bilateral right-sided bronchi and polysplenia associated with bilateral left-sided bronchi. Similarly, the position of the stomach gas bubble should be noted since if it lies on the same side as the cardiac apex and aortic arch the likelihood of congenital heart disease is low, while if it lies on the right side the instance is slightly higher. In dextrocardia without abdominal situs inversus the incidence of heart disease is high, between 75% and 80% (CONDON 1990). A central position of the liver, i.e. situs ambiguous, also carries a higher incidence of complex heart disease. Skeletal anomalies may be associated with clinical syndromes, e.g. eleven ribs, or accessory ossification centres in trisomy 21.

Cardiovascular Disease. Cardiovascular emergencies presenting de novo without a known history of congenital heart disease are rare in children compared with the adult population. Congenital heart disease is outside the scope of this book. The main clinical presentations of cardiovascular emergencies in children are palpitations from arrhythmias, breathlessness due to cardiac failure, headaches or fits from hypertension, chest pain and sudden collapse – often occurring on a sports field. Children with congenital heart disease may present with symptoms of bacterial endocarditis or cerebral abscess. Stroke due to emboli or haemorrhage is infrequent but does occur.

Chest pain is a non-specific symptom and in children rarely results from cardiac causes, more often being musculoskeletal or pulmonic in origin if organic. Pericardial effusion is common following cardiac surgery. Pericardial effusion in children presenting as an emergency is usually infective and most commonly viral but may be tuberculous in endemic areas. It is also seen in connective tissue disorders. Both pericardial effusion and cardiomyopathy are features of Kawasaki disease. Most cardiomyopathies are congenital in children.

Imaging. A chest radiograph is routinely obtained in children presenting with symptoms of pain, palpitations, hypertension or failure. If the child has known congenital heart disease, the findings of cardiomegaly, cardiac contour or situs abnormalities, and hyper- or hypo-pulmonary vascularity, are influenced by this. The radiological findings to note are signs of cardiac failure described elsewhere in this chapter, and alteration in cardiac contour that might indicate cardiomyopathy or pericardial effusion. Comparison with a previous film, if available, is helpful. Cardiac wall motion and pericardial effusion are best assessed by echocardiography. The cause of failure is often supervening infection. Consolidation should be sought. In pericardial effusion the heart attains a globular shape and has an increased transverse diameter. Similar appearances are seen in cardiomyopathy. Echocardiography will distinguish the two. Children with hypertension commonly have a normal chest film. In severe cases there may be cardiac enlargement with a left ventricular pattern and signs of cardiac failure – usually interstitial rather than acute pulmonary oedema. Alteration of the aortic contour with a "double knuckle" sign and the presence of rib notching indicates coarctation.

2.2.1.1.4
LYMPHANGIOMAS (CYSTIC HYGROMA)
Lymphangiomas are classified according to cell type: capillary, cavernous and cystic hygroma. These congenital lesions are probably present at birth and most manifest themselves clinically within the first year due to complications related to the large size and location (GIMENO ARANQUEZ et al. 1996). Primary location in the mediastinum is rare but does occur. Most lymphangiomas extend downwards from the neck (SIEGEL et al. 1989a) and may present as airway compression, especially if there has been

haemorrhage, infection or chylothorax formation (LEMONINE and MONTUPET 1991).

Chest radiographs will show widening of the mediastinum (Fig. 2.17a) and may show displacement and compression of the trachea, often with extension into the neck (Fig. 2.17b). The soft tissue density is homogeneous with a clear curvilinear border. Ultrasound will demonstrate its cystic nature (Fig. 2.17c). There is great variability in size and complexity of the cysts and where the lesion is mainly capillary the numerous slightly dilated capillary lymphatics will appear almost as a solid component owing to the echoes from the walls of the cyst obscuring the fluid component (Fig. 2.17d). If the child is old enough then a Valsalva manoevre may displace the cystic hygroma out of the chest into the neck for better evaluation of its nature, but the extent is better assessed by MRI if available, or if it is not, by CT. CT demonstrates the multilocular cystic mass and, although there may be some displacement of adjacent structures, the mass because of its consistency generally conforms to the mediastinal structures. Contrast enhancement identifies any haemangiomatous areas. MRI demonstrates more anatomical detail characterised by the fluid and solid components and differentiates the lymphangiomatous from the haemangiomatous component. The fluid in the cyst is usually of low signal on T1 weighted images and high signal on T2. However, occasionally there is fat or haemorrhage into the cyst which will give a higher or mixed signal on T1 weighted images. The walls of the cyst usually are of low signal. Pleural effusions may complicate lymphangioma (STOVER et al. 1995).

2.2.1.2
Older Child

In the older child the thymus is small and so is not a problem in the differential diagnosis of mediastinal enlargement. It is usually very obvious whether there is cardiac enlargement or a mass.

2.2.1.2.1
LYMPHOMA
Lymphoma is the third most common neoplastic disease in children but is the commonest anterior mediastinal mass, and is due to a combination of neoplastic infiltration of thymus and mediastinal lymph nodes. Hodgkin's lymphoma accounts for the majority of anterior mediastinal masses although non-Hodgkin's lymphoma is more prevalent (COHEN 1992), accounting for 60% of lymphomas.

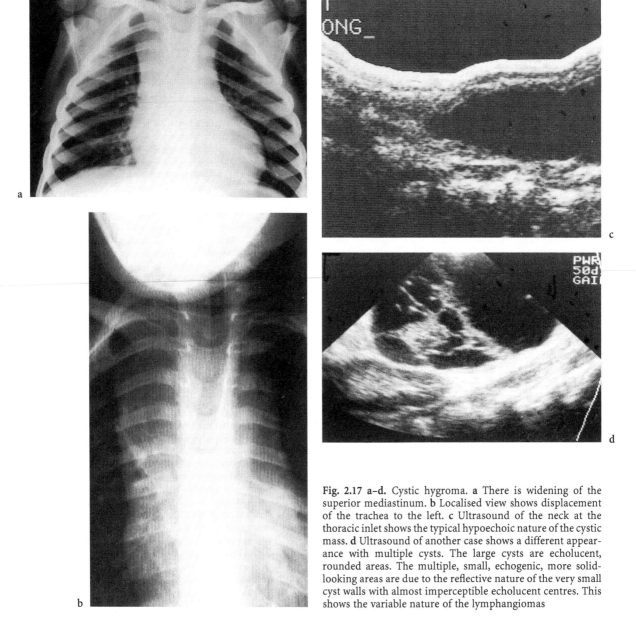

Fig. 2.17 a–d. Cystic hygroma. **a** There is widening of the superior mediastinum. **b** Localised view shows displacement of the trachea to the left. **c** Ultrasound of the neck at the thoracic inlet shows the typical hypoechoic nature of the cystic mass. **d** Ultrasound of another case shows a different appearance with multiple cysts. The large cysts are echolucent, rounded areas. The multiple, small, echogenic, more solid-looking areas are due to the reflective nature of the very small cyst walls with almost imperceptible echolucent centres. This shows the variable nature of the lymphangiomas

Mediastinal involvement in non-Hodgkin's lymphoma, especially of the T-cell type, presents more frequently as an emergency with dyspnoea and cough due to tracheal compression (LEMONINE and MONTUPET 1991) (Figs. 2.18, 2.19), superior vena cava obstruction syndrome and large pleural effusions. Hodgkin's lymphoma occurs in young adults and is rare under 5 years. The typical clinical presentation is with a palpable cervical node. Mediastinal presentation uncommonly occurs as chronic cough due to compression of the airways by nodes or even less frequently by pulmonary infiltration (ALTMAN and SCHWARTZ 1978). More often the mediastinal involvement is found on a child's radiograph done because of the presence of the cervical node. Pleural effusions can occur in both types of lymphoma due to lymphatic obstruction in Hodgkin's disease and pleural invasion in non-Hodgkin's lymphoma. Lymphatic spread from the hilar nodes and interstitial septal involvement produces a characteristic fan-like pattern of radiating streaks (Fig. 2.19). Nodular lesions and subpleural deposits are confined to Hodgkin's disease (ALTMAN and SCHWARTZ 1978). Skeletal involvement due to spread by haema-

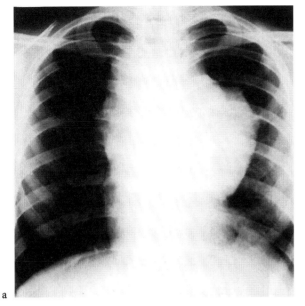

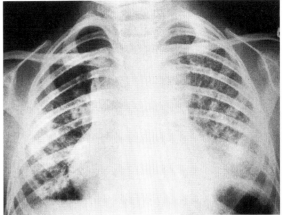

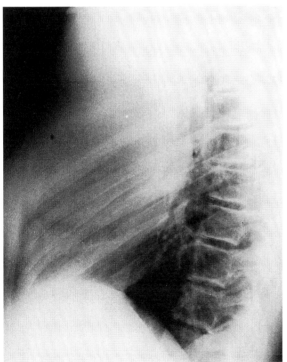

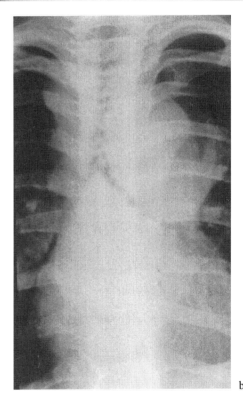

Fig. 2.18 a,b. Lymphoma. a There is widening of the mediastinum with an irregular nodular outline indicative of lymph node enlargement. b The lateral view shows the retrosternal space filled by lymphomatous nodes. There is compression of the trachea and displacement posteriorly

Fig. 2.19 a,b. Lymphoma. a In addition to widening of the mediastinum, there is lymphatic obstruction which produces an interstitial pattern in the lung fields. b Localised views show compression with marked narrowing of the trachea and left main stem bronchus, but these can also be shown by CT or MRI during staging

togenous route or direct invasion (Fig. 2.20) is infrequent in Hodgkin's disease although is occasionally a presenting feature. Infiltration of the mediastinum with cells in acute lymphoblastic

leukaemia may give a similar appearance to non-Hodgkin's lymphoma.

In childhood non-Hodgkin's lymphoma the mediastinum is the second most common primary site. It appears as a large lobulated mediastinal mass in many cases with tracheobronchial compression and often with pleural effusion. CT delineates the mass

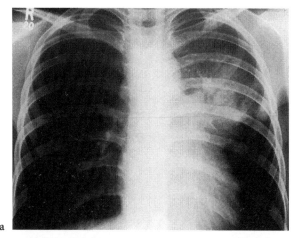

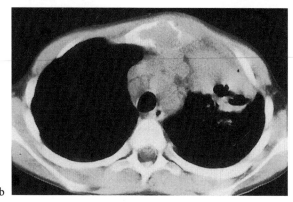

Fig. 2.20 a,b. Hodgkin's disease. **a** This patient presented to Accident and Emergency as an emergency with a cough. The radiograph shows infiltration in the left lung extending from the left parahilar region, which could be mistaken for simple pneumonia. On the lateral projection, there was destructive invasion of the sternum. **b** CT scan shows a mass in the anterior left hemithorax extending into the soft tissues and involving the sternum, which has expanded with bone destruction

and shows its homogeneous nature with clearly defined borders.

In Hodgkin's disease the mass in the mediastinum appears lobulated; tracheobronchial compression occurs but less frequently than in non-Hodgkin's lymphoma. CT may show the lesion to have cystic areas which represent necrotic or haemorrhagic areas within the lymph nodes. CT or MRI will demonstrate the extent of the mass in all lymphomas (Fig. 2.20b) and show subdiaphragmatic involvement. Respiratory compromise due to mediastinal mass can be life threatening and treatment with steroids usually produces dramatic relief. Biopsy should either be delayed or an abutting non-mediastinal site sought otherwise haemorrhage may occur from the distended veins in the mediastinum (Lo Kich and Goodman 1975). All children presenting with mediastinal lymphoma

should have urgent ultrasound of the abdomen to search for renal or splenic involvement.

2.2.1.2.2
GERM CELL TUMOURS
Germ cell tumours arise from primitive germ cell rests and are a rare neoplasm found most commonly in adolescents and young men. On the radiographs these appear as a lobulated unilateral mediastinal mass and on CT there are often areas of low attenuation representing haemorrhage and necrosis which do not enhance with contrast. Invasion of the adjacent tissue planes is a feature of malignancy. Cysts, calcifications and fat are not usually present in malignant germ cell tumours although their presence does not rule out malignancy.

2.2.1.2.3
LANGERHANS CELL HISTIOCYTOSIS
Although the thymus may be the site of localised primary disease it is more frequently involved in the disseminated disease. There may be a large thymic mass which may progress to cavitation. This can be readily identified by CT and if adjacent lung is involved the entry of air into the cysts will also be demonstrated on CT. Rarely calcification may occur (Leonidas 1998).

2.2.1.2.4
OTHER CAUSES OF THE LARGE MEDIASTINUM
Acute mediastinitis is a rare cause of widening of the mediastinum, usually more prominent superiorly, often secondary to oesophageal rupture.

Mediastinal haemorrhage is usually secondary to trauma, iatrogenic or, rarely nowadays, due to a bleeding diathesis.

There is inevitably an overlap between causes of mediastinal widening and focal lesions. Massive lymphadenopathy will cause mediastinal widening whilst mild hilar enlargement will produce a focal enlargement. Some of those conditions that produce widening of the mediastinum have been dealt with in this section as well as in the focal section. The lesions that are more frequently smaller are dealt with in Sect. 2.2.6.

2.2.2
The Bubbly Chest

Common causes of the bubbly chest are shown in Table 2.2, and Fig. 2.21 illustrates the appropriate diagnostic pathway.

Table 2.2. Common causes of the bubbly chest

Unilateral	Bilateral
Neonate/infant	
Congenital cystic adenomatoid malformation	Pulmonary interstitial emphysema
Congenital diaphragmatic hernia	Bronchopulmonary dysplasia
Pneumatocoeles	
Pulmonary interstitial emphysema	
Congenital lung cysts	
Abscesses	
Older child	
Congenital cystic adenomatoid malformation	Cystic fibrosis
Delayed diaphragmatic hernia	Bronchiectasis
Pneumatocoeles – infective	Bronchopulmonary dysplasia
Pneumatocoeles – traumatic	
Bronchiectasis	
Abscesses	

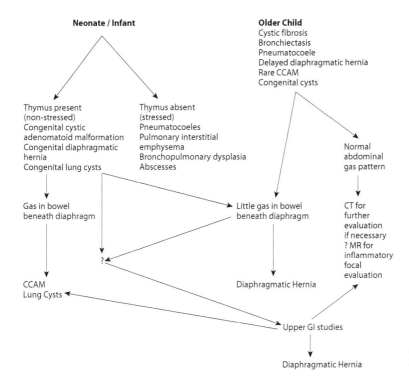

Fig. 2.21. Flow chart illustrating the appropriate diagnostic pathway in the child with a bubbly chest

In stress conditions the thymus involutes rapidly, often within 24 h. In conditions such as congenital diaphragmatic hernia or congenital cystic adenomatous malformation of the lung, the presence of the thymus can help differentiate these from conditions associated with stress such as pneumatocoele secondary to pneumonia, where the thymus is no longer visualised. There are conditions where there is congenital absence of the thymus such as Di George syndrome, but these are exceedingly rare.

2.2.2.1
Unilateral

2.2.2.1.1
CONGENITAL CYSTIC ADENOMATOUS MALFORMATION

This is a rare congenital multicystic lesion produced by proliferation of the terminal bronchi. It is usually confined to one lobe but is occasionally bilateral (STOCKER and MADEWELL 1977). There is no lobar predilection but the middle lobe is less frequently affected. The cysts communicate with the airway and may present with respiratory difficulty due to compression of the remaining lung tissue.

Congenital cystic adenomatous malformation (CCAM) is seen with equal frequency in boys and girls. There are three main types depending on the cyst size and solid component (STOCKER and MADEWELL 1977): (1) main large cyst, (2) multiple small cysts, (3) mainly solid. Respiratory distress is the usual presentation, the time of presentation and the radiological appearance depending on type (SHANJI et al. 1988): type 3 presents at birth and type 2 at 24h, whereas type 1 may present within 4 weeks or even later in life. In type 1 the cyst contains air and may mimic interstitial emphysema, congenital diaphragmatic hernia or lobar emphysema (Fig. 2.22). If the upper abdomen is seen in the chest film then gas-filled loops of bowel seen in the abdomen usually support the diagnosis of CCAM. The presence of a thymus usually excludes acquired disorders such as inflammatory pneumatocoeles. Partially solid or fluid-filled cysts with aerated cysts give an appearance similar to pneumatocoeles or hiatus hernia (Fig. 2.23). CT, although usually unnecessary to make the diagnosis, shows the cystic and solid components.

The majority of cases are diagnosed in the neonatal period. Most present with respiratory distress due to compression of the lung by the malformation, occasionally with a chylous effusion. They rarely present to the Casualty department. Missed or silent lesions will present later in childhood, often due to superadded infection. In the immediate newborn period when the cysts are filled with fluid they may appear as a solid intrapulmonary mass but on presentation to the Casualty department in an older age group they will present either as hyperinflation of the affected lobe or, if there is superadded infection, possibly as partly fluid-filled cystic areas reminiscent of pneumatocoeles. When they are purely air-filled they may resemble fluid-filled loops of bowel or congenital diaphragmatic hernia. Observation of the upper abdomen on the chest film will show loops of bowel which will exclude diaphragmatic hernia.

Sometimes one cyst will predominate and then when this is filled with air, particularly if there is distension, it may mimic congenital lobar emphysema. Occasionally it may rupture and present as a pneumothorax. Type 3 usually presents in the immediate neonatal period as a large soft tissue mass and is therefore unlikely to present to the Casualty department.

Types 2 and 3 have a poor prognosis due to associated anomalies in type 2 and because of the large size in type 3. Lobectomy is the treatment of choice since apart from hypoplasia of the adjacent and contralateral lung due to compression, malignant transformation occurs (ASKIN 1987); this usually takes the form of rhabdomyosarcoma, but bronchiolar

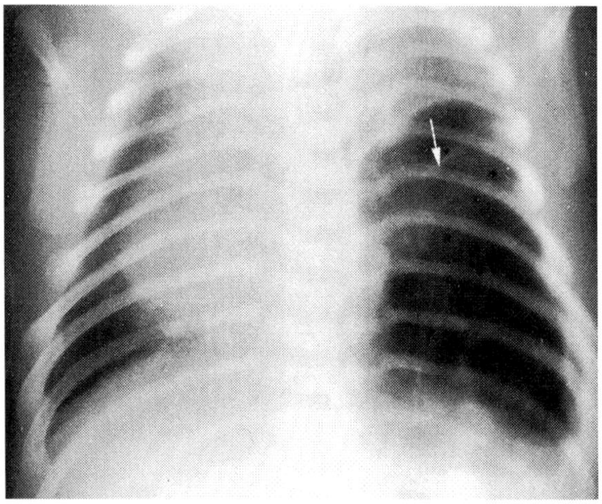

Fig. 2.22. Congenital cystic adenomatoid malformation. There is hyperexpansion of the left lower lobe, with shift of the mediastinum to the right side and compression of the left upper lobe. Within the hypolucent area there are curvilinear opacities (*arrow*) which are the walls of the cystic areas in the lesion. If the film were rather over-penetrated these cystic areas might not be seen, erroneously suggesting congenital lobe emphysema

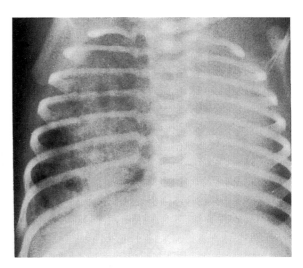

Fig. 2.23. Congenital cystic adenomatoid malformation. This is the mixed type, partly solid and partly cystic, which can be mistaken for partially fluid-filled bowel of a diaphragmatic hernia. Note the normal upper abdomen on this film. If in doubt, do a barium study

alveolar carcinoma has been reported in adults (RIBET et al. 1995). In the early neonatal period, like other conditions that have air trapping later, there may be retained fetal fluid and they may present as an opaque lung. Ultrasonography in utero and in the immediate post-natal period shows fluid-filled cysts in types 1 and 2, and solid structures in type 3. Delayed presentation can occur and may be misinterpreted as pneumonia with pneumatocoeles (Fig. 2.24). Failure to respond to treatment may give the first inkling of the clinical problem.

2.2.2.1.2
CONGENITAL DIAPHRAGMATIC HERNIA

Neonate/infant. Congenital diaphragmatic hernia is of two types: Bochdalek, through a posterior defect in the diaphragm just lateral to the spine, and Morgagni (much less common), retrosternally through an anterior defect just lateral to the midline, usually on the right side.

Congenital diaphragmatic hernia of Bochdalek usually presents at birth, if it is not diagnosed antenatally by ultrasound. The incidence is 1 in 2000 live births (ANDERSON 1986). Clinical presentation is with tachypnoea and distress. On the chest x-ray it appears at birth as an opaque hemithorax due to the fluid-filled loops of bowel. This progresses to air-filled cystic structures as the loops fill with air. When only partially air filled, the loops of bowel may be mistaken for pneumatocoeles in pneumonia but the clinical presentation and presence of the thymus usually differentiates the two conditions. Ultrasound can usually show fluid-filled loops of bowel and Doppler ultrasound the pulsating mesenteric vessels if there is clinical doubt as to the diagnosis. Later, as air fills the bowel, multiple air-filled loops of bowel are seen (Fig. 2.25). These should be traced to below the diaphragm, where there is often a paucity of bowel gas due to the number of loops in the chest. The later appearance with fluid-filled loops of bowel may occur as delayed presentation and cause confusion in an emergency setting. The heart and mediastinum

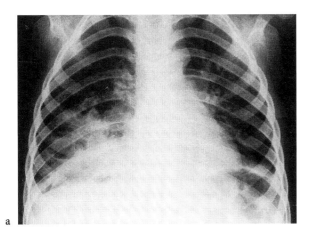

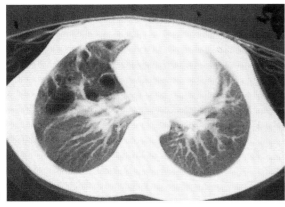

Fig. 2.24 a,b. Congenital cystic adenomatoid malformation. Late presentation at 14 years of age with recurrent respiratory infection. An earlier film post infection had shown only hyperinflation in the right lung. **a** Film taken in an acute phase of infection shows cystic areas with fluid levels. **b** CT scan after resolution of infection shows cystic areas in the right middle lobe

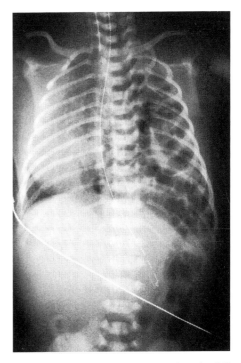

Fig. 2.25. Diaphragmatic hernia. Here the bowel is full of gas and a loop of bowel containing gas is seen extending from the abdomen into the chest, which confirms the diagnosis. The upper abdomen is relatively gasless

are displaced away from the mass. Reduced air or a gasless abdomen is seen sometimes, with a small loop of bowel extending from the abdomen into the chest with non-visualisation of the hemidiaphragm. On the lateral projection the abdomen often appears scaphoid shaped due to the diminished amount of bowel in the abdomen. Left-sided hernia is 5 times more common than right-sided hernia, probably due to the later closure of the pleuroperitoneal canal. On the right some opacification may be due to the herniation of liver into the thorax.

Differentiation from CCAM or sequestration can be made by contrast studies. Air as a contrast agent will show gas-filled loops of bowel but it should not be injected down the nasogastric tube since this may compromise the lung due to the distension of bowel. If confirmation is needed, instillation of water-soluble contrast through the nasogastric tube is appropriate.

As with any congenital space-occupying lesion in the hemithorax, compression of the ipsilateral lung and, if the defect is large, of the contralateral lung due to mediastinal shift, will cause pulmonary hypoplasia. Death is due to the latter. Associated anomalies are cardiovascular disorders, gut malrotation and neural tube defects. They greatly alter the prognosis, especially in cases of congenital heart disease.

Older Child. Congenital diaphragmatic hernia of Bochdalek usually presents in the immediate postnatal period with respiratory distress, but delayed presentation with respiratory distress, recurrent chest infection or small bowel obstruction in the older child is not uncommon and is important as a mistaken diagnosis can lead to death or inappropriate surgery. The cystic appearance with patchy opacification due to partially gas/fluid-filled loops of bowel may easily be mistaken for lower lobe pneumonia with pneumatocoeles (Fig. 2.26) and may lead to death (DELPORT 1996) if not treated. A distended stomach or single loop of bowel may be misinterpreted as a large pneumothorax or lung cyst or, if filled with fluid, an intrathoracic mass.

Children with respiratory symptoms tend to present earlier than those with gastrointestinal symptoms. Right-sided hernias are more often associated with delayed presentation, probably due to the protective tamponade effect of the liver although an association with B-streptococcus pneumonia has been described. It is postulated that the infection may either destroy the hemidiaphragm or provoke the presentation of the hernia through the pre-

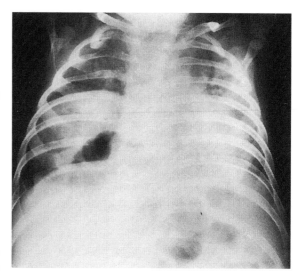

Fig. 2.26. Late presentation of a diaphragmatic hernia in 5 month old. On the right the lower hemithorax is partially filled with liver and gas filled loops of bowel

existing congenital defect in the diaphragm (BANAGALE and WATTERS 1983). An associated pleural effusion is sometimes seen. An earlier previous normal chest radiograph does not exclude the diagnosis.

Morgagni hernia usually presents in the older age group, often as an incidental finding or occasionally with vague abdominal symptoms. Dyspnoea, chest or abdominal pain or discomfort, diarrhoea and vomiting are rare presentations. If there is a large defect, gas-filled loops of bowel will present as cystic lucencies in the hemithorax and, if partly filled with fluid, may mimic pneumatocoeles in a pneumonia (Fig. 2.27a). If the defect is small and contains fluid-filled bowel only, or omentum, it may appear as a soft tissue mass in the right cardiophrenic angle.

The diagnosis is confirmed by barium meal with delayed films if the colon is suspected of being in the hernia (Fig. 2.27b,c), which is often the case in Morgagni hernia. Delayed post-traumatic diaphragmatic hernia due to blunt trauma may present many years after the accident and can result in strangulation of the bowel (VAN DE VEN et al. 1995). Detection of a diaphragmatic hernia may be an incidental finding in a child being radiographed for some other reason such as a chest infection. Occasionally the gastro-oesophageal tract becomes markedly distended with gas and presents more acutely. The radiograph shows multiple cystic areas of fairly uniform dimensions although there occasionally may be one or two large distended cystic areas due to

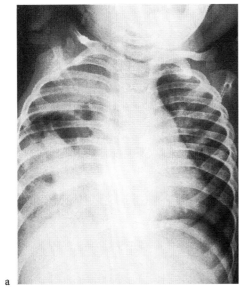

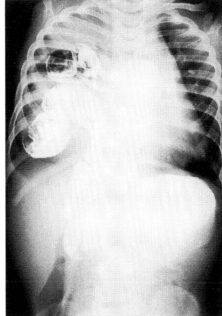

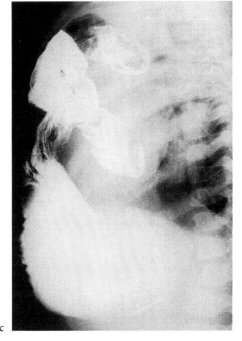

Fig. 2.27 a–c. Right-sided Morgani hernia in a 11/2-year-old. a Multicystic and partly opaque space occupying lesion in the right hemithorax causing compression of the lung and shift of the mediastinum to the left side. b Frontal. Barium meal and follow through showed the stomach and upper small bowel to be in the abdomen but the delayed film shown here demonstrates that the cystic areas are due to loops of bowel. c Lateral. Loops of ileum filled with contrast pass anteriorly through a defect into the lower right thorax

distended stomach or single loop of bowel. If the hernia is large, as it is in most cases, there is very little aerated lung on the ipsilateral side. There is displacement of the mediastinal tract to the contralateral side. On the right side similar appearances may be seen although since the liver may herniate into the right hemithorax, part of the hemithorax will be opaque. Ultrasound can confirm the presence of the liver in the right hemithorax. Further confirmation can be obtained by CT or MRI, though this is rarely necessary.

In differentiating these lesions a plain film is usually sufficient. If the patient is not fit enough to come to the department, ultrasound can show the presence of a diaphragm but small defects cannot be excluded. Oral contrast studies usually differentiate diaphragmatic hernias in difficult cases. If colonic herniation occurs, as in Morgagni hernia, then a water-soluble contrast enema will provide confirmation, although it is probably kinder to the child to get the information by a follow-through examination.

2.2.2.1.3
PNEUMATOCOELES

Pneumatocoeles are the result of expansion of the cystic air spaces caused by the destruction of the walls of distal alveoli in pneumonic consolidation. The organism is usually *Staphylococcus*. Pneumatocoeles occur in up to 60% of children with this infection. More rarely pneumatocoeles are seen with *E. coli, Klebsiella, Pneumococcus, Haemophilus influenza*, tuberculosis and measles virus pneumonias (SHANJI et al. 1988). The pneumatocoeles are produced by inflammatory exudate plugging the distal bronchi, producing a ball valve effect that causes air trapping. The surrounding consolidation prevents collateral air drift and the escape of entrapped air. This progressive increase in the pressure causes the pneumatocoeles and since there is necrotic tissue it occurs later in the disease process, usually in the early healing phase.

Symptoms are usually due to pneumonia but occasionally may present as an acute respiratory emergency due to tension pneumatocoeles or a pneumothorax as a result of rupture of the pneumatocoeles (SHANJI et al. 1988). As the pneumonia resolves, collateral air drift is restored and the pneumatocoeles spontaneously disappear over a period of weeks. Rarely a single pneumatocoele may remain as a thin-walled cyst. If fluid levels persist under antibiotic treatment there is a high risk of continuing infection and abscess formation. Radiologically, pneumatocoeles appear as thin-walled cystic areas of variable size, may change in size on serial radiographs, and in the acute phase are surrounded by consolidated lung (Fig. 2.28), sometimes with fluid levels (Fig. 2.29). Pneumatocoeles occasionally occur after blunt trauma. When there is a history of injury, the diagnosis is easy.

2.2.2.1.4
ABSCESSES

Abscesses are a complication of pneumonia. The majority are caused by aerobic bacteria, of which *Staphylococcus aureus* is commonly the offending organism. The children usually present with a history of weight loss, malaise and cough, often over a period of time. Eventually pain, dyspnoea and sometimes haemoptysis brings the child to Casualty.

Lung abscesses appear on radiographs as thick-walled cavities, often with effusion. Ultrasound will show the cavity wall as a thick echogenic area with more hypoechoic material lying within the cyst due to the particulate matter within the pus-filled cavity.

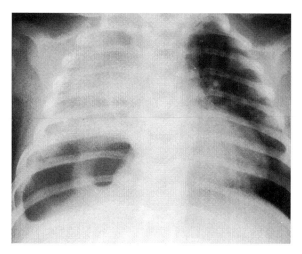

Fig. 2.28. Pneumatocoeles. The right hemithorax is partially opacified with cystic areas at the right base due to pneumonic consolidation and pneumatocoeles

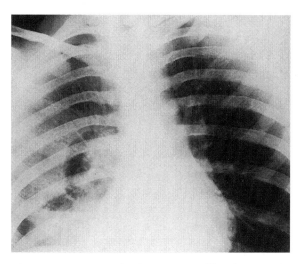

Fig. 2.29. Pneumatocoeles in a 15-year-old asthmatic. The pneumatocoeles are confined to the right lower lobe with fluid levels and occurred in the late phase of pneumatic consolidation, probably exacerbated by an asthmatic attack

Ultrasound will also confirm the intrapulmonary location, based not only on the position of the abscess but also on the fact that it moves with respiration, whereas pleural lesions do not. An abscess appears on the plain film as a round opacity. If there is necrosis or communication with a bronchus, air-fluid levels will be seen (Fig. 2.30a). On the plain film the thickness of the wall can be identified when air is present within the cavity and helps differentiate it from pneumatocoeles, which have very thin walls. Peripheral lesions may be associated with varying

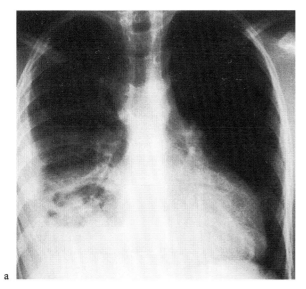

a

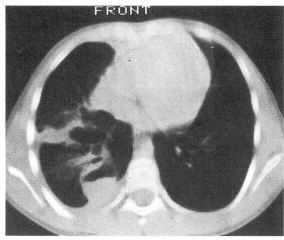

b

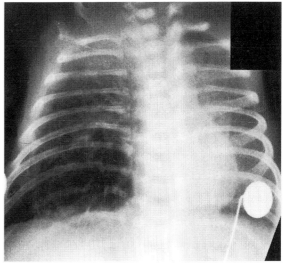

Fig. 2.31. Unilateral interstitial emphysema. This patient was referred from another hospital with a diagnosis of cystic adenomatoid malformation of the right lung. On reviewing the previous film it was evident that the endotracheal tube had entered the right main bronchus, protecting the left lung. This resulted in a localised interstitial emphysema in the right lung, which had become a more chronic form. There is hyperinflation of the right lung with cystic areas and shift of the mediastinum to the left side, compatible with interstitial emphysema

Fig. 2.30 a,b. Abscess. a Frontal projection shows a pleural effusion with opacification of the lower zone, with a fluid level and a thick-walled cavity. b CT scan shows thick-walled cavities with fluid levels

amounts of pleural fluid or pleural thickening. These may be difficult to differentiate from a small amount of loculated pleural fluid on a chest radiograph but are easily distinguished by ultrasound. CT is invaluable for identifying the full extent of the lesion and its location (Fig. 2.30b). Diagnostic aspiration or therapeutic catheter drainage is best done under CT control. Most abscesses respond to antibiotic treatment, and thoracotomy for resection of the abscess is unusual. Abscess formation also occurs following endobronchial obstruction by a foreign body or rarely a tumour and may be the primary presentation of such a lesion.

2.2.2.1.5
UNILATERAL PULMONARY INTERSTITIAL EMPHYSEMA
Pulmonary interstitial emphysema (PIE) occurs in premature ventilated infants, usually with respiratory distress syndrome, and will therefore present in the Special Care Baby Unit. PIE is usually seen as bilateral curvilinear lucencies on the radiographs, although it may appear unilateral if only one lung is predominantly affected. This occurs particularly if the endotracheal tube selectively enters one bronchus. The bronchus to the contralateral lung, being partially obstructed, will protect this lung from emphysema (Fig. 2.31). The appearances are due to air in the lymphatic parenchymal tissues. Although not usually seen in the Casualty department, some cases do present there, having been referred from another hospital because they are thought to be congenital cystic adenomatoid malformation or other pathology.

2.2.2.1.6
CONGENITAL CYSTS
Congenital cysts of the lung produce multicystic areas communicating with the bronchus but these usu-

ally only present as an emergency as tension cysts or are discovered incidentally on a radiograph done for some other purpose.

2.2.2.2
Bilateral

2.2.2.2.1
PULMONARY INTERSTITIAL EMPHYSEMA

Pulmonary interstitial emphysema and bronchopulmonary dysplasia produce the most common bubbly bilateral appearances in neonates. Early or late chronic forms of PIE seen on chest radiographs can be confusing if an appropriate history is not made available (Fig. 2.32).

2.2.2.2.2
CHRONIC BRONCHOPULMONARY DYSPLASIA

Bronchopulmonary dysplasia is iatrogenic, being the result of high ventilation oxygen therapy in a damaged lung, e.g. due to respiratory distress syndrome (RDS), neonatal pneumonia or meconium aspiration (STOCKER and DEHNER 1988). The appearances are more cystic than PIE and much less uniform (Fig. 2.33). It is also much more frequent. Interstitial dilatations vary in size, with some areas of lung apparently little affected.

Bronchopulmonary dysplasia as such is unlikely in itself to present as an emergency but the patient may present with superadded infection. Without an appropriate history being provided to the radiologist the appearances may be very confusing. Without a previous chest x-ray for comparison it can be difficult to decide how much infection contributes to the clinical problem. Occasionally focal areas, if damaged, may dilate and produce respiratory distress, necessitating surgical resection.

As children with bronchopulmonary dysplasia grow older, the lungs also grow and the changes diminish. There is still often hyperinflation and streaky shadowing secondary to areas of fibrosis. Without the history of bronchopulmonary dysplasia, this pattern can be very confusing. Children with bronchopulmonary dysplasia may also have areas of chronic consolidation or collapse. Without a previous film for comparison it is impossible to know if this is recent or due to old disease. Comparison with old films will resolve the problem.

2.2.2.2.3
HISTIOCYTOSIS

Histiocytosis can produce a cyst-like appearance which is extremely rare and in any case seldom

presents as an acute emergency in the neonate; however, older children may present with a pneumothorax.

2.2.2.2.4
BRONCHIECTASIS

Today, bronchiectasis is usually seen in children as a complication of cystic fibrosis or of a missed lobar collapse. It is produced by cystic dilatation of bronchioles damaged by repeated infection. The surrounding parenchyma affected by the same process collapses and contributes to the dilatation. Ensuing fibrosis leads to further traction on the bronchial

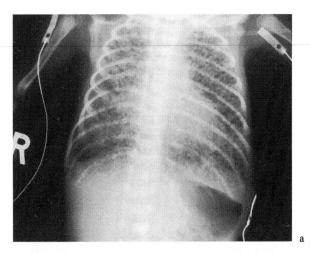

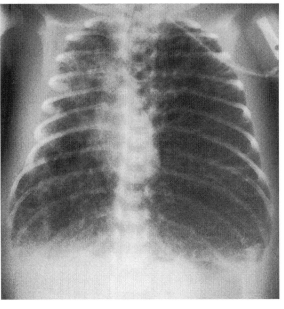

Fig. 2.32. a Interstitial emphysema – early phase. b Late phase in the same patient. Increasing emphysema with marked hyperinflation of the lungs narrowing the cardiac silhouette

walls. Bullae are less common and are seen in cystic fibrosis and chronic bronchitis. Occasionally they rupture and produce a pneumothorax with respiratory distress. Haemoptysis may occur as with any chronic pulmonary infection.

Radiologically bronchiectasis may be localised to one area but CT will usually show a greater extent of the disease. Acute clinical presentation of bronchiectasis is due to secondary infection, haemoptysis or pneumothorax.

2.2.3
Predominantly Hyperlucent Hemithorax

Common causes of predominantly hyperlucent hemithorax are shown in Table 2.3, and Fig. 2.34 illustrates the appropriate diagnostic pathway.

2.2.3.1
Unilateral

2.2.3.1.1
COMPENSATORY EMPHYSEMA

Compensatory emphysema is a very common cause of a hyperlucent lung. It is seen where there is marked reduction in the size of a lobe or contralateral lung. This may be secondary to obstruction such as mucous plugging or foreign body. The hyperlucent area has a decreased pulmonary vascularity on inspiration. It differs from obstructive emphysema in that if an expiratory film is taken there is reduction in volume with increased pulmonary vascularity.

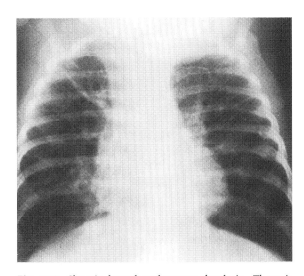

Fig. 2.33. Chronic bronchopulmonary dysplasia. There is general hyperinflation of the lungs and increase in the lung markings with linear fibrosis extending from the hila. Note the old fractures of the left 5th–7th ribs laterally

Table 2.3. Common causes of predominantly hyperlucent hemithorax

Unilateral	Bilateral
neonate and infant	
Emphysema (obstructive or compensatory due to foreign body/mucous plugs etc.)	Emphysema (foreign body/mucous plug)
Pneumothorax/anterior pneumothorax	Bronchiolitis
Lobar emphysema	Whooping cough
Congenital cystic adenomatoid malformation	Cardiac failure
Congenital cyst of the lung (rare single cyst appearance)	Pneumothoraces
Diaphragmatic hernia containing gas-distended stomach	Pulmonary hypoplasia
Large pneumatocoeles	
Poland's syndrome	
Pulmonary hypoplasia	
Pulmonary hypogenetic syndrome	
Older child	
Emphysema (foreign body)	Emphysema (foreign body)
Pneumothorax	Asthma
Pneumatocoeles (large single)	Pneumothoraces
Lung cyst (large single)	
Diaphragmatic hernia containing gas-dilated stomach	
Swyer-James-McLeod syndrome	
Poland's syndrome	
Pulmonary hypoplasia	
Pulmonary hypogenetic syndrome	

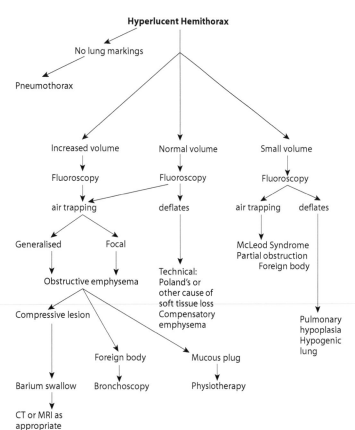

Fig. 2.34. Flow chart illustrating the appropriate diagnostic pathway in cases of hyperlucent hemithorax

2.2.3.1.2

OBSTRUCTIVE EMPHYSEMA

Obstructive emphysema is caused by an endobronchial mass, a foreign body or a mucous plug or by compression of the airway due to masses or vascular rings. More generalised emphysema is seen in bronchospasm secondary to allergic states such as asthma. The pulmonary vascularity in the affected lung is decreased.

Hyperinflation may not be particularly obvious when there is a deep inspiration film. When one suspects that there are hyperinflated lungs then an expiratory film or fluoroscopy will show whether there is air trapping. Where there is air trapping and the segment of lung does not deflate then airway obstruction by a foreign body must be excluded, especially in young children who may not give an appropriate history. Tracheal foreign bodies are more difficult to detect because the lungs are generally uniformly hyperinflated and are particularly dangerous as if they rotate during coughing they may completely obstruct the trachea and lead to asphyxiation.

2.2.3.1.3

PNEUMOTHORAX

Pneumothorax in the newborn infant is usually due to an air leak in RDS (Fig. 2.35) or, more rarely, is secondary to bronchial obstruction and hyperinflation in meconium aspiration. It can be missed or misinterpreted as a pneumomediastinum if there is a small anterior pneumothorax. Appearances differ from older children and adults in that their cross-sectional thorax is more rounded than oval and the AP diameter is greater in the lower thoracic region relative to the upper thorax. In the supine position air collects medially between the anterior edge of the lung and the heart (Fig. 2.36), giving a sharp, very crisp outline to the heart as compared with the older child, in whom it lies laterally and in the apical region.

A pneumothorax in the older child usually presents with pain, particularly on inspiration, and if it is large, with respiratory distress. On the radiograph it produces hyperlucency and increase in size of the ipsilateral hemithorax with contralateral shift of the mediastinum. In the erect position air is seen

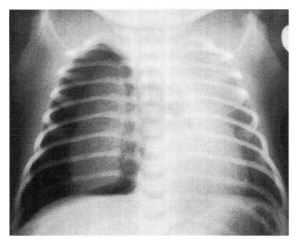

Fig. 2.35. Pneumothorax in a neonate. There is a large pneumothorax on the right side which has shifted the mediastinum to the left. If there is underlying disease in the lung, particularly in the neonatal period, such as RDS, then the lung is stiff and does not necessarily collapse completely, even though there may be tension on the right side displacing the mediastinum to the contralateral side

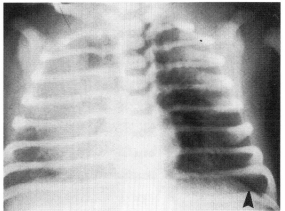

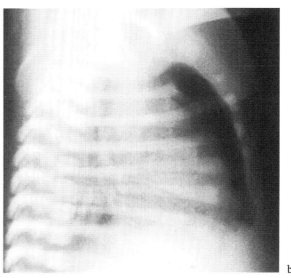

Fig. 2.36 a,b. Anterior pneumothorax. **a** There is a lucency adjacent to the left heart border with a shift of the mediastinum to the right side. There is a lucency just above the left hemi-diaphragm due to subpulmonary air (*arrowhead*), which indicates this is a pneumothorax. **b** The lateral projection shows a retrosternal lucency, confirming the anterior pneumothorax

adjacent to the ipsilateral mediastinum and over the superior surface of that hemidiaphragm, producing a clear-cut edge. An expiratory film increases the apparent size of the pneumothorax. A lateral film shows the air retrosternally and a lateral decubitus with the suspected side elevated will show air adjacent to the upper lateral chest wall. The lateral edge of the lung is seen with air over the apex and blunting of the costophrenic angle with air-fluid levels. In the case of traumatic pneumothorax, the patient is often in a supine position and the air collects anterior to the lung. It is then more difficult to visualise the edge of the lung. In these cases undue sharpness of the mediastinal edge is a tell-tale sign. If the edge is unclear then it is possible to obtain a supine film with a horizontal beam cross table lateral or lateral decubitus, especially in an expiratory phase. This defines the lung edge since air rises to the uppermost part of the chest and outlines the free edge of the lung.

Small pneumothoraces are much more difficult to detect. It is very important to look in the costophrenic angle, where one will see a v-shaped fluid level outlined by air, due to the fluid which normally lies in the intrapleural space becoming visible. This results in fluid levels seen posteriorly and anteriorly, producing a > shape beneath the free lung edge (FELSON 1973). Air may also be seen as a small area of radiolucency (a little "cap") over the lung apex.

Pneumothorax is seen in trauma, closed or penetrating injury, or secondary to rupture of pneumatocoeles. Any obstructive lesion such as foreign bodies, or compressive lesion due to masses or vascular rings, may eventually cause rupture of the alveoli. Pneumothorax can also complicate pulmonary diseases, especially those with hyperinflation such as asthma or cystic fibrosis. Pneumothorax also occurs occasionally in metastatic diseases, particularly when the metastasis is pleural in location, such as in osteogenetic sarcoma and to a lesser extent Wilms' tumour.

Spontaneous pneumothorax occurs less commonly in children than in adults, but increases in frequency with age. The typical habitus of a child presenting with a spontaneous pneumothorax is a tall, thin teenage boy.

When a pneumothorax is under tension it may become life threatening. Unilateral pneumothorax causes depression or inversion of the ipsilateral hemidiaphragm, and marked shift of the mediastinum to the contralateral side (Fig. 2.37). Bilateral pneumothoraces produce eversion of the diaphragm and an elongated heart. One must look very carefully, particularly in an over-penetrated film, to identify a lung edge so as not to miss the pneumothorax, which may not be clearly visible.

2.2.3.1.4
LOBAR EMPHYSEMA

Congenital lobar emphysema usually presents as tachypnoea, dyspnoea or cyanosis in the first few months of life. True congenital emphysema is probably due to an increased number of normally expanded alveoli, i.e. a polyalveolar lobe. This condition occurs predominantly in the upper lobes and is probably due to the more generalised pulmonary loss of elastic recoil. However, in more than 50% of cases there is some form of obstruction (MIKHAILOVA 1996), the most common being intrinsic atresia (ON et al. 1976), bronchial stenosis, cartilage deficiency of the bronchial wall (STOCKER and DEHNER 1988), compression by mediastinal mass or bronchogenic cyst (STOCKER 1988) and dilated vessels in congenital heart disease (HALLER et al. 1979). Most of these causes are not identifiable on a plain film. Radiologically the emphysematous lobe is hyperinflated (Fig. 2.38). The left upper lobe is most frequently affected, followed by the middle lobe and then the right upper lobe. The lower lobes are rarely affected. The expansion can be so great as to be life threatening due to compression of the rest of the lung. In the early stages fetal fluid may be retained; this has been attributed to the polyalveolar lobe (CLEVELAND and WEBER 1993) but may occur in any form of air trapping. The opaque lobe is space-occupying and displaces the mediastinum to the contralateral side (Fig. 2.39a). Gradually over 1–14 days it clears, sometimes with a transient reticular appearance, finally becoming hyperlucent (Fig. 2.39b).

Obstruction of the bronchi causes hyperinflation in various ways: (a) by a ball valve effect when secondary to a foreign body or mucous plug; (b) in bronchomalacia, when there is collapse of the

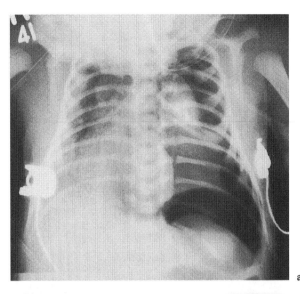

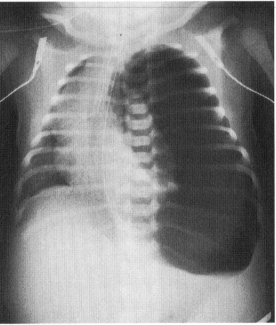

Fig. 2.37 a,b. Tension pneumothorax. **a** A neonate with RDS. There is a tension pneumothorax on the left side. Because the lung is stiff it has not collapsed completely but there is marked shift of the mediastinum to the right side and air can be seen outlining the surfaces of the partially collapsed lung. The left hemidiaphragm is depressed and mildly everted. The shift of the mediastinum is accentuated by the collapse in the right base. **b** Severe tension pneumothorax. The left hemithorax is hyperlucent with no vessels visible and there is shift of the mediastinum across to the right side. The left lung is so collapsed that it cannot be seen and there is compression of the right lung which results in severe respiratory compromise. There is severe depression of the everted left hemidiaphragm

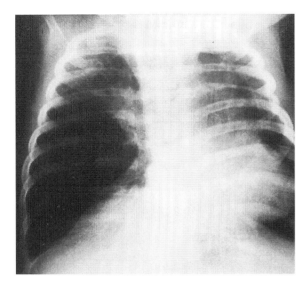

Fig. 2.38. Congenital lobar emphysema. There is hyper-inflation of the right middle lobe, with compression of the right upper lobe and left lower lobe and displacement of the mediastinum to the left side. The appearances are typical of lobar emphysema of the right middle lobe

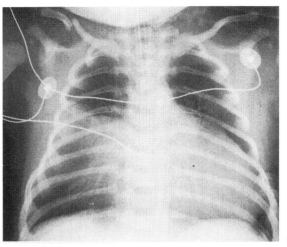

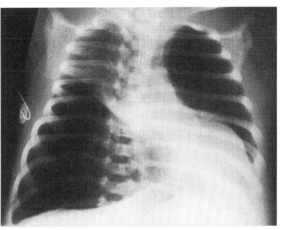

Fig. 2.39 a,b. Lobar emphysema. a In the immediate post-natal period there is opacification in the right middle lobe due to retained fetal fluid. There is only slight shift of the medias-tinum to the left side. The appearances can be misinterpreted as pneumonia. Note the fractured right clavicle due to birth trauma. b Three weeks later there is now obvious hyperlucency and hyperinflation of the right middle lobe, typical of lobar emphysema

bronchus on expiration (DOULL et al. 1996); (c) by collateral drift through the pores of Kohn and the canals of Lambert in bronchial atresia (HALLER et al. 1980) or (d) by external compression such as vascular dilatation in congenital heart disease. Any progressive emphysema or involvement of more than one lobe should alert one to a non-congenital cause such as a foreign body or compressive lesion. This then necessitates a bronchoscopy or barium swallow to detect a mass lesion which may indent the oesophagus as well as the trachea.

The emphysematous lobe will compress the adjacent lobes. This is particularly marked in the right middle lobe, where there may be marked compression of the right upper and lower lobes with bowing upward of the horizontal fissure. This may be misinterpreted as collapse of the two normal lobes with compensatory emphysema in the right middle lobe. To the unwary it may be misinterpreted as a localised pneumothorax. However, if one looks carefully one can see that the vascular markings more widespread than usual. There is usually spreading of the ribs, contralateral shift of the mediastinum and occasionally herniation of the lung across the midline. Screening of the chest will show that there is air trapping in the expiratory phase. If there is still clinical doubt, isotope scans will show diminished perfusion and absence of early ventilation, with delayed films showing air trapping.

2.2.3.1.5
PULMONARY SLING

Pulmonary sling is a rare congenital anomaly due to an aberrant left pulmonary artery arising from the right pulmonary artery and can produce obstructive emphysema (Fig. 2.40a). This is usually in the right lung though occasionally bilateral, but rarely presents as an emergency. On the lateral film there is anterior displacement of and posterior indentation of the trachea. Contrast studies will confirm separation of the trachea from the oesophagus (Fig. 2.40b). Echocardiography can confirm the condition. Bronchography will show the tracheal compression (Fig. 2.40c). MRI demonstrates the lesion and if

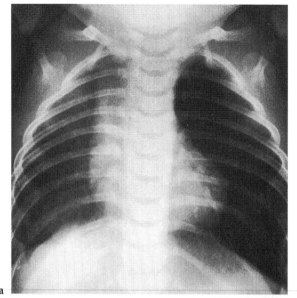

a

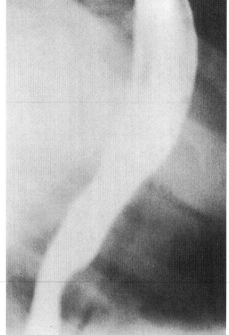

b

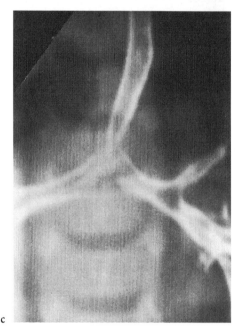

c

Fig. 2.40 a–c. Pulmonary sling. a There is hyperinflation of the lungs, particularly the left lung, with depression of the diaphragm. The film is over-exposed. b Barium swallow shows indentation of the anterior aspect of the oesophagus by the left aberrant pulmonary artery, which separates the oesophagus from the compressed trachea. c Tracheo-bronchogram shows localised compression at the carina with splaying of the main bronchi, which are more horizontal than normal

necessary MRI angiography can be performed, which may obviate the need for conventional contrast angiography.

2.2.3.1.6
CONGENITAL CYSTIC ADENOMATOUS MALFORMATION

Occasionally in type 1 the large cyst dominates or the air trapping in the multiple cysts compresses the wall so that they are difficult to visualise on the radiograph, particularly in an over-penetrated film (Fig. 2.41).

2.2.3.1.7
LUNG CYSTS/PNEUMOCOELES

Pulmonary parenchymal cysts are thought to be developmental (Shanji et al. 1988) but some are acquired as a result of pulmonary infarction (Stocker 1988). Occasionally a pneumatocoele may enlarge and become like a large cyst. Both may produce respiratory distress as a result of a "tension" cyst or rupture causing a pneumothorax. Congenital cysts occur as a result of distal bronchi becoming separate from the rest of the proximal bronchi and usually occur in the lower lobes. If one cyst predominates

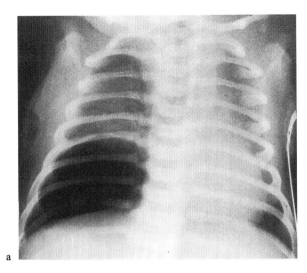

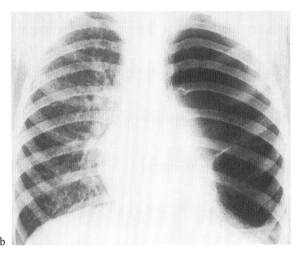

Fig. 2.41 a,b. Congenital cystic adenomatous malformation. a Single cyst. In this case a single cyst predominates which gives the appearance of a solitary cyst or lobar emphysema. b Another patient. Two large cysts occupy the whole of the left hemithorax with severe compression of the left lower lobe. In an over-penetrated film, such a condition may be mistaken for a pneumothorax

and communicates with the bronchus with air trapping there may be rapid expansion. This can present as acute respiratory distress and the appearances of a hyperlucency, which can mimic lobar emphysema (Fig. 2.42a). If very large, cysts can compress the other lobes and mimic a pneumothorax (Fig. 2.42b). A fluid level may be observed within a cyst (Fig. 2.42c).

2.2.3.1.8
ABSCESS CAVITY
If the central cavity is large and empty of fluid it may appear as a large thick-walled cyst (Fig. 2.43).

2.2.3.1.9
SWYER-JAMES-MACLEOD SYNDROME
Swyer-James-Macleod syndrome produces a unilateral hyperlucency on the radiograph due to decreased perfusion and air trapping with a small lung and pulmonary artery (Fig. 2.44). Occasionally only one lobe is affected. Fluoroscopy shows mediastinal shift to the contralateral side on expiration due to air trapping. There is limited movement of the diaphragm on the affected side. Swyer-James-Macleod syndrome is caused by acute bronchiolitis obliterans in infancy but this episode may not be identified clinically. Although the process probably affects all lobes, the condition usually mainly affects only one side, producing the asymmetrical appearance. Usually it is asymptomatic, but dyspnoea on exertion or recurrent chest infections due to bronchiectasis can be its presentation. It is unlikely to present itself acutely but must be recognised on the radiographs when the patient presents with a respiratory tract infection. The patchy change is best demonstrated by HRCT. Mild bronchiectasis is a common CT finding.

Swyer-James-Macleod syndrome can usually be distinguished from other causes of hyperlucency by its reduced lung volume. Only two conditions mimic this. Pulmonary hypoplasia usually has a very small or absent pulmonary artery. A partially occluding radiolucent foreign body will produce a small lung volume, air trapping and diminished vascularity not due to diminutive vessels but due to hypoxic vasoconstriction and can be difficult to distinguish from Swyer-James-Macleod syndrome. When there is doubt, CT should be carried out to resolve the problem. If there is still doubt then bronchoscopy should be carried out.

2.2.3.1.10
POLAND'S SYNDROME
A rare congenital anomaly that one should be aware of is Poland's syndrome, in which absence of the pectoralis major muscle produces a unilateral hyperlucency appearance due to loss of soft tissue. This can be identified by noting the abnormal axillary soft tissue outline, which has a straight border instead of the usual curved one formed by the pectoralis major. Associated anomalies seen on the chest x-ray may include rib and sternal anomalies and occasionally lung herniation. Absence of the nipple and areola has been described and the astute observer may note absence of the soft tissue of the nipple on that side. Skeletal hypoplasia of the hand is an associated anomaly.

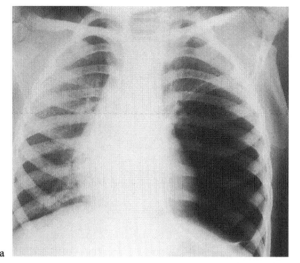

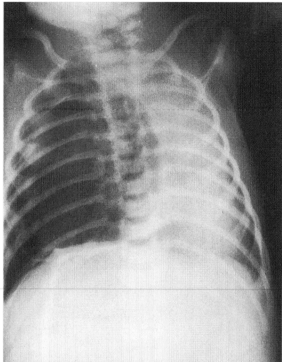

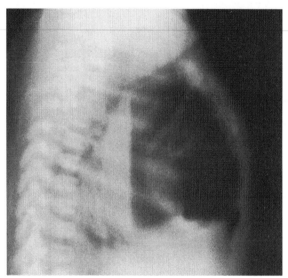

Fig. 2.42 a–c. Congenital cyst. a The thin-walled cyst in the left lower lobe has expanded and almost fills the left hemithorax with shift of the mediastinum to the right side. b Another patient. There is a large congenital cyst on the right side which is hyperinflated, and there is herniation to the left side with marked shift in the mediastinum to the contralateral side. A small drainage tube is seen in situ on the right side. c Lateral projection in the supine position with a horizontal beam shows a fluid level within the cyst

2.2.3.1.11
PULMONARY HYPOPLASIA
This rare condition is usually associated with a malformation such as diaphragmatic hernia or extralobar sequestration, but occasionally occurs as a prime lesion. There is decrease in the volume with a small pulmonary artery. It is more often discovered as an incidental finding rather than presenting as an acute emergency. There is no air trapping on fluoroscopy.

2.2.3.1.12
HYPOGENETIC LUNG SYNDROME
Scimitar syndrome or pulmonary venous lobar syndrome invariably occurs on the right side and appears on the radiograph as a small right lung and hemithorax, often with a curvilinear density formed

by the anomalous vein draining to the inferior vena cava, seen adjacent to the right heart border.

2.2.3.2
Bilateral

2.2.3.2.1
BRONCHIOLITIS
Bronchiolitis is usually caused by respiratory syncytial virus (RSV). It clinically presents between October and January, sometimes as an epidemic form. Though RSV can affect any age group, it is infants under 6 months who suffer the severe illness needing ICU and ventilation. After a short prodromal phase of mild upper respiratory tract infection with cough, the infant becomes acutely ill with wheezing, costal

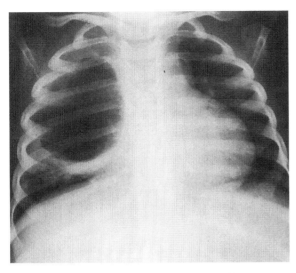

Fig. 2.43. Abscess cavity. The fluid from the abscess cavity is no longer present, leaving a residual thick-walled air-containing cavity

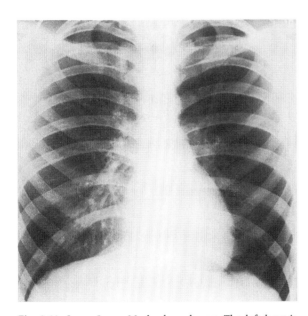

Fig. 2.44. Swyer-James-Macleod syndrome. The left lung is smaller with a smaller left pulmonary artery and attenuation of the vessels, producing a hyperlucent left hemithorax

recession and in severe cases cyanosis. Oedema due to inflammation narrows the peripheral airways, which usually diminish in size in expiration. This will increase secretions and inflammatory exudate with a ball valve effect causing hyperinflation; if complete obstruction occurs, there will be atelectasis (GRISCOM et al. 1978; VAN ALLEN 1932). Intersti-

tial perihilar opacities, subsegmental atelectasis and consolidation occur. When these are adjacent to the heart they produce a shaggy appearance. Although often attributed to pertussis, the appearance is not specific and can be seen in viral infections. Atelectasis is common and, when severe due to mucous plugs, may present as an emergency. Pneumothorax and pneumomediastinum may complicate associated obstructive emphysema. Secondary infections with lobar consolidations occur and may also present as an acute emergency.

Radiologically the lungs are hyperinflated with a flattened or inverted diaphragm and are hyperlucent. Due to the hyperinflation the mediastinum and heart appear narrow. There is peribronchial thickening that is most prominent in the perihilar regions, where small ring shadows or tramline densities extending from hila are apparent. There is often subsegmental atelectasis in the perihilar regions, producing small linear intensities radiating from the hila (Fig. 2.45). Sometimes the central atelectasis produces a shaggy appearance to the heart and may simulate hilar lymphadenopathy. Bacterial contamination often complicates the illness and results in more focal areas of subsegmental consolidation. The child may become toxic clinically. Pulmonary oedema occasionally supervenes. Bronchiolitis obliterans may sometimes be the end result with a unilateral hyperlucent lung.

There is an overlap in the radiographic appearances of bronchiolitis and asthma. Asthma is rare under 3 years of age whereas bronchiolitis is common in infants under 1 year of age. It is possible that a wheezing attack was in fact the first presentation of asthma rather than true bronchiolitis. The appearances are those of hyperinflation only. These appearances are non-specific and can occur in alveolar ventilation associated with acidosis and dehydration. Inhalation of toxic fumes presents with a similar appearance. Cystic fibrosis should also be considered in any infant with recurrent attacks of bronchiolitis.

Bacterial contamination often complicates the illness. The children may become hypoxic. Pulmonary oedema may supervene and progress to adult respiratory distress syndrome.

Most children with bronchiolitis recover completely, but some will progress to chronic pulmonary disease, recurrent pneumonias, atelectatic segments that fail to reinflate and later bronchiectasis and bronchiolitis obliterans causing the Swyer-James-Macleod syndrome.

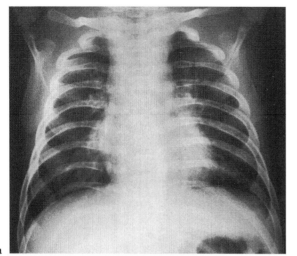

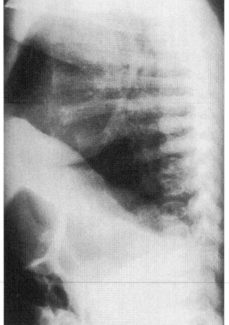

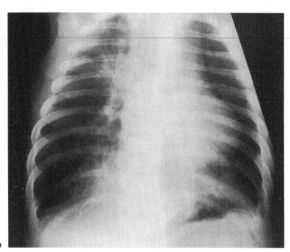

Fig. 2.45 a–c. Bronchiolitis. a Early case. There is mild hyperinflation of the lungs with peribronchial thickening. b Advanced case. There is marked hyperinflation of the lungs with hyperinflated lung tissue seen beneath the heart and inversion of the diaphragm. The streaky opacities from the perihilar region are due to peribronchial thickening and linear atelectasis. c Lateral film. There is hyperinflation of the lungs with increase in the retrosternal air space and eversion of the diaphragm

2.2.3.2.2

WHOOPING COUGH

Whooping cough is caused by *Bordetella pertussis*. It begins with a mild coryza with cough which becomes more persistent; eventually the typical whoop develops. It is now usually only seen in young infants who have not yet been immunised. In the uncomplicated cases there is generalised hyperinflation (Fig. 2.46). The radiological features are non-specific and overlap with those of bronchiolitis. Unilateral lymphadenopathy occurs in some cases. Peribronchial infiltrates and atelectasis produce the "shaggy heart" appearance but are non-specific. Pneumothorax and pneumomediastinum are a complication of emphysema. Lobar collapse due to mucous plugs and secondary infection are complications that may present as acute emergency. The radiographic appearances with linear densities may persist for a month or more. Bronchiectasis can be a late sequela.

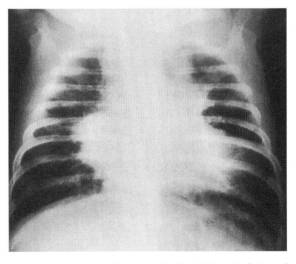

Fig. 2.46. Pertussis. A three month old with hyperinflation of the lungs. There is peribronchial thickening and some linear atelectasis extending from the perihilar regions, giving a shaggy appearance to the heart

2.2.3.2.3
CARDIAC FAILURE
Cardiac failure complicating congenital heart disease may present with mild hyperinflation due to peribronchial oedema that causes narrowing of the bronchi, secretions producing plugs in the bronchi and compression of the airways by enlarged vessels or chambers of the heart (NEWMAN and SANG 1988).

2.2.3.2.4
ASTHMA
Asthma is the commonest single cause of admission of children into hospital. It is the result of an allergic response to a variety of agents in susceptible individuals. It is seldom seen in infants. The reactive response causes constriction of the small muscles of the airways resulting in hyperinflation, mucosal oedema producing peribronchial thickening, and increased secretions causing focal hyperinflation or atelectasis. The collapse must not be mistaken for infection. The majority of children admitted with asthma will not require a chest radiograph and it should only be performed where there is clinical concern, poor response to therapy or suspected localised pathology, e.g. pneumothorax.

In the early stages there is mild hyperinflation. Only by comparison with radiographs when the child is not in an acute attack will the hyperinflation be apparent. Bulging of the soft tissues in the intercostal space may be seen on a good inspiratory film and is an unreliable sign of hyperinflation. True hyperinflation is manifest by flattening of the diaphragm and an increase in the retrosternal space (Fig. 2.47). Peribronchial thickening is seen in the acute attacks and is due to inflammatory cells as a result of the allergic reaction. In chronic conditions this peribronchial thickening may persist even between attacks. Lymphadenopathy is not common unless there is chronic infection but the prominence of the hila may be contributed to by the prominence of the pulmonary vessels and central atelectasis. The main purpose of the radiograph in an asthmatic child is to identify complications such as superadded pneumonia or air leaks, the presence of marked collapse or obstructive emphysema. The attacks may also be complicated by pneumothoraces or more commonly by pneumomediastinum. A pneumomediastinum is seen as air in the parasternal region extending into the soft tissues of the neck. It often outlines the thymus.

A repeat x-ray is usually unnecessary in asthmatics unless there are complications such as pneumonia, severe collapse or air leak. When there is an air leak, the radiographs need to be repeated until there is complete resolution. Extensive atelectasis and pneumonia only need repeat x-rays after about a month to ensure there is complete resolution. Children without focal consolidation or atelectasis do not require repeat radiographs.

2.2.3.2.5
CYSTIC FIBROSIS
The earliest presentation of cystic fibrosis is of a bronchiolitic-type illness, reflecting small airway obstruction seen as overinflated lungs (Fig. 2.48).

2.2.3.2.6
OTHER CAUSES
Bilateral hypoplasia is difficult to diagnose since the changes are symmetrical. Hyperinflation can occur due to rapid ventilation resulting from dehydration or acidosis. An expiratory film usually clarifies the situation.

2.2.4
Mediastinal Lucencies

Common causes of mediastinal lucencies are listed in Table 2.4.

2.2.4.1
Pneumomediastinum

Pneumomediastinum occurs as a result of (a) rupture of the over-distended alveoli in conditions associated with hyperinflation and (b) perforation or rupture of the oesophagus or bronchus caused by trauma, foreign body or, rarely, tumour in the older child. In a small pneumomediastinum the air outlines the thymus and mediastinum. In the infant, where the thymus is large, this may be elevated, producing the so-called angel wings appearance (Fig. 2.49). Air outlining only one border of the heart can be mistaken for a medial pneumothorax. In the older child the thymus is smaller and may only be outlined by a small triangle of tissue or not seen at all, but linear lucent streaks can be seen extending into the

Table 2.4. Common causes of mediastinal lucencies

Pneumomediastinum
Pneumopericardium
Hiatus hernia
Morgani hernia

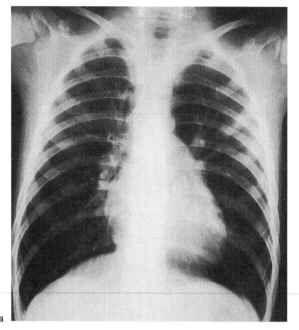

a

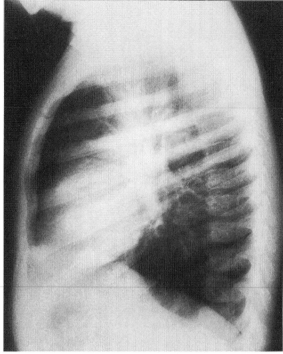

b

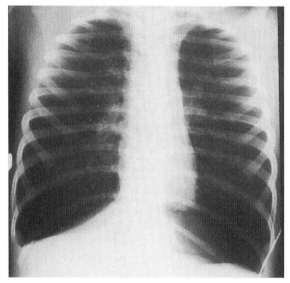

c

Fig. 2.47 a–c. Asthma. a In a moderately severe attack there is hyperinflation of the lungs with inflated lung seen beneath the heart on the left side. There is depression of the diaphragm and peribronchial thickening in the hilar region. b Lateral projection shows diaphragm depression and mild eversion of one hemidiaphragm. There is increased hyperlucency and increased extension of the retrosternal space, which now extends down to the diaphragm. c Status asthmaticus. There is marked hyperinflation of the lungs, with an elongated cardiac silhouette, depression and eversion of the diaphram. The hyperinflation has resulted in an over-exposed radiograph

neck. Air, when it lies subpleurally along the diaphragm, can outline the superior surface of the diaphragm beneath the heart and may easily be missed (Fig. 2.50). Rarely will mediastinal air be so great as to produce tamponade and require surgical intervention.

2.2.4.2
Pneumopericardium

Pericardial air is much less common and is usually seen in patients being ventilated (Fig. 2.51), or in trauma. If the volume of air is large enough, cardiac tamponade can occur and necessitates rapid intervention.

Radiographically pneumopericardium appears as air completely surrounding the heart. This differs from a medial pneumothorax or pneumomediastinum, where the air does not completely surround the heart.

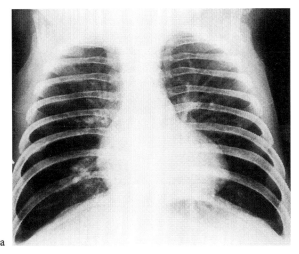

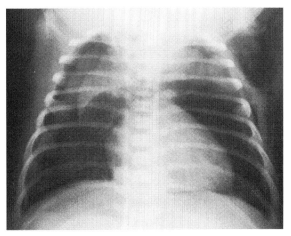

Fig. 2.49. Pneumomediastinum. There is air in the mediastinum with elevation of the two lobes of the thymus, producing the typical "angel's wings" appearance of a pneumomediastinum in an infant. Note small right pneumothorax

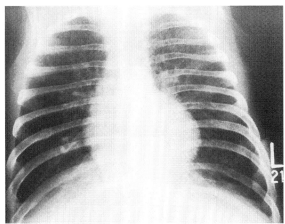

Fig. 2.48 a,b. Cystic fibrosis. a Early appearances. There is mild hyperinflation of the lungs with perihilar peribronchial thickening. b Two weeks later, the same patient presents with increased hyperinflation of the lungs, again with peribronchial thickening. A single attack may be considered as mild bronchiolitis but the repeated attacks with persistent hyperinflation suggest cystic fibrosis

2.2.4.3
Hiatus Hernia

Intrathoracic stomach (Fig. 2.52) and Morgagni hernia can deceive the unwary. It is important not to attribute the patient's condition to a pneumomediastinum which is not present. Hiatus hernia is much less common in children than adults. In children it occurs due to congenital weakness of the oesophageal hiatus. Small hernias are unlikely to be detected on the chest x-ray but larger ones may appear as a mass behind the heart or in the cardiophrenic angle, often with an air-fluid level. Such hernias may be mistaken for a thick-walled ab-

scess although the clinical differentiation is usually obvious. Very occasionally most of the stomach herniates through the hiatus and in a small number of cases this can undergo a volvulus and present acutely with gastrointestinal tract symptoms. The chest radiograph shows a large mass within the cardiac silhouette, although its borders may protude beyond it. There is sometimes a double air-fluid level. Morgagni hernia occurs retrosternally or parasternally through the foramina of Morgagni and occurs more commonly on the right, the left being overlaid by the heart. Morgagni hernias are usually small and often contain omentum only; accordingly they may either not be visualised or be seen as a small soft tissue opacity in the right cardiophrenic angle. Occasionally a portion of the stomach or bowel appears as a lucency, sometimes with a fluid level. When very large they may strangulate and present acutely. Again, contrast studies will confirm the diagnosis and may only show elevation of the segment of bowel, usually the transverse colon, if only omentum is in the hernia.

2.2.5
Predominantly Opaque Hemithorax

Common causes of opaque hemithorax are shown in Table 2.5, and Fig. 2.53 illustrates the appropriate diagnostic pathway.

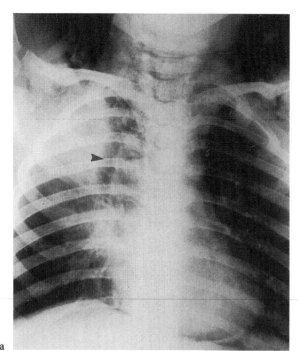

a

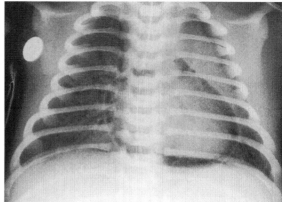

Fig. 2.51. Pneumopericardium. This child with RDS was being ventilated. The whole of the cardiac border is outlined with pericardial air

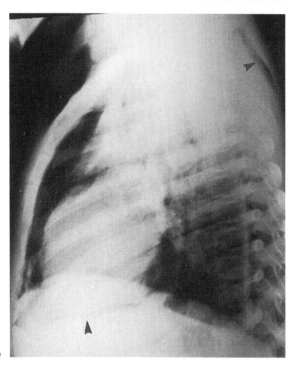

b

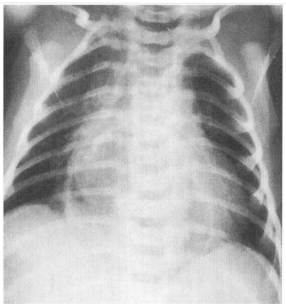

Fig. 2.52. Hiatus hernia containing intrathoracic stomach. A lucency is seen behind the heart with denser curvilinear lines, formed by the walls of the stomach. The walls may be misinterpreted as linear atelectasis and the true nature of the lesion not appreciated

Fig. 2.50 a,b. Mediastinal emphysema. **a** Air is seen in the mediastinum (*arrowhead*) extending into the chest wall, the infraclavicular regions and the neck. A lucency is seen beneath the heart. This is due to air on the superior surface of the diaphragm, elevating the heart. Some of this air may be pericardial on the left side, where it curves around the heart apex. **b** Air is seen retrosternally and a small sliver of air is seen in the posterior chest wall extending towards the neck (*arrowhead*). Air seen inferior to the heart could be due to subpleural air (*arrowhead*)

Table 2.5. Common causes of opaque hemithorax (all age groups)

Pleural effusion
Empyema
Congenital diaphragmatic hernia (fluid-filled loops of bowel)
Agenesis of lung
Atelectasis
Total consolidation – rare
Large tumour – rare

Opaque Hemithorax

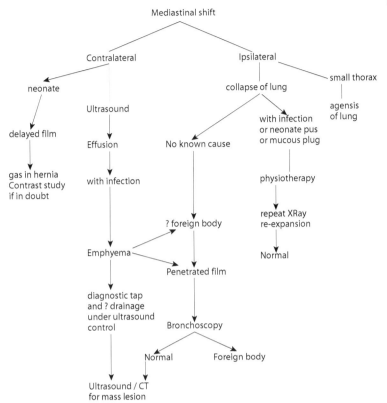

Fig. 2.53. Flow chart illustrating the appropriate diagnostic pathway in cases of opaque hemithorax

2.2.5.1
Pleural Effusions

Pleural effusions are not often so large in the neonate as to compromise lung function or produce a complete opaque hemithorax, but because the fluid distributes over the lung surface they will produce increased density on the affected side (Fig. 2.54). They occur spontaneously soon after birth or following cardiac surgery and are assumed to be due to chylothorax from a thoracic duct leak. They are more frequent on the right but can be bilateral. They have been recorded antenatally by ultrasound. A rare cause of an effusion is lymphangioleiomyomatosis. Chylothoraces usually resolve spontaneously but occasionally need drainage. They are seen in pneumonias, particularly in beta-haemolytic streptococcus in the newborn and staphylococcal pneumonia later. Small effusions will be asymptomatic or there will be symptoms of the underlying cause. When large, they present with tachypnoea, dyspnoea and, if severe, lung compromise with cyanosis.

The most frequent cause of a pleural effusion is infection. In the older child large pleural effusions

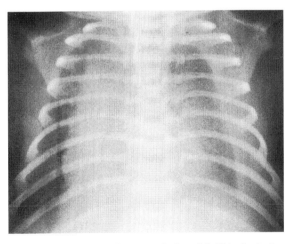

Fig. 2.54. Left pleural effusion. Left pleural fluid is displacing the lung from the lateral chest wall and there is generalised haze on the left side due to the pleural fluid anterior and posterior to the lung. There is a shift of the mediastinum to the right side

can be secondary to malignancy. Lymphoma may appear as a complete opaque hemithorax probably complicated by underlying collapse of the lung, usually with some identifiable mediastinal nodes which can be confirmed by ultrasound, CT or MRI. A penetrated PA film may identify bone destruction if CT is not available. Tuberculosis sometimes presents as an effusion, although rarely a large one. Pleural effusions are also seen in cardiac failure, renal disease, abdominal tumours and infections, and collagen vascular disease. Trauma with haemothorax may occasionally be so large as to cause complete opacification.

Small effusions appear on the radiograph as blunting of the costophrenic angle which can be difficult to differentiate from pleural thickening due to previous infection. Often the positioning of the patient in a lateral decubitus view will show that this is fluid. As the fluid increases it ascends peripherally along the lateral chest wall and on the lateral projection appears as a curved upper border obliterating the posterior costophrenic angle. Eventually there is fluid extending over the apex of the lung.

In the supine position, the fluid extends over the whole surface of the lung, producing a general haziness that can be misinterpreted as pneumonia. There are, however, no air bronchograms, unless there is also an underlying pneumonia. An erect position or preferably a lateral decubitus position, with the dependent side the same side as the effusion, will show the pleural effusion as a collection adjacent to the lateral chest wall. As fluid also accumulates in the fissures it may appear as a wedge on its base or, if small, as a thin opaque line. Loculated fluid, which is not as common in children as adults, may appear as an oval opacity in the fissure and may be misinterpreted as a mass. However, a lateral projection usually clarifies the situation. Subpulmonary effusions can also be difficult to interpret as the fluid collects beneath the lung and gives a configuration like the border of the hemidiaphragm. It can be suspected when the hemidiphragm is unusually high or is flatter than normal and when there is indistinctness of the cardiac silhouette. A lateral decubitus view will show the free fluid. In difficult situations ultrasound can be very useful in confirming the effusion and also as an aid in guiding aspiration. It is also of value in identifying any underlying causative mass. When a malignancy is suspected, urgent CT is indicated, as the mass and its extent are better seen than with ultrasound. Both ultrasound and CT can evaluate any subdiaphragmatic cause, subphrenic inflammation, organ damage in trauma and occasionally a primary malignancy.

Occasionally pneumothorax may complicate a pleural effusion, producing a hydropneumothorax where there is an air-fluid level seen on the chest radiograph. This may also occur with oesophageal or bronchial damage due to trauma or, rarely, in the case of the oesophagus, in severe vomiting episodes.

2.2.5.2
Empyema

Empyema (Fig. 2.55a) is the most common cause of a complete opaque hemithorax and is most commonly a complication of an underlying pneumonia. Radiographically empyema appears as pleural effusions although if the collection is very purulent with much particulate matter, or loculated, then there is very little change in the appearance with changes in the child's position. It may present as an infective consequence of a missed inhaled foreign body and should be considered in any patient who is slow to respond to treatment with antibiotics. Spread from adjacent sites such as subphrenic abscesses or osteomyelitis occasionally occurs. A penetrated PA film will show bone destruction if it is secondary to malignancy. Ultrasound is invaluable in the management of empyema and shows its extent and localisation for percutaneous diagnostic tap or drainage. It distinguishes between a pulmonary abscess and effusion, and allows measurement of the pleural rind. CT can show any associated abscess anatomy for drainage but has little role in uncomplicated empyema, ultrasound being the investigation of choice (Fig. 2.55b). If there is high echogenicity indicating thick pus (Fig. 2.55c), or multiple septa and loculations (Fig. 2.55d), percutaneous drainage may not be possible and open thoracotomy with breakdown of the septa is preferable.

Pleural thickening is frequent and this, with collapse of the underlying lung, will cause failure of the lung to expand on inspiration and be visualised by ultrasound. This does imply a greater degree of involvement pathologically. Children do have a great ability to resolve the pleural thickening but if percutaneous drainage is carried out then the process of recovery may be prolonged. This has to be balanced with the trauma of a thoracotomy. CT scans show the anatomy to better advantage but they are not dynamic and do not show the mobility of the lung. When the effusion is clear on ultrasound with good mobility of the lung and no pleural thickening, percutaneous drainage is usually very effective. Early percutaneous drainage by chest tube carries a low morbidity and mortality and is a viable alternative to surgical management. The presence of

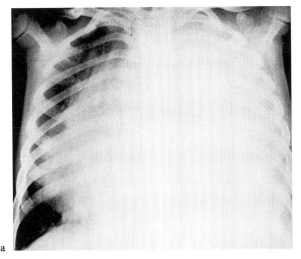

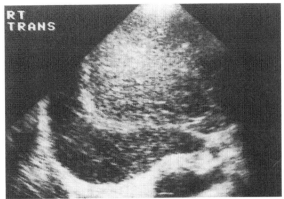

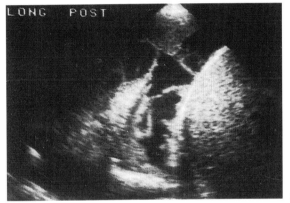

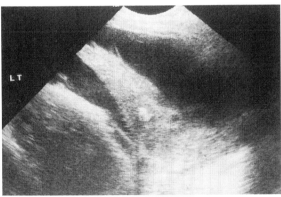

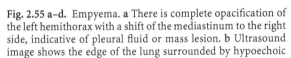

Fig. 2.55 a–d. Empyema. **a** There is complete opacification of the left hemithorax with a shift of the mediastinum to the right side, indicative of pleural fluid or mass lesion. **b** Ultrasound image shows the edge of the lung surrounded by hypoechoic clear fluid. **c** Ultrasound shows echogenic particulate material in the fluid. **d** Ultrasound shows hypoechoic areas of fluid above the diaphragm with numerous septa

pneumatocoeles or mediastinal shift and age greater than 5 years predict a longer duration of drainage. The decision to drain percutaneously or by thoracoscopy or thoracotomy varies between centres.

2.2.5.3
Congenital Diaphragmatic Hernia

Congenital diaphragmatic hernia when the bowel is full of fluid will present with an opaque hemithorax and resembles a large effusion with mediastinal shift. If small pockets of air are seen it may simulate a pneumonia with pneumatocoeles or empyema (Fig. 2.56). If there is little or no gas in the abdomen the index of suspicion for a hernia should be high and, if one is still in doubt, contrast studies must be carried out.

2.2.5.4
Agenesis

Agenesis of a lung is a rare anomaly and is probably due to deficiency of mesenchyma around the developing airway (REID 1977). Degrees of lung hypoplasia are more frequent but do not produce an opaque hemithorax. Pulmonary agenesis with severe hypoplasia may be symptomatic at birth, particularly when right sided (in which case the pronounced shift of the mediastinum leads to compromise of the great vessels), and is often associated with other malformations. More minor degrees of agenesis are usually identified on chest radiographs done for some other cause. They are rarely symptomatic.

Some cases of agenesis are asymptomatic and only become manifest when there is superadded infection. It is important to differentiate it from other

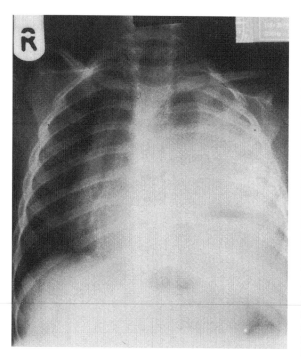

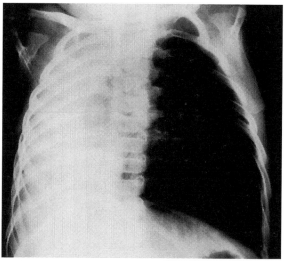

Fig. 2.57. Agenesis of the right lung. There is complete opacification of the right hemithorax with marked ipsilateral mediastinal shift. The right hemithorax is smaller than the left, suggesting that this has been a long-standing process, and therefore a case of agenesis rather than lung collapse. The lucency seen in the superior mediastinum extending across the right side is herniated left lung

Fig. 2.56. Congenital diaphragmatic hernia. There is a largely opaque left hemithorax with just two small pockets of lucency seen, the larger one being in the right apex. There is a moderate shift of the mediastinum to the right side. This appearance represents largely fluid-filled loops of bowel in the left hemithorax with only two small segments containing air; it could easily be mistaken for an empyema with small pockets of loculated air

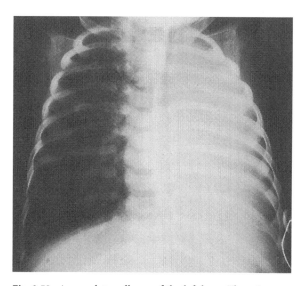

Fig. 2.58. A complete collapse of the left lung. There is complete opacification of the left lung with compensatory emphysema in the right lung. Although the left hemithorax is slightly smaller in volume than the right, this is not as marked as in agenesis

causes of an opaque hemithorax. Radiologically (Fig. 2.57) its appearance differs from that of other causes of opaque hemithorax in that the ipsilateral hemithorax is smaller, with the ribs closer together, and displacement of the mediastinum to the affected side is more marked. The solitary lung is markedly hyperinflated and frequently herniates across to the ipsilateral side. The rotation of the heart may cause loss of the silhouette on the contralateral side, causing a mistaken diagnosis of infection. Complete atelectasis of a normal lung is uncommon and the shift of the mediastinum is usually not as great as with agenesis. In difficult cases bronchoscopy, bronchography or CT will show the atresia of the bronchus, and VQ scanning will demonstrate no perfusion on the affected side. Angiography or MRI angiography will show the absent pulmonary artery.

2.2.5.5
Atelectasis

Complete collapse of the lung (Fig. 2.58) in the infant is often due to mucous plugs, foreign body or a misplaced endotracheal tube. The heart and mediastinum are shifted to the side of the collapse due to the loss of volume and there is elevation of the ipsilateral hemidiaphragm. If there is no infection to suggest mucous plugging then a foreign body should be suspected if there is total lung or lobar collapse.

2.2.5.6
Other Causes

Other causes of complete opacification of the lung are rare. Complete consolidation is very rare and is associated with little or no loss of volume unless there is associated collapse.

In the newborn retained fetal fluid in any condition that will ultimately trap air may present with an opaque area e.g. congenital lobar emphysema, CCAM, pulmonary lymphangiectasia etc. CCAM type 3 is very rare and if sufficient to cause a complete opacification of the hemithorax the neonate probably will not survive due to severe respiratory compromise.

2.2.6
Focal Lesions

Focal lesions are opaque, lucent or a combination of both. They may be responsible for the presenting symptom, e.g. pneumonia, or may be an underlying problem such as a mass causing compression of structures that results in symptoms. Occasionally they are an incidental finding that can be of importance.

Common causes of focal lesions are listed in Table 2.6.

Table 2.6. Common causes of focal lesions (all age groups)

Peripheral:	Round pneumonia
	Pulmonary haematoma
	Neoplasm
	Lung abscess
	Loculated pleural effusion
	Mycotic aneurysm
	Pulmonary embolism infarction
	Fungi
	Hydatid
Paramediastinal:	Round pneumonia
	Neuroblastoma
	Bronchogenic cyst
	Oesophageal duplication cyst
	Neuroenteric cyst
	Mycotic aneurysm
Paradiaphragmatic:	Sequestration
	Diaphragmatic eventration
	Basal subsegmental atelectasis/ consolidation
	Hernia
	Abscess
Hilar:	Lymph nodes
	Vascular
	Mucoid impaction (e.g. cystic fibrosis)

2.2.6.1
Round Pneumonia

Pneumonia in young children differs from that in older children insofar as lobar consolidations are less common. The airways in small children have poor collateral ventilation and the parenchyma is more compact than in adults. Because gravitation influences the infected fluid, the posterior inferior lobe is most commonly involved and the spread from this epicentre produces a round pneumonia (EGGLI and NEWMAN 1993). Air bronchograms are rare. If a round pneumonia presents as a posterior paravertebral region behind the heart (Fig. 2.59) it may mimic a neuroblastoma. In these cases it is wise to start antibiotics and take blood samples for VMAs. Round pneumonias change rapidly in response to treatment and a repeat film after 48h of antibiotics will usually show significant improvement, unlike in patients with true masses, which will not alter. Round pneumonias may lie peripherally and mimic rounded masses (Fig. 2.60) such as solitary metastases. However, most rounded opacities in children with no known malignancy are rarely malignant in origin. Round pneumonias have different contours on the lateral film, unlike true chest masses, and a lateral projection will usually solve a clinical dilemma. Furthermore, usually there is a history of cough, pyrexia and physical signs to differentiate round pneumonias from more sinister lesions.

2.2.6.2
Neuroblastoma

Neuroblastoma occurs in the first 5 years of life and up to 15% of cases occur in the thorax. The paravertebral lesion may be primary or more often extends from the abdomen. Paravertebral neuroblastomas appear as well-circumscribed masses, often with a convex outer border (Fig. 2.61). Those which extend from the abdomen are less well defined. Calcifications, amorphous or irregular, and occasionally curvilinear, occur in 30%. Bony erosions, especially of the posterior ribs, occur. Extension into the spinal canal widens the intervertebral foramen and often presents clinically with cord compression. The chest radiograph may have been taken during general investigation for fever or weight loss, which occur in disseminated disease, or occasionally for pain due to invasion of bone or compression of nerves. A neuroblastoma in the cervical region may compress the trachea and result in respiratory distress (Fig. 2.62). The tumour may be missed if the child is x-rayed with

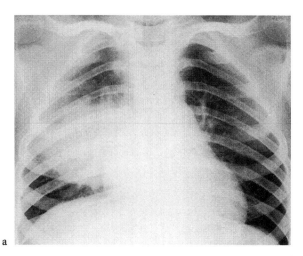

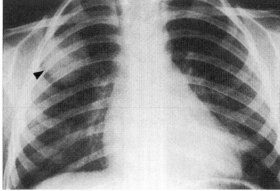

Fig. 2.60. Peripheral round pneumonia. In the right upper zone there is a rounded opacity (*arrowhead*) which is a round pneumonia, but mimics a rounded peripheral mass

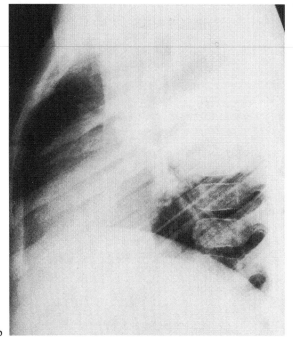

Fig. 2.59 a,b. Round pneumonia. a A round opacity adjacent to the paravertebral region with a slightly indistinct edge gives the impression of a mass lesion. b The lateral projection shows a curvilinear inferior border overlying the vertebra which can be misinterpreted as a round mass

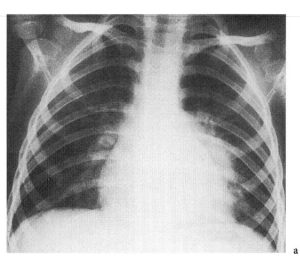

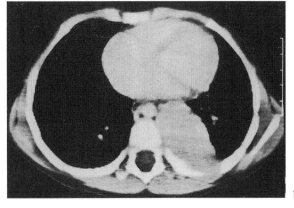

Fig. 2.61 a,b. Neuroblastoma. a A rounded mass is seen adjacent to the left paravertebral region. The lateral portion of the mass extends beyond the confines of the heart. b CT scan shows the left paravertebral neuroblastoma with faint calcification

the chin down, precluding a view of the cervical region. Cervically located neuroblastomas may present with an ipsilateral Horner's syndrome. The tumour may occasionally be seen incidentally on a chest radiograph for respiratory tract investigation. The initial chest radiograph may be diagnostic but the apical lesion may be mistaken for collapsed lobes.

Ultrasound in general has little part in the investigation of thoracic neuroblastoma but in the acute setting apical lesions can be identified as a solid

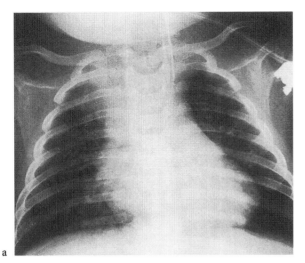

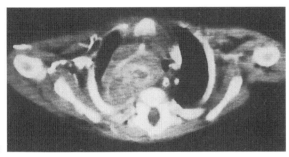

Fig. 2.62 a,b. Apical neuroblastoma. **a** A 5-month-old boy admitted with bronchiolitis. There is an opacity in the right apex with displacement of the trachea to the left side. **b** CT scan with contrast shows a rounded apical lesion which is displacing and compressing the trachea and showing some irregular enhancement. On the unenhanced scan calcification was visible, a common feature in neuroblastoma

mass, often with calcification not visible on the plain radiograph. Furthermore the examination can be performed portably. CT demonstrates calcification better than MRI, but MRI permits evaluation of paravertebral intraspinal extension. On MRI calcifications, if large enough, are visible as signal voids producing black areas in the mass. MRI is the investigation of choice.

Bone scintigraphy and MIBG scans with radiographs of the positive areas are done for staging the extent of disease. Myelography now has no part in the investigation of these disorders.

2.2.6.3
Pulmonary Haematoma

Haematoma may produce a rounded opacity mimicking a mass or rounded pneumonia. It is most commonly secondary to trauma.

2.2.6.4
Bronchogenic Cyst

Bronchogenic cyst is a rare anomaly due to abnormal development and branching of the trachea and bronchus with separation of a segment from the adjacent bronchus. Bronchogenic cysts lie in the middle mediastinum, are the most common of the duplication cysts and, together with enteric and neuroenteric cysts, account for 11% of mediastinal masses in children (KING et al. 1982; RAVITCH 1986). They often contain cartilage. The bronchus and oesophagus arise from the primitive foregut, which is associated with the notochord. Incomplete separation of these two may result in portions of the foregut being sequestered within the developing spinal canal, forming a neuroenteric cyst which is associated with vertebral body anomalies. Out-pouching of the endoderm from the developing oesophagus with incomplete canalisation results in oesophageal duplication cyst.

Bronchogenic cysts consist of non-functioning parenchymal tissue usually without communication with the airway. They lie in the lung parenchyma, usually adjacent to the bronchus or trachea. Hence they can compress the airway, producing respiratory symptoms, although some especially peripheral ones are asymptomatic.

Radiologically bronchogenic cysts appear as a rounded soft tissue density at the level of the carina, hila or lung parenchyma (Fig. 2.63). They remain static in size on serial films unless they become infected, when rapid enlargement can occur. If gas is seen within the mass, especially with a fluid level, communication with the airway or, more rarely, infection should be considered. Compression of the airway can cause localised hyperinflation or less commonly collapse. Localised indentation, usually with posterior displacement of the oesophagus, may be seen on barium swallow but is not specific. Higher placed cysts show anterior displacement with narrowing of the lower trachea. Ultrasound can in some cases provide a definitive diagnosis (MERTEN 1992). Using the suprasternal approach, the lesion appears as a sonolucent mass posterior to the trachea but can be echogenic if it has proteinaceous contents. MRI, because of its multiplanar nature, demonstrates the anatomy in more detail. CT can also show the location of the cyst. Intravenous contrast is necessary, not only to show its relationship to vessels but also to demonstrate the cyst wall, which may not be apparent on an unenhanced scan if the contents are proteinaceous and of the same attenuation as the wall

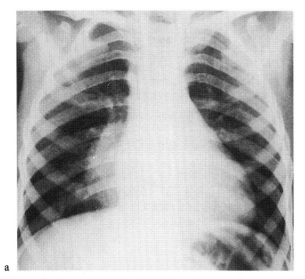

a

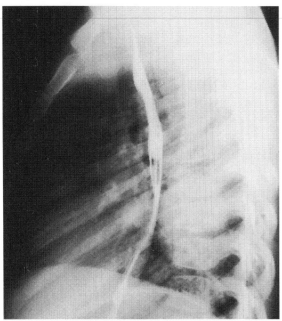

b

Fig. 2.63 a,b. Bronchogenic cyst. **a** A round paravertebral opacity is seen adjacent to the right heart border. **b** The lateral projection shows a rounded opacity in the right paravertebral region posterior to the oesophagus

(MERTEN 1992). Occasionally the cyst wall is of high attenuation on the unenhanced scan. Dystrophic curvilinear calcification is rare. Tissue characteristics on MRI depend on the cyst contents. They usually have a low signal intensity on T1-weighted images and a high signal intensity on T2-weighted images because of the mucous content. The cyst wall enhances with gadolinium.

2.2.6.5
Oesophageal Duplication Cyst

The terms "oesophageal duplication cyst" and "neuroenteric cyst" are often used interchangeably, but the latter should be reserved for those cysts containing neural tissue. Oesophageal duplication cysts form because of failure of tubulation that results in either a second lumen, connecting with the normal lumen, or a separate cystic structure. They occur more commonly on the right side owing to the dextrorotation of the oesophagus. Oesophageal duplication cysts lie in the posterior mediastinum and are usually associated with the lower oesophagus, occasionally occurring within its wall. They compress the oesophagus and, if at a higher level, the trachea (Fig. 2.64a), causing dysphagia or dyspnoea by direct compression and aspiration pneumonia due to impaired swallowing. Some cysts contain gastric mucosa, which can ulcerate and bleed, causing haemoptysis or a sudden increase in cyst size.

Oesophageal duplication cysts appear as a spherical soft tissue mass in the posterior mediastinum, sometimes displacing and compressing the trachea, with hyperinflation of lung or lobe. Barium studies show local indentation of the oesophagus (Fig. 2.64b). Isotope studies will show any ectopic gastric mucosa. CT shows the mass to have low attenuation and its location adjacent to the oesophagus and trachea in the case of higher lesions (Fig. 2.64c). MRI shows the spatial relationship and provides tissue characterisation of the mass. The T1-weighted images have low to intermediate signal unless the cyst contains fat. T2-weighted images have high signal indicating fluid.

Oesophageal duplication cysts may have transdiaphragmatic connections. A search should always be made for a second cyst in the abdomen. Association occurs with diaphragmatic hernia, oesophageal fistula and atresia, other bronchopulmonary foregut malformations and bowel duplication.

2.2.6.6
Neuroenteric Cysts

Neuroenteric cysts contain neural tissue in addition to the intestinal tissue. Located in the middle or posterior mediastinum, often on the right side, they occur in association with vertebral body anomalies

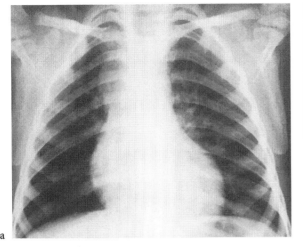

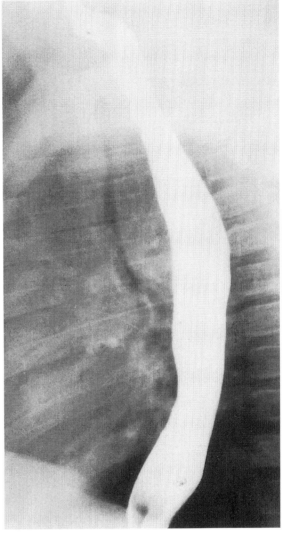

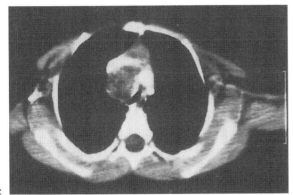

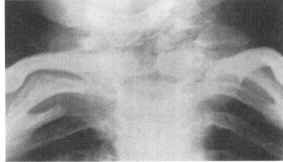

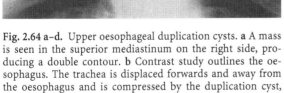

Fig. 2.64 a–d. Upper oesophageal duplication cysts. **a** A mass is seen in the superior mediastinum on the right side, producing a double contour. **b** Contrast study outlines the oesophagus. The trachea is displaced forwards and away from the oesophagus and is compressed by the duplication cyst, causing respiratory complications. **c** CT shows the duplication cyst compressing the trachea. **d** Different patient. Vertebral anomalies with bifid and hemivertebral bodies indicate a neuroenteric cyst

such as bifid or hemivertebral bodies which may cause scoliosis. Intraspinal extension occurs. CT and MRI are required for full evaluation of these lesions. Scintigraphy with technetium-99m sodium pertechnetate will show any gastric mucosa in these and also in enteric duplication cysts.

Neuroenteric and enteric cysts appear as rounded soft tissue opacities in the middle or posterior mediastinum and occasionally cause hyperinflation in a lobe or lung. Vertebral anomalies (Fig. 2.64d) are invariably associated with neuroenteric cysts.

2.2.6.7
Neoplasms

Primary lung neoplasms are rare in children. Most are endobronchial, such as bronchial adenoma, and present radiographically as atelectasis or lobar consolidation which fails to resolve with appropriate treatment. Haemoptysis is often present. Parenchymal tumours such as pulmonary blastoma are exceedingly rare and appear as a rounded peripheral mass. Secondary neoplasms appear as round opacities and are seen most frequently in Wilms' tumour osteosarcoma and soft tissue sarcoma.

In general when the neoplasm is seen on a chest radiograph, the child is already known to have a primary tumour or the primary tumour is obvious. Large deposits may present with airway compromise. Pleural-based lesions may have associated effusions. Pneumothoraces occur in osteosarcoma, or less frequently in Wilms' renal tumour (EGGLI and NEWMAN 1993). Chest wall tumours are rare, accounting for less than 2% of solid tumours, and it would be very unusual for them to present acutely.

Acute presentation to Accident and Emergency is either because of pain, due to associated rib erosion, or breathlessness secondary to a large associated effusion. The underlying cause is seldom suspected initially. Investigation of the child with a large effusion has already been discussed; it should include a penetrated PA film with ultrasound as the initial further procedure.

2.2.6.8
Lung Abscesses

Lung abscesses are usually a complication of pneumonia but may also be secondary to septic emboli or immunocompromise. On the chest radiograph the masses are rounded, have thick irregular walls and often have fluid levels (Fig. 2.65) due to communication with a bronchus. If peripheral, there may be a pleural opacity due to pleural thickening or fluid. The wall of an abscess is much thicker than that in a pneumatocoele. Further assessment by CT or MRI (Fig. 2.65b,c) is usually unnecessary as abscesses re-

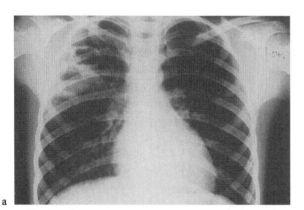

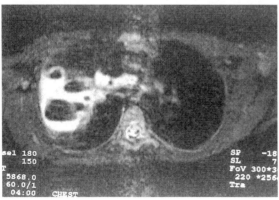

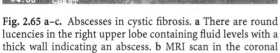

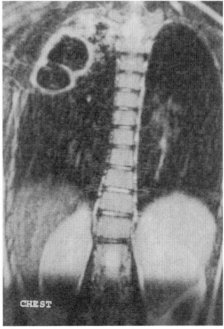

Fig. 2.65 a–c. Abscesses in cystic fibrosis. **a** There are round lucencies in the right upper lobe containing fluid levels with a thick wall indicating an abscess. **b** MRI scan in the coronal plane with T2 sequences shows the thick-walled abscesses. **c** MRI scan in the axial plane with STIR sequences shows the thick-walled abscesses with fluid levels

spond to antibiotics, but is helpful if the response is atypical. Drainage of the abscess under CT control may be needed. Clinical presentation is with pyrexia, cough, dyspnoea, chest pain and occasionally haemoptysis.

2.2.6.9
Loculated Pleural Effusions

Loculated pleural effusions are less common in children than in adults. They are probably due to adhesions in fissures that allow fluid to accumulate focally. Loculated pleural effusions appear as round or oval structures lying in the region of the fissures (Fig. 2.66); while they may mimic a mass they can usually be identified with certainty if both frontal and lateral projections are taken. On an AP view superimposition of the effusion on normal structures may occur and may appear as a hilar mass or a small infiltrate. If the lesion lies peripherally, the fluid nature may be confirmed with ultrasound.

2.2.6.10
Rare Causes

Mycotic aneurysms may be confused with lobar pneumonia. They are usually due to septic emboli, most often from a distant infective focus, usually the heart.

Pulmonary emboli are uncommon but if they occur in children are usually a complication of infected long lines (Fig. 2.67) or sickle cell disease. VQ

scintigraphy aids diagnosis and should be performed in suspected cases. Mismatching defects are seen.

Fungal infection, especially in the immunosuppressed, may present as a focal round lesion.

Pulmonary hamartoma is a rare, benign pulmonary lesion. It rarely produces symptoms and is usually found incidentally on a chest x-ray done for some other cause. The appearances are of a solitary nodule. Although calcification only occurs in 10%, it is said to be pathognomonic, with a "popcorn" pattern.

A pulmonary angioma, unless very large and causing cardiac failure, usually presents as an incidental finding. It may be associated with cutaneous haemangiomata. Pulmonary angiomata appear as a lobulated mass, often with a supplying or draining vessel that is best seen on the lateral film. The lesion may vary in size with respiration. The diagnosis may be confirmed by CT with contrast or MRI; both modalities define the lesion and the associated vessels.

A post-inflammatory pseudotumour is usually an incidental finding on a chest x-ray. Occasionally it may present with respiratory symptoms. It appears as a parenchymal mass which is usually large and sometimes lobulated. Calcification may be present. It is usually amorphous and scattered throughout the mass, although occasionally dense. Post-inflammatory pseudotumour can be readily identified by CT. It has an enhancing margin.

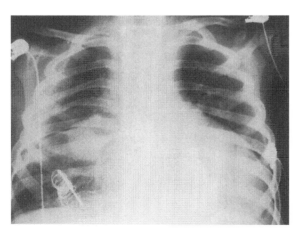

Fig. 2.66. Loculated pleural effusions. The ovoid opacities seen in the right horizontal fissure are typical of loculated pleural fluid

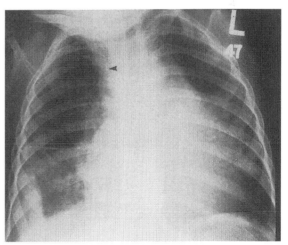

Fig. 2.67. Pulmonary embolism. Peripheral triangular-shaped opacity obliterating the right costophrenic angle with its apex projected towards the hila, very suggestive of pulmonary emboli. Adjacent to the fourth right transverse process is a small high-density area (*arrowhead*) which is the tip of the ventriculocaval shunt – the source of the pulmonary emboli

Hydatid disease, although uncommon, should be considered in patients from endemic areas. If the cyst ruptures into the bronchial tree it produces a typical "water lily" due to the cyst membrane floating on the surface. The child presents acutely with a cough and fever.

Focal lesions lying adjacent to the pericardium, either cysts or fat pads, appear as a soft tissue round density usually in the cardiophrenic angle. If they are fat pads they may well have a rather indistinct border and may have a more lucent appearance than fluid-containing pericardial cysts. If there is doubt as to the nature of the lesion, MRI is indicated.

2.2.6.11
Sequestration

Sequestration is an uncommon congenital anomaly that arises as an accessory lung bud sequestrating abnormal lung tissue either within the normal pulmonary pleura (intralobar sequestration) or within the pleural cavity with its own visceral pleura (extralobar). Intralobar sequestrations lie most commonly in the posterior basal segment while extralobar sequestrations typically lie between the lower lobe and the diaphragm, usually on the left side. Clinically lobar sequestration presents as recurrent pulmonary infections, often with mucopurulent sputum, due to an acquired communication with the bronchial tree secondary to an initial inflammatory process. Extralobar sequestrations are often asymptomatic and discovered incidentally on a chest radiograph. If they communicate with the oesophagus, the child may present to Accident and Emergency in the first year of life with respiratory distress, dysphagia and haematemesis. Therefore any lower lobe mass abutting the left hemidiaphragm should be considered as a sequestration.

The appearance of sequestration on chest x-ray is variable: it may appear as a solid mass, as an air-filled cystic mass (sometimes with fluid levels) or as an abscess depending on communication with the bronchial tree and superadded infections (Fig. 2.68a). The differential diagnosis is pneumonia, empyema, bronchiectasis, eventration and lung abscess. An upper GI contrast study will show any communication with the oesophagus but this is rare. MRI delineates the lesion and will show the inflammatory nature but most importantly it will show its aberrant systemic artery arising from the descending thoracic aorta (Fig. 2.68b). This vessel may sometimes also be demonstrated by ultrasound. Angiography will give greater

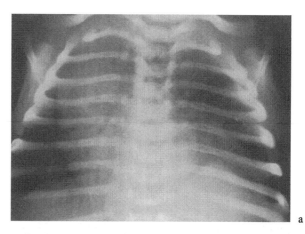

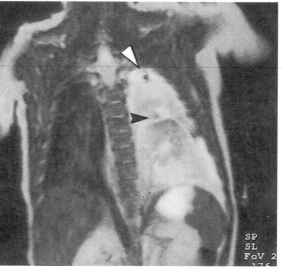

Fig. 2.68 a,b. Sequestration. **a** The left hemidiaphragm has an unusual conical shape. This is associated with a small pleural effusion. **b** Coronal T2-weighted MR image shows a well-circumscribed mass above the left hemidiaphragm and a small vessel ascending into the mass from the aorta. This is typical of the sequestration with its blood supply from the descending aorta. The high signal above the sequestration is due to pleural fluid (*arrowhead*)

detail and in extralobar sequestrations show the supply from the pulmonary arteries. Associated congenital anomalies, especially congenital diaphragmatic hernia and heart disease, occur more commonly in the extralobar type. Sequestrations are often diagnosed in utero but may be completely asymptomatic.

2.2.6.12
Diaphragmatic Eventration

A congenital weakness of the diaphragm may allow herniation of the abdominal organs into the lower

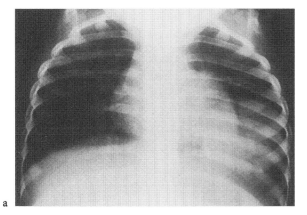

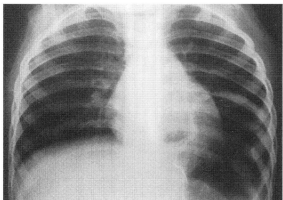

Fig. 2.69 a,b. Eventration. **a** There is an opacity seen at the left base with a rounded upper border which is the upper surface of the eventrated diaphragm. Beneath it there are fluid-filled loops of bowel, giving an opaque appearance. **b** In the same patient air has now entered the loops of bowel, giving a hyperlucent appearance with a curvilinear upper border mimicking the upper border of a cyst

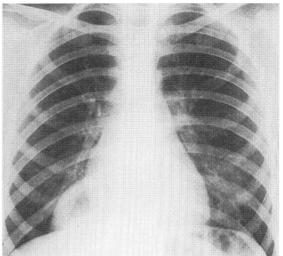

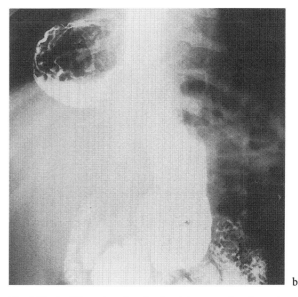

Fig. 2.70 a,b. Hiatus hernia. **a** In the right costophrenic angle there is hyperlucency with a curvilinear thick wall which could be mistaken for an abscess. The right heart border is clearly seen and therefore this lies posteriorly. **b** Barium study shows that the thick-walled cavity is in fact the fundus of the herniated stomach

chest. This causes the hemidiaphragm to bulge upwards. The appearance of the abdominal organs below the upward bulging leaf may be opaque or lucent depending on its content (Fig. 2.69), e.g. solid organ or bowel. Eventrates are mostly asymptomatic but can, if large or bilateral, present with respiratory distress. The main radiological problem is to distinguish between eventration and herniation with a defect in the diaphragm. Initial assessment is by ultrasound, searching for a defect. Further assessment may require GI contrast study or MRI.

2.2.6.13
Hernia

Hiatal hernias in children are rarer than Morgagni or Bochdalek hernias. If fluid filled, especially in the supine position, hernia may appear as a dome-shaped soft tissue mass behind or adjacent to the cardiac silhouette and may mimic an abscess or any other central mediastinal mass. If it contains air it may mimic a thick-walled abscess (Fig. 2.70).

Morgagni hernia may appear as a focal mass in the right costophrenic angle with a lucency if containing air-filled bowel, or as an opaque mass if fluid-filled bowel or omentum only.

Congenital diaphragmatic hernia presenting late and containing stomach or a loop of bowel will appear in the lower hemithorax as a focal mass with a lucent centre or opaque, depending on its contents of air or fluid.

Barium studies rapidly reveal the diagnosis and should be performed in the investigation of lower mediastinal or paramediastinal masses.

2.2.6.14
Hilar Masses

Perihilar and hilar masses are usually due to lymph nodes or vascular enlargement. In general the v-shape between the upper and lower lobe vessels is lost in lymph node enlargement. Bilateral lymph node enlargement is often seen in infections, particularly with simple viral infection. Lymph node enlargement, both unilateral and bilateral, is a common response to infection in children and resolves rapidly with treatment of the infection. If the clinical history is that of acute infection, then the child should be treated. A follow-up film in 1 week should be taken and only if the nodal disease does not then resolve should the question of tuberculosis be raised. To do so on the basis of the initial radiograph would raise unnecessary concern in most children. Nodal disease is a permanent feature of cystic fibrosis, but in these children there is an appropriate history. In cystic fibrosis there may also be mucoid impaction in the distal bronchi, producing finger-like projections from the hila. Although these findings are not acute they may well be seen in radiographs in patients with cystic fibrosis in acute emergency situations when they present with superadded infection. Mucocoele secondary to an atretic bronchus is a rare cause of a hilar mass (Fig. 2.71) and is usually only diagnosed by bronchoscopy. Unilateral paratracheal nodes should be considered to be due to tuberculosis until proved otherwise. Most lymphoma nodes are bilateral and are discussed earlier in this chapter. Aneurysmal dilatation of pulmonary arteries can produce massive hilar opacities mimicking lymphadenopathy (Fig. 2.72). Sarcoidosis is a very rare cause of hilar nodal enlargement in children.

2.2.6.15
Artefacts

Pseudo-masses appearing on the chest film may be due to extrinsic structures such as clothing, hair braids, prominent nipples, skin lesions, developing breasts, rib anomalies or healing fractures. The true nature of the "mass" can often be resolved by (a) an awareness of these artefacts and their characteristic appearances, (b) tracing the contours, which often extend outside the confines of the lungs, (c) correlating the clinical information and x-ray appearances and (d) when doubt persists, repeating the x-ray with clothing removed and using opaque markers on the suspected areas. Although not responsible for the respiratory problems, the appearances must be eliminated as a cause.

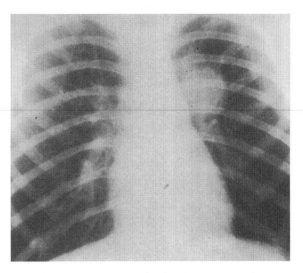

Fig. 2.71. Atretic bronchus filled with mucus, producing a mucocele extending from the left hilar-region

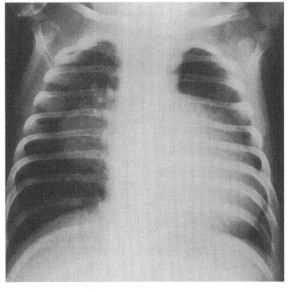

Fig. 2.72. There is aneurysmal dilatation of the right pulmonary artery due to absence of the pulmonary valve. To the unwary this may mimic a large hilar node or other mass

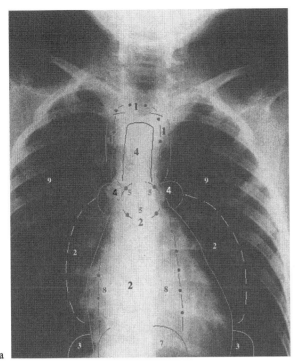

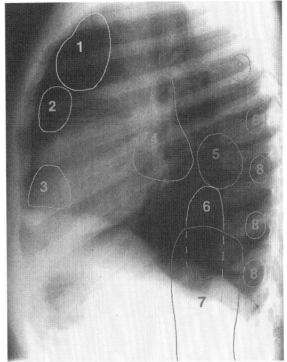

Fig. 2.73. Location of different lesions

Mediastinal lesions – location
1. Cystic hygroma
    Retrosternal goitre (rare)
1, 2. Teratoma
    Reticuloses including leukaemic infiltration
    Extension of cystic hygroma
    Unilateral – round pneumonias
3. *Anterior cardiophrenic angle*
    Pericardial fat pad
    Pericardial cyst
    Hernia of Morgagni (especially on the right)
    Hump of diaphragm
4. *Paratracheal and hilar masses*
    Lymphadenopathy – reticuloses, inflammatory
    Dilated bronchi with mucoid impction – cystic fibrosis,
        mucocoeles
    Vascular
5. Bronchogenic cyst
    Neuroenteric cyst
    Oesophageal duplication cyst

6. Duplication cyst – oesophageal/neuroenteric – on lateral
        film
    Dilated oesophagus – achalasia, stricture – on lateral film
    Lymph nodes
7. Hiatus hernia
    Bochdalek hernia
8. Neurogenic tumours – neuroblastoma, neurofibroma
    Lateral meningocoele
    Paravertebral mass – infection, extramedullary
        haemopoesis
9. Peripheral – Round pneumonia
            Haematoma
            Secondary or rarely primary neoplasm
            Abscess
            Loculated pleural effusion
            Embolism
            Fungi
            Hydatid
            Angioma, hamartoma, pseudotumour –
                rare

The location of the various lesions discussed above is summarised in Fig. 2.73.

2.2.7
Interstitial Disease

Common causes of interstitial disease are listed in Table 2.7.

2.2.7.1
Neonate

Respiratory difficulty presenting in the first few hours of life is due to primary pulmonary pathology: transient tachypnoea of the newborn, respiratory distress syndrome (RDS), neonatal pneumonia or meconium aspiration. The clinical and radiological findings should be correlated. A description of these lesions is outside the scope of this book. Most of

Table 2.7. Common causes of interstitial disease

Neonate
Transient tachypnoea of the newborn
Respiratory distress syndrome
Neonatal pneumonia
Meconium aspiration
TAPVD
Lymphangiectasia
Pulmonary haemorrhage

All age groups
Pneumonia
    Viral
    Bacterial
    Mycoplasmal
    Immunocompromised patients
        Pneumocystis carinii
        Cytomegalovirus
    Aspiration
Pulmonary oedema
Adult respiratory distress syndrome
Cystic fibrosis
Allergy
Pulmonary haemosiderosis

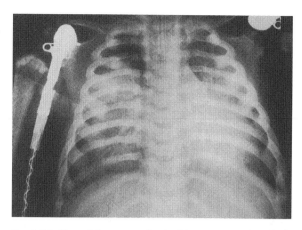

Fig. 2.74. Neonatal pneumonia. In this age group the whole lung is often involved due to intra-uterine infection. There are air bronchograms and fine interstitial opacification which is more confluent in the left base. Note the striations in the upper metaphysis of the right humerus, consistent with intra-uterine infection

these children will not present to an Accident and Emergency department as they are still in the maternity unit. Neonatal respiratory problems that occur after discharge are infection, cardiopulmonary disease and primary lung disease such as fibrosing alveolitis and pulmonary lymphangiectasia. The clinical presentation of all these conditions is tachypnoea. Children with congenital heart disease in general have murmurs and the full extent of the heart disease can be further assessed by echocardiography.

2.2.7.1.1
NEONATAL PNEUMONIA

Infants with congenital infection (Fig. 2.74) often have a history of prolonged delivery and premature rupture of membranes. An RDS pattern that is asymmetrical with an effusion should raise the possibility of beta-haemolytic streptococcus, especially if the lungs are hyperinflated when not ventilated. Lobar consolidations are uncommon in the neonatal period. Patchy infiltrates and diffuse hazy lung can often be mistaken for wet lung, and hazy lungs misinterpreted for RDS, but careful history taking and correlation of the x-ray and clinical findings should avoid confusion.

2.2.7.1.2
VASCULAR CAUSES

Congenital heart disease often presents in the neonatal period with symptoms of failure or is detected on

the routine clinical examination of the neonate. A discussion of congenital heart disease is outside the scope of this book except for a brief discussion of total anomalous pulmonary venous drainage.

Vascular causes of an increased interstitial pattern in the newborn are total anomalous pulmonary venous drainage with obstruction and lymphangiectasia.

Total Anomalous Pulmonary Venous Drainage. Total anomalous pulmonary venous drainage (TAPVD) is an important radiological diagnosis. The infant presents with respiratory distress and cyanosis in the neonatal period. Radiographically there is a fine streaky reticular pattern in the lungs with a normal heart size and contour (Fig. 2.75). Occasionally a pattern of more diffuse opacification reminiscent of pulmonary oedema occurs and mimics RDS, wet lung or pulmonary lymphangiectasia. Children with TAPVD do not have an enlarged heart because the shunt is precardiac. The children have no cardiac murmurs. The anomalous veins may be extremely difficult to demonstrate by echocardiographic studies and the cardiologist may need to be persistent in suggesting the diagnosis. If echo studies are normal, MRI is extremely helpful in demonstrating the anatomy.

Pulmonary Lymphangiectasia. Pulmonary lymphangiectasia is extremely rare. It may be the primary abnormality, although more commonly it is seen as a generalised lymphangiectasia. It occasionally occurs

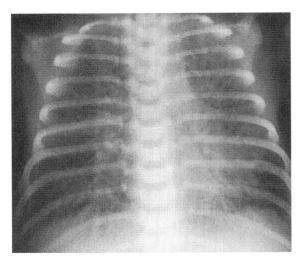

Fig. 2.75. Total anomalous pulmonary venous drainage. There is pulmonary congestion and mild hyperinflation of the lungs with a normal cardiac silhouette which is typical of anomalous obstructed drainage

in cases of congenital heart disease, with severe pulmonary venous obstruction resulting in lymphatic dilatation due to the high pulmonary venous pressures. Radiographically there is a congested reticular nodular appearance due to dilated lymphatics. The appearance is much coarser than in RDS and there is generally hyperinflation.

2.2.7.2
Older Child

Early parenchymal disease manifests itself with indistinctness of the vessels. As the air space becomes involved, small indistinct opacities form and coalesce so that the lungs become diffusely hazy. In pulmonary oedema this often has a bat's wing distribution. In bacterial infection it is usually lobar or segmental with air bronchograms. The air space is filled with oedema fluid, exudate from infection or haemorrhage depending on the aetiology. A coarse reticular pattern such as honeycomb lung is a feature of chronic disease.

2.2.7.2.1
RESPIRATORY TRACT INFECTION
Respiratory tract infection is the commonest acute illness in children and is described as upper or lower respiratory tract infection. Most infections affect the upper respiratory tract. Involvement of the lower respiratory tract is a more serious illness with a greater risk of complication. Upper respiratory tract

infections most commonly occur between 2 and 4 years. Lower respiratory tract infections are more frequent, and potentially more serious, in infants. Viral infections are more frequent than bacterial infections in both groups, especially under 4 years. Respiratory syncitial virus is the most frequently encountered and is responsible for bronchiolitis and pneumonia. Bacterial superadded infection often complicates respiratory syncitial virus infection.

In younger children the main bacterial infections are streptococcus, *Haemophilus influenzae* and pneumococcus. In teenagers *Mycoplasma pneumoniae* is a common and important aetiological agent, followed in frequency by viral and bacterial infections, especially streptococcus and pneumococcus. Children with mycoplasmal pneumonia often have persistent consolidation on the chest radiograph. Clinically they have prolonged and often distressing coughs. Children with streptococcal or pneumococcal pneumonia present acutely. In addition to tachypnoea and recession, pyrexia, cough and wheeze, they may also complain of chest pain. The distinction between viral and bacterial infection is often not possible on a chest radiograph. The value of the radiograph is to exclude any associated consolidation and collapsed segments (MOUTON and PHILLIPS 1992), which, if present, need treatment with antibiotics and physiotherapy when persistent collapse occurs in spite of adequate treatment. Bronchoscopy is indicated to exclude endobronchial obstruction and to aid re-expansion by selective suction and lavage.

2.2.7.2.2
VIRAL PNEUMONIA
Viral pneumonia can be difficult to diagnose in children and the chest radiograph is a routine investigation in suspected cases. A normal radiograph in the early stages does not exclude a pneumonia. The children present appearing ill with fever that is generally milder than in bacterial infections, non-productive cough, dyspnoea, tachypnoea and intercostal recession; often there are also upper respiratory tract symptoms of sore throat, rhinorrhoea and non-specific symptoms of headache and fatigue.

Viral pneumonia is non-specific in appearance but commonly there is peribronchial thickening with hyperinflation (Fig. 2.76). The pattern varies from mild hyperinflation only to perihilar or widespread infiltrates. Perihilar peribronchial infiltrates are the most common pattern. Interstitial infiltrates appear as streaky opacifications extending from the hila and producing a "shaggy" heart. A reticular pattern, a

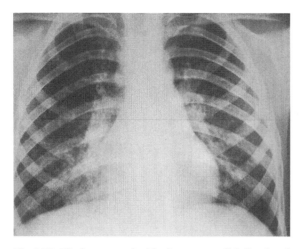

Fig. 2.76. Viral pneumonia. The lungs are well inflated and there are perihilar and peribronchial infiltrates producing peribronchial thickening. There is a nodular pattern throughout the lungs being prominent in the right middle lobe where there is an indistinct right heart border indicating subsegmental collapse/consolidation

diffuse haze, and rarely a miliary pattern are also seen. Lobar consolidations are rare but atelectasis secondary to obstruction from mucosal thickening, secretions and mucous plugs is common and may mimic pneumonic consolidations, though it resolves very rapidly.

Hyperinflation results from mucosal thickening with more focal emphysema due to mucous plugs. Lymphadenopathy is a very variable feature but when present requires a follow-up film after 2 weeks of treatment to ensure resolution. Peripheral infiltrates occur, but if more extensive or with focal lobar consolidation, imply superadded bacterial infection and also require follow-up radiographs. Pleural effusions are uncommon in viral pneumonia and if present are due to heart failure or superadded bacterial infection.

2.2.7.2.3
BRONCHIOLITIS

Bronchiolitis is a seasonal disease occurring primarily in winter months in infants less than 6 months of age. The causative organism is respiratory syncitial virus (RSV); most affected infants are RSV positive, although a smaller number will have a similar illness but be RSV negative. The infants present with fever, tachypnoea and dyspnoea and in severe cases may become extremely hypoxic and require ventilation and on occasion ECMO. The radiographic signs are initially hyperinflation, which may progress to severe hyperinflation, areas of atelectasis and compen-

satory emphysema and the development of interstitial pulmonary oedema. Complications include air leaks, both pneumothoraces and pneumomediastinum. Superimposed bacterial infection is common but collapse due to this cannot be distinguished from collapse due to mucous plugging. The radiographic signs often lag behind the clinical picture.

2.2.7.2.4
BACTERIAL INFECTIONS

With bacterial infections the child usually appears more systemically unwell with higher fever than with viral infections, a productive cough and sometimes chest pain. Wheeze is uncommon in comparison to viral pneumonia. Cyanosis indicates a severe infection with hypoxia due to inadequate oxygen exchange.

The chest radiograph will confirm the diagnosis of pneumonia. Those that present to the Casualty Department are usually ill and unresponsive to treatment.

These pneumonias produce subsegmental or lobar opacities due to either consolidation or collapse. The obliteration of the air space adjacent to a radiopaque structure causes the loss of the border – "the silhouette sign". This is most frequently seen adjacent to the heart border or hemidiaphragm. On the frontal projection the thickness of the air space loss may be so small as not to alter the radiodensity visually, but since it abuts the heart border or diaphragm there will be loss of that part of the border affected (Fig. 2.77a). A lateral film will usually confirm the diagnosis (Fig. 2.77b).

When lobes of the lung collapse in a pneumothorax they become small replicas of themselves and retract to the hilum. The collapse occurring in pneumonia occurs without pleural air and the adjacent structures compensate for the loss of volume, initially by hyperinflation of the adjacent lobes and elevation of the ipsilateral diaphragm, and later by shift of the mediastinum to the ipsilateral side with herniation of the hyperinflated contralateral lung. This herniation will appear on the lateral projection as a lucency anterior to the collapsed opaque lobe. The lobe shape is determined by the adjacent structures and the semi-rigid nature. This pulmonary rigidity will be modfied by the intrapulmonary disease. A predetermined pattern of collapse results, modified by any previous inflammation and adhesions. The surrounding lobes will show a variable degree of hyperlucency due to increased aeration, i.e. compensatory emphysema.

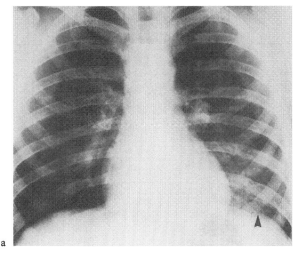

a

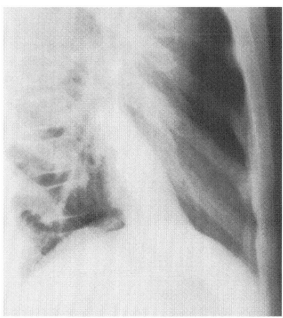

b

Fig. 2.77 a,b. Atelectasis. **a** The left hemidiaphragm is lost medially, the "silhouette sign" (arrow), with a slight haziness and indistinctness of the vessels above. This implies collapse/consolidation over that area of diaphragm. **b** Lateral film. This shows an obvious triangular shaped area of opacity sitting on the diaphragm indicating atelectasis of the anterior segment of the left lower lobe

The loss of air space may be due to consolidation or collapse caused by pus obstructing the bronchi. The appearances of collapse of the various lobes are shown in Figs. 2.78 and 2.79. Upper lobe collapse shows an indistinct upper zone haze on the frontal projection (Fig. 2.80) whilst in the lower lobe there is a wedge-shaped area of tissue usually lying adjacent to the mediastinum. On the left side this lies behind the heart (Fig. 2.81) and is accompanied by loss of all or part of the left hemidiaphragm. If the heart lies on the left hemidiaphragm tangential to the incident beam without air between it and the hemidiaphragm, the left hemidiaphragm border is lost over that region as a normal feature. Only by comparison with previous films can consolidation be detected in this area by virtue of the silhouette sign. Lateral films will clearly confirm the presence of consolidation if there is doubt. Similarly the right heart border is sometimes indistinct due to the bronchopulmonary vessels adjacent to the heart border blending with the cardiac silhouette, giving a false-positive silhouette sign and misdiagnosis as a medial segment middle lobe pneumonia. A lateral view will confirm that the appearances are normal.

In addition to the silhouette sign, consolidation shows as diffuse opacification with air bronchograms (Fig. 2.82). Complications of bacterial pneumonia include effusions, empyema and, particularly with staphylococcal pneumonia, pneumothorax secondary to pneumatocoeles, pyopneumothorax, atelectasis and abscess formation.

Most children with viral pneumonia will not require follow-up radiographs. Those who do not clinically improve on appropriate antibiotic treatment should have a repeat radiograph of the chest to exclude empyema (DRUG and THERAPEUTICS BULLETIN 1997). If the pneumonia was complicated by an effusion or atelectasis it is advisable to have a radiograph after 8 weeks to ensure that the chest radiograph has returned to normal. The appearances on the radiograph lag behind the clinical picture, both at presentation and on recovery, and a radiograph earlier than this may well show residual signs leading to further inappropriate treatment. An uncomplicated pneumonia that has responded to antibiotic therapy does not need a follow-up radiograph (GIBSON et al. 1993). Consolidations may take up to 6 weeks for complete resolution and therefore any radiograph taken earlier may well show signs that are of no clinical significance. Cough should not be considered as an indication for a further x-ray as it often persists after the pneumonia has cleared completely. Any unresponsive pneumonia should alert one to a possibility of a foreign body or rarely an endobronchial tumour, even if the initial radiograph showed no or few signs.

2.2.7.2.5
MYCOPLASMAL PNEUMONIA
This atypical pneumonia is common in school-age children and more prevalent in autumn and winter.

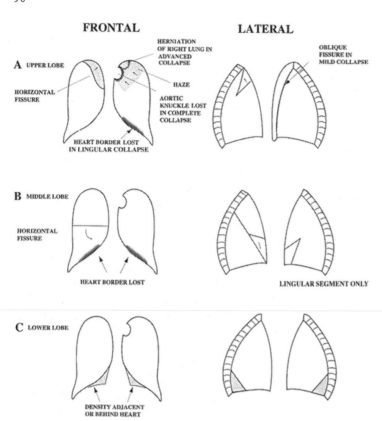

Fig. 2.78. Lobar collapse. Frontal view. There is no horizontal fissure on the left so the collapsing upper lobe appears as an ill-defined haze. Lateral view. Oblique fissure comes to lie as a density adjacent to the anterior chest wall. With further collapse there is herniation of the right lung to the left side (see Fig. 2.79)

The onset is a gradual influenza-like illness with few clinical signs; the illness is milder in the younger child but can progress to become severe. The radiological features are variable. Bilateral involvement, particularly of the lower lobes, is more common than single lobe involvement. The radiographic features are parahilar peribronchial infiltrates, patchy segmental or lobar consolidations that are slow to resolve and lymphadenopathy. These features are non-specific, also occurring in bacterial and, less commonly, viral infections. Pleural effusions are rare. Reticulonodular infiltrates in a lobe have a high specificity for mycoplasmal pneumonia (CASTRIOTA-SCANDBERG et al. 1995). The diagnosis is usually made by the finding of a positive blood test for mycoplasma titres.

2.2.7.2.6

PNEUMONIA IN IMMUNOCOMPROMISED PATIENTS

Immunocompromised children are prone to the development of opportunistic infection. Bronchial washings can identify the causative agent, the most frequent being *Pneumocystis carinii*, cytomegalo virus and *Aspergillus*. The chest radiograph in *Pneumocystis carinii* infection shows a perihilar haze which is progressive, with air bronchograms and hyperinflation. Subcutaneous emphysema and pneumothoraces or even pneumatocoeles develop later. Bronchiolitis obliterans is a recognised complication.

Cytomegalo virus is also seen in immuno deficient states. It can be difficult to differentiate from *Pneumocystis carinii* but the acinar shadows are less prominent and the reticulonodular pattern is more prominent in the outer third of the lung (Fig. 2.83).

2.2.7.2.7

ASPIRATION PNEUMONIA

Aspiration pneumonia may be severe and life threatening due to the inflammatory response to the noxious material, which may become infective or be chemically irritant. It can occur in any unconscious patient, the severely ill patient or those with airway support. In the acute emergency setting it usually presents as a complication of an acute or chronic condition due to aspiration of gastric content or inhalation of foreign material. With the aspiration of

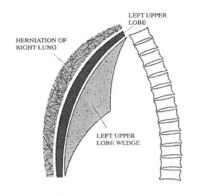

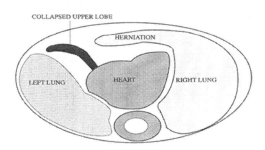

Fig. 2.79. Left upper lobe collapse – lateral projection. In advanced collapse, the upper lobe is seen as a flattened triangle "wedge" against the anterior chest wall. It is seen through the over-expanded (compensatory emphysema) lower lobe. With further collapse the lower lobe cannot compensate for the loss of volume in the upper lobe and there is then herniation of the right lung to the left side anterior to the heart. This appears as a lucency in the retrosternal space

gastric secretions, often termed Mendelson's syndrome, the acute irritant effect of the acid results in pulmonary oedema. The presence of a normal-sized heart generally eliminates a cardiac cause. If the patient is in a posture in which one lung is more dependent than the other, the appearances will be more unilateral. The recovery from aspiration pneumonia is slow and may take a week or more. Aspiration of more solid components such as food particles results in changes which may be more variable with focal atelectasis dependent on the position of the patient at the time of aspiration. The particulate matter lodges in the bronchi, causing atelectasis; the latter is usually segmental in distribution, involving the posterior segments of the upper and lower lobes. If superadded infection intervenes this does not follow the distribution related to gravity. Chronic aspiration will result in fibrosis and bronchiectasis at variable sites.

The young are at higher risk from aspiration of gastric secretions since the acidity and volume are highest in children. In chronic aspiration, respiratory distress may rarely be accompanied by a normal radiograph. In any patient with a history of recurrent pneumonia or persistent unexplained cough the suspicion of aspiration, particularly in relation to gastro-oesophageal reflux, should be raised.

The radiological features are coarse nodules and infiltrates in the newborn and young infant, or more focal opacities in the right upper lobe and apex of the lower lobe due to the supine position. In older children in the upright position, the lower lobes are more frequently involved unless aspiration occurs in a recumbent position. Rarely it may be possible to determine the cause of the aspiration on the chest radiograph, such as in achalasia, when the fluid-filled oesophagus, sometimes with a fluid level, is seen behind the heart and the gas bubble in the stomach is absent (Fig. 2.84). Aspiration pneumonia is more frequent in the neurologically impaired child. A rare cause is an undiagnosed H-type tracheo-oesophageal fistula (TOF). These children may have a very gassy abdomen to suggest the diagnosis. Any child with recurrent infection in the first year of life should have contrast studies with an oesophageal tube or endoscopy to exclude TOF. Older children who have recurrent pneumonia or unexplained chronic cough should be investigated for gastro-oesophageal reflux.

Once aspiration is suspected as a cause of recurrent chest infection, further radiological investigation is indicated. The most sensitive imaging test for reflux is the radionuclide milk scan, but facilities are limited and most children have barium studies. These should include video fluoroscopy of the swallowing mechanism to assess coordination and any tracheal aspiration. Barium studies have a poor sensitivity in the detection of reflux and are carried out mainly for demonstration of an anatomical abnormality such as hiatus hernia and any complication of reflux, e.g. ulceration and strictures. The gold standard for the detection of reflux is pH monitoring.

2.2.7.2.8
NEAR DROWNING

Drowning is the third most common cause of death in children, but this statistic does not reflect the morbidity from near drowning. The appearance of the radiograph in near drowning will depend on the volume of water that has entered the lungs. Laryngeal reflexes may prevent the inhalation of water – so-called dry drowning. In this case the lungs will appear clear. Radiographically the difference be-

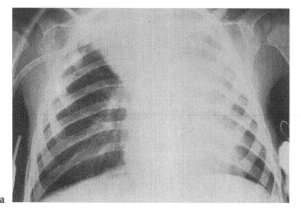

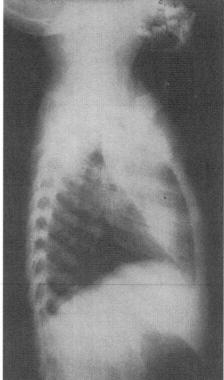

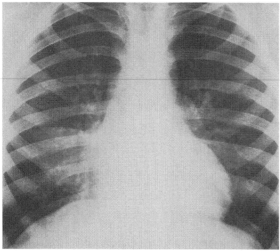

Fig. 2.80 a–c. Upper lobe, lingula and right middle lobe collapse. **a** The upper lobe collapse on the right side produces a wedge-shaped area abutting the superior mediastinum. On the left side there is a generalised haze with loss of the left heart border and aortic knuckle due to collapse of the lingular segment adjacent to the left heart border. **b** Left upper lobe collapse, lateral view. The oblique fissure is displaced forwards by the atelectatic opaque upper lobe. **c** Right middle lobe collapse. The right heart border is indistinct, being equivalent to the lingula collapse on the left side, and there is a faint haze limited by the horizontal fissure, indicating collapse/consolidation in the medial segment

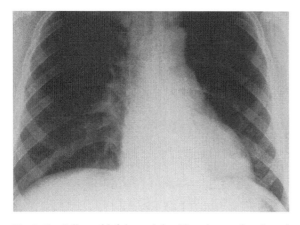

Fig. 2.81. Collapsed left lower lobe. There is a wedge-shaped area of increased density behind the heart with loss of the left hemidiaphragm border over the opacification. Compensatory emphysema is present in the remaining inflated left lung, which produces a hyperlucent area in the left hemithorax

tween fresh and sea water is indistinguishable. The appearances are those of pulmonary oedema with a normal sized heart. The oedema be very patchy in distribution if the water is contaminated, especially with larger particulate material. The degree of oedema and its location will also depend on the volume inhaled, being more central in smaller volumes (Fig. 2.85). The changes resolve over a period of 5–10 days. In some cases the appearances may be normal on admission, so it is always important to observe and repeat radiographs as the condition may worsen over 24h, especially if there has been contaminant material in the water. In a small number of cases superadded infection occurs and may lead to ARDS.

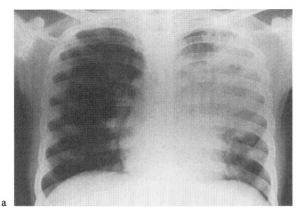

a

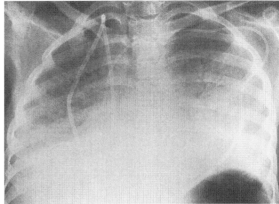

Fig. 2.83. Cytomegalovirus. There is a perihilar alveolar opacification with prominent air bronchograms

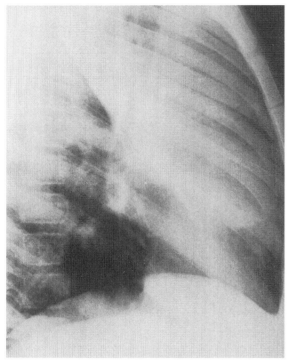

b

Fig. 2.82 a,b. Left upper lobe pneumonia. a There is opacification in the left upper lobe with faint air bronchograms, which are seen as branching radiolucencies. There is loss of the upper left heart border due to the adjacent consolidation in the lingula segment. b The lateral projection shows the oblique fissure in its upper portion outlined by a consolidation anterior to it

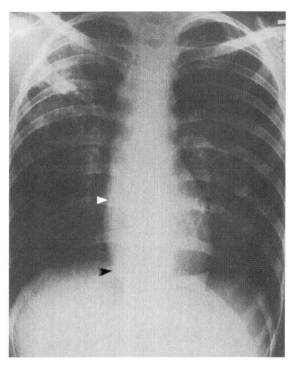

Fig. 2.84. Aspiration pneumonia due to achalasia of the cardia. There are small infiltrates in the right upper lobe with a double contour to the right heart border due to the dilated oesophagus (*arrowhead*). Note that there is no gastric air bubble

2.2.7.2.9
PULMONARY OEDEMA

The most common cause of pulmonary oedema is an increase in the pulmonary venous pressure secondary to left-sided cardiac failure. In the early stage of failure the fluid accumulates in the interstitial spaces. The fluid within the perivascular sheaths produces loss of the clear definition of the pulmonary vascular markings. This is seen particularly prominently in the very young child and is a less valuable sign in the older child. Similarly the walls of the bronchi seen end-on may appear thickened and ill-defined. The increasing fluid in the interlobar septa produce Kerley A and B lines. The B lines appear as short, fine, transverse, radiodense lines

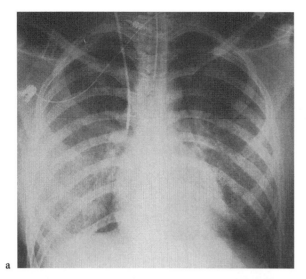

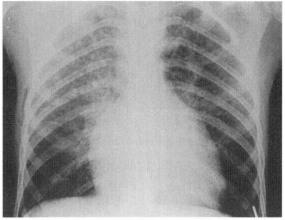

Fig. 2.86. Cardiac failure. Cardiomegaly, prominent indistinct pulmonary vessels and perihilar haziness are present. Septal lines are seen as linear opacities radiating from the hila. There is mild hyperinflation of the lungs. A little air is seen in the soft tissues of the right lateral border due to previous thoracotomy

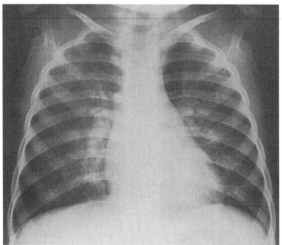

Fig. 2.85 a,b. Near drowning. a There is bilateral pulmonary oedema which is uneven in distribution reflecting the distribution of the inhaled water. This is more prominent on the right side particularly at the right base where there is loss of the right hemidiaphragm which may represent a more focal degree of collapse due to some inhaled particulate matter. b In this case there is a smaller volume inhaled and the alveolar oedema is confined to the perihilar regions

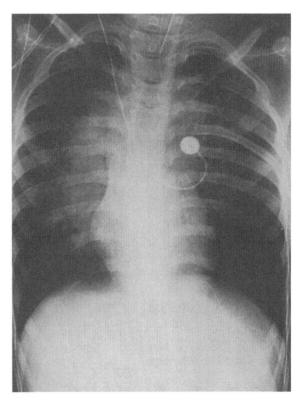

Fig. 2.87. Acute pulmonary oedema. The distribution of the alveolar oedema extends from the perihilar regions and produces the typical "bat's wing" configuration

perpendicular to the pleural surface, most easily seen in the costophrenic sulci and anteriorly in the retrosternal space. The A lines are longer opacities extending from the hilar region (Fig. 2.86). Interstitial oedema usually precedes alveolar oedema unless there is very sudden cardiac decompensation. Fluid in the alveolar spaces produces acinar shadows. These are irregular, poorly defined, small patches of opacification scattered throughout the lung. The medial regions of the lungs become particularly affected. As the fluid increases these shadows coalesce,

with the peripheral areas being spared. This produces a central perihilar opacification producing the so-called bat's wing or butterfly pattern (Fig. 2.87). Associated findings are cardiomegaly, pleural effusions and superior mediastinal widening due to venous congestion.

Occasionally the pulmonary oedema may be unilateral and asymmetric. This sometimes occurs due to some pre-existing condition on the ipsilateral or contralateral side. Ipsilateral pulmonary oedema may occur due to the patient's prolonged posture with the dependent lung being involved, or in left to right shunt where the blood flow is not of uniform distribution. Contralaterally, unilateral pulmonary oedema is seen where there is a reduced pulmonary blood flow to one lung, as occurs with pulmonary artery anomalies (Swyer-James-Macleod syndrome being the most common in children).

Non-cardiac causes include acute infections (Fig. 2.88), glomerulonephritis, inhalation of noxious gases or fluids, collagen vascular diseases, allergic response, shock lung, raised intracranial pressure and iatrogenic causes. In these latter conditions the heart size may often be normal. Non-cardiogenic pulmonary oedema tends to present as alveolar oedema.

2.2.7.2.10

ADULT RESPIRATORY DISTRESS SYNDROME
ARDS is due to generalised capillary damage occurring in patients without any pre-existing lung disease. It has a wide range of clinical causes, the most common being sepsis and gastric aspiration. It is divided into three stages:

Stage 1 (12–24 h): increasing hypoxia and lung stiffness result in acute respiratory failure requiring mechanical ventilation.
Stage 2 (1–5 days): increasing hypoxia despite oxygen and ventilatory support.
Stage 3 (5 days +): microvascular destruction and infarction.

In the early stages up to 12 h the chest radiograph is usually normal unless there is a precipitating cause such as pneumonia or aspiration. In stage 1, that is 12–24 h, there are patchy ill-defined opacities throughout the lungs. The appearance may mimic pulmonary oedema of cardiac origin except that the heart size is usually normal and the oedema is more peripheral in distribution. From 24 h to 4 days areas of consolidation coalesce to produce diffuse alveolar opacification of the whole lung, differentiating it from cardiogenic pulmonary oedema with its bat's wing distribution. A further differentiating point is the presence of air bronchograms. Pleural effusions are uncommon. From 4 to 7 days the consolidation becomes inhomogeneous due to the reduction in

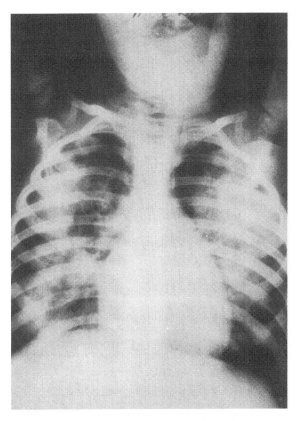

Fig. 2.88. Patchy pulmonary alveolar oedema that is more confluent on the left side in this case due to influenzal pneumonia

pulmonary oedema. Superimposed bacterial pneumonia may occur at this time to form more focal areas of consolidation. From 7 days the lungs remain abnormal, often with a reticular or bubbly pattern. Severe ARDS is often complicated by widespread pulmonary vascular thrombosis and infarction (MORGAN and GOODMAN 1991).

Mortality from ARDS is high, mostly due to respiratory-related complications. Those who do survive have surprisingly little long-term impairment of lung function although many have residual pulmonary opacities and evidence of hyperinflation. A coarse reticular pattern is seen in some survivors (FRASER et al. 1990).

There are radiographic features which help in differentiating between hydrostatic and increased permeability oedema. Hydrostatic oedema, which is mostly due to cardiac failure, is characterised by redistribution of the blood flow to the upper lobe veins, uneven distribution of the pulmonary oedema, cardiomegaly and normal or increased vascular pedicle size. Pleural effusions and peribronchial cuffing are frequent, but septal lines are not common. In renal or overhydration oedema, the pulmonary blood flow pattern is normal but the vessels are increased, with cardiomegaly and vascular pedicle widening. The oedema is usually central in location. Peribronchial cuffing and pleural effusions are common. Capillary oedema seen in ARDS is peripheral in distribution initially. When it becomes confluent it is widespread but patchy, with normal blood flow distribution. The heart size and vascular pedicles are normal. Septal lines are not seen and peribronchial cuffing and pleural effusions are rare (FRASER et al. 1990).

2.2.7.2.11
CYSTIC FIBROSIS

Cystic fibrosis is one of the most common incurable diseases of childhood and may present to the emergency department at any stage of disease. It is inherited as an autosomal recessive trait. The basic abnormality is that the secretion from the exocrine glands is viscous and causes blockage of ducts in the tracheobronchial tree. Often the first presentation is of recurrent cough or wheeze, recurrent pneumonias or persistent pansinusitis. Later in the disease children present with the complications of bronchiectasis with atelectasis, pneumothorax and haemoptysis.

Radiographically, early in the disease the chest is normal but during the first year of life hyperinflation of the lungs is seen (Fig. 2.89a), often with lobar segmental atelectasis particularly in the upper lobes. Any child presenting with repeated atelectasis with or without hyperinflation of the lungs should be investigated for cystic fibrosis (Fig. 2.89b). As the disease progresses it is complicated by superadded infection producing thickened bronchial walls seen either as small ring shadows in cross-section or linear shadows when seen longitudinally (Figs. 2.90, 2.91). Bronchiectasis and cyst formation become manifest as rounded opacities on the radiographs. With further progression these cystic areas coalesce to form larger cysts which may appear as lucencies when filled with air or dense when filled with secretions or pus. When the bronchiectatic proximal bronchi are filled with fluid they appear as finger-like projections extending from the hila. Hilar lymphadenopathy ensues as the disease progresses and causes very prominent hilar shadows. Enlarged bronchial arteries providing collateral circulation may contribute to the opacities seen on the radiographs. Erosion through the arteries may cause haemoptysis and lead to emergency presentation,

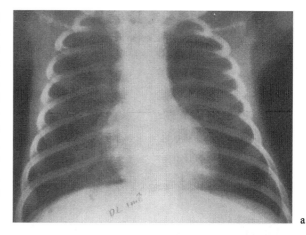

a

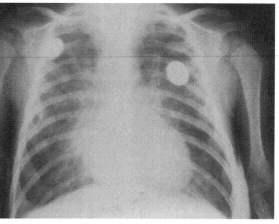

b

Fig. 2.89 a,b. Cystic fibrosis. These images show the progressive changes in cystic fibrosis over a period of 3 months. **a** At 1 month of age there is mild hyperinflation of the lungs with very early peribronchial thickening. **b** At 3 months there is a greater degree of hyperinflation and peribronchial thickening is more prominent; subsegmental linear atelectasis now extends from the perihilar regions

although this is very rarely sufficiently severe to cause death. Similarly, subpleural cysts may rupture, leading to a pneumothorax.

The main complication that leads to presentation in Accident and Emergency or acute exacerbation is infection, often with deterioration in respiratory reserve. The chest x-ray may show pneumonia, atelectasis and rarely lung abscesses and right heart failure due to pulmonary hypertension. Pulmonary hypertension and cor pulmonale should be carefully looked for in cystic fibrosis. In severe cystic fibrosis the marked overinflation of the lungs produces a small cardiac silhouette, although the main pulmonary artery is usually enlarged. In these children if the heart is normal in size or enlarged it may indicate cardiac decompensation.

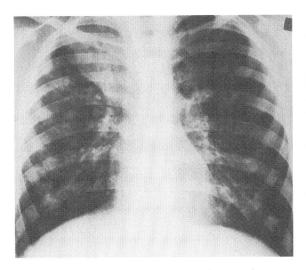

Fig. 2.90. Cystic fibrosis: older patient. The typical appearance of well-established changes of cystic fibrosis is seen. Marked perihilar peribronchial thickening extends into the periphery. There is collapse in the right upper lobe with dilated air bronchograms within it. Note that the heart shadow is small due to the hyperinflated lungs

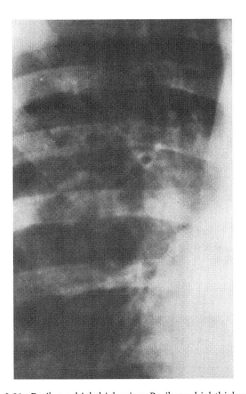

Fig. 2.91. Peribronchial thickening. Peribronchial thickening can be assessed by comparing the size of the bronchus with that of the companion vessel. The ring shadow of the dilated bronchus is seen with a thickened wall adjacent to the normal-sized vessel seen end on (white). The vessels should normally be the same size but peribronchial thickening leads to an increase in size of the bronchus

Most children with cystic fibrosis are followed up with chest radiographs. Fine-section CT can assess the distribution and severity of the bronchiectasis, particularly if there is one segment involved requiring surgery. Expiratory high-resolution CT will show air trapping in children in whom there is discrepancy between the clinical history and chest x-ray, and this explains the reduced falling peak flow in the pressure with little radiographic change.

There should be a high index of suspicion of cystic fibrosis in any child with recurrent respiratory problems; this is particularly so in those with hyperinflated lungs and atelectasis, (especially if there is thickening of the bronchial walls). A positive sweat test is simple to do and is diagnostically accurate, provided it is correctly performed. Gene probes are now routinely used to confirm the diagnosis and carrier states. Patients who are carriers may have asthma-like illnesses.

2.2.7.2.12
ALLERGIC LUNG DISEASE
Allergic lung disease presents as a bronchiolitis-type pneumonia in the young and as a pneumonia or asthma-like illness in the older child. The diagnosis is difficult if there is not a clear history of exposure to an allergen. The radiographic appearances are variable. In a typical case, there is alveolar shadowing with hyperinflation. The alveolar shadowing is unusual in small children.

The appearances are more often those of hyperinflation. This may be associated with atelectasis and, if bilateral, an interstitial pneumonic pattern involving more predominantly the lower lobes.

The causative allergen may be difficult to identify since the changes may occur days after exposure. Any recurrent pneumonia in a young infant without adequate explanation should raise the possibility of allergy.

2.2.7.2.13
CONNECTIVE TISSUE DISEASE
Pulmonary manifestations of connective tissue disease in children are rare and tend to occur in the teenage child. In systemic lupus, air space shadowing predominates. This is seen on CT as a ground glass appearance mainly in the middle and lower zones with some interstitial thickening. The children may present to Accident and Emergency with a history of progressive diminution in effort tolerance due to restrictive lung disease.

In systemic sclerosis, basal fibrotic changes predominate. Complications include air leaks and the child may present with a pneumothorax or subcutaneous emphysema.

2.2.7.2.14
FIBROSING ALVEOLITIS

Fibrosing alveolitis is a rare condition in children and is different to that seen in adults. The child clinically presents with tachypnoea and may be hypoxic. The symptoms are present from birth. Radiographically, the most typical pattern is one of air space shadowing which is diffuse and is often initially interpreted as acute infection. With progression, the pattern changes to hyperinflation with atelectasis due to fibrosis.

2.2.7.2.15
PULMONARY HAEMOSIDEROSIS

Pulmonary haemosiderosis is a rare disorder occurring secondary to chronic recurrent intrapulmonary haemorrhage of a diffuse alveolar nature. In infants and children it is most often primary, while in adolescents it is usually secondary to some other haemorrhagic or vascular disorder. It presents clinically with recurrent episodes of pneumonia, respiratory symptoms of cough, wheeze and dyspnoea and often an iron deficiency anaemia. It may also present with acute haemoptysis.

Ultimately death may result from haemorrhage or respiratory failure. The radiographic appearances are variable and change from indistinct bilateral infiltrates to massive alveolar opacification similar to that of pulmonary oedema. Obstruction of the bronchi by blood may result in atelectasis and emphysema. The natural history is one of recovery with repeated episodes of bleeding. Initially the chest x-ray may return to normal but with repeated bleeding a more chronic pattern ensues with a miliary or reticulonodular pattern and reactive lymph node enlargement.

2.2.7.2.16
TUBERCULOSIS

Pulmonary tuberculosis (TB) is once again becoming more common and is often asymptomatic when discovered as a result of contact tracing. Clinical presentation is with fever, anorexia, weight loss, general malaise and cough. In children most TB is primary. The radiographs reveal ill-defined consolidation which may be subsegmental or lobar and involve any lobe, and in most cases is associated with hilar or paratracheal lymphadenopathy, which is usually unilateral. Occasionally the bronchi are compressed by the nodes, or stenosed, leading to atelectasis or

obstructive emphysema. Pleural effusions may occur but are not common. Post-primary TB has a different pattern. Typically the disease is in the upper lobes or apical segment of the lower lobes.

Initially there is consolidation, then cavitation with progressive loss of volume and fibrosis. Following treatment focal calcification and fibrosis ensue. Tubercular bronchopneumonia may superimpose on cavitating disease. Miliary tuberculosis due to haematogenous spread is more common in post-primary disease and produces the typical multiple small discrete foci throughout the lungs. Children with AIDS are at increased risk of TB.

2.2.7.2.17
MISCELLANEOUS PNEUMONIAS

The radiographic appearance of varicella (chicken pox) is one of an ill-defined nodular pattern distributed through both lungs, often with hilar lymphadenopathy. Intrapulmonary calcified nodules may be seen. Measles pneumonia (rubeola) produces an increase in the interstitial lung markings, predominantly in the perihilar regions. These may coalesce to form patchy consolidations, but lobar consolidations are due to superadded infection. There is usually mild hyperinflation. Atelectasis and hilar lymphadenopathy are frequently observed.

2.3
Foreign Bodies

Aspiration of foreign bodies occurs most often in small children, over 50% of cases occurring below the age of 3 years (DAVIS 1996) and 80% under 10 years (WEISSBERG and SCHWARTZ 1987). The mortality is greater in the younger age group, presumably due to the small size of the airways. In one series about 80% of those who died were under 4 years old (MITTLEMAN 1984). Most inhaled foreign bodies are radiolucent. They are most frequently of vegetable origin; this is important because left in situ they set up an inflammatory response. The inhalation of grasses may be responsible for coughs and wheezes in the summer. Laryngeal foreign body aspiration usually but not always has a history of choking and may present with stridor, wheeze, cough, episodes of cyanosis and apnoea. There may be vomiting and difficulty in swallowing, which also occurs with oesophageal foreign bodies.

Intrabronchial foreign bodies are more frequently encountered and are less likely to be initially fatal. However, there is a greater chance of the diagnosis being missed and delayed presentation is much more common. With delayed presentation there are additional signs of fever and unresolved or recurrent pneumonia and cough, sometimes accompanied by haemoptysis. One must remember that if there has been trauma, particularly if the skull radiograph shows missing teeth, then as a precautionary measure radiographs of the chest should be obtained to detect any inhaled fragments of teeth.

Laryngeal obstruction is one of the most common causes of accidental death in children under 1 year old. Clinical presentation is with stridor, cough and acute respiratory distress (MOUTON and PHILLIPS 1992). Unsuspected foreign bodies in the lower airways may present more insidiously with cough and respiratory tract infections. Mediastinal and subcutaneous emphysema may occasionally be the presentation (SAOJ et al. 1995) but is seen more frequently with oesophageal foreign bodies. Oesophageal foreign bodies may present late with respiratory symptoms either due to extrinsic pressure on the airways by the direct mass effect or secondary to mediastinal abscess formation. A positive history of choking is more frequent in cases of aspirated rather than ingested foreign bodies.

The diagnosis of an inhaled foreign body can be elusive and persistence is important even with a negative history of foreign body ingestion or inhalation (REILLY et al. 1997). Most inhaled foreign bodies are radiolucent. They are often of vegetable matter. Peanuts, because of their oil content, set up intense inflammatory responses, thus narrowing the airways further and often resulting in permanent bronchial stenosis; however, any vegetable matter is more likely to produce a direct inflammatory response than an inert object such as a bead. Consolidation develops distal to the endobronchial obstruction. Most oesophageal foreign bodies (usually coins) are opaque. It must always be remembered that a negative chest radiograph does not exclude a foreign body. Air trapping, atelectasis and infection are not specific for foreign bodies and occur in any lesion causing obstruction. Asthma and infection can mimic appearances suggestive of a foreign body (SVEDSTÖM et al. 1989).

The inhaled foreign body, if not reactive, may be discovered incidentally if radiopaque. Aspirated staples, because of their hook-like spikes, can migrate peripherally. Most foreign bodies are radiolucent and set up an inflammatory response and the changes seen are usually due to bronchial obstruction. Inhalation is almost invariably into the lower lobes. In children the incidence of aspiration into the right and left is equal, probably due to the equality of the right and left bronchial angles in children compared with adults. The typical radiological finding in uncomplicated non-opaque foreign body aspiration is of ipsilateral obstructive emphysema seen maximally on an expiratory film. It cannot be over-emphasised that the inspiratory film may be normal. This is in part due to over-distension but is also contributed to by reduced vascularity due to hypoxic vasoconstriction. Atelectasis at presentation is uncommon, presumably due to collateral air drift.

The initial investigation in all suspected inhaled foreign bodies should be a PA chest with paired inspiration and expiration films to show the obstructive emphysema, if these are possible. If obstruction is shown and the history is appropriate, the child should be referred for bronchoscopy. In some cases the child will be admitted to the ICU while awaiting bronchoscopy as there is a considerable danger that a foreign body may dislodge with coughing and become impacted in the trachea or larynx and lead to respiratory obstruction. If paired inspiration and expiration films are not feasible due to lack of co-operation, the child should undergo fluoroscopy. Air trapping is then easy to identify. Paradoxical movement, probably due to inhibitory reflex initiated by the foreign body in the main bronchus, may occur even without any other visible sign at fluoroscopy. If the patient is too young to co-operate for an expiratory film and fluoroscopy cannot be done urgently, then a lateral decubitus film should be obtained.

On the dependent side the mediastinum will compress the normal lung unless there is air trapping. If there is doubt, bilateral decubitus views should be obtained.

If the foreign body is known to be opaque, the initial radiographs should include a lateral film of the neck, which may show the foreign body (Figs. 2.92, 2.93). Calcified laryngeal cartilages in teenagers and normal calcifications, especially the stylo-hyoid ligament (which may resemble a fish bone) and the triticeal cartilage, are commonly mistaken for foreign bodies in those not familiar with children. A lateral view of the chest to locate the site where the foreign body is lodged can be taken if necessary. The film may show collapse due to obstruction or localised hyperinflation with or without a radiopaque foreign body and sometimes lucencies in a button representing holes for the thread may be the only indication of a foreign body. It is always important to obtain an expiratory film or fluoroscopy to show air trapping.

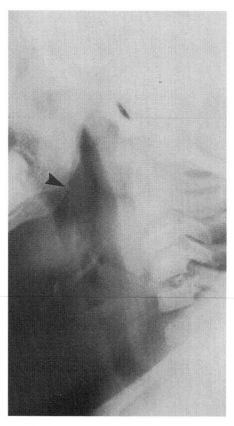

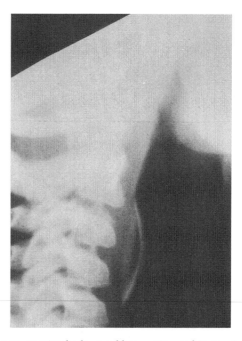

Fig. 2.93. Foreign body. A rubber suction pad is seen in the upper oesophagus

Fig. 2.92. Foreign body. A fish bone is seen in the hypopharynx just anterior to the epiglottis (*arrow*)

The inhaled opaque foreign body may be seen on the PA radiograph and be shown in the upper airway or trachea causing generalised hyperinflation (Fig. 2.94) or lodged in the lower airway with (Fig. 2.95) or without obstructive emphysema (Fig. 2.96).

Radiolucent foreign bodies present with hyperinflation (Fig. 2.97) or occasionally with collapse. A combination of both may indicate a fragmented foreign body. Such an appearance, however, may be seen with any intraluminal lesion producing either a ball-valve effect, causing hyperinflation, or complete obstruction, causing collapse. Asthma and infection with mucous plugs or pus will mimic foreign bodies.

In the presence of normal radiographs and a strong history, bronchoscopy is also indicated as not all inhaled foreign bodies lead to radiographic signs. Both rigid and flexible bronchoscopy should be available.

Missed foreign bodies may manifest as collapsed lobes or empyema (Fig. 2.98) and in these cases CT occasionally demonstrates the opacity not visualised on the plain film. Bronchiectasis may be a late manifestation of missed foreign body.

Though radio-isotope perfusion studies may show abnormality when radiographic findings are inconclusive, partial occlusion, especially in the acute presentation, may produce a normal study. In general such studies are not indicated. Bronchoscopy is the definitive investigation.

An opaque foreign body in the upper oesophagus may require a lateral film for localisation if it overlies the trachea and there is doubt as to its exact site.

Foreign body in the oesophagus may be demonstrated by contrast studies. Iso-osmolar non-ionic contrast should be used in these circumstances of delayed diagnosis since perforation may have occurred (Fig. 2.99). The common sites for entrapment of foreign bodies are the narrowed regions of the cricopharyngeal muscle, the aortic knuckle, and less commonly the gastro-oesophageal junction.

In cases of suspected ingestion of a foreign body it is always important to take the chest radiograph before the abdominal film. If the abdominal film is taken first and shows no foreign body, and then the chest radiograph is taken and no foreign body is seen, one might assume that no foreign body has been ingested. However, it is possible for a foreign body to be lodged in the oesophagus during the exposure of the abdominal film and then to drop into

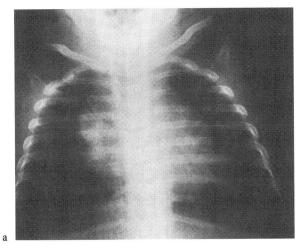

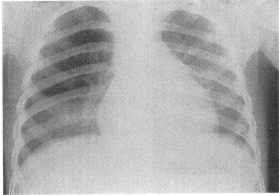

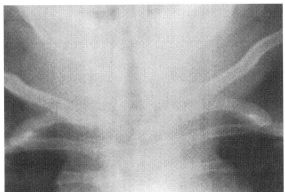

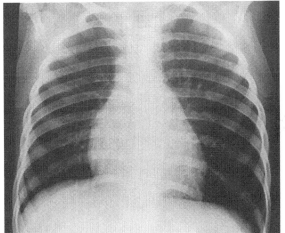

Fig. 2.94 a,b. Foreign body. **a** A curvilinear opacity, a meat bone, is seen in the upper trachea overlying the T1 vertebral body with hyperinflation of the lungs. **b** Localised view of the upper trachea showing the curvilinear foreign body

the stomach during the interval required for positioning for the chest film. It will then not be seen on the chest film, and the wrong conclusion reached of no ingested foreign body.

If no cause is found radiographically for a foreign body in a patient with a history of choking then bronchoscopy should be performed (BARMIOS FONTOBA et al. 1997). Similarly, oesophageal foreign bodies may present late as upper respiratory tract infection or croup (MACPHERSON et al. 1996). There should be a high index of suspicion of an oesophageal foreign body in patients with pre-existing pathology of the oesophagus such as a repaired tracheo-oesophageal fistula, and a history of unexplained or recurrent upper respiratory tract infection. The foreign body can be removed by endoscopy or by fluoroscopically guided balloon extraction (DOKLER et al. 1995). The latter technique is not freely available, is unpleasant and requires skill

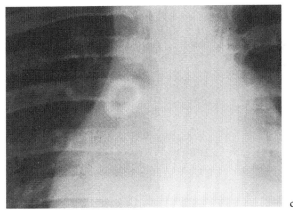

Fig. 2.95 a–c. Radiopaque foreign body in left main bronchus. **a** Film taken at the referring hospital showed deflation in the left lung, thought to be due to the foreign body. The film, however, is under-penetrated and taken in a partial expiratory phase with the left lung deflating normally and the right lung not deflating. **b** A penetrated full inspiratory film shows, in fact, that the left lung expands normally but there is failure to expand on the right side due to a radiopaque foreign body seen in the left main bronchus. **c** Localised views show the rounded opacity in the right main bronchus which was due to the inhaled antenna from the toy "Po of the Tellytubbies"

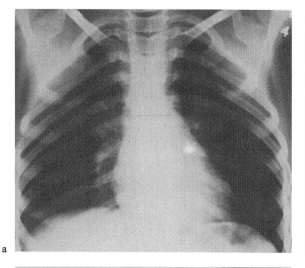

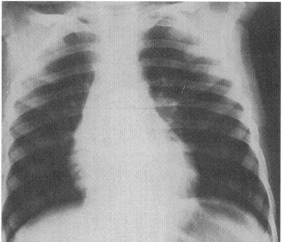

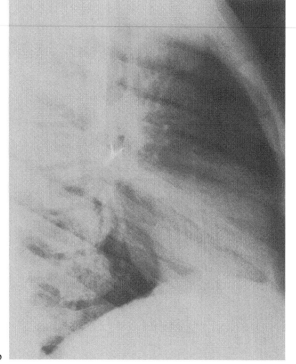

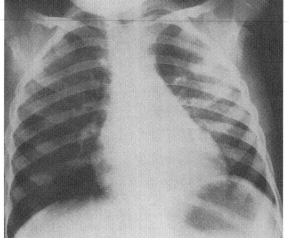

Fig. 2.97 a,b. Peanut in the right main bronchus. a The inspiratory film shows that the right side is less inflated than the left. On this single film it is uncertain whether there is air trapping on the left with slight shift of the mediastinum to the right or whether there is poor aeration on the right. b Expiratory film shows there is now normal deflation on the left side whereas the right side remains inflated and the mediastinum is now more central. A peanut was found in the right main bronchus

Fig. 2.96 a,b. Foreign body. a A radiopaque foreign body. A drawing pin is seen in the left main bronchus. There is mild hyperinflation of the left lung. b Lateral projection confirms the location of the drawing pin in the left main bronchus

and is not recommended. There is a danger that during removal the foreign body may be inhaled.

2.4
Trauma

Only a small number of children with trauma have thoracic injury, but the injuries tend to be of a seri-ous nature. Severe thoracic trauma mostly results from motor vehicle accidents, either as an occupant or pedestrian. There is a high mortality in arterial injury (ROUSE et al. 1992). The extraskeletal thoracic injuries of child abuse, though rare, are the most severe, with a mortality of 50% (PECLET et al. 1990).

The routine trauma series in children includes a lateral cervical spine, a chest x-ray and an abdominal x-ray. The chest radiograph should be taken early, but only after life-threatening lesions such as tension pneumothorax and haemorrhage have been treated. Associated injuries to other parts of the body are

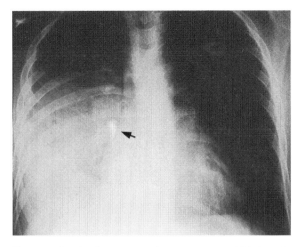

Fig. 2.98. Foreign body presenting as empyema. This is a 12-year-old boy who presented with a chest infection with no history of inhalation of foreign bodies. The radiopaque foreign body is seen in the region of the bronchus to the right lower lobe, probably at the bifurcation to the middle lobe. There is a pleural effusion with collapse/consolidation of the right middle and lower lobe. This is a delayed presentation of a foreign body with empyema

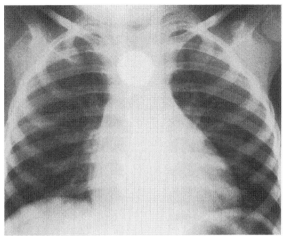

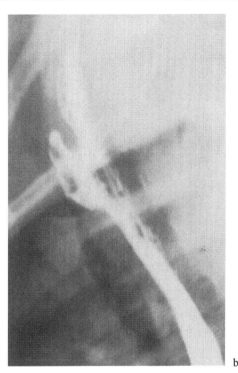

Fig. 2.99 a,b. Foreign body in the oesophagus. a A radiopaque coin is seen overlying the upper mediastinum. The coin would be too large to be in the trachea. No history of ingestion of foreign body was elicited. b Contrast study in the lateral projection shows that the penny has eroded the anterior portion of the oesophagus. It lies in the soft tissues, forming a mediastinal abscess, compressing the trachea and causing respiratory difficulty

common and can be assessed once the child is stable. In handling the child, especially if unconscious, it is important to be aware that there may be injury to the cervical spine, and if this has not been excluded a spinal collar should be applied in Casualty before the patient is x-rayed. Ideally, the trauma patient should be radiographed in the erect position as not only do erect radiographs show fluid levels or subphrenic gas, but the mediastinum can be better assessed. In the supine position there is apparent widening (Swischuk 1996), which may be misinterpreted as indicating aortic damage or other vascular injury, or oesophageal rupture, which is not always accompanied by an air leak. However, though ideal, erect radiographs are seldom achievable. Most films are supine and familiarity with these is essential. Decubitus views will help to resolve questions of free air but in practice most children with severe trauma undergo CT, and most problems are resolved this way.

Pulmonary contusion is most commonly found due to blunt trauma although the extent is underestimated on plain radiographs. CT is much more sensitive and should be done as soon as the patient is stable. Pulmonary contusion is usually due to a serious blunt chest trauma. The contusion itself is due to a leakage of blood into the interstitial spaces of the lung. As it occupies air space, it appears like consolidation and the blood plus increased secretions result in occlusion of the bronchi and atelectasis. Radiographically the contusions appear as patchy infiltrates or large areas of consolidation with atelectasis (Figs. 2.100, 2.101). If vessels are ruptured, pulmonary haematoma results in indistinct opacities on radiographs, often ovoid or rounded in nature. These may cavitate. Haematomata appear as initially indistinct opacities and then become more discrete over a few days before complete resolution. Lung

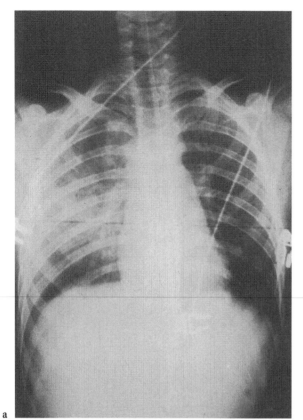

a

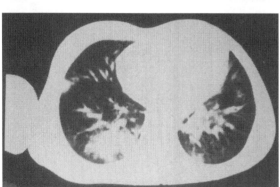

b

Fig. 2.100 a,b. Pulmonary contusion. a On the right side there is alveolar opacification due to fluid extending into the air spaces. b On multiple section the CT scan shows much more extensive involvement. In addition to the opacification posteriorly on the right side due to interstitial blood there is peribronchial blood behind the heart on the left side. There is also more peripheral focal opacification posteriorly on the left and laterally on the right

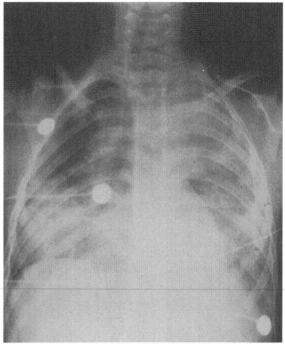

a

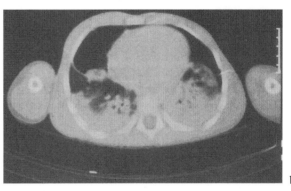

b

Fig. 2.101 a,b. Pulmonary contusion. a Extensive alveolar opacifications seen with an uneven distribution, generalised on the left side with loss of the left hemidiaphragm border and more focal medially on the right side in the right lower zone. The right heart border is lost due to adjacent fluid-filled lung. b CT scan shows that there is extensive collapse and fluid-filled lung seen posteriorly with air bronchograms

lacerations, in addition to atelectasis and consolidations due to bleeding, may also show interstitial air or a hydropneumothorax due to air leak. The patient may present with shortness of breath and pain, often with a cough and sometimes haemoptysis. The x-ray appearances of lung parenchyma injury, similar to pneumonias, lag behind the clinical condition and therefore one must be wary of using the radiograph as a direct indication of the patient's condition and prognosis.

2.4.1
Traumatic Lung Cysts

Traumatic lung cysts have a similar radiological appearance to pneumatocoeles and are often re-

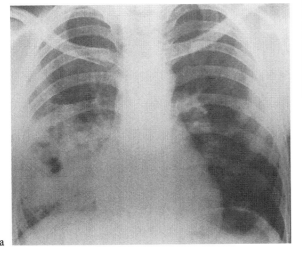

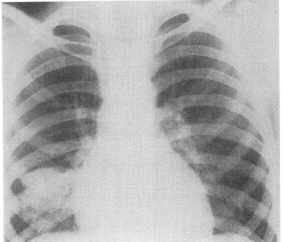

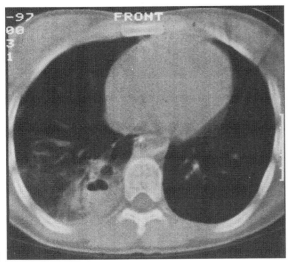

Fig. 2.102 a–c. An 11-year-old presenting with history of blunt trauma. a Pulmonary contusion with pneumatoceles and fluid levels. b Three weeks later the pneumatoceles and lung contusions have cleared, leaving a rounded haematoma. c CT scan (different patient) showing, in the right paravertebral region occupation of the alveolar air spaces by blood. Air bronchograms are seen laterally and pneumatocoeles more medially

ferred to as traumatic pneumatocoeles. They are usually due to blunt trauma without associated rib fracture. The aetiology is thought to be fracture of small bronchi due to sudden compression restricting the air outflow at the same time as compressing the lung. This causes distal lung tissue to burst in a balloon-like manner. They appear on a chest x-ray (Fig. 2.102) or CT within 1–3 days of injury as the pulmonary contusion or haematoma resolves and, like inflammatory pneumatocoeles, resolve spontaneously within 2–16 weeks (SHANJI et al. 1988). Rupture will cause a pneumothorax.

2.4.2
Rib Fractures

Rib fractures due to trauma, with the exception of non-accidental injury, are uncommon in children,

probably due to the flexible nature of ribs in children. Single rib fractures carry a low risk of serious injury. Multiple rib fractures carry a high mortality reflecting the seriousness of the injury and are often associated with head injury. Rib fractures in very young children are mostly associated with child abuse and are exceedingly rare in response to accidental trauma.

2.4.3
Tracheobronchial Injuries

Tracheobronchial injuries are rare and, if proximal, cause mediastinal and cervical emphysema. More distal damage is intrapleural and causes a pneumothorax. Patients with trauma who have hoarseness or stridor in addition to dyspnoea, cough and haemoptysis should be suspected of having tracheobronchial injury. These signs, with a pneumothorax or mediastinal subcutaneous emphysema, should alert one to the possibility of tracheobronchial injury and fibre-optic bronchoscopy should be carried out to assess the injuries.

2.4.4
Pneumothorax

Pneumothorax may be secondary to injury to the lung, airways or oesophagus, or be due to direct penetration of the chest; lack of response to drainage may indicate tracheal or bronchial tear. A pneumomediastinum may be associated with the pneumothorax or be an isolated finding. A pneumopericardium can cause cardiac tamponade.

A tension pneumothorax in addition to the hyperlucent hemithorax on the chest radiograph can produce dramatic shifts of the mediastinum. Lung contusion and haematoma may, however, prevent total collapse of the lung and it is possible to have a marked tension pneumothorax without the ipsilateral lung being totally collapsed. Mediastinal shift can impair venous return. Mediastinal compression caused by the shift secondary to pneumothorax can significantly decrease cardiac output, especially if accompanied by cardiac tamponade due to pericardial blood. Rapid treatment by insertion of a cannula or drain is needed. The radiograph differentiates a pneumothorax from a haemothorax and lung contusion, which may clinically mimic a tension pneumothorax (CHRISTOPHER et al. 1997). Pleural fluid, although uncommon, suggests a haemothorax and if large carries a high mortality.

A large opaque hemithorax is not always due to a haemothorax. Rupture of the hemidiaphragm can allow the liver to herniate into the chest, giving an opaque hemithorax appearance on the chest film (WIRBEL and MUTSCHLER 1997). Once suspected, it is imperative to perform a CT scan before placing a drainage tube. Ultrasound may give some help by showing fluid in the chest cavity, but CT is more sensitive.

2.4.5
Haemopericardium

Cardiac silhouette enlargement implies haemopericardium and impending cardiac tamponade. The heart shape becomes globular. Widening of the mediastinum may indicate haemorrhage secondary

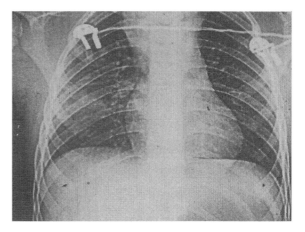

Fig. 2.103. Widening of the superior mediastinum which was shown to be due to a venous tear (superior vena cara) rather than aortic rupture

to aortic rupture or venous tears (Fig. 2.103). Aortic rupture in children is frequently rapidly fatal, so that in practice a widened mediastinum is more frequently due to venous than arterial tears. Mediastinal haematomas are usually accompanied by displacement of the trachea and oesophagus (often outlined by the nasogastric tube), depression of the main stem bronchus, presence of a left apical pleural fluid due to leakage of blood from the mediastinum (SWISCHUK 1996), obscuration of the aortic knuckle if left sided, and loss of the paraspinal shadow. A large associated haemothorax is often present. Fractures of the sternum and first ribs are associated injuries. These injuries are usually seen in motor vehicle accidents, often due to impact on the steering wheel, and therefore are rarely seen in children. The incidence increases with age as children become front seat passengers or drivers.

Fractures of the sternum due to severe direct trauma are best seen on the lateral projection and pre- and retrosternal soft tissue swelling is often seen due to oedema and haematoma. Fracture of the sternum is often associated with cardiac injury, and its silhouette should be carefully scrutinised. If there is any suspicion of vascular damage, a dynamic contrast-enhanced CT scan should be carried out, which will confirm or refute the presence of haematoma. Angiography is still the most sensitive method of confirmation of aortic damage if there is time to perform it and is indicated in delayed presentation when an abnormal mediastinal contour is detected. CT is the most sensitive method of assessing thoracic trauma, particularly pulmonary and pleural space damage. The irregular infiltrates, nodular or confluent, and homogeneous consolidations seen on the chest x-ray within hours of injury may be due to lung contusion, but CT reveals many of these to be due to lacerations surrounded by haemorrhage. Air fluid in cavities, paravertebral opacities, pneumothorax and associated bony injuries are more clearly defined on CT than on the chest film (WAGNER and AMIESON 1989).

2.4.6
Oesophageal Rupture

Except in cases of direct injury, oesophageal rupture is extremely rare; this is especially so in children, and so it can be easily missed. When rupture occurs it usually involves the lower third of the oesophagus and the contents enter the mediastinum, aided by the negative pressures of inspiration. Pneumomediastinum, pneumothorax and pleural effusions are radiographic signs and, especially if there is substernal pain extending into the neck or shoulders, these should raise the suspicion of oesophageal injury in the appropriate clinical setting. A water-soluble contrast swallow, if the patient's condition permits, will confirm the diagnosis. Most oesophageal ruptures in children are iatrogenic and caused during the passage of a nasogastric tube or occur as the result of impaction of a foreign body or during endoscopic removal.

2.4.7
Traumatic Diaphragmatic Rupture

Diaphragmatic rupture is rare in children but may be seen in association with other significant injuries, often thoracic aortic damage, resulting in death (ESTERA et al. 1979). In the massively traumatised patient the signs are often masked by other injuries. The diagnosis of diaphragmatic rupture is difficult both clinically and radiologically. Recognition is imperative as catastrophic complications due usually to rupture of trapped herniated bowel which becomes ischaemic or, more rarely, torsion of herniated liver, may occur at any time following diaphragmatic damage.

Diaphragmatic rupture is most frequently caused by compressive blunt trauma to the abdomen but is also described with penetrating trauma. The chest radiograph may show gas-filled loops of bowel in the chest cavity but often, due to accompanying haematoma, the hemithorax is largely opaque. Care-

ful scrutiny of the position of the nasogastric tube tip may show this to be above the diaphragm if there is stomach herniation. Left diaphragmatic hernias are more common due to the protective effect of the liver on the right side. Even if no bowel is seen above the diaphragm, an elevated or abnormal contour to the left hemidiaphragm, particularly when associated with basal opacities and pneumothorax, should raise the possibility of diaphragm rupture.

Computed tomography may show the rupture and air in the bowel loops above the diaphragm. It will also show associated organ damage, if present, and is the examination of choice. If CT is negative, equivocal or unavailable, water-soluble contrast studies, if the patient's condition permits, are extremely helpful and can show the herniated hollow viscus. The bowel enters and exits through a single site and the contriction at this site will appear as a loop of contrast-filled bowel with a tight constriction at the site. If the obstruction is complete, there will be a beak shape beneath the diaphragm due to complete constriction and obstruction of the viscus. If only the omentum herniates, then there is usually angulation and elevation of the affected bowel segment. In right diaphragmatic rupture where only the liver herniates, the plain radiograph may only show a soft tissue opacity with a complex upper border above the right hemidiaphragm. CT is important to identify fluid-filled loops of bowel and other herniated abdominal viscera. A contrast-filled and folded herniated stomach may appear as two semicircular loops of contrast separated by a band of soft tissue attenuation resembling a sandwich (CACERES et al. 1995). Gastric obstruction is rare. A herniated liver may be partially inverted with a suprahepatic position of the gallbladder. There is interruption of the diaphragm contour but this is not always seen (CATASCA and SIEGAL 1995). A high signal from omental fat may help in identifying a small hernia.

Upper and lower gastrointestinal series should be performed before discharge in all patients with serious body injury in whom diaphragmatic rupture has not already been excluded by previous studies (MANSOUR 1997). Ultrasound, although not giving the same detail as CT, can be valuable in the assessment as it can be performed quickly and portably in Casualty; however, it may not be possible to obtain a good view since access is often limited by dressings, pain etc. In addition to assessing fluid in the chest or pericardium, ultrasound can demonstrate integrity of diaphragm, although small defects may be missed.

Diaphragm rupture may appear acutely or be delayed, but usually it is seen within the first 2 weeks of injury. In children, motor vehicle accidents account for the majority of acquired diaphragmatic hernias. Delayed presentation after this may be due to obstruction or strangulation. Sudden breathlessness any time after initial injury should raise the possibility of diaphragm rupture. Plain radiographs show gas in the bowel above the diaphragm in a true hernia. Apparent elevation of the left hemidiaphragm due to gas-distended stomach or gas in loops of bowel is another sign. Less commonly, herniation can occur on the right. There is then elevation of the right hemidiaphragm with opaque liver and/or gas-filled loops of bowel in the right chest cavity.

Barium studies, CT and MRI can define the diaphragmatic defect and the herniated contents in the chest.

2.4.8
Imaging of Trauma

The chest radiograph in trauma patients is valuable but has diagnostic limitations and a number of intrathoracic injuries can be missed (SIVIT et al. 1989). The clinical significance of these missed injuries is variable; in particular small pneumothoraces may be overlooked and contusion underestimated. The initial radiograph should be assessed for any skeletal injury which may direct one to the underlying soft tissue damage. Rib fractures may be difficult to detect when fresh but a local subpleural haematoma is suggestive. They become more obvious when callus forms 6–10 days after the initial injury. Pulmonary contusions are seen as nodular or confluent consolidations that become denser and larger over 48 h and then slowly resolve, sometimes appearing as a transient mass. Pulmonary haematoma appears as an oval rounded mass, more discrete than contusions, and is slow to resolve (Fig. 2.102b), occasionally cavitating. Traumatic pneumatocoeles are usually of little clinical significance as they rarely rupture to produce a pneumothorax. Bronchial damage results in a pneumothorax or atelectasis which may be massive. Widening of the mediastinum and cardiovascular silhouette implies cardiovascular damage and must be excluded by CT, chest x-ray or angiography as appropriate. Pericardial rupture, although very rare, causes displacement of the heart to the left side.

Pneumomediastinum can occur in non-penetrating and penetrating injuries and is occasionally due to oesophageal rupture. Penetrating injuries in addition may result in air in the great vessels. The presence of foreign bodies, inhaled or in the soft tissues, should be sought in trauma situations. When the plain radiograph is inconclusive or when clinical signs suggest intrathoracic injury, CT should be performed with dynamic contrast enhancement. Ultrasound, although less sensitive than CT, is invaluable since it is portable and can show the contents of an opaque hemithorax. It is very important to differentiate between fluid and viscera, particularly if drainage is being contemplated. The late effects of pulmonary injury can be functionally assessed by VQ lung scintigraphy.

Transthoracic and transoesophageal echocardiography has a place in children's thoracic trauma. Echocardiography can detect pericardial effusion and cardiac damage, and even traumatic intrapericardial diaphragmatic hernia containing stomach has been diagnosed in the emergency department, though in the adult (COLLIVER et al. 1997). Myocardial damage can be assessed by radio-isotope studies. As with all trauma, CT is the mainstay of investigation.

2.5
Stridor

Stridor is a harsh, hissing or whistling sound produced by turbulence of air flow through a partial obstruction, creating vibrations of the surrounding tissues. The airways in young children are small with less structural support than those in adults. The mucosal lining is also very sensitive to insult and will rapidly swell. Hence a greater degree of narrowing occurs in children than in adults. If this narrowing impedes ventilation sufficiently, stridor will result. Masses or other lesions, be they intrinsic or extrinsic, will also have a more profound effect in children. Inspiratory stridor is generally a sign of supraglottic lesions, while expiratory stridor typically indicates an intrathoracic cause. This information should be included on the request form so that the radiologist can direct attention to the most appropriate region. Associated with stridor are variable findings of cough, dyspnoea, cyanosis and recurrent respiratory tract infections.

Radiological investigations (Table 2.8) should start with simple non-invasive studies, only increasing in complexity if a definitive diagnosis is not obtained (Fig. 2.104). Speed and minimal disturbance are of paramount importance as any child with stridor may be precipitated into respiratory arrest. High-kV AP and lateral views of the chest and neck will enhance the airway soft tissue anatomy and help

Table 2.8. Radiological investigation of stridor

Soft tissue, neck: (neck extended)	Lateral:	True lateral
		Inspiratory phase
		Screen if necessary
	AP:	High-kV technique – air column enhanced
Chest: (chin up)	AP:	Position of trachea
		Hyperinflation – local or generalised
		Mediastinal masses
	Lateral:	Compression of trachea, separation from oesophagus (F.B. calcifications etc.)
	Screening/tomography:	If necessary
Barium studies		Displacement
		Foreign bodies especially radiolucent
Tracheobronchography		Stenoses, tracheal size, tracheomalacia and congenital bronchial malformation
CT		Mediastinal masses
		Tracheal size
		Abnormal vessels
MRI		Particularly in differentiating normal from abnormal thymus
Ultrasound		Masses – neck and mediastinum – cystic vs solid and identification of normal thymus
Isotope		Ectopic thyroid etc.
Angiogram		Digital subtraction etc. for abnormal vessels

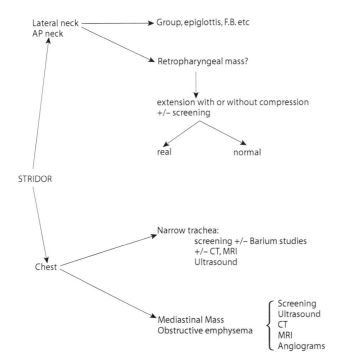

Fig. 2.104. Flow chart illustrating the diagnostic pathway for the investigation of stridor

localise the cause of the stridor, e.g. inflammatory oedema, foreign bodies or masses. It is important that the chest x-rays are exposed with the chin elevated. A chin overlying the lung apex will obscure AP views of the trachea. The trachea in children is floppy. Radiography exposed with the chin down may give a false impression of displacement by a mass. The Valsalva manoeuvre in a co-operative child will rarely demonstrate laryngocoeles. AP and lateral chest films demonstrate tracheal displacement, compression, masses or associated lung abnormalities. Tracheomalacia may be identified by fluoroscopy or bronchoscopy. Barium swallow can show displacements and compression due to masses. In carefully selected cases tracheobronchography with water-soluble iso-osmolar non-ionic contrast may be more appropriate than CT for showing tracheal size and focal stenoses. This should be combined with bronchoscopy.

Computed tomography can miss focal stenoses unless ultra-fast CT is used (BRODY et al. 1991). Spiral CT with reconstruction is better than single-slice CT but breath-holding in a child with stridor is difficult and in a young child impossible, so this technique is not ideal. CT with intravenous contrast enhancement will demonstrate extrinsic masses and abnormal vessels but not intrinsic tracheal pathology.

Magnetic resonance imaging can evaluate tracheal narrowing and the cause of extrinsic compression (HOFFMAN et al. 1991) and is of value in assessing mediastinal masses and distinguishing these from a normal large thymus. It is consequently to be preferred to CT. CT and MRI are unlikely to be indicated in an emergency setting other than to identify the cause of a mass seen on the plain radiograph. Ultrasound can identify causes of space-occupying lesions in the mediastinum and larynx but requires appropriate expertise (GAREL et al. 1991). The causes of stridor are numerous (Table 2.9) but the more common ones presenting as an emergency are acute inflammatory conditions, sometimes tracheomalacia, aspiration and foreign bodies.

2.5.1
Acute Epiglottitis

Acute epiglottitis is caused by *Haemophilus influenzae* type B, most commonly in children between 3 and 6 years old. In addition to expiratory stridor, dysphagia is present owing to the supraglottic oedema. Lateral radiographs of the neck may

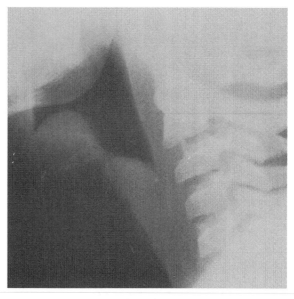

Fig. 2.105. Epiglottitis. The lateral projection shows marked thickening due to oedema and loss of the normal configuration of the epiglottis and the aryepiglottic fold

confirm the diagnosis but are not indicated in the management as complete obstruction of the epiglottis can be precipitated by handling of the neck of the child in an attempt to get the radiograph. Direct visualisation of the cherry red epiglottis by those with appropriate expertise and ability to perform intervention and tracheostomy is preferable if confirmation of the diagnosis is needed, but this is seldom indicated as the clinical features are typical. If, however, a lateral film has been taken for stridor, the epiglottis may be seen to be markedly thickened due to oedema, with the aryepiglottic fold extending to the subglottic space and hypopharyngeal overdistension (Fig. 2.105). In all cases of stridor in which radiography is performed, a lateral film of the airway is mandatory since the AP film may show only subglottic narrowing and be misinterpreted as showing croup rather than epiglottitis or other conditions which may enlarge the epiglottis, such as oedema, haemorrhage or cyst. In all these conditions the child with stridor may lose the normal cervical lordosis.

2.5.2
Croup

Croup has a variety of causes, the most common of which is acute laryngotracheobronchitis due to a virus, usually parainfluenza and less commonly respiratory syncitial virus. Recurrent croup is prob-

Table 2.9. Causes of stridor

Intrinsic	
Supraglottic:	
1. Congenital:	Cysts – aryepiglottic, dermoid
	Thyroglossal duct, lingual thyroid
	Flabby epiglottis
2. Inflammatory:	Epiglottitis – bacterial, viral or allergic
Glottic and subglottic:	
1. Congenital:	Haemangioma, paralysis of vocal cord
	Stenoses, laryngomalacia
	Laryngeal cyst, papilloma
2. Trauma:	Birth injury
	Post surgery or intubation
	Stenosis or granuloma
3. Inflammatory:	Viral croup
	Laryngitis
	Abscess
	Oedema (allergic)
4. Foreign body	
5. Metabolic:	Hypocalcaemia
6. Neoplastic:	Rhabdomyosarcoma etc.
7. Neurogenic	
8. Aspiration	
Trachea:	
1. Congenital:	Haemangioma or lymphangioma
	Tracheomalacia
	Cartilage ring abnormalities – segmental malacia.
	Stenoses – primary or associated with tracheo-oesophageal fistula (TOF)
2. Inflammatory:	Laryngotracheitis
3. Foreign bodies	
4. Neoplastic	
5. Post-operative:	Intubation, tracheostomy
	Following repair of tracheo-oesophageal fistula
Extrinsic	
1. Congenital:	Vascular compression
	Oesophageal atresia
	Tracheo-oesophageal fistula
	Ectopic thyroid
	Congenital goitre
	Duplication cyst (oesophageal)
	Cystic hygroma
2. Inflammatory:	Retropharyngeal (or retro-oesophageal) abscess
3. Foreign body:	Within oesophagus, primary or secondary to abscess formation
4. Tumours:	Mediastinal teratoma
	Lymphoma
	Thyroid, neuroblastoma
5. Post surgical	

ably due to atopy or bacterial tracheitis. It is a disease of infants and young children, occurring between 6 months and 3 years. It often develops or worsens in the evening and is often associated with a viral lower respiratory tract infection. Inspiratory and expiratory high-kV films will show the vocal cords indistinct and thickened. On the AP projection there is tapering of the trachea due to subglottic oedema and spasm; on the lateral view narrowing of the subglottic space is observed with marked over-distension of the hypopharynx in inspiration that is much greater than in epiglottitis (Fig. 2.106). The narrowing of the subglottic portion of the trachea due to collapse during inspiration is less prominent in expiration and may in fact disappear completely. The tapering caused by thickened vocal cords, however, will always remain and is best seen on the frontal projection. The child's head should be sup-

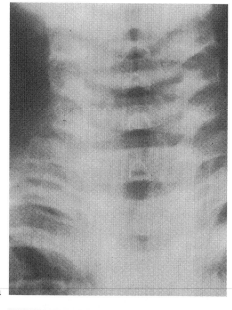

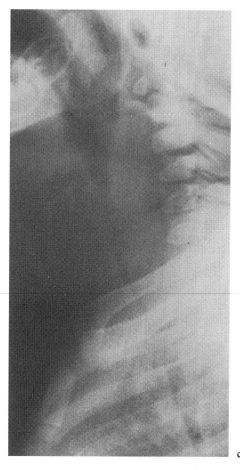

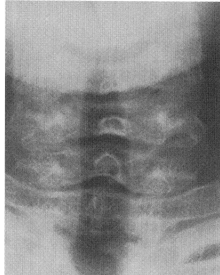

Fig. 2.106 a–c. Croup. **a** The frontal projection shows the typical tapering of the trachea. **b** Normal trachea for comparison. This shows the normal wide trachea with the prominent shoulder formed by the inferior aspect of the vocal cords. **c** Lateral projection shows narrowing in the subglottic space with gaseous distension of the hypopharynx

ported in extension as flexion may cause complete obstruction. More unusual features include a bacterial membrane in addition to irregular oedema, and occasionally a detached membrane that can look like a foreign body (STRIFE 1988).

2.5.3
Retropharyngeal Mass

Retropharyngeal abscess may be a complication of bacterial pharyngitis or be secondary to a penetrat-ing injury or foreign body. It appears as a swelling of the posterior pharyngeal wall. The neck is held in hyperextension. Occasionally, gas or an air-fluid level may be seen in the soft tissues. Haemorrhage into the soft tissues in children with a bleeding disorder or haemorrhage into a previous existing pathology such as cystic hygroma can present as an acute retropharyngeal mass or subglottic compression (Fig. 2.107), or stridor due to contralateral displacement of the trachea.

Inhaled foreign bodies may cause stridor directly by laryngeal oedema. A penetrating injury to the

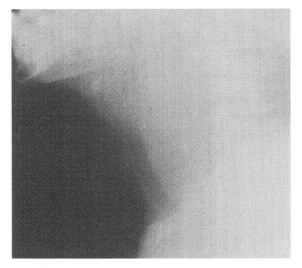

Fig. 2.107. Prevertebral mass. This prevertebral mass was caused by haemorrhage in a haemophiliac

retropharynx in children is typically due to an object such as a lollipop stick or pencil. Deliberately inflicted trauma in child abuse may be due to finger penetration and may present with a history of bleeding from the mouth or a mediastinal or retropharyngeal abscess.

2.5.4
Tracheomalacia

Tracheomalacia is due to a weakness of the tracheal wall cartilage. It may be (a) primary, (b) associated with tracheo-oesophageal fistula, (c) secondary to compression by masses, (d) secondary to cardiovascular anomalies with vascular rings, or (e) associated with congenital syndromes or systemic disease (BENJAMIN 1984). It is frequent in children with Down's syndrome, who often have a very stormy first 2 years of life with recurrent infections. Primary tracheomalacia may present in the premature child. Presentation to the Casualty Department is usually in the mature infant who presents with unexplained respiratory distress and stridor, often with a "barking" cough and occasionally apnoea. Bronchoscopy is required to confirm the diagnosis. Those less critically ill can be examined by inspiration/expiration films in AP and lateral projections and fluoroscopy (Fig. 2.108). These show marked narrowing in the AP diameter in expiration. Moderate narrowing of the trachea at the thoracic inlet is common in normal young children. In children in whom tracheomalacia is associated with cardiovascular anomalies, onset is

usually more gradual, but apnoeic episodes during feeding may cause acute presentation. This is particularly seen in innominate artery compression syndrome, which causes significant anterior tracheal indentation associated with collapse of the trachea, readily identified on fluoroscopy. A double aortic arch is the commonest associated vascular ring anomaly and, in addition to respiratory problems, may present with feeding problems. The chest radiograph shows the presence of a right aortic arch. Barium studies will show bilateral compression on the frontal projection and posterior indentation on the lateral projection. MRI will confirm the aberrant anatomy. Traecheomalacia is associated with tracheo-oesophageal fistula. In children with symptoms of tracheomalacia following anastomosis and repair of the fistula, contrast study of the oesophagus with a naso-oesophageal tube will show the tracheomalacia and the tracheal compression caused by proximal pouch dilatation.

2.5.5
Laryngomalacia

Laryngomalacia (congenital flaccid larynx) presents in the neonatal period with stridor, which diminishes with activity. It is usually assessed by laryngoscopy.

2.5.6
Other Causes

Tracheal cysts and granuloma following tracheostomy are unlikely to present acutely. If sudden stridor develops following tracheostomy it is more likely to be due to extrinsic pressure caused by haematoma or, if delayed, by false aneurysm formation (DRYDEN et al. 1993). Subglottic haemangioma has a pathognomonic appearance, with asymmetry of the subglottic walls being seen on AP views. It can also be demonstrated by ultrasound and is found in patients with cutaneous haemangiomas. Papillomas produce multiple soft tissue shadows encroaching on the lumen of the vestibular slit and may be seen in the rest of the upper airways. Laryngeal papillomatosis may be associated with oesophageal lesions which are demonstrated by barium studies. Stenoses, congenital or as a result of tracheostomy, rarely present acutely.

In the investigation of stridor, the plain radiograph will differentiate many conditions and familiarity with the normal appearances is important.

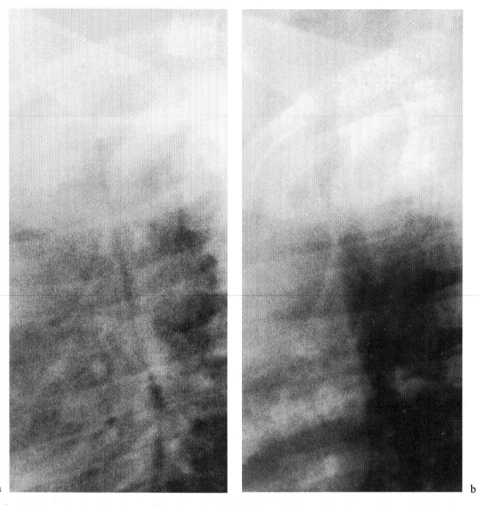

a   b

Fig. 2.108 a,b. Tracheomalacia. **a** Expiratory film shows marked collapse of the trachea. **b** In quiet respiration the trachea is of normal dimensions

Fluoroscopy, apart from identifying the cause of stridor, e.g. tracheomalacia, may show signs of partial obstruction to air flow with widening of the mediastinum in inspiration. The more invasive techniques will elucidate the causes in most patients, but should be used selectively following discussion between radiologist and physician.

References

Adams EJ, Ignotus PI (1993) Sonography of the thymus in healthy children, frequency of visualization, size and appearance. AJR 161(1):153–155

Altman AJ, Schwartz AD (1978) Malignant diseases of infancy, childhood and adolescence. Saunders, Philadelphia, pp 244–254

Anderson KD (1986) Congenital diaphragmatic hernia. In: Welch KJ et al. (eds) Paediatric surgery, 4th edn. Chicago Year Book, Chicago, p 589

Askin FB (1987) Congenital and developmental anomalies. In: Dehner LP (ed) Pediatric surgical pathology, 2nd edn. Williams and Wilkins, Baltimore, pp 247–256

Banagale RC, Watters RH (1983) Delayed right sided diaphragmatic hernia following group B-streptococcal infection: a discussion of its pathogenosis, with a review of the literature Hum Pathol 14:67–69

Barmios Fontoba JE, Gutierrez C, Lluna J, Vila JL, Poquet J, Ruiz-Company S (1997) Bronchial foreign body: should bronchoscopy be performed in all patients with a choking crisis? Paediatr Surg Int 12:(2–3) 118–120

Bees NR, Richards SW, Fearne C, Drake DP, Dicks-Mireaux C (1997) Neonatal thymic haemorrhage. Br J Radiol 70:210–212

Benjamin B (1984) Tracheomalacia in infants and children. Ann Otol Rhinol Laryngol 93:438–442

Bode V, Scheidt W (1988) Change in thymic size during and following cytotoxic therapy in young patients. Pediatr Radiol 18:20–23

Brody AS, Kuhn JP, Glen Seidel F, Brodsky LS (1991) Airway evaluation in children with use of ultrafast CT: Pitfalls and Recommendations. Radiology 178:181–184

Caceres J, Mata JM, Castaner E, Villanueva A (1995) CT recognition of traumatic herniation of the stomach: the "sandwich" sign. J Thorac Imaging 10(2):150–152

Carty H (1990) Ultrasound of the normal thymus in the infant. A simple method of resolving a clinical dilemma. Br J Radiol 63:737

Castriota-Scandberg A, Popolizio T, Sacco M, Coppi M, Scarle MG, Cammisa M (1995) Diagnosis of mycoplasma pneumonia in children: which is the role of the thoracic radiography? Radiol Med 89(6):782–786

Catasca JV, Siegal MJ (1995) Post traumatic diaphragmatic herniation. CT findings in two children. Paediatr Radiol 25(4):262–264

Christopher NC, Mellick LB, Gibbs Andrews H (1997) Pediatric trauma. Paediatrics 5(2):30–40

Cleveland RM, Weber B (1993) Retained fetal lung liquid in congenital lobar emphysema: a possible predicter of polyalveolar lobe. Paediatr Radiol 23(4):291–295

Cohen MD (1992) Imaging of children with cancer. Mosby, St Louis, pp 342–134

Colliver C, Oller DW, Rose G, Brewer D (1997) Traumatic intraperitoneal diaphragmatic hernia diagnosed by echocardiography. J Trauma 42(1):115–117

Condon VR (1990) The heart and great vessels. In: Silverman FN, Kuhn JP (eds) Essentials of Caffey's pediatric X-ray diagnosis. Chicago Year Book, Chicago, p 383

Davis CM (1996) Inhaled foreign bodies in children. An analysis of 40 dases. Arch Dis Child 41:402

Delport SD (1996) Aftermath of failed diagnosis of late-presenting congenital diaphragmatic hernias. South Afr J Surg 34(2):69–72; discussion 72–73

Dokler ML, Bradshaw J, Mollitt DL, Tepas JJ 3rd (1995) Selective management of pediatric oesophageal foreign bodies. Am Surg 61(2):132–134

Doull IJ, Connett GJ, Warner JO (1996) Bronchoscopic appearances of congenital lobar emphysema. Paediatr Pulmonol 21(3):195–197

Drug and Therapeutics Bulletin (1997) Intrapleural streptokinase for empyema. DT B 35:95–96

Dryden CM, Pinder M, Pace NA, Dougall JR (1993) Stridor after tracheostomy. Br J Intensive Care 55–56

Eggli KD, Newman B (1993) Nodules, masses and pseudomasses in the pediatric lung. Radiol Clin North Am 31(3):651–666

Estera AS, Platt MR, Mills LJ (1979) Traumatic injuries of the diaphragm. Chest 75:306–313

Felson B (1973) Chest. Roentgenology. Saunders, Philadelphia, pp 366–399

Fraser RG, Pare JAP, Pare PD, Fraser RS, Genereux GP (1990) Pulmonary hypertension and edema in diagnosis of diseases of the chest, 3rd edn, vol III, pp 1823–1968

Garel C, Hassan M, Legrand I, Elmaleh M, Narcy PH (1991) Laryngeal ultrasonography in infants and children: pathological findings. Pediatr Radiol 21:164–167

Gibson NA, Hollman AS, Paton JY (1993) Value of radiological follow up in childhood pneumonia. BMJ 307:1117

Gimeno Aranguez M, Colomar Palmer P, Gonzalez-Mediero I, Ollero Caprani JM (1996) The clinical and morphological aspects of lymphangioma: a review of 145 cases. Anal Esp Pediatr 45(1):25–28

Griscom NT, Wohl MEB, Kirkpatrick JA Jr (1978) Lower respiratory infections: how infants differ from adults. Radiol Clin North Am 16(3):367–387

Haller JA Jr, Golladay ES, Pickard LR, Tepas JJ 3rd, Shorter NA, Shermeta DW (1979) Surgical management of lung bud anomalies: lobar emphysema, bronchogenic cyst, cystic adenomatoid malformation and intralobar sequestration. Am Thoracic Surg 28:33–43

Haller JA, Tepas JJ 3rd, White JJ, Pickard LR, Robotham JL (1980) The natural history of bronchial atresia: Serial observations of a case from birth to operative correction. J Thorac Cardiovasc Surg 79:868–872

Hasselbatch H, Jeppensen DL, Evsboll AK, Lisse IM, Nielsen MB (1997) Sonographic measurement of thymic size in healthy neonates. Relation to clinical variables. Acta Radiol 38(1):95–98

Hoffman U, Hoffman D, Vogl T, Wilimzig C, Mantel K (1991) Magnetic resonance imaging as a new diagnostic criterium in paediatric airway obstruction. Prog Paediatr Surg 27:221–230

King RM, Telander RL, Smithson WA, Banks PM, Han HT (1982) Primary mediastinal tumours in children. J Paediar Surg 17:512–520

Lemonine G, Montupet P (1991) Mediastinal tumours in infancy and childhood. In: Fallis JC et al (eds) Pediatric thoracic surgery. Elsevier, New York, p 258

Leonidas JC (1998) The thymus: from past misconceptions to present recognition. Pediatr Radiol 28:275–282

Levitt RL, Husbond JE, Glazer HS (1984) CT of primary germ cell tumours of the mediastinum. AJR 142:73–78

Lo Kich JJ, Goodman R (1975) Superior vena cava syndrome. Clinical management. JAMA 231:58

Macpherson RI, Hill JG, Othersen HB, Tagge EP, Smith CD (1996) Esophageal foreign bodies in children: diagnosis, treatment and complications. AJR 166(4):919–924

Mansour KA (1997) Trauma to the diaphragm. Chest Surg Clin North Am 7(2):373–383

Merten DF (1992) Diagnostic imaging of mediastinal masses in children. AJR 158:825–832

Meza MP, Benson M, Slovis TL (1993) Imaging of mediastinal masses in children. Radiol Clin North Am 31(3):583–604

Mikhailova V (1996) Congenital lobar emphysema in childhood. Khirurgia 49(3):8–12

Mittleman RE (1984) Fatal choking in infants and children. Am J Forens Med Pathol 5:201

Morgan PW, Goodman LR (1991) Pulmonary oedema and adult respiratory distress syndrome. RCNA 29(5):943–963

Morton RJ, Phillips BM (1992) Accidents and emergencies in children. Oxford University Press, Oxford, pp 191–200

Newman B, Sang K (1988) Abnormal pulmonary aeration in infants and children. Radiol Clin North Am 26(2):323–339

Obaro RC (1996) Case report: true massive thymic hyperplasia. Radiology 51:62–64

Oermann CM, Moore RH (1996) Foolers: things that look like pneumonia in children (review). Semin Respir Infect 11(3):204–213

Oh KS, Dorst JP, White JJ, Haller JA, Johnson BA, Byrne WD (1976) The syndrome of bronchial atresia or stenosis with mucocele and focal hyperinflation of the lung. Johns Hopkins Med J 138:48–53

Oh KS, Newman B, Bender TM, Bowen A (1988) Radiological evaluation of the diaphragm. Radiol Clin North Am 26(2):355–364

Peclet MH, Newman KD, Eichelberger MR, Gotschall CS, Garcia VF, Bowman LM (1990) Thoracic trauma in children. An indicator of increased mortality. J Paediatr Surg 25:961

Pedroza Melendez A, Larenas-Linnemann D (1997) Thymus hyperplasia, differential diagnosis in wheezing infant. Allergol Immunopathol 25(2):59–62

Ravitch MM (1986) Mediastinal cysts and tumours. In: Welch KJ et al. (eds) Paediatric surgery, 4th edn. Chicago Year Book Medical, Chicago, pp 602–618

Reid L (1977) The lung: its growth and remodelling in health and disease. AJR 129:777–778

Reilly J, Thompson J, MacArthur C, et al. (1997) Pediatric aerodigestive foreign body injuries are complications related to timeliness of diagnosis. Laryngoscopy 107(1): 17–20

Ribet ME, Copin MC, Soots JG, Gosselin BH (1995) Bronchioloalveolar carcinoma and congenital cystic adenomatoid malformation. Anals Thorac Surg 60(4): 1126–1128

Rouse TM, Eichelberger MR (1992) Trends in paediatric trauma management. RCNA 72(6):1347–1364

Saoj R, Ramchandra C, S'Cruz AJ (1995) Subcutaneous emphysema: an unusual presentation of foreign body in the airway. J Paediatr Surg 30(6):860–862

Shanji FM, Sachs JH, Perkins DG (1988) Cystic disease of the lung. Surg Clin North Am 68:581–618

Siegel MJ, Glazer HS, St. Amour TE, Rosenthal DD (1989a) Lymphangiomas in children. MR imaging. Radiology 170:467

Siegel MJ, Glazer HS, Wiener JL, Molina PL (1989b) Normal and abnormal thymus in childhood. MR imaging. Radiology 172:367

Sivit CJ, Taylor GA, Eichelberger MR (1989) Chest injury in children with blunt abdominal trauma. Evaluation with CT. Radiology 171:815–818

St. Amour TE, Siegel MJ, Glazer HS, Nadel SN (1987) CT appearance of normal and abnormal thymus in childhood. Comput Assist Tomogr 11:645

Stocker JT (1988) Congenital and developmental disease. In: Dail DH, Hammar SP (eds) Pulmonary pathology. Springer, Berlin Heidelberg New York, pp 41–71

Stocker JT, Dehner LP (1988) Acquired neonatal and paediatric disease. In: Dail DH, Hammar SP (eds) Pulmonary pathology. Springer, Berlin Heidelberg New York, pp 73–127

Stocker JT, Madewell JE (1977) Congenital cystic adenomatoid malformation of the lung: Classification and morphologic spectrum. Hum Pathol 8:155

Stover B, Lanbenberger J, Hennig J, Niemeyer C, Ruckauer K, Brandis M (1995) Value of RARE-MRI sequences in the diagnosis of lymphangiomatosis in children. Magn Reson Imaging 13(3):481–488

Strife JL (1988) Upper airways and tracheal obstruction in infants and children. Radiol Clin North Am 26(2):309–322

Sty JR, Wells RG, Starshak RK, Gregg DC (1992) Diagnostic imaging of infants and children, vol III: the chest. Aspen, Gaithersburg Md., pp 105–231

Svedström E, Puhakka H, Kero P (1989) How accurate is chest radiography in the diagnosis of tracheobronchial foreign bodies in children. Paediatr Radiol 19:520–522

Swischuk LE (1996) Wide mediastinum after motor vehicle accident. Paediatr Emerg Care 12(5):382–384

Van Allen CM (1932) Obstructive pulmonary emphysema and collateral respiration. Surg Gynecol Obstet 55:303–307

Van Mossevelde PW, Svevrijnen R, Hitge-Boetes C, Monnens L (1993) Two children with stridor and a thymus in the posterior mediastinum. Tijilschr Kindergeneesk 61(3): 108–112

Van de Ven K, Vanclooster P, de Gheldere C, Meersman A, Verhelst F (1995) Strangulation: a late presentation of right-sided diaphragmatic rupture. Aeta Chir Belg 95(5): 226–228

Wagner RB, Jamieson PM (1989) Pulmonary contusion. Surg Clin North Am 69(1):31–40

Weissberg D, Schwartz I (1987) Foreign bodies in the tracheobronchial tree. Chest 91:730

Wirbel RJ, Mutschler WE (1997) Right sided diaphragmatic rupture with intrathoracic displacement of the entire right lobe of liver. Unfallchimig 100(3):249–252

3 Radiology of Paediatric Gastrointestinal Emergencies

D. Grier

CONTENTS

3.1 Introduction

This chapter is divided into three sections by age: neonatal abdominal problems, those of the infant and small child and those of older children. Each section will discuss the approach to imaging of common emergency presentations, with a short overview of the imaging of specific conditions.

Acute gastrointestinal emergencies are common throughout childhood, the differential diagnosis depending as much on the age of the child as on the clinical findings. In most instances acute gastrointestinal symptoms have their origin within the gastrointestinal tract, but a minority will be caused by disease elsewhere, e.g. lower lobe pneumonia or sickle crisis. Occasionally presentation with non-gastrointestinal symptoms may cause delay in diagnosis, e.g. lethargy and coma in intussusception.

When imaging children with acute presentations it is helpful to be aware of the the likely differential diagnosis so as to be able to optimise imaging investigations. Dialogue with the referring clinician is important so that imaging is performed in a safe and appropriate manner with the minimum of distress to the child and parents.

D. Grier, FRCR, Consultant Radiologist, Bristol Royal Hospital for Sick Children, St. Michael's Hill, Bristol, Avon, BS2 8BJ, UK

Children are more sensitive than adults to the deleterious effects of ionising radiation because of their longer life expectancy and because they are still developing. This should not detract from the use of ionising radiation, but means that sound principles (justification and optimisation) should apply. Ultrasound has become important in the acute paediatric abdomen: the smaller size of children compared with adults makes the examination more productive. There are several conditions peculiar to children where the radiologist has the opportunity to effect a cure.

Management of acutely unwell children begins with a competent clinical evaluation, which in many cases allows for subsequent management without the need for imaging. When there is genuine diagnostic confusion, imaging is invaluable in either narrowing the differential diagnosis or confirming a diagnosis. Its routine use to exclude conditions is generally unhelpful as "negative" radiology has distinct limitations and in the acute abdomen should never override clinical findings. However, there are certain instances where imaging can confidently exclude important conditions, e.g. intussusception and malrotation.

One of the major determinants of morbidity and mortality in children with gastrointestinal emergencies is diagnostic delay and it should be the role of imaging to direct management in an efficient manner.

3.2
Overview

3.2.1
Imaging Modalities

Imaging acute gastrointestinal disorders in children involves the judicious use of plain films, ultrasound and fluoroscopy. The vast majority of problems can be solved using these techniques, with computed tomography and nuclear medicine being useful in certain well-defined circumstances such as in blunt abdominal trauma and gastrointestinal bleeding respectively.

3.2.1.1
Plain Radiography

Abdominal radiography is frequently performed in children with acute gastrointestinal symptoms, though up to half such examinations may be unhelpful and limiting radiography to patients with specific "high-yield" clinical findings may result in considerable savings with no important diagnostic loss (ROTHROCK et al. 1992). Such indications include previous abdominal surgery, suspected foreign body ingestion, abdominal distension, peritoneal signs and abnormal bowel sounds. It is important to consider the potential clinical impact of radiographs before they are obtained. Even in the presence of major abdominal disease, films are often normal or show only non-specific abnormalities and their routine use in many acute abdominal conditions is questionable, especially where more accurate diagnostic tests are available, such as ultrasound.

In most situations supine radiographs provide all of the important information, readily showing bowel gas distribution, patterns of dilatation, calcification and pneumatosis and they are of greater quality than erect or decubitus films. Air-fluid levels will not be visible on supine films but their demonstration adds little to the clinical management of most children except in the early neonatal period. The lung bases as well as the inguinal area should be included so as not to overlook important extra-abdominal findings.

The detection of free intraperitoneal gas is an important indication for horizontal beam films, with the erect chest radiograph being the most sensitive. However, in very ill children a lateral decubitus (right side up) or a "shoot through" lateral radiograph are useful alternatives. Sensitivity is increased by positioning the patient 10 min prior to exposure to allow time for gas movement to take place.

3.2.1.2
Ultrasound

Ultrasound is increasingly useful in the evaluation of children with acute abdominal disorders (HAYDEN 1996). Its advantages are portability, speed and lack of ionising radiation, making it ideal for use in sick children (BARR 1994). In experienced hands it permits a comprehensive examination of the abdomen with high accuracy in the diagnosis of intussusception, hypertrophic pyloric stenosis and appendicitis and it should be the first imaging modality when any of these conditions is suspected. Bowel ultrasound using a linear array transducer of 5–10 MHz is able to detect and localise bowel involvement in a variety of inflammatory and infective conditions. The rest of the abdomen should be imaged with a curvilinear or sector probe of between 3.5 and 7.5 MHz, depending on the size of the child. The whole abdomen should always be examined as remote complications, e.g. abscess, may be detected or an alternate explanation for symptoms discovered.

3.2.1.3
Contrast Examinations

Contrast studies of the gastrointestinal tract are required for the evaluation of many acute gastrointestinal conditions. They are best performed by those used to examining children, adopting a tailored approach so that the clinical question is answered with minimal discomfort and exposure to ionising radiation. A variety of contrast agents is available, including barium, air and water-soluble contrast media, with the choice depending on the clinical circumstances.

3.2.1.4
Computed Tomography

Computed tomography is valuable in blunt abdominal trauma in children and in the evaluation of complex intra-abdominal sepsis, though it involves a large dose of ionising radiation, the administration of intravenous iodinated contrast medium and frequently sedation or anaesthesia.

3.2.1.5
Magnetic Resonance Imaging

Magnetic resonance imaging, whilst invaluable in paediatric imaging, has at present no role to play in acute gastrointestinal conditions. This is partly because of the difficulty in scanning young and sick children who may require sedation or anaesthesia and its lack of availability, but also because most problems can be solved rapidly without it.

3.2.1.6
Nuclear Medicine

Pertechnetate scanning for the detection of Meckel's diverticula is probably the most common abdominal nuclear medicine examination performed in children (O'HARA 1996). Labelled red cell scanning and sulphur colloid scans are helpful in the localisation

and detection of obscure gastrointestinal bleeding (ROBINSON 1993).

3.2.1.7
Interventional Techniques

Arteriography to localise and embolize a source of gastrointestinal bleeding and percutaneous drainage of intra-abdominal fluid collections may be required but a description of these procedures is beyond the scope of this chapter.

3.2.2
Presentations of Gastrointestinal Emergencies in Children

Common presenting symptoms of children with acute gastrointestinal emergencies are listed in Table 3.1. Abdominal pain has many possible causes, many of which arise outside of the gastrointestinal tract. Non-organic pain needs also to be considered so that inappropriate investigations and treatment are not unnecessarily instituted. Clinical expression and localisation of pain are difficult in the younger child, adding to diagnostic difficulty.

The pattern of pain may be helpful, as in acute appendicitis, but it is often non-specific. Visceral pain tends to be midline and poorly localised, whilst peritoneal pain is better localised causing guarding, rigidity and rebound tenderness. Lateralised rather than central pain is a significant feature which should lead to imaging to exclude organic causes, particularly renal. Referred pain is common and may be misleading, with diaphragmatic irritation causing shoulder tip pain and lower lobe pneumonia causing abdominal pain.

Vomiting is ubiquitous in childhood and whilst a feature of obstruction and gastroenteritis, may also be caused by severe pain, urinary tract and other infections, metabolic and toxic conditions

Table 3.1. Common gastrointestinal symptoms in childhood

Pain
Vomiting
Diarrhoea
Distension
Mass
Jaundice
Bleeding
Failure to pass meconium
Constipation

and fever. Central nervous system disorders (e.g. hydrocephalus, tumours, abdominal "migraine" and Reye's syndrome) may present with vomiting as the major symptom, diverting attention from the underlying cause (JOHNS 1995). Bilious vomiting in children must always be taken seriously and at any age should suggest the possibility of malrotation and volvulus. Failure to pass meconium within the first 24–48 h of life is abnormal; it may be due to bowel obstruction and requires radiographic evaluation. In older children "constipation", a clinical diagnosis, is a significant problem and may cause severe abdominal pain. However, severe constipation may be painless and care should always be taken to consider other causes before ascribing abdominal pain to constipation.

Abdominal distension may be due to bowel dilatation because of obstruction, gastroenteritis, paralytic ileus due to sepsis or drugs, severe ascites or pneumoperitoneum. Abdominal masses in children do not usually present acutely unless complicated by haemorrhage, infection or torsion of a vascular pedicle, e.g. ovarian cyst. Renal enlargement, usually hydronephrosis or pyonephrosis, is the commonest "mass" at all ages, though duplication cysts, mesenteric cysts and choledochal cysts may also present as a mass. Ultrasound is the most useful initial imaging modality, establishing the site of origin of the mass and frequently allowing a specific diagnosis to be made. Plain radiography is less helpful and rarely specific, though the presence of calcification may narrow a differential diagnosis.

Jaundice in neonates, especially preterm babies, is usually physiological, being due to immaturity of liver enzymes, and in most cases responds to conservative medical management. Non-gastrointestinal causes of jaundice (sepsis, hypothyroidism) are more common than intrinsic abnormalities of the biliary tract. Jaundice with pale acholic stools in the first 2 months of life should always be investigated to exclude biliary atresia. Sonography of the liver and biliary tract is the most useful initial imaging investigation, providing a rational base for further management.

Gastrointestinal bleeding is often dramatic but rarely life threatening in children and usually ceases spontaneously, though an exception is bleeding from oesophageal varices. Haematemesis and melaena suggest a source proximal to the ligament of Treitz, whereas bright red rectal bleeding signifies more distal pathology. Bleeding from a Meckel's diverticulum is often between these two extremes with dark blood and clots, often sufficient to lower the

Table 3.2. Causes of vomiting in the neonatal period

Malrotation and volvulus
Gastro-oesophageal reflux
Sepsis
Gastroenteritis
Neonatal obstruction
Hiatus hernia

haemoglobin acutely. The differential diagnosis ranges from benign and common (anal fissure, polyps) to life-threatening conditions such as necrotising enterocolitis, intussusception and small bowel volvulus.

3.2.3
Management of Children in the Radiology Department

Imaging must be relevant and designed to answer specific questions and so initiate a change in management. Children and their parents should be approached and dealt with calmly and sympathetically and procedures explained to them when possible. It is important that staff are familiar and comfortable when working with sick children, as lack of confidence is easily transmitted to children. Parents should accompany their children whenever possible and a quiet and warm environment permits greatest cooperation and relaxation, particularly in young infants and neonates, who may rapidly lose body heat. Sufficient immobilisation must be provided for young children so that repeat films are kept to a minimum.

The presence of the requesting clinician during complex examinations is helpful and makes for efficient communication of findings, as well as ensuring that the clinical question has been addressed before the child leaves the department.

3.3
The Neonate

Vomiting is common in the neonatal period (Table 3.2) and is most often due to gastro-oesophageal reflux related to immaturity of the lower oesophageal sphincter. Its significance and the need for radiological investigation have to be considered in the clinical context. Bilious emesis is an important finding and must always be taken seriously: the possibility of malrotation and volvulus necessitates a contrast

Table 3.3. Causes of abdominal distension and obstruction in the neonate

Intestinal atresia/stenosis/web
Hirschsprung's disease
Meconium ileus
Immature left colon
Anorectal anomalies
Incarcerated inguinal hernia
Intussusception
Duplication cyst
Malrotation and volvulus
Ascites
Pneumoperitoneum
Sepsis
Drugs
Metabolic disturbance
Necrotising enterocolitis

Table 3.4. Causes of jaundice in the neonate

Neonatal hepatitis
Physiological
Biliary atresia
Choledochal cyst
Bile plug
Bile duct perforation
Hypothyroidism
Sepsis

Table 3.5. Causes of gastrointestinal bleeding in the neonate

Swallowed maternal blood
Necrotising enterocolitis
Malrotation and volvulus
Oesophagitis
Milk allergy
Peptic ulceration
Hirschsprung's disease (enterocolitis)

Table 3.6. Causes of an abdominal mass in the neonate

Choledochal cyst
Liver cysts
Duplication cyst
Mesenteric cyst/lymphangioma
Teratoma
Haemangioendothelioma (liver)
Meconium pseudocyst
Genitourinary causes
    Renal (hydronephrosis, cystic disease, mesoblastic
      nephroma)
    Adrenal (haemorrhage, neuroblastoma)
    Ovarian cyst

study of the upper gastrointestinal tract if no other cause is evident. Most term infants will pass meconium in the first 24 h of life and 99% do so by 48 h, with failure to do so leading to progressive abdominal distension which may be due to obstruction or atresia. Other causes of distension include pneumoperitoneum, ascites, masses, paralytic ileus (sepsis, drugs, postoperative) and necrotising enterocolitis (Table 3.3).

Choking with feeds, often with cyanosis and respiratory distress, must always be investigated urgently. When this is due to unrecognised oesophageal atresia the baby will also be mucousy and drooly at the mouth due to inability to swallow secretions. Similar respiratory symptoms and choking may also be caused by a diaphragmatic hernia, aspiration secondary to gastro-oesophageal reflux, distal obstruction, "H"-type tracheo-oesophageal fistula, laryngeal cleft, vascular rings or pharyngeal incoordination.

Jaundice in the neonatal period (Table 3.4) is usually physiological and responds to medical therapy. When there is conjugated or worsening hyperbilirubinaemia or when a mass is palpable, ultrasound is helpful. Bleeding is uncommon but may be due to a variety of conditions (Table 3.5).

Trauma is uncommon in the neonatal period, but when encountered, non-accidental injury should be considered. Birth trauma may cause rupture of the liver or spleen and iatrogenic trauma may arise from the passage of nasogastric tubes.

Abdominal masses are rare (Table 3.6), are often detected prenatally and are best evaluated by ultrasound, which will determine the site of origin and nature in the majority of cases.

3.3.1
Abdominal Radiographs

Abdominal radiographs are important in the evaluation of many neonatal gastrointestinal problems. Supine films (Fig. 3.1) will demonstrate bowel distribution and calibre, pneumatosis, calcification and a moderate pneumoperitoneum. Horizontal beam films are valuable for the detection of small amounts of free gas and in differentiating gas admixed with intraluminal contents from pneumatosis. They will also display air-fluid levels, which may help to differentiate various causes of neonatal bowel obstruction (CARTY and BRERETON 1983). A chest radiograph is essential if there is suspicion of oesophageal atresia, with separate chest and abdominal radiographs being preferable to one inclusive film ("babygram"), as exposure and collimation can be optimised for each.

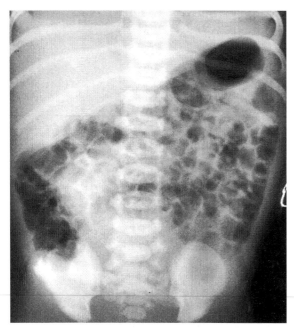

Table 3.7. Signs of free intraperitoneal gas on supine abdominal radiographs

Upper abdominal lucency
Visible falciform ligament
Gas in subhepatic and subphrenic spaces
Central abdominal lucency (football sign)
Visualisation of both sides of the bowel wall (Rigler's sign)
Visible umbilical arteries (lateral umbilical ligaments)
Scrotal gas
"Triangles" of gas between loops of bowel

Table 3.8. Causes of free intraperitoneal gas in neonates

Perforated viscus
   Spontaneous
   Obstruction/volvulus
   Necrotising enterocolitis
Laparotomy
Ventilation (air leak)
Pneumatosis

Fig. 3.1. Normal neonatal abdomen. Gas is present within stomach and multiple loops of bowel. Differentiation of small from large bowel is not possible, as the haustral pattern of the latter has not yet developed. No rectal gas is visible, either because it has not yet reached this level or because the rectum is dependent and fluid filled

Gas enters the stomach and proximal small bowel soon after delivery, is present in distal ileum 5–11 h later (CARTY and BRERETON 1983) and reaches the rectum by 24 h. Obstruction may be overlooked if sufficient time has not elapsed for gas to pass distally. Nasogastric suction may confound appearances by decompressing bowel and rectal gas may be introduced by a thermometer or gloved finger so its presence does not exclude obstruction.

A prominent but normal loop of bowel is sometimes present in the lower right abdomen with an inverted "U" appearance, caused by gas in a redundant sigmoid loop (JOHNSON and ROBINSON 1984). A similar finding may be present in the left upper quadrant due to air trapping at the splenic flexure: prone or decubitus films will clarify findings in difficult cases.

Signs of a pneumoperitoneum (Fig. 3.2) on supine films may be subtle (Table 3.7) and in difficult cases a horizontal beam film is necessary. A right side up (left lateral) decubitus film is preferable though a lateral "shoot through" may be the only option in an unstable neonate who cannot be moved. Causes of a pneumoperitoneum are given in Table 3.8.

When bowel obstruction is a consideration, the number and distribution of dilated loops may indicate its approximate level. However, colon and small bowel may be indistinguishable in the early neonatal period as they are of similar calibre and as the colon lacks haustral markings, is more centrally located than in older children and contains no solid faecal residue. When the small bowel is dilated, its calibre may equal or exceed that of the colon.

Air-fluid levels are common on horizontal beam radiographs when there is bowel dilatation from any cause, though they are often sparse or absent in meconium ileus and meconium plug syndrome.

Multifocal peritoneal calcification is characteristic of meconium peritonitis (Fig. 3.3) and may be located on bowel serosa or in any of the potential peritoneal spaces. It may extend into the scrotum. Intraluminal calcification may accompany high anorectal anomalies where there is a fistula to the urinary tract and is also a feature of multiple gastrointestinal atresias. Other causes of calcification are listed in Table 3.9.

A mass may displace adjacent loops of bowel, though radiographic findings are often non-specific and ultrasound is more useful. Calcification within the mass is suggestive of a meconium pseudocyst, though duplication cysts, teratoma and neuroblastoma may also calcify.

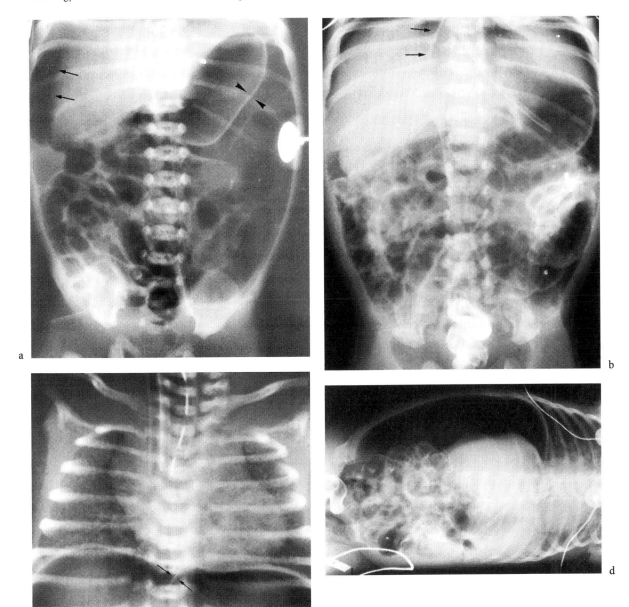

Fig. 3.2 a–d. Pneumoperitoneum. **a** Supine abdominal radiograph demonstrating an abnormal lucency in the upper abdomen with gas outlining the right lobe of the liver (*arrows*); gas also outlines both sides of the wall of the stomach and bowel loops – Rigler's sign (*arrowheads*). An umbilical arterial catheter is present. **b** Supine radiograph showing free gas outlining the stomach and loops of bowel. The falciform ligament (*ar-* *rows*) is visible in the upper abdomen. **c** Chest radiograph showing large sub-diaphragmatic collections of free air in this ventilated neonate, who also has oesophageal atresia. The falciform ligament (*arrows*) is just visible. **d** Left lateral decubitus radiograph showing a large pneumoperitoneum with wide separation of the right lobe of the liver and the lateral abdominal wall

If anorectal atresia is suspected it is usual to delay abdominal radiography for up to 24 h to allow time for gas to define the level of obstruction. When evaluating neonatal films it should be remembered that multiple anomalies may coexist (CARTY and BRERETON 1983).

3.3.2
Contrast Gastrointestinal Studies

Contrast gastrointestinal studies are best performed in a specialist paediatric centre, with close liaison between clinician and radiologist allowing the ex-

Table 3.9. Causes of intra-abdominal calcification in the neonatal period

Meconium peritonitis
Meconium pseudocyst
Intraluminal calcification
    High anorectal anomalies
    Multiple gastrointestinal atresias
Adrenal haemorrhage
Duplication cyst
Tumours
    Neuroblastoma
    Teratoma

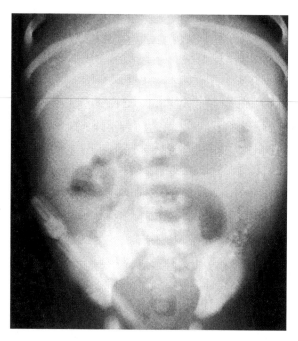

Fig. 3.3. Meconium peritonitis. Plain radiograph showing multifocal calcification throughout the abdomen, and mild gaseous distension of several loops of bowel centrally

amination to be tailored to the clinical problem. Staff who are used to managing small, often sick and fragile neonates, attention to warmth, radiation protection, fluid balance and the ability to be able to deal rapidly with the underlying condition or with any complications of the procedure (e.g. perforation) are important considerations.

A choice of contrast media is available, including barium, low-osmolar non-ionic and conventional ionic contrast media. Barium is cheap and safe, allowing good bowel opacification and for most studies should be diluted to 50% with water. It is relatively non-toxic if aspirated into the lungs but has been reported to cause peritoneal and mediastinal granuloma if perforation occurs. For this reason a low-osmolar non-ionic contrast medium with an iodine concentration of 180–200 mg /ml is preferred if perforation is possible; being near isotonic, this will not cause significant fluid or electrolyte disturbance. Similarly, if a contrast examination of defunctioned bowel distal to a stoma is performed, low-osmolar water-soluble contrast medium should be used as there is a risk of unevacuated barium consolidating into a particularly hard and tenacious "bariumoma" which may cause problems at later surgical procedures. Conventional ionic water-soluble contrast media (e.g. Gastrografin) should only be used in neonates with caution when their therapeutic effect is required, as they are variably hypertonic and may deplete the circulating volume, leading to circulatory collapse. When used, intravenous fluid replacement will need to be increased and carefully monitored.

3.3.3
Imaging Strategies

Many conditions in this age cause bowel obstruction and from a radiological viewpoint may be divided into "high" lesions affecting the oesophagus, stomach, duodenum or proximal small bowel, and "low" lesions involving the distal small bowel, colon and anus. The former usually require no further imaging beyond plain radiographs whilst the latter need a contrast enema to determine the level and nature of obstruction.

High obstructions usually present in the early neonatal period and may be diagnosed by plain radiography alone without recourse to contrast studies. Inability to pass a nasogastric tube suggests oesophageal atresia and a frontal chest radiograph should be obtained with the tube inserted gently as far as possible. Coiling of the tube and failure to advance it past the level of T3/4 confirms the presence of atresia (Fig. 3.4). A retrosternal lucency is often visible due to the distended upper oesophageal pouch. A fistula from the trachea to the distal oesophagus is usually present (85%), allowing air to pass distally, causing mild distension of the stomach and small bowel.

If a tube can be passed into the stomach a supine abdominal radiograph is obtained and the level of any obstruction inferred from the bowel gas pattern. A "single bubble" indicates gastric outlet obstruction (Fig. 3.5), a "double bubble" duodenal obstruction (Fig. 3.6) and a "triple bubble" proximal jejunal obstruction (Fig. 3.7), always assuming that sufficient time has elapsed for gas to have reached the level of obstruction. If the findings are equivocal, a further

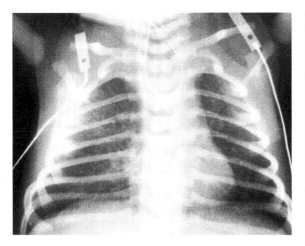

Fig. 3.4. Oesophageal atresia. Chest radiograph with Repoygle tube coiled in the proximal oesophageal pouch

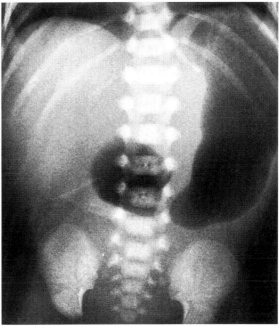

Fig. 3.6. Duodenal atresia. Plain supine radiograph shows gaseous distension of the stomach and duodenal cap ("double bubble"). There is no distal bowel gas

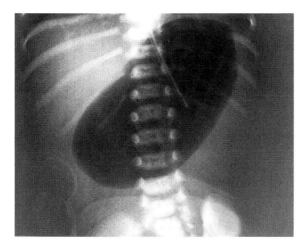

Fig. 3.5. Pyloric atresia. Supine radiograph after injection of 20 ml of air through the oesophageal tube shows a distended stomach with no distal gas

Table 3.10. Causes of low obstruction in a neonate

Meconium ileus
Meconium plug syndrome
Meconium peritonitis
Ileal, colonic and rectal atresia/stenosis
Hirschsprung's disease
Immature left colon
Malrotation and volvulus
Duplication cyst
Omphalomesenteric remnants
Inguinal hernia
Internal hernia/mesenteric defect
Necrotising enterocolitis
Sepsis
Drugs
Paralytic ileus

radiograph should be taken after injecting 10–20 ml of air through the tube. Complete obstruction is present when dilated proximal bowel is present with no distal gas. A horizontal beam film will show air-fluid levels according to the number of dilated bowel loops but the diagnosis of obstruction is usually clinically obvious and the supine film sufficiently diagnostic so they are not routinely obtained. Incomplete obstruction is suggested by variably dilated proximal bowel with gas in normal-calibre distal bowel and requires further imaging to identify its cause as this pattern is common in malrotation and volvulus, when to delay surgery could be fatal.

In this circumstance dilute barium (50% w/v) or a low-osmolar non-ionic water-soluble contrast medium should be injected under fluoroscopic guidance into the stomach through a nasogastric tube and films obtained to show the position of the duodeno-jejunal junction. Once the examination is diagnostic, residual contrast medium should be removed from the stomach if there is a nasogastric tube in position to reduce the risk of aspiration. Delayed images may be required if obstruction is more distal.

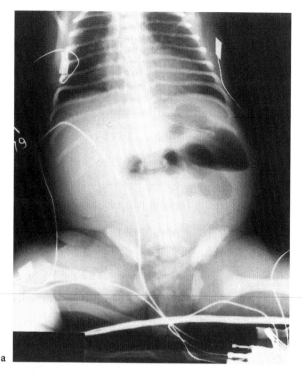

a

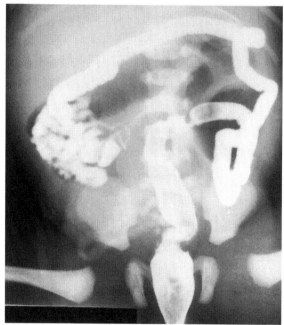

b

Fig. 3.7 a–b. Jejunal atresia. **a** Erect radiograph shows several dilated bowel loops in the upper abdomen, containing air-fluid levels, and no distal gas (high obstruction). **b** A contrast enema shows a small unused colon with reflux into collapsed distal ileum. Note the disparity in size between colon and dilated proximal bowel

Multiple dilated bowel loops on a supine film indicates low obstruction, which has a large number of mechanical and functional causes (Table 3.10). An ileus caused by sepsis should always be considered as this is the commonest cause of a negative laparotomy in this age group (Fig. 3.8) (CARTY and BRERETON 1983). Anorectal anomalies, distal ileal atresias, Hirschsprung's disease and meconium ileus are common causes of low obstruction whereas colonic atresia and immature left colon are rare. At all levels stenoses are less frequent than atresias.

An attempt may be made to differentiate "functional" obstruction due to Hirschsprung's disease, meconium ileus and meconium plug syndrome from atresias on plain films (HUSSAIN et al. 1991) though radiographic findings are not specific and overlap. Prominent colonic distension with conspicuous air-fluid levels and less marked dilatation of small bowel is often present in Hirschprung's disease, whereas bowel loops of varying calibre and a paucity of air-fluid levels are characteristic of meconium ileus and immature left colon (meconium plug syndrome). Atresias have more uniform bowel dilatation and multiple air-fluid levels, often with focal bulbous distension of the loop proximal to the atresia.

A contrast enema is required to determine the nature of low obstruction. A soft catheter should be passed into the rectum and contrast injected gently and slowly by syringe. Although gravity infusion is in principle a safer way of delivering contrast medium, the poor compliance of the neonatal colon (particularly in meconium ileus) makes this method impractical. The examination should be started with gentle injection, the catheter lying low in the colon and unrestrained. If the child repeatedly evacuates contrast, then firm taping of the buttocks, further insertion of the catheter and ultimately balloon inflation may be necessary to instil adequate contrast and make a diagnosis. Dilute barium is an excellent contrast medium, though in sick neonates and in those in whom perforation is possible a low-osmolar non-ionic contrast medium is preferred. If the appearances of meconium ileus or immature left colon are demonstrated, a therapeutic enema with Gastrografin can be performed with appropriate precautions.

Ultrasound of the neonatal abdomen may be helpful, particularly if radiographs show a gasless appearance (Table 3.11). Dilated fluid filled bowel, pneumatosis or free fluid may be identified. Occasionally a specific diagnosis can be made, e.g. the fluid-filled double bubble in duodenal atresia or dilated colon in colonic atresia. A gasless abdomen is

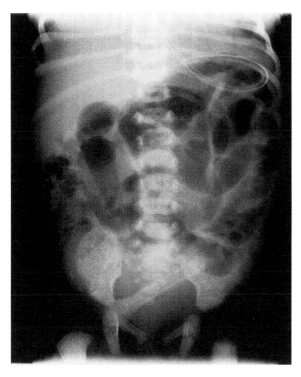

Fig. 3.8. Sepsis. Supine radiograph showing multiple dilated gas-filled loops of bowel simulating a low obstruction pattern in this neonate with meningitis

Table 3.11. Causes of gasless abdomen in neonates

Normal (soon after delivery)
Oesophageal atresia (no fistula)
Sedation
Asphyxia
Malrotation and volvulus
Severe vomiting
Closed loop obstruction
Nasogastric decompression
Ascites

Table 3.12. Frequency of different types of oesophageal atresia/tracheo-oesophageal fistula

OA with fistula to distal oesophagus	85%
OA – no fistula	10%
'H'-type tracheo-oesophageal fistula	5%
OA – proximal fistula	<1%
OA – proximal and distal fistula	<1%

OA, Oesophageal atresia.

3.3.4
Oesophageal Atresia and Tracheo-oesophageal Fistula

Oesophageal atresia and tracheo-oesophageal fistula occur in 1:3000–5000 live births and should be suspected in a newborn with drooling of saliva, cyanosis and choking with feeds (MCALISTER and KRONEMER 1996). They should always be suspected if there is a history of polyhydramnios, and are usually diagnosed in the first day of life.

Chest radiographs may show mildly hyperinflated lungs, with peribronchial and segmental opacities due to aspiration. The diagnosis is confirmed by obstruction to the passage of a nasogastric tube in the proximal oesophagus (Fig. 3.4). A tube of at least 8 F should be used as smaller tubes may occasionally coil in the proximal oesophagus in the absence of obstruction. A lateral film may show compression and anterior displacement of the trachea by the dilated pouch. There is usually a fistula (85%) from the trachea to the distal oesophagus (Table 3.12), allowing air to enter the stomach; the stomach is therefore often mildly distended, though gas is absent if there is no fistula or if it is obstructed (GOH et al. 1991). Passage of a tube into the stomach in the setting of a neonate thought to have oesophageal atresia suggests an "H"-type fistula or laryngeal cleft and warrants further investigation.

An "H"-type tracheo-oesophageal fistula is difficult to diagnose clinically. Chest radiographs show mild pulmonary hyperinflation with increased interstitial markings or right upper lobe atelectasis as a result of aspiration and bowel distension due to excess swallowed air. A tube oesophagogram is the most sensitive imaging technique for detecting an "H"-type fistula (MCALISTER and KRONEMER 1996) and is also useful in the postoperative infant if a recurrent or residual fistula is suspected (Fig. 3.9), though endoscopy may be as useful in this situation. The child with an "H"-type fistula may present as an emergency, often in the newborn period, either

a rare finding in malrotation and volvulus, but the diagnosis may be suggested by the finding of abnormal orientation of the superior mesenteric vessels with the vein lying in front of or to the left of the artery. The "whirlpool" sign, as shown with colour Doppler, is characteristic of malrotation and volvulus and is caused by the superior mesenteric vein spiralling around the artery in the twisted mesentery.

There follows a brief discussion of a number of specific acute gastrointestinal conditions principally affecting neonates with the emphasis on those likely to present after the first few days of life.

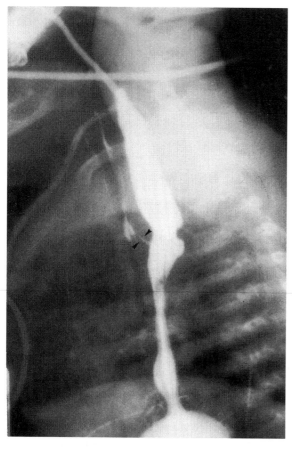

Fig. 3.9. "H"-type tracheo-oesophageal fistula. Lateral film from an oesophageal tubogram demonstrates a fistula (*arrowheads*) between the upper oesophagus and the trachea

Table 3.13. VACTERL spectrum of associated anomalies

Vertebral
Anorectal
Cardiac
Tracheal
OEsophageal
Renal/radial
Limb

(usually bilious) as most (85%) atresias are distal to the ampulla of Vater. Atresia is 4 times as common as stenosis. Both are due to failure of recanalisation of the duodenum between weeks 8 and 10 of gestation.

Plain films show gaseous distension of the stomach and of the proximal duodenum with no distal bowel gas ("double bubble"). Duodenal dilatation is usually marked but if the findings are not typical 10–20 ml of air may be injected into the stomach to distend the duodenal cap and confirm that none passes distally (Fig. 3.6). There is no role for the use of contrast studies when the classical appearances are present.

If the duodenal cap is only slightly distended and there is distal gas, incomplete duodenal obstruction may be present. As it is not possible to differentiate stenosis from malrotation on plain films a contrast study is required, and should be done urgently.

Associated anomalies are common, with malrotation present in 20%–40% of cases: this cannot be diagnosed prior to surgery in the presence of atresia. Congenital heart disease (20%), annular pancreas (30%) and Down's syndrome (30%) and components of the VACTERL spectrum of anomalies may also be found. Contrast studies after surgery may show an abnormal duodeno-jejunal junction which may be related to surgery rather than to a pre-existing anomaly and so does not necessarily indicate a propensity for volvulus (ZERIN and POLLEY 1994).

3.3.6
Malrotation and Midgut Volvulus

Malrotation is a most important congenital abnormality of the gastrointestinal tract, which if the diagnosis is not made swiftly is life threatening as it predisposes to duodenal obstruction and midgut volvulus. In the first trimester the fetal midgut elongates in an extra-abdominal location and then re-enters the abdomen. Its proximal (duodeno-jejunal) and distal (ileo-caecal) components rotate

with a history of choking when fed or with a history of recurrent chest infections with an acute exacerbation.

More than 50% of affected infants have coexistent anomalies in other systems (VACTERL, Table 3.13), and the prognosis depends to a large extent on these and any associated prematurity. Oesophageal stenosis is less common than atresia, though they may coexist (THOMASON and GAY 1987; NEWMAN and BENDER 1997), and usually causes fusiform narrowing at the junction of the middle and distal thirds of the oesophagus.

3.3.5
Duodenal Atresia

Duodenal atresia occurs in 1:3500 live births, presenting early in the neonatal period with vomiting

270° anticlockwise around the axis of the superior mesenteric artery. The duodeno-jejunal junction becomes fixed to the posterior abdominal wall in the left upper abdomen and the ileocaecal junction descends to the right iliac fossa. Interruption of this process may occur at either end, leading to malrotation. In the normal neonate the root of the small bowel mesentery extends from the duodeno-jejunal junction to the distal ileum, providing a broad base and protecting against volvulus, but in malrotation the mesenteric root is shortened with increased likelihood for volvulus and variable obstruction and vascular compromise of bowel. Dense fibrous peritoneal reflections (Ladd's bands) extend from the caecum to the liver or posterior abdominal wall in an attempt to stabilise caecal position and may obstruct the duodenum.

Malrotation is an expected accompaniment of congenital diaphragmatic hernia, gastroschisis, exomphalos and various cardiac syndromes associated with visceral heterotaxy. In children with treated diaphragmatic hernia there appears to be no increased incidence of volvulus compared with isolated malrotation (LEVIN et al. 1995), though volvulus may occur in other conditions such as atrial isomerism (SHARLAND et al. 1989). Malrotation has also been reported in identical twins (BURTON et al. 1993; CROWLEY and BAWLE 1996).

Most (75%) patients with malrotation present in the first month of life with bilious vomiting, which may be associated with abdominal pain and variable abdominal distension. Symptoms may be intermittent, reflecting partial twisting and untwisting of the midgut, but unrelieved volvulus leads to bowel ischaemia, necrosis, bleeding and shock. Older children may have less obvious symptoms such as failure to thrive, anorexia, nausea and diarrhoea and vomiting is less often bilious (JACKSON et al. 1989; SCHEY et al. 1993; POWELL et al. 1989). The key to management is to consider the diagnosis in any child with bilious vomiting and to exclude it by contrast studies of the upper gastrointestinal tract. Obstruction is usually in the third part of the duodenum and is usually due to volvulus or occasionally Ladd's bands. Morbidity and mortality are related to younger age, presence of bowel necrosis and associated anomalies (MESSINEO et al. 1992).

Plain radiographs are often non-specific and may be normal even in the presence of volvulus, so they should never be the end point in imaging an infant who is suspected of malrotation. There may be mild gaseous distension of the stomach and the proximal duodenum with reduced distal gas reflecting partial duodenal obstruction (Fig. 3.10). The duodenal cap may have a triangular appearance (POTTS et al. 1985) and duodenal dilatation is less prominent than in duodenal atresia. Small bowel may be visible in the right flank and may show wall thickening and pneumatosis if there is necrosis (BERDON et al. 1970). Some infants with volvulus have an almost completely gasless pattern, whilst others have a picture of distal obstruction. The former suggests that small bowel vascularity may not be completely compromised as gas is able to be resorbed, whereas the latter implies inability to absorb gas because of severe vascular compromise (KASSNER and KOTTMEIER 1975).

If malrotation is suspected an upper gastrointestinal contrast study should be performed. The duodeno-jejunal junction (ligament of Treitz) should be to the left of the spine at the same level as the duodenal bulb (LONG et al. 1996). In malrotation its position is variable but generally lies inferior and to the right of this. About 3% of patients with malrotation will have a normally located duodeno-jejunal junction with malrotation relating to caecal position, and so in these patients it may be useful to follow contrast through to the caecum (BERDON et al. 1970; SCHEY et al. 1993; LONG et al. 1996).

Volvulus is characterised by a "corkscrew" appearance of the duodenum and proximal small bowel as they spiral around the superior mesenteric vessels (Fig. 3.10). In the presence of complete duodenal obstruction, volvulus will not be detected but should be assumed to be present. An abnormal location of the duodeno-jejunal junction is not always due to malrotation as longstanding bowel dilatation from other causes may displace it (TAYLOR and LITTLEWOOD TEELE 1985) and manual palpation and feeding tubes may temporarily distort normal appearances (KATZ et al. 1987). A sharp "Z"-like angulation of the distal duodenum and proximal jejunum is associated with the presence of peritoneal bands (ABLOW et al. 1983).

Contrast enemas are able only to identify caecal position, which is variable in normal patients, and so they have no routine role in suspected malrotation. In malrotation the caecum usually lies in the right upper quadrant, midline or to the left of the spine; however, in a significant number (20%) it is normally located, and unless reflux of contrast into distal small bowel demonstrates twisting or beaking, volvulus will not be identified (SIEGEL et al. 1980).

Ultrasound may show a dilated fluid-filled duodenal loop (Fig. 3.11) with beaking and hyperperis-

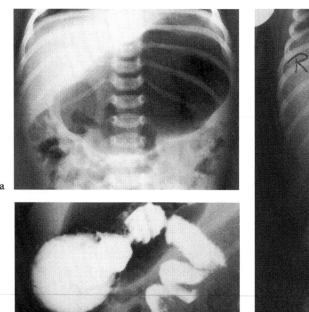

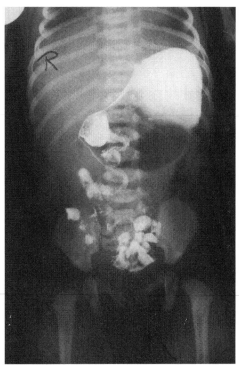

Fig. 3.10 a–c. Malrotation and volvulus. **a** Supine radiograph shows gaseous distension of the stomach and proximal duodenum, with normal-calibre distal bowel. **b,c** A barium meal demonstrates mild distension of the proximal duode- num due to partial obstruction with a corkscrew or spiral appearance of the distal duodenum indicating midgut volvu- lus

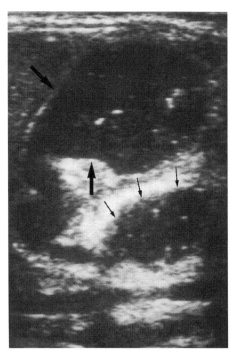

Fig. 3.11. Malrotation and volvulus. Ultrasound of the upper abdomen showing fluid within the gastric antrum (*large arrow*) and in the dilated proximal duodenum (*small arrows*)

talsis, thick-walled small bowel loops in the right flank and free intraperitoneal fluid (LEONIDAS et al. 1991). Malposition of the superior mesenteric vein anterior or to the left of the artery is present in most patients with malrotation (Fig. 3.12) (GAINES et al. 1987) but is neither sensitive nor specific enough to be used as the sole criterion (ZERIN and DIPIETRO 1992), and a normal arrangement (to the right of the artery) does not exclude malrotation (DUFOUR et al. 1992). If an abnormal arrangement is discovered during sonography for other reasons, a contrast study is mandatory (WEINBERGER et al. 1992).

A "whirlpool" appearance of the superior mesen- teric vein rotating clockwise around the axis of the superior mesenteric artery has been described in midgut volvulus on ultrasound and computed to- mography (SHIMANUKI et al. 1996; PRACOS et al. 1992) and appears specific as long as the direction is clockwise. The artery may have a hyperdynamic pul- sating appearance (SMET et al. 1991). However, at present the upper gastrointestinal contrast study re- mains the gold standard for identifying malrotation and volvulus.

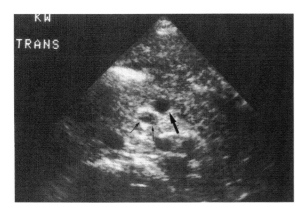

Fig. 3.12. Malrotation. Ultrasound of the upper abdomen showing the superior mesenteric vein (*large arrow*) anterior and to the left of the superior mesenteric artery (*small arrows*)

Surgical treatment includes resection of compromised bowel and division of Ladd's bands. The bowel is positioned in the abdomen in the position of non-rotation with the caecum in the left iliac fossa. An appendicectomy is usually performed, because of the possibility of an abnormally located appendix causing confusion should it later become inflamed. It is generally accepted that all children who have malrotation, even in the absence of symptoms, should have surgery as the risk of volvulus remains lifelong (POWELL et al. 1989).

3.3.7
Small Bowel Atresia

The small bowel is the commonest location for gastrointestinal atresias (1:750 live births), with the ileum slightly more commonly affected than the jejunum. They are due to a prenatal vascular insult leading to obliteration of the small bowel lumen. Jejunal atresias usually present in the first 24 h of life with bilious vomiting and variable but less marked distension compared with ileal atresias, which present slightly later. Meconium may be passed initially before features of obstruction develop. In jejunal atresia supine radiographs show modest distension of the stomach and dilatation of a few loops of bowel (Fig. 3.7), whilst ileal atresias show a low obstruction pattern with multiple dilated loops. Bowel loops are usually of similar calibre, though the loop immediately proximal to the atresia often has a bulbous appearance (GAISIE et al. 1980; JOHNSON and ROBINSON 1984) and air-fluid levels will be prominent on horizontal beam films.

Contrast studies are not generally required in jejunal atresia but a contrast enema will be required to differentiate ileal atresia from other causes of low obstruction. A range of appearances may be encountered from a normal-calibre colon containing meconium plugs with proximal atresias, to a small empty colon (microcolon) with distal atresias. The colon may contain some meconium plugs, and reflux of contrast usually occurs into collapsed distal ileum and stops at the level of atresia. Small bowel stenosis is much less common than atresia and causes less in the way of bowel distension. Gas is seen beyond the level of stenosis in normal-calibre bowel. If stenosis is suspected, an upper gastrointestinal contrast study and follow through should be performed, and any calibre change is usually seen at the level of stenosis.

Two complicated types of ileal atresia are recognised. In "apple-peel" syndrome there is absence of most of the ileum and of the superior mesenteric artery. The small bowel mesentery is deficient, with residual distal small bowel spiralled around vessels related to the right colon (SEASHORE et al. 1987). This entity accounts for less than 5% of atresias and has a familial basis though its mode of inheritance is not clear. Plain films show high obstruction with dilatation of the stomach, duodenum and proximal jejunum and contrast enema shows a microcolon with a spiral appearance of the distal ileum suggestive of volvulus (SCHIAVETTI et al. 1984). The caecum may be located high in the right side of the abdomen. Some of these cases are associated with malrotation and may be due to intrauterine volvulus and necrosis of the midgut. Overall survival of infants with apple-peel small bowel is less than 50% (SEASHORE et al. 1987).

Multiple small and large bowel atresias with intraluminal calcification has an autosomal recessive inheritance (GUTTMAN et al. 1973; POMBO et al. 1982). Calcification has a spherical or elongated appearance and is often dense. The contrast enema is as described for uncomplicated ileal atresias, unless colonic obstruction (due to colonic atresia) prevents demonstration of the distal ileum.

Overall the prognosis for small bowel atresias regardless of anatomical type depends on the amount of viable bowel present.

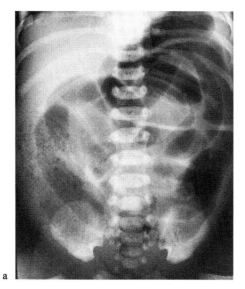
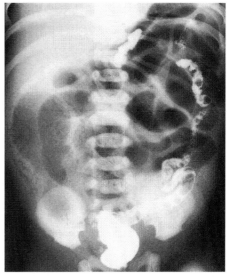
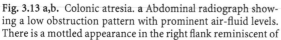

Fig. 3.13 a,b. Colonic atresia. **a** Abdominal radiograph showing a low obstruction pattern with prominent air-fluid levels. There is a mottled appearance in the right flank reminiscent of but not specific for meconium ileus. **b** A contrast enema shows a small unused colon terminating in the upper abdomen

3.3.8
Colonic Atresia

The colon is the least common site of atresia (POWELL and RAFFENSPERGER 1982; WINTERS et al. 1992), with an incidence of approximately 1:40 000 live births (MCALISTER and KRONEMER 1996). Colonic atresia is associated with other intestinal atresias, gastroschisis, exomphalos and malrotation (POWELL and RAFFENSPERGER 1982) and is due to an intrauterine vascular insult. Presentation may be delayed for several days with distension and vomiting predominating. The proximal colon (transverse and right) is more commonly affected than the distal colon (WINTERS et al. 1992).

Radiographs show a low obstruction pattern with multiple air-fluid levels and often a very distended segment of bowel containing a conspicuous air-fluid level in the right flank corresponding to a dilated caecum and ascending colon, which may be massive if the ileocaecal valve is competent (Fig. 3.13). Contrast enemas show a microcolon with a blind ending at the level of the atresia, often with a club or windsock appearance (Fig. 3.13). Ultrasound may suggest the diagnosis by showing distended fluid-filled bowel with haustral markings which may be visible before bowel gas reaches the level of atresia on plain films (PASTO et al. 1984).

3.3.9
Anorectal Anomalies

Anorectal atresias occur in about 1:5000 live births and are due to failure of descent and separation of the hind gut and the genitourinary tract. They are associated with the VACTERL spectrum of congenital anomalies, with vertebral (60%), cardiac (15%) and genitourinary tract (40%) anomalies predominating. Currarino's triad is the association of an anorectal anomaly, sacral bone defects and a presacral mass which may be an anterior meningocoele, a teratoma or a duplication cyst. Anorectal anomalies are conventionally divided into high and low lesions with distal bowel terminating above and below the levator sling respectively.

The diagnosis is clinical and usually allows differentiation of high from low lesions. High lesions are commoner in girls and have a greater incidence of associated anomalies.

Plain radiographs should be delayed for 24 h if possible to allow time for gas to reach and distend distal bowel. A supine film shows a low obstruction pattern (Fig. 3.14). Gas within the urinary bladder or calcification in bowel suggests a recto-urethral fistula and therefore a high lesion. A prone lateral film is obtained with barium paste or a metal object marking the anal pit so that the relationship of distal

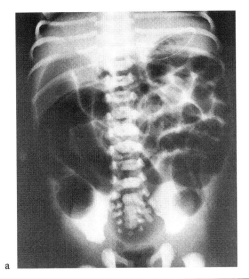

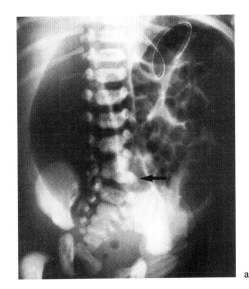

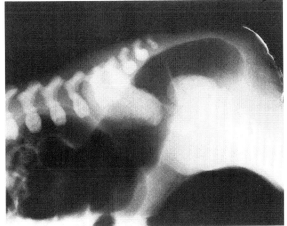

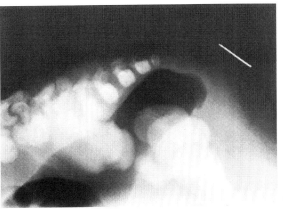

Fig. 3.14 a,b. Low anorectal anomaly. Supine radiograph (a) and prone lateral film (b) show a low obstruction pattern with distal gas extending to within 1 cm of the natal cleft marked with barium paste

Fig. 3.15 a,b. High anorectal anomaly. a Supine radiograph showing a low obstruction pattern with multiple dilated loops of bowel. Note the accessory left sided hemivertebra fused to L5 (*arrow*), causing an acute lumbosacral tilt. b Prone lateral radiograph demonstrating air-filled distal bowel terminating greater than 1 cm from the anal pit (metal marker)

bowel gas to skin can be assessed. Gas extending to within 10 mm of the skin supports a low lesion (Figs. 3.14, 3.15). The "M" line of Cremin has been used to locate the level of the pelvic floor and lies midway between and parallel to a line joining the pubic bones to the sacrococcygeal articulation and one drawn tangential to the inferior border of the ischia. Bowel gas terminating above this line suggests a high lesion and below it a low lesion.

Neither method is completely accurate as reduced distal bowel gas or meconium within the distal loop may simulate a high lesion, and over-distension of distal bowel may cause a high lesion to appear spuriously low. The spine, hips and heart should be imaged in view of the association of anorectal

malformations with other congenital anomalies (VACTERL).

3.3.10
Meconium Ileus

Meconium ileus is the earliest clinical manifestation of cystic fibrosis, occurring in about 15% of affected children (AGRONS et al. 1996). Abnormal small bowel secretions cause viscid meconium which cannot be propelled into the colon, leading to distal small bowel obstruction. Failure to pass meconium, bilious vomiting and abdominal distension occur,

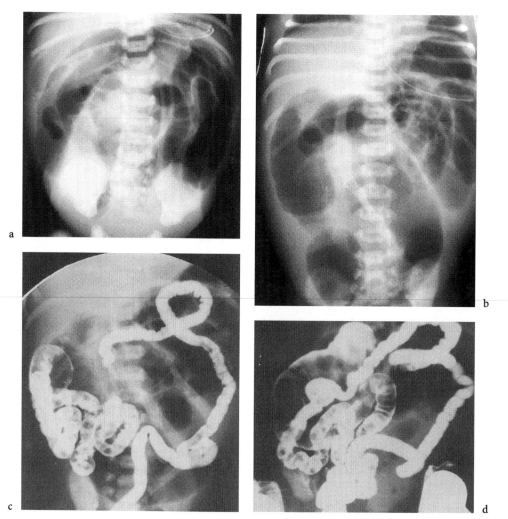

Fig. 3.16 a–d. Meconium ileus. Supine (a) And erect (b) radiographs show a low obstruction pattern with varying calibre of dilated bowel and a paucity of air-fluid levels. Water-soluble enema (c,d) demonstrates a microcolon, with reflux into distal small bowel outlining impacted meconium

with the last-mentioned often present at delivery (ZIEGLER 1994).

Plain radiographs show a low obstructive pattern with variable calibre of dilated loops compared with atresias (Fig. 3.16a,b). There are few or no air-fluid levels because the thick immiscible meconium prevents their formation (BUONOMO 1997), though if obstruction is unrelieved for any length of time they may form in more dilated proximal small bowel. A mottled appearance in the right flank, due to small bubbles of gas trapped in the meconium, is suggestive of but not specific for meconium ileus (STRINGER 1989). More often than not the pattern is simply that of distal obstruction indistinguishable from any other cause although the characteristic bulbous dilatation of atresias is absent (CARTY and BRERETON 1983).

A contrast enema shows a microcolon which is often non-compliant and difficult to fill. If contrast refluxes into distal ileum, multiple intraluminal filling defects (inspissated meconium) will be identified (Fig. 3.16c,d) (MCALISTER and KRONEMER 1996).

Non-operative management of uncomplicated meconium ileus may be attempted by refluxing water-soluble contrast media proximal to the occluding plugs into dilated small bowel. Care must be taken with fluid balance during and after the procedure if hypertonic water-soluble contrast media are used in order to prevent depletion of the intravascular circulating volume (NOBLETT 1969), and the ability to proceed immediately to surgery if complications supervene is important (EIN et al. 1987).

Gastrografin or other ionic water-soluble contrast media have been used to good effect, though there is some evidence that it is not the hypertonicity of the contrast medium but rather additives such as Tween 80 (formerly a component of Gastrografin) that are most important in relieving obstruction (KAO and FRANKEN 1995). A success rate of 50%–60% is expected in cases of uncomplicated meconium ileus (DOCHERTY et al. 1992; KAO and FRANKEN 1995), but it is not unusual to have to repeat the enema one or more times to completely evacuate the inspissated meconium (BUONOMO 1997) and there is a small risk (2.75%–5%) of perforation (DOCHERTY et al. 1992). Meconium ileus is complicated by intrauterine perforation, volvulus, atresia and pseudocyst formation in about 50% of cases (AGRONS et al. 1996). Suggestive plain film findings include calcification, prominent air-fluid levels and a mass (Fig. 3.17). Prenatal perforations may seal spontaneously, form a pseudocyst or cause a generalised chemical peritonitis. Peritoneal calcification is not specific for cystic fibrosis and is actually commoner with other causes of intrauterine perforation (FINKEL and SLOVIS 1982). Bowel wall calcification is probably commoner than previously thought in patients with meconium ileus (LANG et al. 1997).

3.3.11
Immature Left Colon

Immature left colon is an uncommon cause of functional obstruction occurring in infants of diabetic mothers, those born by caesarean section and premature neonates. There is delayed passage of meconium, distension and vomiting, though these infants are generally less unwell than those with mechanical obstruction.

Plain radiographs show a low obstruction pattern though air-fluid levels are inconspicuous (Fig. 3.18a). A contrast enema will show a small rectum and left colon, though rectal and sigmoid colon calibre are in normal proportion (cf. Hirschsprung's disease). A funnelled appearance is seen near the splenic flexure, with mild dilatation of the right and transverse colon and a more abrupt and proximal transition than in Hirschsprung's disease (Fig. 3.18b). Usually there is variable evacuation of meconium plugs following the enema, after which symptoms subside (BUONOMO 1997). In a few patients there is either a poor response to the enema or the

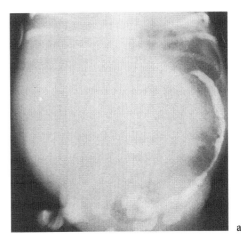

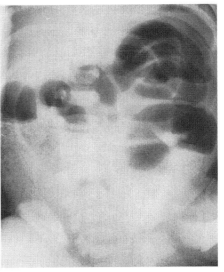

Fig. 3.17 a,b. Complicated meconium ileus. a Abdominal radiograph shows a large soft tissue mass in the right abdomen displacing bowel to the left, with contrast outlining a small unused colon. b Erect radiograph demonstrates a mottled appearance in the right flank suggestive of meconium ileus and multiple air-fluid levels

appearances are suggestive of Hirschsprung's disease, in which case a suction rectal biopsy is indicated (BERDON et al. 1977).

3.3.12
Hirschsprung's Disease

Hirschsprung's disease causes functional bowel obstruction and is due to failure of relaxation of aganglionic distal bowel. In the majority of cases (75%) aganglionosis extends from the anus to the rectosigmoid region with normal proximal innervation and the condition is sporadic. In the remainder

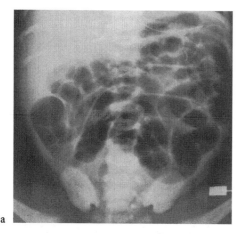

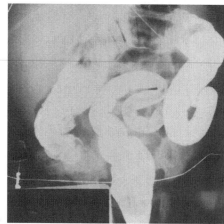

Fig. 3.18 a,b. Immature left colon. **a** Erect radiograph demonstrates a low obstruction pattern with many gas-filled dilated loops of bowel and no air-fluid levels. **b** A contrast enema outlines a small-calibre sigmoid and descending colon, with a transition to a mildly dilated proximal colon at the splenic flexure. The larger calibre of the rectum compared with the sigmoid colon differentiates this from Hirschsprung's disease

it extends more proximally, with 8%–10% involving the whole colon and occasionally the small bowel, and is known as long segment disease. Boys are affected more often than girls in the commoner short segment type, but sex incidence is equal in long segment disease (DE CAMPO et al. 1984), in which there is often a family history.

Most cases (85%) present within the first month of life, with abdominal distension, vomiting and variable constipation. A later presentation is less common and most of these children will be found in retrospect to have had delayed passage of meconium in the neonatal period. There is an association with Down's syndrome (5%) and an enterocolitis occurs in between 10% and 30% of infants, causing severe bloody diarrhoea which may be fatal (VINTON 1994).

Perforation, usually of the terminal ileum or right colon, may occur in up to 3% of patients in the neonatal period (BRERETON and STRINGER 1991) and is commoner with total colonic disease. The diagnosis depends on clinical suspicion followed by suction rectal biopsy.

Abdominal radiographs show a distal obstructive appearance, sometimes with colonic dilatation out of proportion to small bowel (CARTY and BRERETON 1983). There is less marked small bowel dilatation compared with other causes of low obstruction and colonic air-fluid levels are prominent (Fig. 3.19a,b). Absence of rectal gas on supine radiographs has been considered suggestive of Hirschsprung's disease but is more common in neonates with sepsis or necrotising enterocolitis (BRADLEY and PILLINK 1991). A pneumoperitoneum may be present if perforation has occurred (NEWMAN et al. 1987). In total colonic aganglionosis there may be paucity of colonic gas and a non-specific low obstruction pattern (DE CAMPO et al. 1984).

Contrast enemas show a narrow rectum, often with spastic contractions and a transition zone proximal to which is dilated bowel (ROSENFIELD et al. 1984). In normal neonates the rectum is larger in calibre than the sigmoid colon but in Hirschsprung's disease the reverse is true (Fig. 3.19c). Mucosal oedema and ulceration proximal to the transition zone indicate coexistent enterocolitis. The transition zone is usually in the mid sigmoid colon but may be absent in young neonates and rectal examination or biopsy may obscure it. Enemas have a false-negative rate of 20%–30%, so a rectal biopsy is required when the enema appears normal. Water-soluble (isosmolar) contrast may be substituted for barium in ill neonates (O'DONOVAN et al. 1996) with no loss of diagnostic accuracy.

No obvious abnormality is present in the majority (85%) of patients with total colonic involvement, though foreshortening of the colon, decreased redundancy of the flexures and subtle spasm may be identified (DE CAMPO et al. 1984).

Post-evacuation films may be useful in identifying the level of a subtle transition zone. The presence of considerable residual barium on delayed films (24 and 48hs), whilst consistent with Hirschsprung's disease, may also be seen in sepsis and hypothyroidism. With the use of suction rectal biopsy to confirm the diagnosis, delayed films are no longer required. Late presentation of classical Hirschprung's disease is unusual today. Occasionally the diagnosis is missed – the child presenting as an emergency with enterocolitis and bloody diarrhoea.

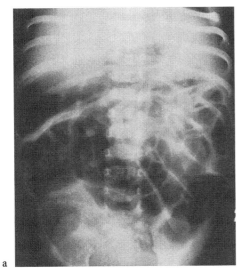

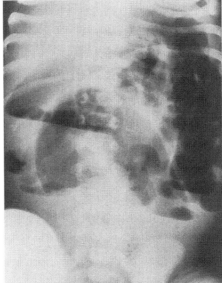

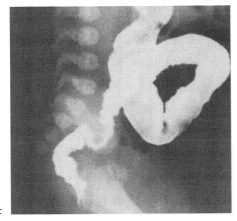

Fig. 3.19 a–c. Hirschsprung's disease. Supine (**a**) and erect (**b**) radiographs showing a low obstruction pattern with prominent distension of colon which contains air-fluid levels, and an early lateral image from a contrast enema (**c**) showing a narrow and slightly irregular rectum and distal sigmoid colon. The descending and proximal sigmoid colon are of normal calibre

This is then a surgical emergency and no special imaging is required. Older children may also present refractory constipation and gross faecal loading of the colon on plain radiographs. There may be some secondary small bowel dilatation but rarely obstruction. In acquired constipation the maximal faecal loading is distally in the sigmoid colon and rectum with relative proximal sparing. A contrast enema will usually show the typical cone or transition zone in classical Hirschsprung's disease. Very short segment disease or hypoganglionosis cannot be diagnosed with imaging, the enema showing faecal loading but no demonstrable transition zone.

3.3.13
Necrotising Enterocolitis

Necrotising enterocolitis occurs almost entirely in premature neonates, with more than 90% being less than 36 weeks' gestation. It may rarely be seen in term infants, particularly in those with congenital heart disease. It is the commonest acquired neonatal gastrointestinal emergency, with prematurity, low birth weight and coexistent cardiac and respiratory abnormalities being predisposing factors, compromising the immature gut and impairing its resistance to bacterial invasion (VINTON 1994; UKEN et al. 1988).

Abdominal distension, tenderness, vomiting and rectal bleeding soon after the initiation of feeding, usually in the first week of life, are typical. There is a predilection for involvement of the distal ileum and the right colon.

Plain radiographs are initially non-specific, showing mild gaseous distension of bowel, though on sequential films the normal changeable appearance of bowel loops is lost with one or more loops becoming "fixed". Wall thickening manifest by increased separation of bowel loops is an early sign, as is loss of the

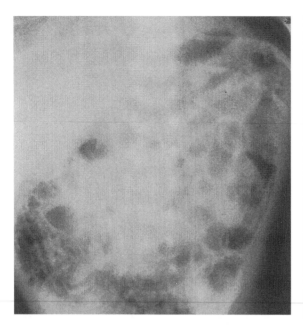

Fig. 3.20. Necrotising enterocolitis. Supine radiograph shows "bubbly" intramural lucencies in the right flank and linear pneumatosis in the left flank

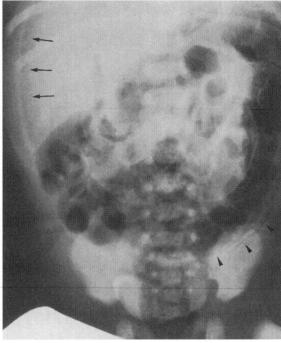

Fig. 3.21. Necrotising enterocolitis and pneumoperitoneum. Supine radiograph shows mild gaseous dilatation of bowel with prominent left-sided pneumatosis (*arrowheads*), with the right lobe of the liver outlined by free gas (*arrows*)

normal sharp bowel outline (CARTY and BRERETON 1983), and with progressive disease generalised bowel dilatation develops.

Intramural air may be seen as either linear or cystic lucencies. The former are more easily recognised as the latter may be simulated or obscured by gas admixed with bowel contents (Fig. 3.20): horizontal beam films are helpful in making this distinction (JOHNSON 1988). Portal venous gas is seen in less than 10% of cases and heralds severe but not necessarily fatal disease. Perforation may occur (Fig. 3.21), most often in the terminal ileum: necrotising enterocolitis accounts for about half of all cases of neonatal perforation (BRERETON and STRINGER 1991).

Bowel wall thickening and free intraperitoneal fluid may be identified by ultrasound, with pneumatosis producing patchy areas of increased echogenicity within the bowel wall. Sonography is more sensitive than plain radiographs for the detection of portal venous gas. Contrast enemas are generally not performed during the acute phase as the risk of perforation and septicaemia may outweigh any advantage. If done, they will demonstrate mucosal ulceration and oedema, spasm and occasionally intramural extravasation of contrast in affected areas (UKEN et al. 1988).

Treatment entails withholding oral feeds, administration of broad-spectrum antibiotics and general supportive care, though surgery is required for perforation. No single organism has been implicated in the pathogenesis of necrotising enterocolitis, and though many neonates have gram-negative septicaemia, it is likely this is a secondary phenomenon.

Late complications of necrotising enterocolitis include colonic and small bowel strictures which typically present 4–6 weeks after the acute episode and may require resection. Not infrequently presentation is as an emergency with obstruction but strictures may also present more insidiously with failure to thrive. A water-soluble contrast enema will outline such strictures and may need to be performed through stomas and per rectum.

3.3.14
Omphalomesenteric Remnants

The omphalomesenteric duct links the distal ileum to the umbilicus, joining the developing midgut to the yolk sac in utero. Its persistence as a fibrous band (MOORE 1996) may cause bowel obstruction by direct compression, internal hernia, closed loop ob-

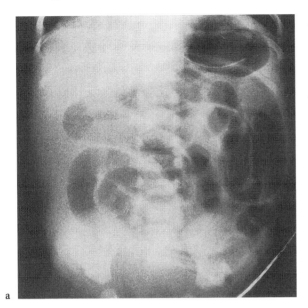

a

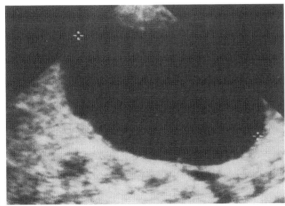

b

Fig. 3.22 a,b. Cystic omphalomesenteric remnants. a Plain radiograph shows a low obstruction pattern. b Ultrasound demonstrates a well-defined anechoic cystic lesion

struction or volvulus. It is very difficult to determine the cause of obstruction prior to surgery, but as the infant is so obviously obstructed and requires surgery this is irrelevant. Occasionally a cystic lesion is identified with ultrasound but differentiation of a Meckel's diverticulum from a small duplication cyst may be difficult (GOYAL and BELLAH 1993).

Plain radiographs show a pattern of low bowel obstruction (Fig. 3.22a). Portal venous gas has been reported secondary to volvulus of small bowel around the band (GAISIE et al. 1985) and discharge of bowel contents from the umbilicus or ileal prolapse may occur if the duct remains patent. An associated cyst may be detected with ultrasound (Fig. 3.22b).

3.3.15
Internal Hernia

Internal hernias cause variable bowel obstruction and may be due to mesenteric defects or peritoneal bands. Radiographs may show a low obstructive pattern or localised dilatation of one or more loops of bowel depending on the level of involved bowel. Contrast studies may suggest an internal hernia but more often simply document the level of obstruction. Diagnosis is usually made intraoperatively.

3.3.16
Gastric Volvulus

Gastric volvulus is an uncommon cause of bowel obstruction in children because the stomach is generally well fixed within the abdomen (ANDIRAN et al. 1995) but it may be catastrophic if not recognised. Presentation is with sudden onset of vomiting, retching and pain, which becomes increasingly severe. Upper abdominal distension may be noted and it may be impossible to pass an oesophageal tube into the stomach.

Plain radiographs show a dilated stomach, which may contain two air-fluid levels on erect films if volvulus is mesentero-axial and one level if it is organo-axial (ZIPROKOWSKI and TEELE 1979), with a beak in the antropyloric region (CAMPBELL 1979). Contrast studies show a normally located oesophagogastric junction, with inversion of the stomach so that the antrum is superior to the fundus, and the antrum may be twisted and is usually obstructed. There is an association with "wandering spleen" and asplenia, presumably due to a deficient gastrosplenic ligament (GARCIA et al. 1994).

3.3.17
Functional Obstruction

Functional obstruction is a common entity in which prematurity, sepsis or metabolic derangements contribute to impaired bowel peristalsis, leading to delayed passage of meconium and variable abdominal distension. There is no mechanical obstruction or intrinsic abnormality of the colon differentiating this entity from Hirschprung's disease or immature left colon.

The clinical findings of distension, failure to pass meconium and bilious vomiting require radiographic evaluation. Plain radiographs show a low obstruction pattern with no specific diagnostic features. A water-soluble contrast enema outlines a normal calibre rectum and colon with no transition zone or cone typical of Hirschsprung's disease or immature left colon. The colon usually contains multiple meconium plugs which are often evacuated during or soon after the examination. Symptoms generally subside following the enema with treatment of any underlying sepsis or metabolic abnormalities.

3.3.18
Biliary Disorders

Jaundice in the neonate is most commonly due to immaturity of the liver enzymes resulting in inability to excrete adequate amounts of bilirubin and as such it is largely unconjugated. Treatment is by phototherapy and exchange transfusion if severe. If jaundice is persistent or worsening or there is conjugated hyperbilirubinaemia, an underlying cause must be sought. Ultrasound is the best initial imaging modality with the aim being to identify a gallbladder and exclude bile duct dilatation. This is the only investigation indicated urgently: further management and imaging will follow the normal pattern in jaundiced neonates, usually including hepatobiliary scintigraphy.

Spontaneous bile duct perforation is a rare entity presenting with variable abdominal distension, jaundice and acholic stool (O'HALLER 1991). Ultrasound shows free intraperitoneal fluid but no bile duct dilatation. A definitive diagnosis may be obtained by hepatobiliary scintigraphy showing accumulation of tracer in the peritoneum or by aspiration of ascitic fluid. Drainage of the ascitic fluid may result in spontaneous closure, but surgery is required if a leak persists.

Biliary obstruction may be caused by intraluminal sludge in an otherwise normal biliary tract (bile plug syndrome). It has conventionally been treated surgically though some cases may resolve spontaneously (LANG and PINCKNEY 1991). Ultrasound will show variable dilatation of the bile ducts containing echogenic sludge. Inspissated bile is a similar condition in patients with an underlying illness (e.g. cystic fibrosis) leading to alteration of the composition of bile. Gallstones are uncommon in neonates and have been reported to resolve spontaneously without need for specific therapy (KELLER et al. 1985). Predisposing causes include total parenteral nutrition, short

Table 3.14. Classification of choledochal cysts

Type 1: fusiform dilatation of common bile duct
Type 2: saccular diverticulum of common duct
Type 3: saccular cyst in medial wall of duodenum
Type 4: multifocal intrahepatic bile duct ectasia (Caroli's disease)

gut syndrome, frusemide, prolonged fasting and phototherapy.

3.3.19
Choledochal Cyst

Choledochal cysts (Table 3.14) are related to an anomalous insertion of the pancreatic duct into the common bile duct proximal to the ampulla of Vater, allowing reflux of pancreatic secretions into the bile duct, thereby causing inflammation and dilatation. There is an association with biliary atresia in the neonatal period and so jaundice should not automatically be attributed to the cyst (TORRIS et al. 1990).

One-third of patients present in the first year of life, with most of the remainder presenting in the first decade (STRINGER et al. 1995). Persistent jaundice is the commonest finding in the neonatal period, but in older children recurrent attacks of pain, vomiting and jaundice are more frequent. A right upper quadrant mass may be palpated, though this is uncommon and the cyst is detected by ultrasound (AKHAN et al. 1994; STRINGER et al. 1995). An upper abdominal cyst may have been detected antenatally and subsequently confirmed postnatally in asymptomatic neonates.

Ultrasound is the most useful initial imaging modality, showing a well-defined right upper quadrant cyst, separate from the gallbladder, in type 2 and 3 choledochal cysts. Type 1 cysts (80%–90%) are characterised as fusiform dilatation of the extrahepatic bile duct. In type 4 cysts, multiple focal intrahepatic cysts are present with variable abnormalities affecting the extrahepatic biliary tree. Sludge, debris and calculi may be seen within choledochal cysts. Hepatobiliary scintigraphy with technetium-99m hepato-iminodiacetic acid (HIDA) confirms communication with the biliary tree and serves to exclude biliary atresia, which is a recognised association of choledochal cyst in neonates.

Complications include cholangitis, pancreatitis, calculi and cholangiocarcinoma (KIM et al. 1995) and for this reason surgery with cyst excision and a choledocho-enterostomy is performed.

3.4
The Infant and Young Child

Common emergencies seen in infants and young children include hypertrophic pyloric stenosis, intussusception, gastroenteritis and ingestion of foreign objects. Trauma and Henoch-Schönlein purpura are important but are less common.

Abdominal pain may be caused by a variety of mechanical and inflammatory conditions (Table 3.15) though localisation of pain may still be difficult at this age. Vomiting is a non-specific symptom in children and may be due to disease within or outside the gastrointestinal tract. Increasingly forceful projectile vomiting is typical of hypertrophic pyloric stenosis. As in the neonate, bilious vomiting should always be taken seriously because of the possibility of malrotation and volvulus (Table 3.16). Some causes of gastrointestinal bleeding (Table 3.17) require no imaging (anal fissures) but others dictate prompt investigation and treatment (intussusception and malrotation).

Infectious hepatitis and haematological disorders are the commonest causes of jaundice, and gallstones and structural abnormalities of the biliary tree are less frequent (Table 3.18), though emergency presentation with jaundice is unusual at this age. Ultrasound is the most useful initial imaging investigation. Hydronephrosis is the commonest abdominal "mass" at any age (Table 3.19) although faecal residue may simulate a mass and lead to requests for further imaging. Ultrasound should be the first imaging modality when a mass is encountered.

Table 3.15. Causes of abdominal pain in infants and young children

Trauma
Ingested foreign body
Obstruction (hernia/adhesion)
Gastroenteritis
Intussusception
Mesenteric adenitis
Peptic ulcer
Henoch-Schönlein purpura
Appendicitis
Constipation
Incarcerated inguinal hernia
Ischaemia (sickle cell/volvulus)
Non-gastrointestinal causes
    Pneumonia
    Streptococcal pharyngitis
    Urinary tract infection

Table 3.16. Causes of vomiting in infants and young children

Gastro-oesophageal reflux
Hiatus hernia
Malrotation
Intussusception
Gastroenteritis
Obstruction
Pneumonia
Strictures/adhesions
Hypertrophic pyloric stenosis
Intestinal stenoses and webs
Incarcerated inguinal hernia
Non-gastrointestinal causes
    Pneumonia
    Urinary tract infection
    Diabetes mellitus
    Encephalitis/meningitis

Table 3.17. Causes of gastrointestinal bleeding in infants and young children

Colitis (idiopathic and infective)
Polyp
Gastroenteritis
Intussusception
Meckel's diverticulum
Henoch-Schönlein purpura
Anal fissure
Haemorrhoid
Vascular anomaly/angiodysplasia
Haemolytic uraemic syndrome
Hirschsprung's disease
Duplication cyst
Foreign body
Oesophageal/gastric varices
Peptic ulceration
Malrotation and volvulus

Table 3.18. Causes of jaundice in infants and young children

Parenchymal liver disease
Cholelithiasis
Haematological disorders
Infective hepatitis
Choledochal cyst
Drugs
Total parenteral nutrition

Table 3.19. Causes of masses in infants and young children

Cyst
Intussusception
Abscess
Hepatosplenomegaly
Hydrops of gallbladder
Constipation
Mesenteric cyst/lymphangioma
Faecal impaction
Tumour
    Neuroblastoma
    Wilms' tumour
    Rhabdomyosarcoma
    Hepatoblastoma
Non-gastrointestinal
    Hydronephrosis
    Renal cyst
    Ovarian cyst

Table 3.20. Causes of small bowel dilatation in infants and young children

Adhesions
Incarcerated hernia
Intussusception
Midgut volvulus
Henoch-Schönlein purpura
Appendicitis
Gastroenteritis

Table 3.21. Causes of gasless abdomen in infants and young children

Severe vomiting
Nasogastric aspiration
Ascites
Midgut volvulus
Intussusception
Closed loop obstruction
Sedation/paralysis

3.4.1
Abdominal Radiographs

Imaging of acute emergencies can usually be managed by a combination of plain radiography, ultrasound and fluoroscopy, with only occasional recourse to computed tomography and nuclear medicine.

Abdominal radiography may be restricted to a supine film unless free intraperitoneal gas is suspected, when a horizontal beam film (left side down decubitus, erect chest or lateral "shoot through") is required. Horizontal beam films may also be helpful in the detection of pneumatosis and air-fluid levels but in most other circumstances provide no extra information over supine radiographs.

The film should include the lung bases and inguinal regions so that basal pneumonia and herniae will not be overlooked. Gas is usually present in the stomach and colon, with the latter being identified by the presence of faecal material and haustra. Variable amounts of gas are present in the small bowel, which lies centrally and has a smaller calibre than the colon. The lower border of the liver may be identified, as may the outline of the spleen and kidneys.

Bowel dilatation may result from a number of causes, with its distribution helping to identify the aetiology. Generalised dilatation of small and large bowel may be due to gastroenteritis, paralytic ileus, drugs or sepsis. Small bowel dilatation (Table 3.20) with decreased or absent colonic and rectal gas suggests mechanical obstruction and bowel wall thickening suggests inflammation or ischaemia. Horizontal beam films will show air-fluid levels when bowel is dilated and occasionally their distribution is helpful. Air-fluid levels of varying lengths and at

Table 3.22. Causes of pneumatosis in infancy and beyond

Bronchopulmonary dysplasia
Malrotation/volvulus
Iron ingestion
Nesidioblastosis
Steroid therapy
Congenital heart disease
Short bowel syndrome
Viral gastroenteritis
Hirschsprung's disease
Hypertrophic pyloric stenosis
Neutropenic colitis/typhlitis
Cystic fibrosis

similar levels support functional obstruction such as an ileus, whereas in mechanical obstruction they tend to be shorter and more variably located. However, findings must always be interpreted in the light of clinical findings if errors are to be avoided.

A gasless abdomen is uncommon and may simply reflect severe vomiting or fluid-filled obstructed bowel or be due to other serious intra-abdominal pathology (Table 3.21). Pneumatosis is very rare outside of the neonatal period but may be caused by a large number of processes (Table 3.22).

3.4.2
Imaging Strategies

Plain films are essential in the assessment of infants and young children with suspected mechanical bowel obstruction, perforation or trauma. They are important in documenting the presence and location of ingested foreign bodies (mostly coins) and in cases of suspected caustic ingestion are required to detect perforation of the oesophagus (pleural effusion, pneumothorax, pneumomediastinum) or stomach. They are often requested for non-specific abdominal pain though the diagnostic yield is low. They may exclude obstruction but in many other conditions more useful information is rapidly provided by ultrasound, especially when hypertrophic pyloric stenosis, intussusception and acute appendicitis are considerations. Abdominal and bowel ultrasound in skilled hands is a very useful technique in children and even in the presence of an ileus or bowel obstruction, the use of graded abdominal compression will allow a comprehensive examination of bowel, mesentery and peritoneum. As normal radiographs do not mean there is no serious intra-abdominal pathology some would argue that ultrasound should be the first investigation. However, local circumstances and access to ultrasound vary, and radiographs are still performed as clinicians are generally more familiar and comfortable with them in emergency presentations.

Reduction of intussusception and suspected malrotation are the commonest indications for fluoroscopy. Technetium-99m pertechnetate imaging in young children with rectal bleeding is the technique of choice for the localisation of a Meckel's diverticulum. Computed tomography of the abdomen is the most useful examination in the assessment of severe blunt abdominal trauma and the evaluation of complex abdominal masses and fluid collections; it may also be used as a supplement to ultrasound if tenderness, bowel gas or dressings prevent a full examination.

3.4.3
Duplication Cyst

Duplication cysts are lined with gastrointestinal mucosa and smooth muscle and lie adjacent to bowel on its mesenteric border. The majority (82%) are cystic and do not communicate with the bowel lumen but a small number are tubular (usually colonic) and may communicate with adjacent bowel. The commonest locations are small bowel (50%) and oesophagus (20%), with the colon (13%), duodenum (10%) and stomach (5%) being less commonly affected (MACPHERSON 1993).

Most cysts present by the age of 1 year with vomiting or recurrent abdominal pain. A palpable mass may be present but is less common (IYER and

MAHOUR 1995). Intra-abdominal duplications may form a lead point for intussusception. Infection or internal haemorrhage from contained ectopic gastric mucosa may cause pain and lead to enlargement and subsequent detection of a mass. Ectopic gastric mucosa is most frequent in oesophageal duplications.

Most oesophageal duplications are located in the distal third and are often asymptomatic, though high duplications may cause dysphagia or stridor and so present early. Tubular duplications are common in the colon and are associated with genitourinary anomalies (YOUSEFZADEH et al. 1983). About 7% of duplications are multiple (MACPHERSON 1993).

Chest radiographs may show an oesophageal duplication cyst as a mediastinal soft tissue mass with compression and displacement of the trachea. Contrast studies demonstrate variable indentation or narrowing of the oesophageal lumen. With abdominal duplications, plain films may show a soft tissue mass with displacement of loops of bowel, less commonly obstruction and rarely mural calcification (ALFORD et al. 1980). Ultrasound will confirm the cystic nature of the mass and may offer a specific diagnosis if the wall has an inner echogenic (KANGARLOO et al. 1979) and an outer hypoechoic layer (MOCCIA et al. 1981), the former representing mucosa and the latter smooth muscle (BARR et al. 1990). Peristalsis may also be seen (SPOTTSWOOD 1994), helping distinguish duplication from choledochal, mesenteric, pancreatic and ovarian cysts. Fluid within the cyst is usually anechoic, but if haemorrhage or infection has supervened, it may be variably echogenic.

Contrast studies of the gastrointestinal tract may be required to fully evaluate duplications. Such studies may show mass effect upon the adjacent bowel, often with a "claw" or beak-like appearance (BLAKE 1984), and communicating tubular duplications may be opacified. Cross-sectional imaging with computed tomography is useful, particularly in the chest and pelvis. Technetium-99m pertechnetate imaging may be helpful in complicated cases, especially where the cyst is non-communicating, as up to 20% of duplication cysts contain ectopic gastric mucosa (MACPHERSON 1993).

3.4.4
Hypertrophic Pyloric Stenosis

Increasingly forceful non-bilious vomiting in an infant of 4–6 weeks of age suggests hypertrophic pyloric stenosis. This is a condition of unknown aetiology that causes thickening of the smooth muscle of the pylorus, producing gastric outlet obstruction. It occurs in 1:3000 live births and is 4 times as common in boys as in girls. There is a family history in up to 16% of cases (POON et al. 1996). Affected infants vomit soon after feeding, often in a projectile fashion, and appear hungry; prominent gastric peristaltic waves may be present. Weight loss, dehydration, hypochloraemic metabolic alkalosis and lethargy ensue. The diagnosis is made by clinical examination during a test feed in most (80%) cases, when a typical olive is felt (HERNANZ-SCHULMAN et al. 1994). In these cases no further imaging is needed and treat-

ment is surgical following correction of dehydration and metabolic anomalies.

Imaging is useful when the test feed is normal (VAN DER SCHOUW et al. 1994; GODBOLE et al. 1996) and in patients with an atypical history. Plain radiographs may show gaseous distension of the stomach with a paucity of distal gas but are generally unhelpful and should not be routinely obtained (Fig. 3.23a). Drainage by nasogastric tube may decompress the stomach and obscure this appearance, as may forceful vomiting.

Ultrasound has now supplanted the use of contrast studies where expertise is available, allowing direct

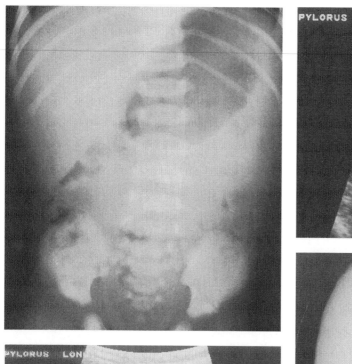

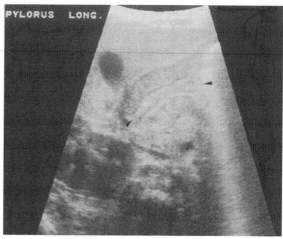

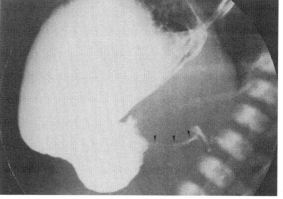

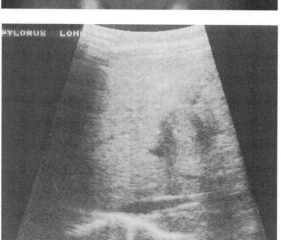

Fig. 3.23 a–d. Hypertrophic pyloric stenosis. **a** Plain radiograph shows moderate gaseous distension of the stomach and reduced distal gas. **b,c** Ultrasound shows elongation of the pylorus (*between arrowheads*) with concentric muscle thickening in the longitudinal and transverse projections. **d** A barium meal shows an elongated, narrowed and curved pyloric canal (*arrowheads*) with a mass effect upon the gastric antrum

visualisation of the thickened pyloric muscle. In transverse section it has a "target" appearance with echogenic central mucosa and peripheral muscle of lower echogenicity (Fig. 3.23b,c). Muscle thickness greater than 2.5 mm and a pyloric canal length greater than 16 mm are diagnostic (Neilson and Hollman 1994). The sensitivity of ultrasound is 97%, the specificity 99% and the positive predictive value 99%. Additional findings include non-relaxation of the pylorus, prominent gastric peristalsis and failure to detect fluid passing from the stomach into the duodenum. Problems may arise in infants who present at a younger age, or who were born preterm, where although the morphological appearances are those of hypertrophic pyloric stenosis, muscle thickness and canal length do not meet the above criteria. In these circumstances the pyloric muscle index may be helpful (Carver et al. 1988), but experience of the sonographer in observing the ancillary signs is probably more important. If the examination is equivocal a repeat scan in 24–48 h is often diagnostic.

Pitfalls include over-distension of the stomach, which displaces the pylorus posteriorly, making it difficult to find; in such cases nasogastric aspiration of the stomach is recommended. An empty stomach with a collapsed antrum may simulate an abnormal pylorus, but allowing the infant to ingest small amounts of clear fluid to distend the antrum in a controlled fashion will usually clarify the situation. If there is a nasogastric tube in place the stomach should be emptied at the end of the examination. It is good practice to examine the whole abdomen in infants suspected of having hypertrophic pyloric stenosis, especially if the pylorus appears normal, as other causes of vomiting may be identified.

If ultrasound is normal or equivocal and hypertrophic pyloric stenosis is still suspected, an upper gastrointestinal contrast study should be considered. This will confirm the diagnosis or identify an alternative cause for vomiting. Elongation and curvature of the pyloric canal with a string appearance and mass effect upon the antrum and base of the duodenal cap are typical findings (Fig. 3.23d). There may be considerable delay in gastric emptying and patience is required if the typical features are not to be missed. Gastro-oesophageal reflux is commonly seen in the presence of hypertrophic pyloric stenosis.

3.4.5
Inguinal Hernia

Inguinal hernia occurs in about 1%–2% of live births and is due to persistence of the processus vaginalis.

This is patent in 80%–90% of newborn infants, closing by the age of 2 years, but in a minority it persists throughout childhood, predisposing to inguinal hernia. There is a higher incidence of inguinal hernia in preterm infants and those of low birth weight, with up to 50% of preterm infants having bilateral herniae. Males are more commonly affected than females in a 4:1 ratio. Half of all herniae present by the age of 6 months. They may present as asymptomatic inguinal lumps or with pain and vomiting due to obstruction if incarceration has occurred. In skilled hands manual reduction of an apparently irreducible hernia is usually possible but urgent surgery is occasionally required.

Plain films have little role to play in the management of inguinal herniae. Occasionally the clinician may have difficulty in distinguishing a hydrocoele from a hernia or in deciding whether a hernia has been fully reduced, in which case a plain radiograph may be helpful in showing bowel gas in the inguinal region (Fig. 3.24). However, bowel may only contain fluid and so the absence of gas in the inguinal region does not exclude the presence of a hernia. In established obstruction, small bowel dilatation may be seen. If on clinical examination a groin swelling is not appreciated as a hernia, ultrasound may be re-

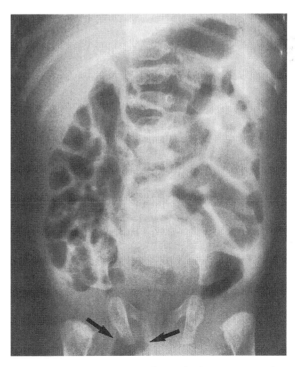

Fig. 3.24. Inguinal hernia. Radiograph showing gas within bowel in the right inguinal region, associated with generalised mild small bowel dilatation indicating obstruction

quested. It may show the defect in the inguinal canal containing herniated bowel, omentum or fluid. There is no place for contrast studies of the gastrointestinal tract as a routine investigation. Occasionally, however, a study done for other reasons will show small bowel in the inguinal canal.

3.4.6
Mesenteric Cyst

The abdomen is an uncommon location for a lymphangioma but they may occur in the mesentery and retroperitoneum. These children may present as an emergency with a mass, pain and occasionally vomiting (Ros at al. 1987), especially if there is haemorrhage or infection within the cyst. A more chronic presentation is simply with longstanding abdominal distension, especially if the lesion is retroperitoneal.

Plain radiographs show displacement of bowel loops and occasionally obstruction, especially if there is a volvulus around the mass. Ultrasound demonstrates a cystic mass which is usually multilocular. Cysts may show varying degrees of echogenicity due to debris, haemorrhage or infection (Fig. 3.25). When the cyst is unilocular a single wall is a helpful finding in differentiation from a duplication cyst. Computed tomography may show enhancement of septa and cyst walls and will better demonstrate retroperitoneal extension. Contrast studies will show displacement of adjacent bowel but other than this are normal unless obstruction is present. Lymphangiomas may vary in size markedly over the course of time because of

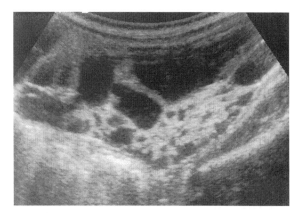

Fig. 3.25. Mesenteric cyst/lymphangioma. Ultrasound of the right flank showing a multicystic mass which was intimately related to several loops of bowel

alterations in lymph drainage or in response to infection.

3.4.7
Ingestion of Foreign Bodies

Ingestion of foreign bodies is typically a problem of young children owing to their inquisitiveness and propensity for putting objects into their mouths. Most occur in children under 5 years, with coins being the commonest ingested objects (CAMPBELL et al. 1983; TOWBIN et al. 1989; HARNED et al. 1997). At least (80%) of ingested bodies, sharp or blunt, will pass into the stomach (Fig. 3.26) and onward without mishap. Impaction is usually in the oesophagus, with 70% located above the thoracic inlet at the level of the cricopharyngeus muscle and most of the remainder at the gastro-oesophageal junction.

Delay in diagnosis and removal of impacted objects is associated with increased morbidity. Approximately 20%–35% of children with impacted coins are asymptomatic (SCHUNK et al. 1989; CARAVATI et al. 1989). Dysphagia and drooling are usually prominent in those with a short history of impaction whilst respiratory symptoms (cough, stridor) predominate in longstanding cases (MACPHERSON et al. 1996; HARNED et al. 1997). Impaction at unusual sites in the oesophagus suggests the presence of a pre-existing abnormality and complications of impaction include perforation, stricture, diverticula formation and airway narrowing (Fig. 3.27).

Imaging has an important role in children who may have ingested foreign bodies, including those who are asymptomatic (SCHUNK et al. 1989). Most metallic objects are readily visible on radiographs, with coins being differentiated from ingested disc batteries by the en-face double density and bevelled profile of the latter (MAVES et al. 1986). Plastic and aluminium objects may not be visible on plain films (EGGLI et al. 1986; HERMAN and McALISTER 1991) so further evaluation is needed if one of these may have been ingested and radiography is negative.

A lateral radiograph of the soft tissues of the neck and a frontal film of the chest and upper abdomen are required even in the absence of symptoms. Oedema and narrowing of the cervical trachea may be present if an object is impacted at the thoracic inlet (Fig. 3.28) and more than one object may be detected. Mediastinal gas is an indicator of oesophageal perforation. It is important to recognise disc

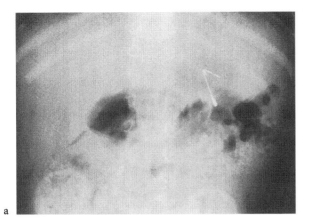

a

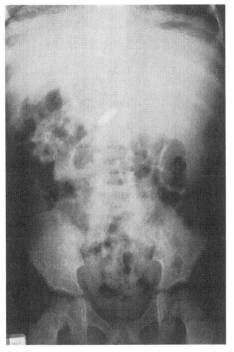

b

Fig. 3.26 a,b. Ingested foreign body. Plain radiograph shows an open safety pin (a) and a coin within the stomach. (b) Incidental unrelated splenomegaly is present due to portal hypertension

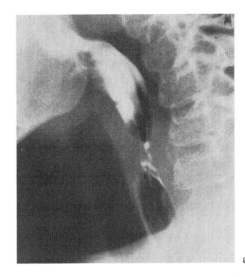

a

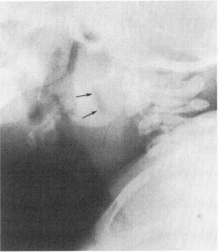

b

Fig. 3.27 a,b. Complications of foreign body ingestion. a An upper oesophageal stricture and b traumatic pharyngeal perforation and retropharyngeal abscess with widening of the retropharyngeal soft tissues with several linear air collections (*arrows*)

batteries as they are generally removed even if they have reached the stomach, as they may corrode and leak and cause severe caustic burns. A child who has swallowed a foreign body may complain of a sensation of sticking in the throat due to oesophageal oedema, even after the object has been proven to lie within the stomach. Once in the stomach, foreign bodies are generally allowed to pass naturally and there is no indication for follow-up radiographs as long as the child remains asymptomatic.

Retrieval of impacted objects from the oesophagus should be undertaken promptly to prevent

complications (Fig. 3.28) and in the United Kingdom this is achieved by oesophagoscopy under general anaesthesia. In North America extraction of foreign bodies using a Foley catheter under fluoroscopic guidance has been popular (CAMPBELL et al. 1983; KIRKS et al. 1992) though concerns about safety have led to its recent decline (MEYER 1991). If it is to be attempted the object should be blunt and present for less than 24h with no evidence of tracheal narrowing (TOWBIN et al. 1989). The airway must be protected and the object retrieved swiftly from the pharynx in order to avoid airway obstruction.

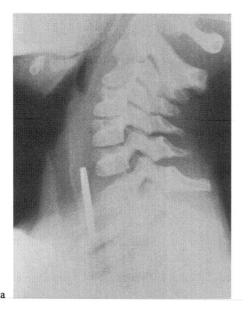
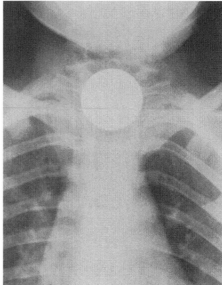

Fig. 3.28 a,b. Impacted oesophageal foreign body. **a** Lateral and **b** frontal radiographs of the neck showing an impacted coin just above the thoracic inlet with slight narrowing of the cervical trachea

3.4.8
Heavy Metal Ingestion

Heavy metal ingestion is now extremely uncommon since the introduction of modern leadless pencils but may cause abdominal pain and in the long-term neurological or haematological abnormalities. Plain abdominal radiographs may show scattered metallic densities projected over the gastrointestinal tract, and chronic ingestion of lead (or other heavy metal) can cause metaphyseal sclerosis which may be identified in the iliac crests and proximal femora.

3.4.9
Caustic Ingestion

Caustic ingestion may cause severe mucosal inflammation with ulceration, necrosis, perforation and later extensive stricture formation. Damage to the oesophagus tends to be worse than to the stomach as gastric secretions partly neutralise ingested alkali.

Chest radiographs in the acute phase may show a dilated air-filled atonic oesophagus if damage is severe and pneumomediastinum or hydropneumothorax if perforation has occurred. Endoscopy is used for assessment of the extent and severity of damage to the upper gastrointestinal mucosa and contrast studies are generally not required. If such studies are performed, water-soluble contrast media

should be used and may show ulceration and perforation. They are useful to document established strictures in the healing phase, which may require serial dilatation over a period of 12 months or more.

3.4.10
Intussusception

Idiopathic intussusception typically occurs between 6 and 18 months of age and is due to intraluminal prolapse of a segment of bowel which is then propelled distally by peristalsis. About 85% of cases arise in the distal ileum and pass into the colon (ileo-colic), but a small number arise either in the colon (colo-colic) or within the ileum (ileo-ileal), often related to a pathological lead point such as a duplication cyst (STONE et al. 1980; NORTON et al. 1993). Intussusception causes variable bowel obstruction and ischaemia which may lead to necrosis and perforation.

Typical symptoms include colicky abdominal pain in 80% of affected children, vomiting in about 75% and the passage of "redcurrant jelly" stool in 60%. True rectal bleeding is a late event indicating mucosal compromise. About 10% of patients present with diarrhoea and vomiting mimicking gastroenteritis and sometimes lethargy and drowsiness lead to consideration of meningitis or septicaemia. A tender mass is palpable in about 80% of children though

Table 3.23. Lead points and conditions predisposing to intussusception

Duplication cyst
Meckel's diverticulum
Polyp
Lymphoma/leukaemia
Henoch-Schönlein purpura
Cystic fibrosis
Haemolytic uraemic syndrome
Haemangioma
Lymphangioma
Lipoma
Other tumours
Bezoars
Intestinal parasites

Table 3.24. Plain film signs in intussusception

Soft tissue mass outline by colonic gas
Mass containing mottled lucencies
Gasless right flank
Non-visualisation of the tip of the caecum
Non-visualisation of the liver border
Small bowel obstruction
Gasless abdomen
Normal
Free air

clinical examination may be difficult, particularly during bouts of crying.

Idiopathic intussusception is caused by hypertrophy of Peyer's patches in the distal ileum. The latter act as a lead point. The incidence of idiopathic intussusception is increased in spring and autumn, suggesting a viral aetiology. Chronic presentations with recurrent abdominal pain may occur (WATSON and BISSET 1994) and do not preclude non-operative reduction, though a pathological lead point or underlying predisposing condition (e.g. cystic fibrosis) is more likely (HOLMES et al. 1991). Indeed, it is not uncommon to see transient intussusceptions of the small bowel in children with cystic fibrosis. Overall the incidence of lead points is less than 5%; lead points are commoner in those under 3 months and over 3 years of age, and the commonest is a Meckel's diverticulum (Table 3.23).

The diagnosis of intussusception may be confirmed by plain radiography if a soft tissue mass surrounded by colonic air is identified (Fig. 3.29). The presence of small lucencies due to fat within a soft tissue mass is highly suggestive of intussusception, as is a circular soft tissue mass with peripheral lucency (RATCLIFFE et al. 1992; LEE 1994; DANEMAN and ACTON 1996). Secondary small bowel obstruction may be present. In about 25% of patients plain radiographs are normal (ALFORD et al. 1992), in 50% the features are suggestive (SARGENT et al. 1994) and in the remainder the findings are non-specific. The more signs that are present, the more likely an intussusception (MERADJI et al. 1993; YANG et al. 1995) but there is considerable intra- and inter-observer variation in their interpretation (Table 3.24).The role of plain radiographs in suspected intussusception has been recently questioned (SARGENT et al. 1994; DANEMAN and ALTOW 1996), especially in view of the increased use of ultrasound, which has sensitivities and specificities of almost 100% (PRACOS et al. 1987; VERSCHELDEN et al. 1992) in both confirming and excluding the presence of intussusception (Fig. 3.30). Even if the plain radiograph is diagnostic, ultrasound should still be performed as pathological lead points may be identified and absence of detectable blood flow on colour Doppler may have implications for the likelihood of non-operative reduction.

A high frequency (5–7.5 MHz) linear array probe should be used. The characteristic sonographic appearance of intussusception was originally described as a target in cross-section. It has a hyperechoic centre and hypoechoic periphery, with a "pseudo-kidney" appearance in longitudinal section (SWISCHUK et al. 1985). The use of high-resolution scanners has refined these appearances into a series of concentric rings representing the intussuscipiens and the entering and returning limbs of the intussusceptum (HAYDEN 1996). A "crescent in doughnut" configuration has been described (DELPOZO et al. 1996a) in which the apex of the intussusception and its trailing mesentery can be identified, the latter causing a curvilinear echogenicity on transverse scans (DANEMAN and ALTON 1996). There appears to be no correlation between the size of the intussusception and its reducibility. Absent blood flow on colour Doppler may indicate those with compromised bowel for whom surgery and bowel resection will be required whilst its presence suggests non-operative reduction is more likely to be successful (LIM et al. 1994; LAGALLA et al. 1994). The accuracy of these findings remains to be determined (KONG et al. 1997). Evidence of trapped fluid between the walls of the entering and returning limbs of the intussusceptum is associated with a lower reduction rate and an increased incidence of bowel compromise (DELPOZO et al. 1996b). Small amounts of free intraperitoneal fluid are, however, common, especially where there is small bowel obstruction, and do not affect management. Ultrasound may detect pathological

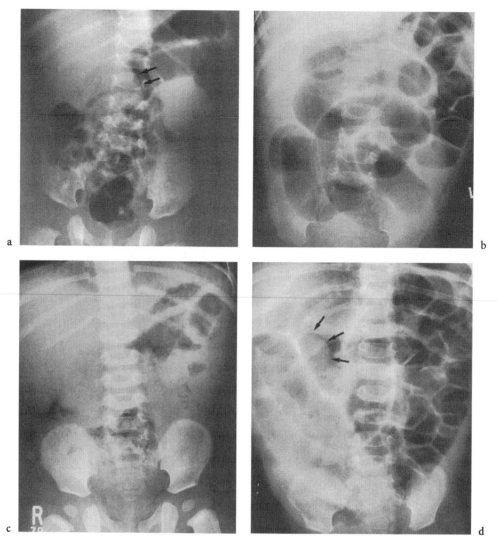

Fig. 3.29 a–d. Intussusception. Plain radiographs showing suggestive appearances. **a** A soft tissue mass in the transverse colon, producing an abrupt "cut-off" (*arrows*). **b** Multiple dilated loops of small bowel indicating high-grade obstruction. **c** a paucity of bowel gas in the right flank. **d** Partial small bowel obstruction with a soft tissue mass visible in the right upper abdomen (*arrows*)

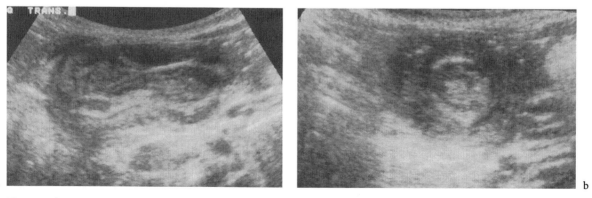

Fig. 3.30 a,b. Intussusception. Transverse (**a**) and longitudinal (**b**) ultrasound scans showing the characteristic appearance of multiple concentric rings and eccentric central echogenicity (invaginated mesenteric fat)

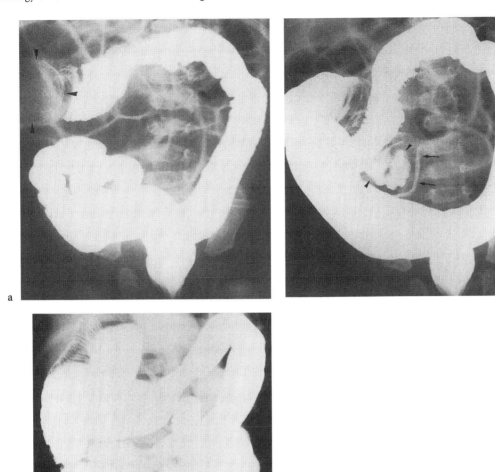

Fig. 3.31 a–c. Intussusception. Barium enema showing **a** coiled spring appearance of an intussusception in the proximal transverse colon (*arrowheads*), **b** partial reduction, with filling of the caecal pole (*arrowheads*) and appendix (*arrows*) but no reflux into terminal ileum and **c** complete reduction with reflux into multiple loops of ileum

lead points such as duplication cysts and inverted Meckel's diverticula (DANEMAN et al. 1997).

Non-operative reduction has been the preferred method of management of intussusception for many years, with surgery reserved for those cases which cannot be reduced or those patients too unwell to undergo an attempt. Until recently hydrostatic reduction by barium enema was the most popular method in Europe and North America (Fig. 3.31), though it is now being replaced by pneumatic reduction (Fig. 3.32) (STEIN et al. 1992; GU et al. 1988). In South-east Asia ultrasound-guided hydrostatic reduction using water or water-soluble contrast medium is popular (CHAN et al. 1997; CHOI et al. 1994; PEH et al. 1996; ROHRSCHNEIDER and TROGER 1995). Both pneumatic and ultrasound-guided methods are reported to have greater reduction rates compared with barium, but there are no controlled studies confirming this. A practical advantage of the use of pneumatic reduction is that it is quick, dry and less messy and so the infant is at less risk of cooling.

Absolute contraindications to attempted reduction by any technique are perforation, peritonitis and the inability to satisfactorily resuscitate the child. The most important factor in predicting outcome appears to be duration of symptoms, with

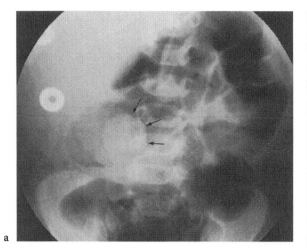

a

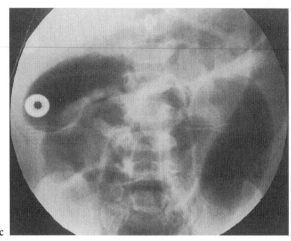

c

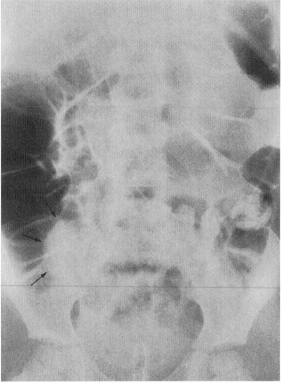

b

Fig. 3.32 a–c. Intussusception. Air enema showing **a** intussusception in the transverse colon outline by air (*arrows*) and **b** residual soft tissue "mass" due to an oedematous ileocaecal valve (*arrows*) in the ileocaecal region with reflux of air into distal ileum. **c** A further attempt resulted in abolition of this mass with reflux of air into the terminal ileum

those greater than 48 h more likely to have failed reduction, perforation and need for bowel resection (STEIN et al. 1992), though this of itself does not preclude attempted non-operative reduction. Rectal bleeding, an ileo-ileocolic intussusception and small bowel obstruction are also considered important adverse determinants of outcome (MCDERMOTT et al. 1994), but are not absolute contraindications to careful attempted non-operative reduction.

When performing reduction with barium the reservoir should be 3 feet above the table. Pressure is applied for as long as the intussusception is moving retrogradely but only for 3 min if there is no progress, and a total of three attempts may be made. This "rule of threes" is modified slightly when using air in that a maximum pressure of 120 mmHg is applied. A 5-foot column is utilised when water or a water-soluble contrast medium (under ultrasound control) is employed.

Complete reduction is confirmed by reflux of air, barium or water into the terminal ileum and disappearance of the soft tissue mass. Differentiation of a non-reduced intussusception from oedema of the ileocaecal valve (which may be marked) may be aided by ultrasound and clinical observation if the infant is stable or by a repeat enema after several hours.

Non-reduction of an intussusception by the above criteria used to be considered an indication for surgery. It is now recognised that in a stable child a repeat enema after 4–6 h may permit reduction of up to 50% of these cases, probably because some of the oedema and venous congestion of the intussusceptum and ileocaecal valve has subsided (SAXTON et al. 1994; CONNOLLY et al. 1995). The use of air following an unsuccessful attempt with barium seems to be safe (DANEMAN and ALTON 1996) though success rates may be less than if air is the initial modality. Some intussusceptions will spontaneously resolve (SWISCHUK et al. 1994), perhaps explaining why some "irreducible" intussusceptions will have undergone reduction between the radiology department and the operating theatre. Some of these probably represent those reduced during induction of anaesthesia and those not appreciated to have been reduced in the radiology department.

An expectant approach can be taken to infants in whom the soft tissue mass is abolished by enema without the demonstration of reflux into the distal ileum (EIN et al. 1994; PIERRO et al. 1993). Sonography may be reassuring in this situation as it may confirm absence of residual intussusception and show the typical thickened appearance of the ileocaecal valve and variable wall thickening of the distal ileum (ROHRSCHNEIDER et al. 1994). An unsuspected lead point may be identified. If concern about successful reduction persists, a repeat enema can be performed.

Identification of lead points may be less easy with pneumatic reduction (MILLER et al. 1995) than with barium, which is a good reason to perform ultrasound prior to attempted reduction (STRINGER et al. 1992). A lead point may not prevent successful reduction (DON et al. 1992; MILLER et al. 1995), though even incomplete reduction will facilitate subsequent surgery as less bowel handling will be required.

Perforation of the colon is a real possibility whichever method is used to reduce intussusception. There is good evidence that perforations occurring during pneumatic reduction are smaller, easier to repair and result in less faecal contamination of the peritoneal cavity than those occurring during reduction with barium (SHIELS et al. 1993; DANEMAN et al. 1995). Barium has the added disadvantage of inducing peritoneal granulomata and adhesions and is less easily removed from the peritoneal cavity. A specific complication of pneumatic reduction is a tension pneumoperitoneum for which a large-bore needle must be available for immediate decompression. The incidence of perforation is approximately 0.5% with both techniques but it is likely that many already exist within necrotic bowel and are simply uncovered during intussusception reduction (BRAMSON and BLICKMAN 1992).

Between 5% and 10% of intussusceptions will recur (after surgical and non-operative reduction). There is no contraindication to repeat non-operative reduction (FECTEAU et al. 1996), though there is a slightly lower success rate in those initially reduced surgically compared with those reduced non-operatively. Of intussusceptions that recur, one-

third do so in the first 24h and nearly one-half between 3 and 6 months, with lead points found in up to 10% of these patients. With further recurrence (1%–2%), serious consideration must be given to the possibility of an underlying lead point and many surgeons would elect to operate at this time. If non-operative reduction is successful, a diligent search for a predisposing cause using ultrasound, barium follow through, barium enema and a Meckel's scan is worthwhile.

Although many centres use sedation prior to attempted reduction there is no convincing evidence of its utility in increasing the reduction rate. Sedation may be counterproductive with pneumatic reduction in that allowing the child to strain and perform Valsalva manoeuvres during the procedure allows transient episodes of increased intraluminal pressure (>120 mmHg) with no increase in transmural pressure and so may aid reduction (SHIELS et al. 1991). However, a narcotic such as morphine means less discomfort for the infant during the procedure and is advocated. Muscle relaxants such as glucagon have no role to play. The risk of bacteraemia during intussusception reduction appears to be low (SOMEKH et al. 1996), but prophylactic antibiotics should be given to those at risk of endocarditis.

Reported success rates of non-operative management are variable because of different techniques and selection criteria, but a rate of 75%–80% is reasonable if attempts are made on all infants except those for whom immediate surgery is indicated. Given the speed and cleanliness of air reduction and its potential for a reduction in radiation dose (PERSLIDEN et al. 1996) it is likely to continue to be adopted in preference to barium.

3.4.11
Henoch-Schölein Purpura

Henoch-Schölein purpura is an idiopathic inflammatory disorder causing a small-vessel vasculitis. It affects skin, joints, kidneys and bowel, with gastrointestinal symptoms usually following the onset of rash and arthralgia, although in a minority they may occur first and so lead to diagnostic difficulty. Abdominal symptoms occur in most patients (COUTURE et al. 1992), with pain (60%) and bleeding (50%) being prominent. The diagnosis is made on clinical findings of purpuric rash affecting the buttocks and lower extremities and transient arthralgias

(GLASIER et al. 1981). The typical age is 3–7 years and there is a male predominance.

The initial radiological investigation is the plain radiograph, which may show bowel wall thickening due to haemorrhage and oedema tending preferentially to affect the duodenum and jejunum (GLASIER et al. 1981; DOYLE and MULLANY 1986). Small bowel obstruction due to haemorrhage or intussusception may occur (COUTURE et al. 1992). Most of these cases are ileo-ileal and so are not amenable to hydrostatic or pneumatic reduction, though some will resolve spontaneously. Perforation is rare and will be indicated by the presence of free intraperitoneal gas. There is an increased incidence of appendicitis in Henoch-Schölein purpura.

Ultrasound done to investigate the cause of the abdominal pain shows bowel wall thickening (HAYDEN 1996; BOMELBURG et al. 1991; COUTURE et al. 1992; HU et al. 1991) which may be focal or diffuse, as well as free fluid, mesenteric lymphadenopathy, decreased peristalsis and gallbladder wall thickening (PERRY et al. 1990). Ileo-ileal intussusception may be identified and when it appears "loose", periodic sonographic observation may permit conservative management (HU et al. 1991; CONNOLLY and O'HALPIN 1994). The sensitivity of ultrasound for the detection of bowel wall thickening is probably greater than that of plain films and it usually obviates the need for contrast studies and provides an ideal modality for follow-up. This is especially important in a condition which may have a relapsing course.

Contrast studies are not routinely indicated. If performed because of diagnostic uncertainty following plain films and ultrasound, they show eccentric mucosal thickening most marked in the duodenum and proximal jejunum (Fig. 3.33) (DOYLE and MULLANY 1986) with variable separation of bowel loops reflecting wall thickening. Thumbprinting in the colon indicates oedema and haemorrhage.

3.4.12
Anal Fissure

Anal fissure is a very common cause of rectal bleeding at all ages; it also leads to pain on defaecation and is associated with constipation. Visual inspection of the anal canal will confirm the diagnosis and imaging is not required.

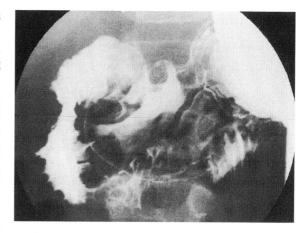

Fig. 3.33. Henoch-Schönlein purpura. Barium meal shows thickening of duodenal folds and annular narrowing of the second part of the duodenum

3.4.13
Infection

Gastroenteritis is common in this age group and presents no diagnostic difficulty when typical features of diarrhoea, vomiting and mild abdominal pain are present. Problems may arise if pain is severe and there is marked abdominal tenderness or prominent rectal bleeding, when an acute abdomen or intussusception may be considered.

Viral infection is more frequent than bacterial infection, with rotavirus, adenovirus and the Norwalk agent (LIEBERMAN 1994) being common causes in children. Imaging is usually not required in straightforward cases but may be helpful in those with severe disease or atypical clinical findings. Plain radiographs are often normal (Fig. 3.34) but may show mild dilatation of small and large bowel (Figs. 3.35, 3.36), often with multiple short air-fluid levels if erect films are obtained. Gastroenteritis is a rare cause of pneumatosis (Fig. 3.37) (CAPITANIO and GREENBERG 1991).

Ultrasound is helpful in gastroenteritis in excluding entities such as intussusception or appendicitis and will show fluid-filled hyperperistaltic loops of bowel with little or no evidence of wall thickening. Some free fluid may be present and transient small bowel intussusception is occasionally encountered (HAYDEN 1996). Colour Doppler usually shows no increase in bowel wall blood flow (QUILLIN and SIEGEL 1993, 1994a).

Bacterial infection of the gut is less common and tends to affect older children. It may result in severe

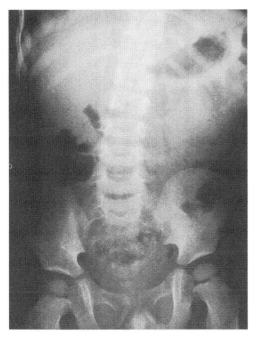

Fig. 3.34. Gastroenteritis. Normal plain abdominal radiograph

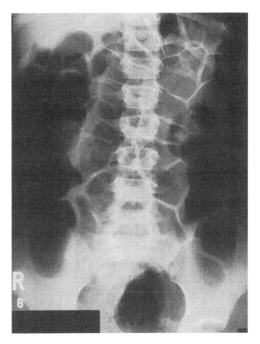

Fig. 3.36. Gastroenteritis. Plain abdominal radiograph showing marked gaseous distension of the large bowel

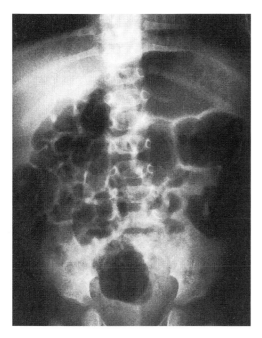

Fig. 3.35. Gastroenteritis. Plain abdominal radiograph showing modest gaseous distension of the small and large bowel

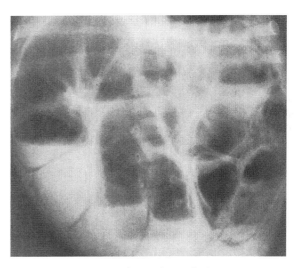

Fig. 3.37. Pneumatosis. Plain radiograph showing extensive linear pneumatosis of bowel in an infant with gastroenteritis. Multiple air-fluid levels are present in dilated loops of bowel

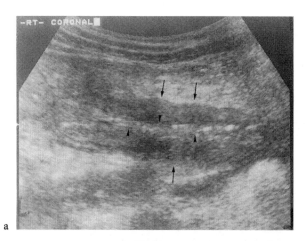

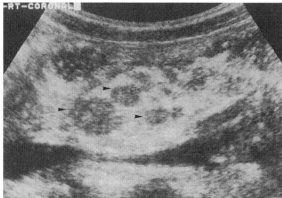

Fig. 3.39. "Mesenteric adenitis". Ultrasound shows multiple enlarged lymph nodes (*arrowheads*) at the base of the mesentery, anterior to the inferior vena cava

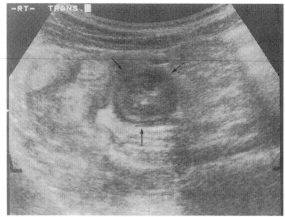

Fig. 3.38 a,b. Infective terminal ileitis. Longitudinal (a) and transverse (b) sonograms showing thickened hypoechoic bowel wall (*arrows*) and compressed echogenic central mucosa (*arrowheads*)

abdominal pain, in addition to diarrhoea and vomiting, which may be sufficient to simulate an acute abdomen. Common organisms include *Salmonella enteritidis*, *Campylobacter jejuni* and *Yersinia enterocolitica*.

Plain radiographs may be obtained when symptoms are severe and simulate other pathology. They may be normal or show a localised ileus or rarely a toxic megacolon if there is severe colitis. Ultrasound is helpful when an acute abdomen is a consideration and may demonstrate wall thickening of the affected bowel (Fig. 3.38), most often the terminal ileum and right colon (PUYLAERT et al. 1988, 1989; HAYDEN 1996; MATSUMOTO et al. 1991). Mesenteric lymphadenopathy is common (Fig. 3.39). The bowel wall may exhibit increased mucosal blood flow on colour Doppler (QUILLIN and SIEGEL 1993, 1994a). A similar appearance may be caused by Crohn's disease

and typhlitis, though clinical and sonographic follow-up should help differentiate the conditions. Increased blood flow in Crohn's disease tends to be transmural (QUILLIN and SIEGEL 1994a).

3.4.14
Gastro-oesophageal Reflux

Gastro-oesophageal reflux is a common occurrence in neonates and young infants, which in the vast majority of cases is physiological and not pathological. A poorly developed lower oesophageal sphincter and a short intra-abdominal course of the oesophagus allow relatively easy retrograde passage of gastric contents into the oesophagus. During the first year of life the incidence of gastro-oesophageal reflux declines rapidly as the lower sphincter matures. The incidence of reflux is highest in neurologically impaired children, in those who have had repair of oesophageal atresia and in preterm infants.

Symptoms include vomiting, which occurs soon after feeds, aspiration, recurrent chest infections, failure to thrive and pain and dysphagia due to peptic oesophageal ulceration and stricture. Diagnosis is usually by 24h pH probe monitoring with imaging reserved for detecting anatomical abnormalities such as hiatus hernia and malrotation or complications such as peptic stricture.Infants occasionally present as an emergency because of severe vomiting which is clinically confused with hypertrophic pyloric stenosis. The reflux may be detected during ultrasound examination for this condition, but is usually observed on contrast studies undertaken for investigation of the vomiting after a normal ultra-sound scan.

3.4.15
Congenital Diaphragmatic Hernia

A small proportion (5%) of patients with congenital diaphragmatic herniae present after the neonatal period and may cause diagnostic confusion. Whilst respiratory symptoms predominate, a significant number will have gastrointestinal symptoms (BERMAN et al. 1988), including recurrent vomiting, diarrhoea and failure to thrive. These children usually present as outpatients rather than as emergencies. The main exception to this is when there is an intercurrent chest infection or bowel herniation through a right-sided defect previously plugged by liver. The child then presents with increased respiratory difficulty, or if there is strangulation or obstruction of herniated bowel, with pain and vomiting.

Plain films may be diagnostic, showing bowel passing from the abdomen into the thorax (Fig. 3.40), but confusion with staphylococcal pneumonia, pneumatocoeles, gastric volvulus and pneumothorax may occur (SIEGEL et al. 1981). The presence of a scaphoid abdomen with little bowel gas is helpful and erect radiographs may show air-fluid levels within intrathoracic bowel. Many patients will have had previously normal chest radiographs.

Confirmation with barium studies is essential if there is any diagnostic confusion so as to prevent inappropriate therapy. Sonography may be useful, showing absence of the diaphragm and the presence of bowel in the pleural cavity. Bochdalek herniae are commoner than Morgagni herniae with most of the former left-sided and the latter right-sided (BERMAN et al. 1988).

3.4.16
Meckel's Diverticulum

A Meckel's diverticulum arises from the anti-mesenteric border of the distal ileum. It represents a remnant of the omphalomesenteric duct joining the fetal midgut to the yolk sac (Table 3.25). It is present in approximately 2% of individuals (GHAHREMANI 1986), is 5 cm long, has a broad base and contains all layers of bowel wall. Most Meckel's diverticula are asymptomatic, but in up to 15%–25% of affected in-

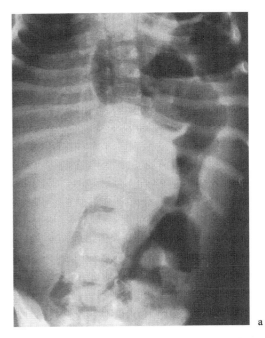

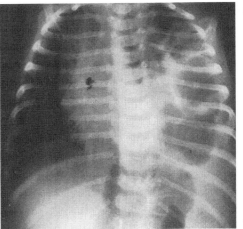

Fig. 3.40 a,b. Diaphragmatic hernia. Supine abdominal (a) and chest (b) radiographs show dilated gas-filled bowel in the left flank extending into the left hemithorax. There is some mediastinal deviation to the right

dividuals, usually those in whom the Meckel's diverticulum contains ectopic gastric mucosa, it may present clinically. More than 50% of patients who become symptomatic do so before the age of 2 years.

The main complications of Meckel's diverticula in this age are bleeding and obstruction, usually due to an intussusception or more seriously a volvulus around the diverticulum or related omphalomesenteric band. Diverticulitis, clinically indistinguishable from appendicitis, stone formation and perforation are commoner presentations in older children and young adults.

Table 3.25. Complications of omphalomesenteric remnants

Intussusception
Bleeding
Neonatal obstruction
   Bands
   Volvulus/internal hernia
Diverticulitis
Perforation
Stone formation
Umbilical fistula
Cyst

Rectal bleeding is the most frequent emergency presentation of a Meckel's diverticulum, typically occurring under the age of 2 years (O'HARA 1996). Bleeding is usually painless, bright red and self-limiting and arises from ulceration of adjacent ileum due to acid secretion by ectopic gastric mucosa.

The most useful imaging investigation is a technetium-99m pertechnetate isotope scan. Images of the abdomen acquired over 1 h following injection show normal tracer accumulation in the stomach and some urinary excretion. A Meckel's diverticulum shows progressive tracer uptake mirroring gastric activity and is usually located in the lower right abdomen (Fig. 3.41). The examination is 90% accurate in children (SFAKIANAKIS and CONWAY 1981; COONEY et al. 1982), with false-positives caused by duplication cysts, haemangiomas, intussusception , ectopic kidney and inflammatory bowel disease (COONEY et al. 1982). False-negatives may occur if the amount of ectopic gastric mucosa is too little to detect with the gamma camera or if the diverticulum overlies bladder. A lower abdominal image with the bladder empty or a lateral view may be useful. Angiography may be required in rare instances; this may be positive even in the absence of active bleeding (ROUTH et al. 1990).

Obstruction and pain may be caused by intussusception associated with inversion of the diverticulum. Rarely the diverticulum prolapses into an inguinal hernial sac (Littre's hernia). If obstruction occurs, plain radiographs will show varying degrees of small bowel dilatation, but do not usually permit a specific diagnosis. A giant Meckel's diverticulum may appear as an isolated, often spherical gas collection and may contain an air-fluid level with no evidence of generalised small bowel dilatation. Occasionally a calcified concretion may be identified in the lower abdomen representing a stone within the diverticulum, and rarely a polypoid intraluminal soft tissue mass is visible due to an inverted diver-

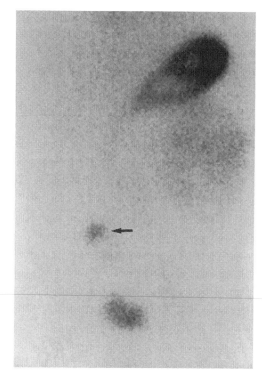

Fig. 3.41. Meckel"s diverticulum. A pertechnetate scan shows a distinct focus of abnormal tracer uptake in the right lower abdomen (*arrow*)

ticulum (JOHNSON et al. 1993). The detection of the diverticulum on small bowel contrast studies is quite specific but unusual: if inverted it may appear as a polypoid intraluminal filling defect (GAISIE et al. 1993).

Ultrasound may assume a greater role in the management of children with gastrointestinal bleeding in the future as Meckel's diverticula associated with intussusception and bleeding have been identified (FINK et al. 1995). A blind-ending short segment (3–4 cm) of thick-walled gut appears characteristic and may be detected even when it acts as a lead point for an intussusception (HAYDEN 1996).

3.4.17
Wandering Spleen

Wandering spleen is a very uncommon entity and is due to malfixation of the spleen because of lax or absent supporting ligaments. It typically presents in infancy as an acute abdomen with severe pain. Torsion of the splenic pedicle leads to ischaemia and ultimately infarction.

Plain radiographs show a variable bowel gas pattern, with the diagnosis suggested by the presence of a soft tissue mass and absence of the normal splenic outline in the left upper abdomen.

Sonography may confirm absence of the spleen from its normal position and its presence in the mid abdomen, where it is variably enlarged and hypoechoic with reduced or absent blood flow on Doppler. Computed tomography may be required if the spleen cannot be identified with ultrasound because of overlying bowel gas (HERMAN and SIEGEL 1991b).

3.5
The Older Child

Acute gastrointestinal emergencies in older children overlap those of adults, with acute appendicitis, mesenteric adenitis and trauma being common. Pain may be due to inflammatory conditions, obstruction or trauma (Table 3.26) and is generally better localised than in younger children. However, it may also be caused by a variety of non-gastrointestinal conditions (Table 3.27). Vomiting is frequently associated with pain in children, particularly in bowel obstruction, but like pain, may be due to a large number of other non-gastrointestinal conditions

such as diabetes mellitus, pyelonephritis, raised intracranial pressure and poisoning (Table 3.28). Gastrointestinal bleeding is less common and, as in younger children, is usually self-limiting, though a cause is more frequently identified. The nature of the bleeding (haematemesis, rectal bleeding or melaena) may help narrow the differential diagnosis, as may other symptoms such as pain or the presence of a mass (Table 3.29).

Endoscopy is the most sensitive technique for the diagnosis of upper gastrointestinal bleeding. Colonoscopy or double-contrast barium enemas are equally accurate in the evaluation of colonic bleeding, the former having the advantage that biopsy can be performed, though it requires sedation or anaesthesia. Nuclear medicine investigation techniques using either technetium-99m sulphur colloid or labelled red blood cells are useful in the localisation of obscure but active gastrointestinal bleeding (ROBINSON 1993). If a Meckel's scan is to be performed it should precede the labelled red cell scan as circulating stannous compounds may affect extraction of pertechnetate by gastric mucosa.

Table 3.26. Causes of abdominal pain in the older child

Acute appendicitis
Peptic ulcer
Trauma
Mesenteric adenitis
Cholelithiasis
Hernia
Obstruction
Pancreatitis
Intussusception
Inflammatory bowel disease
Non-gastrointestinal causes (see Table 3.27)

Table 3.27. Non-gastrointestinal causes of an acute abdomen

Lower lobe pneumonia
Diabetic ketoacidosis
Streptococcal pharyngitis
Sickle crisis
Urinary tract infection
Renal colic
Poisoning (heavy metal)
Porphyria
Abdominal migraine
Sepsis (causing ileus)
Primary peritonitis

Table 3.28. Causes of vomiting in the older child

Gastro-oesophageal reflux
Hiatus hernia
Peptic ulcer
Pancreatitis
Gastroenteritis
Malrotation
Mesenteric adenitis
Sepsis
Appendicitis
Bezoar
Drugs
Non-gastrointestinal causes see (see Table 3.27)

Table 3.29. Causes of gastrointestinal bleeding in older children

Meckel's diverticulum
Inflammatory bowel disease
Infectious colitis
Anal fissure
Haemorrhoids
Vascular anomaly
Polyp
Henoch-Schönlein purpura
Intussusception
Lymphoid nodular hyperplasia
Mallory-Weiss tear
Foreign body ingestion
Oesophageal/gastric varices
Peptic ulceration

Table 3.30. Causes of intra-abdominal calcification

Renal calculi
Gallstones
Pancreatic calcification (hereditary pancreatitis)
Meconium peritonitis
Meconium pseudocyst
Intraluminal calcification with atresias
Fistulae to genitourinary tract
Appendicolith
Meckel's diverticulum concretion
Duplication cyst
Adrenal haemorrhage
Hepatoblastoma
Hepatoma
Teratoma
Neuroblastoma

Table 3.31. Causes of bone changes on abdominal radiographs

Fractures
Rickets
Sickle cell anaemia (vertebra, femoral head)
Segmentation anomalies (VACTERL)
Avascular necrosis
Hip dislocation
Dense metaphyseal lines (heavy metal poisoning)
Lucent metaphyses (leukaemia, metastases)

Angiography may be required in the face of continued or recurrent haemorrhage.

3.5.1
Imaging Strategies

Abdominal radiographs allow easier differentiation between small and large bowel in older children than in younger children because of the larger calibre, peripheral distribution and faecal content of the large bowel in older children. Colonic haustra are better developed and more clearly seen, particularly in the right colon, and valvulae conniventes are more easily appreciated in small bowel. Normal small bowel does not exceed 2.0–2.5 cm in diameter and even when dilated does not usually exceed the calibre of large bowel. A colonic calibre greater than 6.0 cm in diameter is always abnormal and when combined with mucosal and haustral thickening indicates a toxic megacolon, though a toxic megacolon may be present with lesser degrees of colonic distension. Dilatation is a feature of obstruction, severe gastroenteritis and paralytic ileus with thickening of valvulae, haustra or bowel wall indicating inflammation or ischaemia.

Radiographs should include the lung bases and the inguinal regions. As in younger children, the supine film provides most of the necessary information required for clinical management. Erect chest radiographs are more sensitive in the detection of free intraperitoneal gas than are erect abdominal films, though a right side up decubitus abdominal film is valuable in patients too ill for an erect chest film. A search for calcification should be made, particularly in the region of the kidneys, ureters, urinary bladder, pancreas and gallbladder (Table 3.30). Bone abnor-malities may provide a clue to an underlying condition, e.g. sickle cell anaemia or lead ingestion (Table 3.31).

Intramural gas (pneumatosis) may be identified by recognition of linear or bubbly lucencies adjacent to but peripheral to intraluminal gas. Gas in the biliary tree may be differentiated from portal venous gas by its central location. Portal venous gas tends to be more peripherally located. In difficult cases ultrasound may be helpful in making this distinction.

Ultrasound has much to offer and requires little in the way of patient preparation other than a full bladder. Clear fluids may be introduced into the stomach by mouth or nasogastric tube if one is present to aid visualisation of the stomach or pancreas. Gas may also be evacuated from the stomach through a tube, though one should not be inserted simply for the purposes of the ultrasound examination without a clinical indication. Ultrasound offers reassurance and is as helpful in excluding major pathology as it is in confirming it.

3.5.2
Acute Appendicitis

Acute appendicitis has an incidence of 2–4 per 1000 per year, with a peak at about 12 years. It is not uncommon in younger children but is rare in infancy. A characteristic clinical picture is of peri-umbilical pain which moves to the right iliac fossa as focal peritoneal irritation develops, with subsequent vomiting. This presentation is less common in younger children, in whom onset and progression may be more rapid and perforation more likely, occurring in up to 80% of patients under 5 years of age (POLLACK 1996; GRAHM and ROKORNY 1980). Very young children are unable to vocalise their symptoms or localise pain and other commoner conditions such as gastroenteritis or intussusception may initially be suspected, leading to delay in diagnosis

(LUND and MURPHY 1994). Diarrhoea may be the presenting symptom of an associated pelvic abscess following perforation. In older girls it may be difficult to distinguish between ovarian pain and appendicitis and ultrasound is particularly helpful in these patients. In young children urinary tract infection is often the initial clinical diagnosis. Further confusion may occur if leucocytes are found in the urine, as may be seen in young children with appendicitis even in the absence of bacteriuria.

In most (80%) patients clinical evaluation is all that is required to make the diagnosis. Although a period of observation has been shown to be helpful with no increased morbidity (DOLGIN et al. 1992),

Table 3.32. Plain films signs in acute appendicitis

Lumbar scoliosis (concave to right)
Blurring of properitoneal flank stripe and psoas
Paucity of bowel gas in right iliac fossa
Distal small bowel obstruction
Sentinel dilated bowel loop
Appendicolith
Colon "cut-off"
Free air (very rare)
Pneumatosis

imaging has a role both in confirming the diagnosis and in suggesting alternative conditions, and without imaging the negative laparotomy rate may approach 25% (CERES et al. 1990).

Plain abdominal radiographs are often obtained in children suspected of acute appendicitis and a large number of signs have been described (Table 3.32). The most specific plain film finding is the presence of a calcified appendicolith, whose detection in a patient clinically suspected of acute appendicitis effectively confirms the diagnosis (Fig. 3.42). However, this is present only in a minority of patients (<10%). None of the other signs are very sensitive, none directly visualises the inflamed appendix (SHIMKIN 1978; VAUDAGNA and McCOET 1975; DIDONATO 1976) and normal films (present in up to 50%) do not exclude the diagnosis (FRANKEN et al. 1989).

Perforation occurs in up to 40% of patients though free gas is uncommon, probably because the omentum effectively seals off the appendix from the rest of the peritoneal cavity early in the disease. A dilated transverse colon with non-visualisation of the ascending colon (colon "cut-off") may be seen with perforation (SWISCHUK and HAYDEN 1980), as

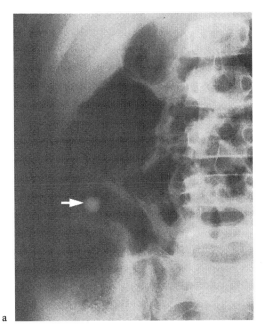
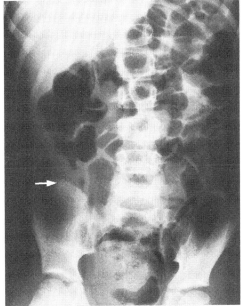

a   b

Fig. 3.42 a,b. Acute appendicitis. Plain radiographs showing a a round calcified appendicolith just superior to the iliac crest (arrow) and b absence of caecal gas and slight mass effect upon the gas-filled ascending colon. A small calcified appendicolith is projected over the iliac blade (arrow)

can disproportionate jejunal dilatation (RIGGS and
PARVEY 1976).

Ultrasound is now the most useful imaging modality in the evaluation of children in whom appendicitis is suspected (PUYLAERT 1986; HAYDEN 1996).
Diagnosis relies on the use of a high-frequency (5–
10 MHz) linear array transducer and the application
of gradual but firm compression of the lower right
abdomen, displacing bowel loops out of the field of
view. Criteria for adequate compression include the
ability to see the psoas muscle and the iliac vessels
clearly, with near apposition of the anterior and posterior abdominal walls. The examination should always include the liver, spleen, kidneys, pancreas,
gallbladder and urinary bladder as well as a search
for free or localised fluid within the abdomen and
pelvis.

The sonographic appearance of acute appendicitis
is a blind-ending, non-compressible tubular structure measuring at least 6 mm in diameter (Figs. 3.43,
3.44) (HAYDEN 1996). Peri-appendiceal fluid and an
appendicolith may be identified. Colour Doppler
imaging may show increased blood flow within the
appendix wall, increasing its conspicuity (QUILLIN
and SIEGEL 1992, 1994b). Reported rates for sensitivity and specificity are between 85% and 95% (KAO
et al. 1989; VIGNAULT et al. 1990; SIVIT et al. 1992b;
SIVIT 1993; PATRIQUIN et al. 1996). A true retrocaecal appendix, an inflamed but gas-containing appendix and appendicitis confined to the tip (LIM et al.
1996) may be very difficult to identify. A localised
ileus in the right iliac fossa is often present. Free fluid
may be present in the pelvis and right paracolic gutter in up to 29% of cases but is found in a similar
proportion among those without appendicitis (SIVIT
1993). Self-localisation by the patient has been suggested as an aid to increased sensitivity
(CHESBOROUGH et al. 1993). The normal appendix
may be identified in up to 50% of patients with
careful technique, allowing confident exclusion of
the diagnosis (SIVIT et al. 1992b, RIOUX 1992). Following perforation the above findings are present in
only about 30% of cases (QUILLIN et al. 1992;
HAYDEN 1996), with the presence of peri-appendiceal fluid a useful sign (QUILLIN et al. 1992). A
decompressed appendix related to a complex "mass"
is present in another 30% (Fig. 3.45) but in the remainder only a mass or localised or free
fluid may be seen (HAYDEN 1996). Colour Doppler
may be helpful if a hyperaemic localised fluid collection (peri-appendiceal or pelvic) is identified, indicating perforation and abscess formation (QUILLIN
and SIEGEL 1995). Remote complications such as

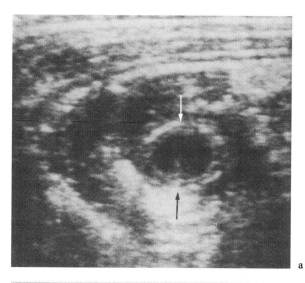

a

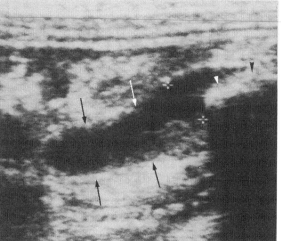

b

Fig. 3.43 a,b. Acute appendicitis. Transverse (**a**) and longitudinal (**b**) ultrasound of the right lower abdomen shows a
blind-ending, non-compressible tubular structure (*arrows*),
which contains an echogenic appendicolith near its tip that
casts an acoustic shadow (*arrowheads*)

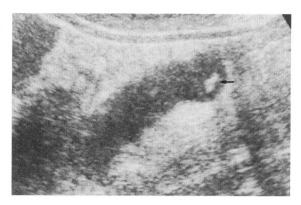

Fig. 3.44. Acute appendicitis. Longitudinal ultrasound scan of
the right abdomen showing a tubular structure with a small
appendicolith at its tip (*arrow*)

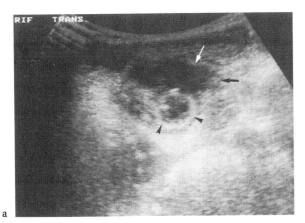

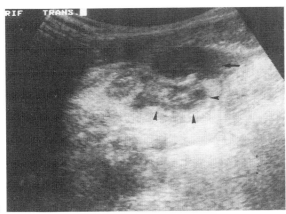

Fig. 3.45 a,b. Acute appendicitis with localised perforation. Transverse (a) and longitudinal (b) ultrasound showing a partly decompressed appendix (*arrowheads*) with an adjacent low-attenuation collection (*arrows*) representing a localised abscess

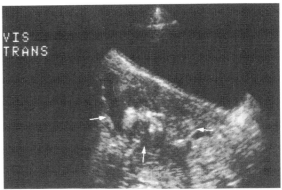

Fig. 3.46. Acute appendicitis. Pelvic ultrasound showing a complex collection posterior to the bladder (*arrows*) representing an abscess

ternative diagnosis in children suspected of having appendicitis (GAENSLER et al. 1989; SIMONOVSKY 1995; SIVIT et al. 1992b), identifying gallbladder, renal and pancreatic abnormalities, and in adolescent girls it is able to evaluate the pelvis for ovarian pathology such as cysts. Inflammatory bowel disease due to infection or Crohn's disease may be suggested by finding thickening of the wall of the terminal ileum.

Fluid collections (mostly pelvic) may be found in up to 5% of patients following appendicectomy. The majority require no specific treatment and resolve spontaneously though clinical features of sepsis unresponsive to antibiotics indicate the need for drainage (BAKER et al. 1986).

3.5.3
Abdominal Emergencies in Children with Cystic Fibrosis

Abdominal complaints are increasingly encountered in children with cystic fibrosis, some children having more intestinal than respiratory problems. Abdominal pain is common and may be caused by meconium ileus equivalent, intussusception, liver and gallbladder disease and fibrosing colonopathy. These children may also present with conditions unrelated to cystic fibrosis, as does the normal population. Emergency presentations include pain, vomiting, intestinal obstruction and, rarely, bleeding from oesophageal varices.

pelvic abscess (Fig. 3.46), liver abscess and portal vein thrombosis may be identified (SLOVIS et al. 1989).

Computed tomography is accurate in the detection of acute appendicitis both in adults (KURTIN et al. 1995) and in children and may be at least as sensitive and specific as ultrasound (FRIEDLAND and SIEGEL 1997). In uncomplicated cases it offers no advantage over ultrasound, especially as the radiation dose is high, but it is probably more sensitive for the detection of complex intraperitoneal fluid collections following perforation.

The barium enema is now of historic interest as only non-specific indirect signs (mass effect on the caecum, spasm of the terminal ileum, non-filling of the appendix) are detected (DEMOS and FLISAK 1986; FEDYSHIN et al. 1984). Perforation and peritoneal soiling with barium are reported complications (SHUST et al. 1993). Ultrasound may provide an al-

Meconium ileus equivalent, also known as distal intestinal obstruction syndrome, is so called because obstruction caused by viscid intestinal contents, usu-

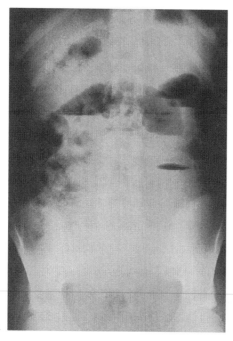 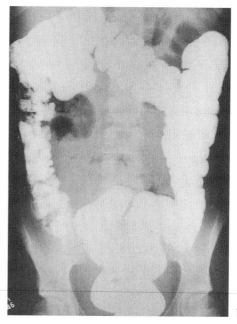

Fig. 3.47 a,b. Meconium ileus equivalent. **a** Plain abdominal radiograph showing a mottled appearance in the right flank with a few small bowel air-fluid levels. **b** Water-soluble con- trast enema showing inspissated faecal material in the ascend- ing colon

ally in the right colon and terminal ileum, is reminiscent of meconium ileus of neonates. It occurs in 10%–15% of patients with cystic fibrosis (AGRONS et al. 1996) and may be precipitated by failure to take pancreatic supplements, respiratory infection or dehydration (GROSS et al. 1985). Symptoms include abdominal pain, distension, constipation and vomiting, and a mass in the right lower abdomen may be present.

Plain radiographs show variable small bowel dilatation and a mottled appearance in the right flank due to inspissated bowel contents in the distal ileum and right colon (PILLING and STEINER 1981). A water-soluble enema performed with Gastrografin outlines these filling defects and may be therapeutic, facilitating expulsion of this material (Fig. 3.47). An equally effective method is to administer Gastrografin orally in a single dose (O'HALLORAN et al. 1986).

Ultrasound may suggest the diagnosis of meconium ileus equivalent by the presence of packed intestinal contents and proximal fluid-filled loops of bowel, often with vigorous peristalsis. If intussusception is identified by ultrasound an attempt may be made to reduce it non-operatively if the general condition of the child is satisfactory and providing it is not ileo-ileal.

Fibrosing colonopathy is a recently recognised entity in children with cystic fibrosis and may lead to intestinal obstruction (SMYTH et al. 1994). Strictures with marked submucosal fibrosis develop, usually in the proximal colon (AGRONS et al. 1996). Presentation is with intestinal obstruction. Contrast enemas show variable colonic narrowing, mucosal irregularity, wall thickening and loss of haustration. Colonic wall thickening may also be identified by ultrasound. The condition is believed to be associated with the use of high-strength pancreatic supplements. Surgery may be required to resect the stricture. Thickening of the colonic wall may be identified sonographically in some otherwise asymptomatic patients with cystic fibrosis, possibly representing an earlier stage of this condition.

3.5.4
Abdominal Trauma

In the last decade management of blunt abdominal trauma in children has altered from immediate exploratory surgery to a more conservative approach based upon improved imaging of the abdomen (COX and KUHN 1996). Surgery is still indicated for

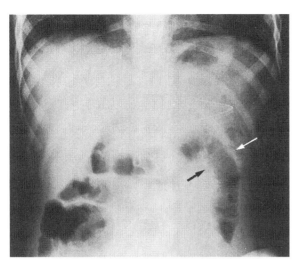

Fig. 3.48. Abdominal trauma. Plain radiograph showing prominent gaseous distension of the splenic flexure due to an ileus (*arrows*).

those with penetrating injuries and those who are haemodynamically unstable but evaluation by computed tomography has become important for the remainder.

Visceral injury is more common than bowel rupture, but prompt recognition of the latter is important to expedite surgery. Imaging will not necessarily influence the decision to operate on a child with blunt trauma, but allows for subsequent conservative management to be rationally based on the pattern and severity of injury (SIVIT and KAUFMAN 1995).

Plain films have a limited but important role in abdominal trauma. They should include a supine abdominal radiograph and if possible an erect chest film. If the latter is not possible and perforation is suspected, a decubitus abdominal film with the right side elevated should be obtained. Free intraperitoneal gas may be due to perforation of a hollow viscus, a penetrating injury or rarely an air leak from mechanical ventilation. Pelvic, rib (Fig. 3.48) or spinal fractures may be identified but radiographs cannot provide direct evidence of visceral, gut or mesenteric injury and may be normal in the presence of severe injury.

Significant abdominal trauma is a likely sequela of road traffic accidents, crush injuries and severe falls. The presence of abdominal wall bruising or gross haematuria, a marker of hepatic and splenic injury as well as renal trauma, is an important indication for imaging the abdomen. A history of a mechanism of injury that is frequently associated with internal organ injury is also an indication for imaging even in the absence of signs of severe trauma.

Whilst sonography has its advocates (FILIATRAULT and GAREL 1995) its value in the acute situation is not generally accepted (SIVIT and KAUFMAN 1995). It is more useful in the follow-up of patients and in the detection of delayed complications of trauma and surgery, e.g. pancreatic pseudocysts and other fluid collections. It has poorer sensitivity than computed tomography for the detection of visceral and bowel injury in the acute phase.

Computed tomography is the modality of choice for imaging blunt paediatric abdominal trauma (KIRKS et al. 1992). Detection of liver, splenic and renal injury is straightforward but identification of pancreatic, mesenteric and bowel damage is more difficult (COX and KUHN 1996). The abdomen should be evaluated from the dome of the diaphragm to the bladder base with dynamic intravenous contrast enhancement. A low-osmolar non-ionic contrast medium with an iodine content of 300 mg/ml at a dose of 2 ml/kg (maximum 100 ml) allows optimal differentiation of organs from adjacent soft tissues, detection of devitalised organs or segments and visualisation of intraparenchymal haematomas. Rarely, a source of haemorrhage is directly identified (TAYLOR et al. 1994). A slice thickness of 8–10 mm is appropriate in most instances, with contiguous scans through the upper abdomen. Helical scanners permit contiguous images of the rest of the abdomen but with conventional scanners an interslice gap may be required. Delayed images, particularly of the kidneys and urinary bladder, are useful if there is suspicion of disruption of the urinary tract. If a urinary catheter is present it should be clamped prior to the start of the scan.

Oral contrast medium may more clearly define bowel wall thickening and intramural haematomas, and occasionally spill into the peritoneal cavity will indicate perforation (COX and KUHN 1996). However, severely injured children usually have some degree of ileus and so contrast medium introduced into the stomach may not completely opacify the small bowel and there is a small risk of aspiration, particularly if sedation or anaesthesia is employed. In addition it will be more difficult to identify extravasation of intravenous contrast medium and bowel wall enhancement. If oral contrast is to be used then dilute water-soluble contrast medium (1:40) is appropriate. Water is a better alternative to optimise distension of the upper gastrointestinal tract but in practice neither is routinely used.

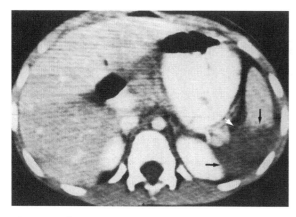

Fig. 3.49. Splenic injury. Computed tomography showing disruption and non-enhancement of the posterior aspect of the spleen (*arrows*) with adjacent free fluid

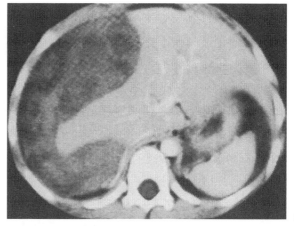

a

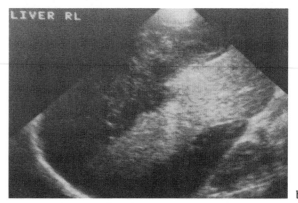

b

Fig. 3.51 a,b. Hepatic trauma. **a** Computed tomography demonstrates a complicated low-attenuation subcapsular haematoma surrounding and compressing the right lobe of the liver (by courtesy of Dr. T.R. Brown, Musgrove Park Hospital, Taunton). **b** Ultrasound shows a similar appearance

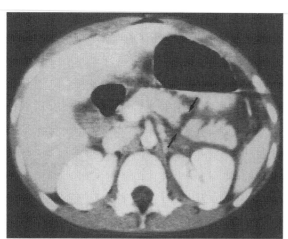

a

b

Fig. 3.50 a,b. Pancreatic trauma. Computed tomography demonstrates complete transection of the body of the pancreas (**a**) and contusion with a small lesser sac fluid collection (**b**) (*arrowheads*)

Injuries to the liver, spleen and kidneys are usually clearly apparent with contusion, haematoma, laceration or fracture evident by virtue of irregular focal low-density non-enhancing parenchymal abnormalities or disruption of the normal contour of the organ (Figs. 3.49–3.51). Areas of devitalisation will not enhance and usually have segmental or peripheral locations, well demarcated from perfused tissue.

Pancreatic trauma is relatively uncommon (2% of abdominal injuries) and may be difficult to identify acutely, though indirect signs such as fluid in the lesser sac and anterior pararenal space are helpful (SIVIT et al. 1992a). Pseudocyst formation is a relatively common delayed complication of severe pancreatic injury and may be managed percutaneously, though if drainage continues endoscopic or magnetic resonance pancreatography will be required to determine the integrity of the pancreatic duct.

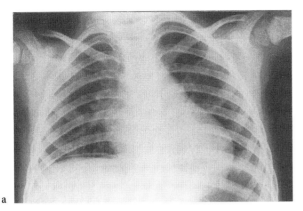

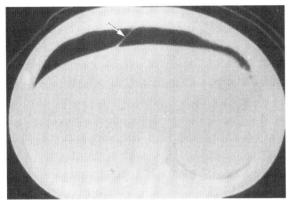

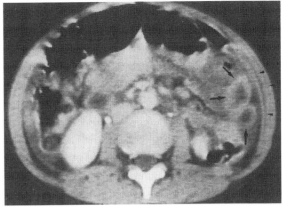

Fig. 3.53. Abdominal trauma. Computed tomography of the abdomen showing bowel wall thickening and intense enhancement in the left flank (*arrows*) with free fluid. There is also some fluid between the muscles of the abdominal wall (*arrowheads*): jejunal perforation

Fig. 3.52 a,b. Pneumoperitoneum. a Erect chest radiograph showing gas under the right hemidiaphragm. b Computed tomography of the upper abdomen viewed on lung windows showing intraperitoneal gas outlining the falciform ligament (*arrow*)

Extraluminal gas (Fig. 3.52), if seen, is suggestive of bowel perforation but is not in isolation sufficiently sensitive or specific as it is present in only approximately 50% of patients with perforation. It may arise from other causes such as pneumomediastinum from trauma or ventilation or from peritoneal lavage. Prior diagnostic peritoneal lavage will also lead to free intra-abdominal fluid and cause confusion and so should not be performed if computed tomography is to be undertaken. Free intraperitoneal fluid (especially if the Hounsfield number is close to 0, suggesting bowel contents rather than blood) focal bowel wall thickening (Fig. 3.53) and mural enhancement are significant findings (SIVIT et al. 1994; JAMIESON et al. 1996; COX and KUHN 1996), which even in the absence of free gas suggest perforation. Focal or generalised bowel dilatation may be present and there may be increased attenuation of the adjacent mesentery. Extraluminal oral contrast medium, though specific for perforation, is extremely uncommon (COX and KUHN 1996). It is im-

portant to recognise perforation as the clinical findings of peritonitis may be delayed for several hours. Using the above criteria some children may be operated upon who have only mesenteric injury but this appears reasonable if those with perforation are not to be denied prompt treatment.

Mesenteric injury ranges from haematoma to avulsion of mesenteric vessels with the potential for bowel ischaemia and the development of ischaemic bowel perforation or stricture. Findings on computed tomography include streakiness of the mesenteric fat, a mesenteric mass due to haematoma, haemoperitoneum and rarely a sentinel clot with higher than soft tissue attenuation at the site of bleeding (COX and KUHN 1996).

The commonest sites of bowel injury due to blunt trauma are the duodenum and small bowel. The latter is especially vulnerable adjacent to fixation points in the proximal jejunum and distal ileum. Damage is mediated by shear or compression forces or a sudden rise in intraluminal pressure (COX and KUHN 1996). Incomplete bowel rupture may occur and is caused by submucosal shearing. The bowel wall may remain intact though later stricture formation may occur. If the latter is suspected it is best imaged by contrast studies of the gastrointestinal tract. Herniation of a loop of bowel through a mesenteric rupture also leads to symptoms of subacute obstruction and is also best imaged by careful contrast studies.

Detection of duodenal perforation is aided by visualisation of extraluminal gas or oral contrast medium in the right anterior pararenal space (KUNIN et al. 1993). Duodenal haematoma may

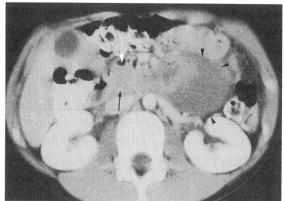

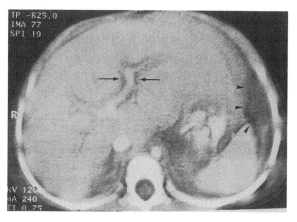

Fig. 3.55. Abdominal trauma. Computed tomography showing periportal low attenuation or "tracking" (*arrows*) in this patient with blunt abdominal trauma but no evidence of hepatic injury. The aorta is reduced in calibre and there is free fluid in the left upper quadrant (*arrowheads*)

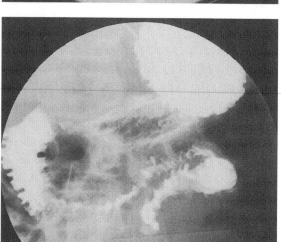

Fig. 3.54 a,b. Duodenal haematoma. **a** Computed tomography shows thickened folds in the third part of the duodenum (*arrows*), with an adjacent retroperitoneal fluid collection (*arrowheads*). **b** A contrast study shows extensive narrowing of the lumen of the third and fourth parts of the duodenum and of the proximal jejunum, with mucosal thickening

be identified as focal wall thickening with variable luminal narrowing, may be associated with retroperitoneal fluid and may slowly enlarge, leading to progressive obstruction (Fig. 3.54). It may also be identified on ultrasound as a mass lesion in the right upper abdomen eccentrically surrounding and protruding into the dilated fluid-filled duodenal lumen. A duodenal haematoma is a well-recognised complication of non-accidental injury and any child presenting with such a lesion should be carefully examined with this in mind. A common clinical history in such children is that the injury was allegedly caused by a fall down stairs, but children do not sustain duodenal injury by this mechanism. In non-accidental injury the history is usually longer and vomiting, weight loss and dehydration are prominent. The distinction between perforating and non-

perforating duodenal injuries is important as the latter are managed conservatively whilst the former require prompt surgery.

A subgroup of children with blunt abdominal trauma will show the "hypoperfusion shock bowel" appearance. This consists of delayed and dense nephrograms, small calibre aorta and vena cava, bowel dilatation with marked wall enhancement and decreased pancreatic and splenic enhancement due to splanchnic vasoconstriction. These patients, although appearing stable, have a very precarious haemodynamic state and a high mortality (Cox and Kuhn 1996; Sivit et al. 1994).

Hepatic periportal low attenuation is found in up to 20% of children undergoing computed tomography following blunt abdominal trauma (Patrick et al. 1992) and was initially considered an important marker for severe liver injury, even in the absence of visible parenchymal abnormalities (Fig. 3.55). It was thought to represent blood or lymph tracking along the path of the portal vein and its branches (Macrander et al. 1989; Siegel and Herman 1992). However, it has also been described in liver transplantation and malignancy and is attributed to lymphatic distension (Siegel and Herman 1992). Though present in a significant number of patients with hepatic trauma, it is commoner in those with no imaging evidence of liver injury (Sivit et al. 1993b). It is likely to be related to elevation of central venous pressure in children who have had aggressive fluid replacement because of hypotension or hypovolaemia, probably mediated by rapid expansion of central venous volume, third space

Table 3.33. Causes of pancreatitis in childhood

Trauma
Drugs (L-asparaginase, steroids)
Mumps
Hereditary pancreatitis
Gallstones
Shock
Sepsis
Reye's syndrome
Haemolytic uraemic syndrome
Pancreatic duct anomalies

effects and distension of periportal lymphatics (SHANMUGANATHAN et al. 1993).

3.5.5
Pancreatitis

Pancreatitis is rare in childhood, with trauma accounting for most cases (YEUNG et al. 1996) and intrinsic structural abnormalities, e.g. pancreas divisum and gallstones, responsible for only a small proportion (Table 3.33).

The acute presentation of children with pancreatitis is with pain (95%) and vomiting (56%). The symptoms are non-specific. The diagnosis in children is difficult as clinical findings may be vague and elevation of serum amylase is not specific, the level also being raised in choledochal cyst and mumps.

Plain radiographs may rarely show pancreatic calcification, characteristic of hereditary pancreatitis. There may be mild dilatation of the duodenum and proximal small bowel, reflecting a localised ileus (DAVIS 1980), and a generalised paucity of gas elsewhere, especially if disease is severe. The colon "cut-off" sign is very rare in children.

The diagnosis of pancreatitis may be suggested by ultrasound, which is helpful both at presentation and during follow-up (FLEISCHER et al. 1983; SIEGEL et al. 1987). Enlargement of the gland and reduction in its echogenicity are useful signs of inflammation but are usually present only in those with severe disease. Bile duct dilatation, choledochal cysts, pancreatic pseudocysts (Fig. 3.56) and gallstones may be detected, though the latter are less common than in adults. If bowel gas hampers visualisation of the pancreas, computed tomography is indicated in suspected cases (HERMAN and SIEGEL 1991a). Pancreatic enlargement is a helpful but uncommon finding (29%) suggesting severe inflammation (KING et al. 1995). Extrapancreatic fluid collections are

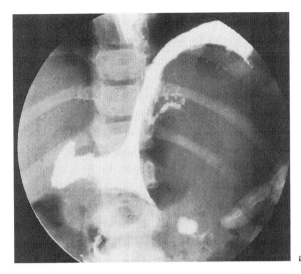

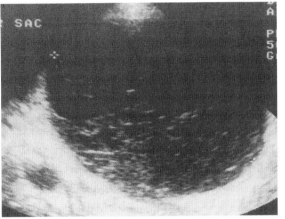

Fig. 3.56 a,b. Pancreatic pseudocyst. **a** Barium meal shows significant indentation of the greater curvature of the stomach by an extrinsic mass. **b** Ultrasound demonstrates a complex cystic mass in the lesser sac

more frequent than intrapancreatic collections, the commonest sites being the anterior pararenal space, the lesser sac, the lesser omentum and the transverse mesocolon. Most of these resolve spontaneously and only rarely require drainage. Pseudocyst complicates acute pancreatitis in between 10% and 23% and may extend a considerable distance from the pancreas and even into the mediastinum, though the majority of cases are confined to the abdomen (YEUNG et al. 1996; HERMAN and SIEGEL 1991a).

3.5.6
Immunocompromised Host

An acute abdomen may complicate treatment of childhood malignancy or bone marrow transplantation and imaging has an important role in ensuring appropriate treatment. Intussusception, neutropenic colitis (typhlitis) and graft versus host disease may occur, as may any condition that might occur in non-immunocompromised individuals, e.g. acute appendicitis. Neutropenic colitis causes severe abdominal pain, often localised to the right iliac fossa, diarrhoea and fever (MCNAMARA et al. 1986). The children are neutropenic because of chemotherapy or non-engraftment following bone marrow transplantation (DONNELLY 1996). Bacterial invasion of bowel wall leads to inflammation and oedema which may progress to haemorrhage, necrosis or perforation.

Plain radiographs show non-specific colonic wall thickening, a paucity of bowel gas in the right flank, small bowel dilatation and occasionally pneumatosis (Fig. 3.57), with free gas indicating perforation. Ultrasound and computed tomography are helpful in excluding other conditions and in showing wall thickening of the caecum and ascending colon (BENYA et al. 1993). Pneumatosis is not specific for typhlitis, as it may occur in patients on high-dose steroid therapy, with infections, after irradiation and in graft versus host disease.

Treatment is primarily conservative, with surgery reserved for those who deteriorate, perforate or have uncontrolled haemorrhage.

Intussusception may occur in patients with leukaemia and lymphoma and may cause similar clinical findings to typhlitis. Plain film appearances may be characteristic but are often non-specific, and ultrasound is of value in being able to directly visualise the intussusception (GAVAN and HENDRY 1994) and exclude other pathology. If the general condition of the child is satisfactory an attempt at non-operative reduction may be made.

3.5.7
Peptic Ulceration

Peptic ulceration is an increasingly recognised problem in children (MEZOFF and BALISTRERI 1995; DRUMM et al. 1988; VINTON 1994) and may be primary or secondary to a pre-existing illness or drug ingestion (MEZOFF and BALISTRERI 1995). Duodenal ulcers are commoner than gastric ulcers in both groups (DRUMM et al. 1988). Children with primary peptic ulcers are usually over 10 years of age and have a higher incidence of affected relatives (50%) than those with secondary ulceration. In many the disease pursues a chronic course into adult life. Pain may be non-specific, though the presence of nocturnal waking or bleeding suggests the diagnosis. Stress ulcers are seen in younger children and account for 80% of all ulcers in infancy and early childhood. Bleeding is commoner in this group (MEZOFF and BALISTRERI 1995).

Symptoms in older children are similar to those in adults, with periodic abdominal pain relieved by food in the case of duodenal ulceration or aggravated by food with gastric ulceration. In younger children, vomiting, non-specific abdominal pain or bleeding may be the presenting feature. An acute abdomen or perforation is extremely rare (MOON et al. 1997). Endoscopy is a more sensitive method of diagnosis than imaging with single-contrast barium studies, which detect only 66% of duodenal and 14% of gastric ulcers (DRUMM et al. 1988). The use of double-contrast techniques may increase sensitivity but this has not been satisfactorily evaluated in children. Plain films have little to offer except in the rare case when perforation is suspected.

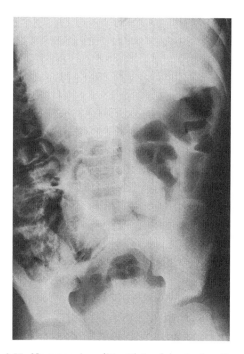

Fig. 3.57. Neutropenic colitis. Plain abdominal radiograph showing extensive intramural air in a dilated right colon

3.5.8
Polyps and Polyposis Syndromes

Intestinal polyps are usually solitary but are occasionally part of a polyposis syndrome. Hamartomatous polyps (solitary and Peutz-Jaeger's syndrome) are benign, but adenomatous polyps have malignant potential.

Juvenile polyps account for about 90% of all childhood polyps, typically causing episodes of bright rectal bleeding and occasionally pain or intussusception. The typical age is 3 years and over and only occasionally is bleeding profuse enough to simulate a Meckel's diverticulum. Most juvenile polyps are located in the distal colon, are solitary and may undergo spontaneous "auto-amputation". When the diagnosis is suspected, confirmation may be obtained by double-contrast barium enema or colonoscopy. The advantage of the former is there is no need for sedation or anaesthesia, but colonoscopy allows snaring of the polyp, providing therapy and a histological diagnosis. Whichever technique is employed, the entire colon should be examined as occasionally polyps are multiple.

Peutz-Jegher's syndrome is an autosomal dominant condition consisting of multiple hamartomatous polyps in the small bowel with less marked involvement of the stomach and colon, whilst juvenile polyposis coli consists of multiple large bowel hamartomatous polyps (VINTON 1994). There are also several syndromes of adenomatous polyposis (familial adenomatous polyposis, Gardner's syndrome) which have malignant potential (VINTON 1994).

Emergency presentation with any of the polyposis syndromes is with symptoms of intestinal obstruction, colicky or recurrent abdominal pain due to either intermittent obstruction or intussusception and more rarely vomiting if polyps obstruct the jejunum. The investigation and management are the same as for any child presenting with an acute abdomen, i.e. plain abdominal radiographs, ultrasound and then contrast studies if necessary.

3.5.9
Haemolytic Uraemic Syndrome

Haemolytic uraemic syndrome is associated with gastroenteritis due to *E. coli* (0157:H7) (SIEGLER 1995), which causes a colitic illness with bloody diarrhoea, fever, abdominal pain and vomiting. Toxins produced in the gut induce a microangiopathic haemolytic anaemia, thrombocytopenia and varying degrees of renal failure.

Plain films may show dilated small and large bowel with air-fluid levels as in gastroenteritis, mucosal oedema of the colon (thumb-printing) and

in severe cases a toxic megacolon. Contrast studies are generally not indicated but if performed show mucosal oedema and spasm affecting the entire colon (FRIEDLAND et al. 1995). Ultrasound demonstrates colonic wall thickening, which is often rather echogenic and frequently hypovascular on colour Doppler (FRIEDLAND et al. 1995). Free intraperitoneal fluid may be seen, as will a complicating intussusception. The kidneys are frequently affected in the acute stage, with appearances varying from normal to marked parenchymal echogenicity. Late obstruction due to stricture may occur months after the acute onset and require surgical resection.

3.5.10
Inflammatory Bowel Disease

Approximately 25% of cases of inflammatory bowel disease present in childhood, with Crohn's disease slightly more common than ulcerative colitis. Recurrent abdominal pain, diarrhoea and variable rectal bleeding are typical of Crohn's disease, which may occasionally present as an acute abdomen. The ileocaecal region is most commonly affected but children have a higher incidence of involvement of proximal small bowel and colon compared with adults.

Ulcerative colitis always involves the rectum and extends a variable distance proximally in the colon. Disease confined to the rectum is present in about 20%, and disease confined to the distal colon in 20%; pancolitis is present in the remaining cases. Diarrhoea, rectal bleeding and mucous are typical symptoms of ulcerative colitis, often with cramping pains relieved by defaecation. A fulminant presentation is uncommon though toxic megacolon may complicate the course of the disease (VON ALLMEN et al. 1995). Up to 25% of children may require surgery for refractory disease or complication.

Both conditions may cause weight loss and failure to gain height with minimal or no gastrointestinal symptoms, and occasionally arthritis and other non-gastrointestinal manifestations may be the first symptoms. Emergency presentation is usually because of an increase in severity of symptoms, or in children with Crohn's disease because of symptoms related to fistulae or obstruction. Most children present less acutely to the out-patient clinic. With severe colitis, differentiation of Crohn's disease from ulcerative colitis may not be possible and the most important differential diagnosis is the exclusion of an infective colitis (salmonella, shigella, campylobacter) by stool culture.

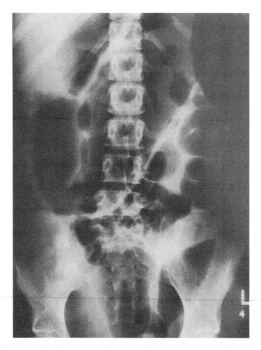

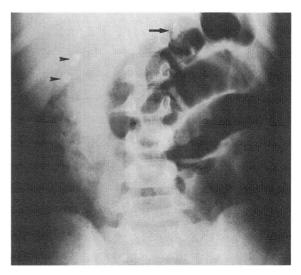

Fig. 3.59. Crohn's disease. Plain radiograph showing calcified gallstones in the right upper quadrant (*arrowheads*), with proximal small bowel dilatation and a paucity of distal gas. Adrenal calcification is also present due to previous neonatal adrenal haemorrhage (*arrow*)

Fig. 3.58. Toxic megacolon in ulcerative colitis. The transverse colon is extremely dilated with mucosal thickening

The diagnosis of inflammatory bowel disease is suggested by history and must be confirmed by biopsy, with imaging demonstrating the extent of disease and complications in the acute phase. Plain films are usually normal in quiescent or mildly active disease. In acute exacerbations they may show bowel wall thickening with absent faecal residue in acutely inflamed colon because of spasm. Lack of stool in the entire colon suggests a pancolitis (AIDEYAN and SMITH 1996). Toxic megacolon is identified by marked dilatation of the colon (>6 cm), with visible mucosal oedema and ulceration, mucosal islands and thumbprinting (Fig. 3.58). If mucosal changes are visible, a toxic colon is still present even if the calibre of the colon is less than 6 cm. A toxic megacolon may also be caused by pseudomembranous colitis, infectious colitis and ischaemia. Plain films may also demonstrate extra-intestinal manifestations of inflammatory bowel disease such as gallstones (Fig. 3.59), arthritis and sacro-iliitis.

An instant (unprepared) enema is valuable in defining the extent of any colitis provided toxic megacolon is first excluded. No bowel preparation is required as inflamed colon is usually empty of faecal matter. Elective upper and lower gastrointestinal studies will define the extent, location and nature of disease and detect complications such as strictures

and fistulae. A small bowel examination may be required in Crohn's disease to document disease extent as small bowel endoscopy is not feasible.

Labelled white cell scanning will document location and activity of bowel inflammation in children and is useful in both diagnosis and follow-up of children with inflammatory bowel disease (Fig. 3.60), with a reduced radiation dose compared with barium studies (Fig. 3.61) (JEWELL et al. 1996).

Bowel wall thickening may be identified on ultrasound and computed tomography (FAURE et al. 1997), and increased bowel wall blood flow may be detectable with colour Doppler in Crohn's disease (QUILLIN and SIEGEL 1993). Since up to 20% of patients with Crohn disease may initially present with symptoms suggestive of acute appendicitis, the sonographic demonstration of thick-walled ileum (often hypervascular) with decreased peristalsis may be useful (HAYDEN 1996).

3.5.11
Mesenteric Adenitis

Mesenteric adenitis is not a single pathological entity but a clinical "diagnosis" applied to children who have abdominal pain, fever and vomiting who do not have gastroenteritis or acute appendicitis. A proportion of these children are suspected clinically to have acute appendicitis but at laparotomy a normal ap-

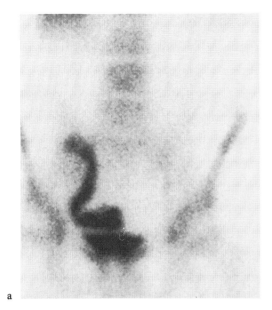

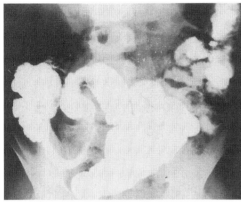

Fig. 3.60 a,b. Crohn's disease. a Technetium-99m hexamethylpropylene amine oxime scan showing abnormal activity in the distal ileum. b Late film from a barium follow through showing fixed narrowing of the distal ileum with separation of adjacent loops indicating bowel wall and mesenteric thickening

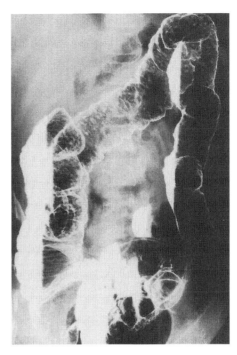

Fig. 3.61. Ulcerative colitis. Barium enema showing mucosal ulceration throughout the colon, most marked in the transverse colon

pendix is found along with non-specific mesenteric lymph node enlargement. There may be a small amount of ascites. The condition is probably caused by a variety of self-limiting infective and inflammatory processes.

Since the introduction of abdominal ultrasound for the diagnosis of acute appendicitis, enlarged mesenteric nodes (Fig. 3.39) may be observed in patients with and without appendicitis (SIVIT et al. 1993a). Patients with bacterial and viral gastroenteritis may have prominent lymphadenopathy and nodes may also be seen in asymptomatic children, so their finding must be interpreted in the appropriate clinical context.

3.5.12
Bezoar

Bezoars are rare and are derived from various indigestible substances which remain in the stomach and small bowel, forming a mass. Symptoms include pain, nausea, vomiting, constipation and occasionally a palpable mass.

Phytobezoars derived from poorly digested skins and seeds of vegetables are commonest and are frequently associated with obstruction (CHOI and KANG 1988; VERSTANDIG et al. 1989). Trichobezoars form from hair and are common in children with learning difficulties (SHARMA and SHARMA 1992). Lactobezoars, associated with high strength milk feeds, are now exceedingly rare.

Plain abdominal radiographs may show a mottled "mass" or filling defect in the stomach (Fig. 3.62a), often forming a cast of its lumen, or evidence of small bowel obstruction. Confirmation may require an upper gastrointestinal contrast study (Fig. 3.62b) or endoscopy and treatment is removal via gastrotomy unless the bezoar can be fragmented mechanically without opening bowel.

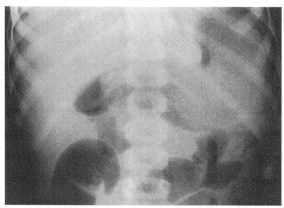

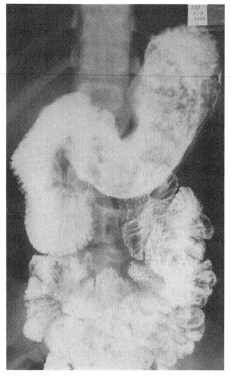

Fig. 3.62 a,b. Gastric bezoar. **a** Erect and supine abdominal radiographs and **b** barium study showing a mottled filling defect within the lumen of the stomach, extending into the proximal jejunum

Complications of bezoars include obstruction, bleeding and perforation (SHARMA and SHARMA 1992).

3.5.13
Constipation

Constipation is a common childhood problem and is essentially a clinical diagnosis with the infrequent passage of small hard stools. It is occasionally associated with severe pain during attempted defaecation, leading to reluctance to pass stool and so exacerbating the problem in young children, whilst older children may develop soiling due to overflow incontinence. Marked constipation and faecal loading may cause acute severe abdominal pain leading to an emergency presentation and may be a contributory factor for urinary tract infection (BLETHYN et al. 1995). Spurious diarrhoea may result from overflow incontinence. Impacted faeces may be palpated as an abdominal or pelvic mass.

In more than 95% of cases constipation is "idiopathic" but even in these cases local factors such as anal fissure may complicate and worsen symptoms. Management comprises a combination of disimpaction, laxatives and behavioural therapy. In a carefully selected group of children imaging is required to look for evidence of a predisposing cause such as Hirschsprung's disease.

The routine use of plain abdominal films to "diagnose" constipation is unhelpful (BEWLEY et al. 1989) though they may be a useful adjunct in the evaluation of a patient with no evidence of a faecal mass on abdominal or rectal examination. Spinal and sacral anomalies may suggest an underlying neurological cause, and delayed ossification of the femoral capital epiphyses may indicate hypothyroidism. Faecal loading as displayed by plain radiographs (Fig. 3.63) does not equate to constipation. Ultrasound may be useful in those children with an abdominal mass, differentiating a true from a faecal mass.

3.5.14
Biliary Disorders

Gallbladder and biliary disease in children is less frequent than in adults, with acute calculous and acalculous cholecystitis, gallbladder hydrops and complications of choledochal cysts the most common entities.

Right upper quadrant pain, fever and tenderness are suggestive symptoms. These and jaundice are the usual emergency presentations. Jaundice is less common than in adults and even in the presence of gallstones is more likely to be related to an underlying haematological disorder. Crohn's disease and terminal ileal resection predispose to gallstone formation by interruption of the enterohepatic circulation of bile salts.

Most (90%) gallstones are not radiopaque so plain radiographs have no role in the evaluation of biliary tract disease in children. Gallstones are increasingly

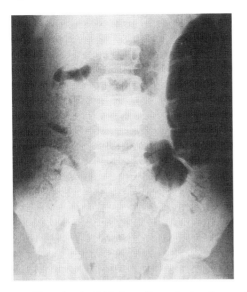

Fig. 3.63. "Constipation". Plain radiograph showing marked faecal loading of the colon

recognised in children and haemolytic anaemia is an important cause (O'HALLER 1991). Once biliary disease is suspected, ultrasound of the liver and biliary tree is the most useful modality. This may be performed as an emergency examination without the child fasting and repeated during fasting if necessary. There is high sensitivity (98%) for the detection of gallstones, which are identified as mobile echogenic foci within the gallbladder lumen casting acoustic shadows. When the gallbladder is inflamed, usually due to temporary impaction of a stone at its neck, it may become distended and thick walled and pericholecystic fluid may be identified (O'HALLER 1991). Bile duct stones are very rare in children compared with their incidence in adults, though as in adults they are often difficult to visualise by ultrasound, with a dilated common bile duct often being the only suggestive sign.

Sonography may reveal abnormalities without the biliary tree as a cause of jaundice such as decreased liver parenchymal reflectivity in viral hepatitis and increased echogenicity in fibrosis or cirrhosis. Masses at the porta hepatis may also be identified and include nodes, tumour, pancreatic pseudocyst and choledochal cyst. The last-mentioned is identified as a cystic mass usually with dilatation of the left and right intrahepatic bile ducts but not of the smaller intrahepatic ducts. In all other cases of obstructive jaundice the intrahepatic ducts are also dilated.

In acalculous cholecystitis a distended thick-walled gallbladder is present but no calculi are identified. This is usually an accompaniment of severe systemic disease and rarely requires treatment in its own right (CRANKSON et al. 1992). Underlying conditions include severe sepsis and trauma, the mechanism being biliary stasis leading to gallbladder distension and inflammation. Acute hydrops of the gallbladder refers to non-inflammatory distension and is a feature of the mucocutaneous syndrome (Kawasaki disease), where partial obstruction of the cystic duct may be produced by lymphadenopathy (CHUNG et al. 1996).

The use of hepatobiliary scintigraphy in the evaluation of acute cholecystitis is popular in North America but is not routinely performed in the United Kingdom. It is useful in evaluating congenital anomalies such as biliary atresia, and spontaneous bile duct perforation in the neonate, choledochal cysts and the situation following surgery or trauma to the biliary tree.

3.5.15
Adhesive Obstruction

Bowel obstruction due to adhesions should be a consideration in any child who has previously had abdominal surgery and presents with colicky abdominal pain, distension and vomiting. Adhesions form in 2%–15% of children following laparotomy, with most cases of adhesive obstruction presenting in the first few months after surgery and 80% by 2 years. A significant proportion will require lysis of the adhesions and about 5% of children will develop recurrent adhesive obstruction.

Plain abdominal radiographs show variable small bowel dilatation (Fig. 3.64) and a paucity or absence of distal bowel gas depending on the completeness and duration of obstruction. If an erect film is obtained the number of dilated loops and fluid levels reflects the level of obstruction. Where there is incomplete obstruction and the cause is not apparent, a contrast study of the small bowel may be considered, though this provides little extra information over the plain radiographs in most cases. Ultrasound may allow detection of other causes such as intussusception or mass but is of little use in established adhesive obstruction.

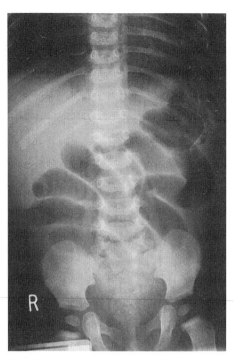

Fig. 3.64. Adhesive obstruction. Supine abdominal radiograph showing small bowel dilatation in an infant who presented with distension and vomiting several months after a laparotomy

3.5.16
Gonadal Disorders

Although not within the remit of this chapter, torsion, infarction and inflammatory conditions of the gonads and adjacent structures may cause severe abdominal pain. A high clinical index of suspicion is required together with thorough examination of the scrotum in boys and consideration of ovarian pathology in girls. Both torsion of the testicle and inflammatory epididymitis are most prevalent in pubertal boys. Where epididymitis is likely surgery may be avoided if sonography demonstrates an enlarged epididymis with increased flow on Doppler.

3.5.17
Colonic Volvulus

Colonic volvulus in childhood is a rare cause of bowel obstruction (ANDERSEN et al. 1981), most often affecting the sigmoid colon and less commonly the right colon. Abdominal pain and vomiting are the commonest presenting features though they

may be intermittent (MELLOR and DRAKE 1994; MERCADO-DEANE et al. 1995). Plain radiographs may be normal if taken following resolution of symptoms when volvulus has subsided, but may show non-specific intestinal obstruction or marked sigmoid or caecal dilatation if taken acutely. In sigmoid volvulus obstruction tends to be at the level of the proximal twist and so enormous gaseous distension of the sigmoid loop is less common than in adults. A contrast enema may show a beaked appearance of the distal sigmoid colon associated with partial or complete obstruction (ANDERSEN et al. 1981).

In caecal volvulus there may be a prominent air-fluid level on plain films and beaking in the ascending colon with occasional filling of the distended caecum during an enema (KIRKS et al. 1981). The enema may prove therapeutic with detorsion of the volved bowel occurring during or shortly after the examination (MELLOR and DRAKE 1994). Surgery is required for those cases which do not resolve spontaneously and for those patients with recurrent episodes.

3.6
Summary

The causes of acute paediatric gastrointestinal symptoms are legion, but a sound clinical evaluation together with the age of the child enables a working differential diagnosis to be established in most cases. In these circumstances imaging is most effectively used to confirm the diagnosis and to exclude other important conditions. The use of ultrasound in the acute paediatric abdomen has increased in importance over the past decade, and in many instances it is the only imaging modality required. Plain radiographs still have an important role to play, particularly in the neonate and where perforation is suspected, but they should not automatically be obtained when conditions like hypertrophic pyloric stenosis, intussusception and acute appendicitis are thought likely on clinical grounds. Contrast studies and computed tomography, though less frequently required, are nevertheless important tools with defined roles, with the former offering the possibility of treatment in intussusception and meconium ileus.

Acknowledgements. I am grateful to Mr. R. Spicer and Dr. L. Goldsworthy for their helpful comments during the preparation of this chapter.

References

Ablow RC, Hoffer FA, Seashore JH, et al. (1983) Z-shaped duodeno-jejunal loop: sign of mesenteric fixation anomaly and congenital bands. AJR 141:461–464

Agrons GA, Corse WR, Markowitz RI, et al. (1996) Gastrointestinal complications of cystic fibrosis: a radiologic-pathologic correlation. Radiographics 16:871–893

Aideyan UO, Smith WL (1996) Inflammatory bowel disease in children. Radiol Clin North Am 34:885–902

Akhan O, Demirkazik FB, Ozman MN, et al. (1994) Choledochal cysts: ultrasonographic findings and correlation with other imaging findings. Abdom imaging 19:243–247

Alford BA, McIlhenny J (1992) The child with acute abdominal pain and vomiting. Radiol Clin North Am 30:441–453

Alford BA, Armstrong P, Franken EA, et al. (1980) Calcification associated with duodenal duplications in children. Radiology 134:647–648

Andersen JF, Eklof O, Thomasson B (1981) Large bowel volvulus in children: review of a case material and the literature. Pediatr Radiol 11:129–138

Andiran F, Tanyel FC, Balkanci E, et al. (1995) Acute abdomen due to gastric volvulus: diagnostic value of a single plain radiograph. Pediatr Radiol 25:S240

Baker DE, Silver TM, Coran AG, et al. (1986) Post appendicectomy fluid collections in children: incidence, nature and evolution evaluated using ultrasound. Radiology 161:341–344

Barr LL (1994) Sonography in the infant with acute abdominal symptoms. Semin Ultrasound CT MR 15:275–289

Barr LL, Hayden CK, Stansberry SD, et al. (1990) Enteric duplication cysts in children: are their ultrasonographic wall characteristics diagnostic? Pediatr Radiol 20:326–328

Benya EC, Sivit CJ, Quinones R (1993) Abdominal complications after bone marrow transplantation in children: sonographic and CT findings. AJR 161:1023–1027

Berdon WE, Baker DH, Bull S, et al. (1970) Midgut malrotation and volvulus: which films are most helpful? Radiology 96:375–383

Berdon WE, Slovis TL, Campbell JD, et al. (1977) Neonatal small left colon syndrome: its relationship to aganglionosis and meconium plug syndrome. Radiology 125:457–462

Berman L, Stringer DA, Ein S, et al. (1988) Childhood diaphragmatic hernias presenting after the neonatal period. Clin Radiol 39:237–244

Bewley A, Clancy MJ, Hall JRW (1989) The erroneous use by an accident and emergency department of plain abdominal radiographs in the diagnosis of constipation. Arch Emerg Med 6:257–258

Blake NS (1984) Beak sign in duodenal duplication cyst. Pediatr Radiol 14:232–233

Blethyn AJ, Jones KV, Newcombe R, et al. (1995) Radiological assessment of constipation. Arch Dis Child 75:532–533

Bomelburg T, Claasen U, von Lengerke HJ (1991) Intestinal ultrasonographic findings in Schönlein-Henoch syndrome. Eur J Pediatr 150:158–160

Bradley MJ, Pilling D (1991) The empty rectum on plain X-ray. Does it have any significance in the neonate? Clin Radiol 43:265–267

Bramson RT, Blickman JG (1992) Perforation during hydrostatic reduction of intussusception: proposed mechanism and review of the literature. J Pediatr Surg 27:589–591

Brereton RJ, Stringer MD (1991) Paediatric emergencies (review). Baillieres Clin Gastroenterol 5:913–930

Buonomo C (1997) Neonatal gastrointestinal emergencies. Radiol Clin North Am 35:845–863

Burton EM, Strange ME, Pitts RM (1993) Malrotation in twins: a rare occurrence. Pediatr Radiol 23:603–604

Campbell JB (1979) Neonatal gastric volvulus. AJR 132:723–725

Campbell JB, Quattromani FL, Foley LC (1983) Foley catheter removal of blunt oesophageal foreign bodies. Experience with 100 consecutive children. Pediatr Radiol 13:116–119

Capitanio MA, Greenberg SB (1991) Pneumatosis intestinalis in two infants with rotavirus gastroenteritis. Pediatr Radiol 21:361–362

Caravati EM, Bennett DL, McElwee NE (1989) Pediatric coin ingestion: a prospective study on the utility of routine roentgenograms. Am J Dis Child 143:549–550

Carty H, Brereton RJ (1983) The distended neonate. Clin Radiol 34:367–380

Carver RA, Okorie M, Steiner GM, et al. (1988) Infantile hypertrophic pyloric stenosis – diagnosis from the pyloric muscle index. Clin Radiol 38:625–627

Ceres L, Alonso I, Lopez P, et al. (1990) Ultrasound study of acute appendicitis in children with emphasis upon the diagnosis of retrocaecal appendicitis. Pediatr Radiol 20:258–261

Chan KL, Saing H, Peh WCG, et al. (1997) Childhood intussusception: ultrasound guided Hartmann's solution reduction or barium enema reduction? J Pediatr Surg 32:3–6

Chesborough RM, Burkhard TK, Balsara ZN, et al. (1993) Self localisation in ultrasound of acute appendicitis: an addition to graded compression. Radiology 187:349–351

Choi SO, Park WH, Woo SK (1994) Ultrasound guided water enema: an alternative method of non-operative treatment for childhood intussusception. J Pediatr Surg 29:498–500

Choi SO, Kang JS (1988) Gastrointestinal phytobezoars in childhood. J Pediatr Surg 23:338–341

Chung CJ, Rayder S, Meyers W, et al. (1996) Kawasaki disease presenting as focal colitis. Pediatr Radiol 26:455–457

Connolly B, O'Halpin D (1994) Sonographic evaluation of the abdomen in Henoch-Schönlein purpura. Clin Radiol 49:320–323

Connolly B, Alton DJ, Ein SH, et al. (1995) Partially reduced intussusception: when are repeated delayed reduction attempts appropriate? Pediatr Radiol 25:104–107

Cooney DR, Duszynski DO, Camboa E, et al. (1982) The abdominal technetium scan (a decade of experience). J Pediatr Surg 17:611–619

Couture A, Veryac C, Baud C, et al. (1992) Evaluation of abdominal pain in Henoch-Schönlein syndrome by high frequency ultrasound. Pediatr Radiol 22:12–17

Cox TD, Kuhn JP (1996) Computed tomography of bowel trauma in the paediatric patient. Radiol Clin North Am 34:807–818

Crankson S, Nazer H, Jacobson B (1992) Acute hydrops of the gallbladder in childhood. Eur J Paediatr 151:318–320

Crowley JJ, Bawle E (1996) Small bowel malrotation in each of a pair of identical twins. Pediatr Radiol 26:127–128

Daneman A, Alton DJ (1996) Intussusception. Issues and controversies related to diagnosis and reduction. Radiol Clin North Am 34:743–756

Daneman A, Alton DJ, Ein S, et al. (1995) Perforation during attempted intussusception reduction in children – a comparison of perforation with barium and air. Pediatr Radiol 25:81–88

Daneman A, Myers M, Shuckett B, et al. (1997) Sonographic appearances of inverted Meckel diverticulum with intussusception. Pediatr Radiol 27:295–298

Davis S, Parbhoo SP, Gibson MJ (1980) The plain abdominal radiograph in acute pancreatitis. Clin Radiol 31:97–93

De Campo JF, Mayne V, Boldt DW, et al. (1984) Radiological findings in total aganglionosis coli. Pediatr Radiol 14:205–209

del-Pozo G, Albillos JC, Tejedor D (1996a) Intussusception: ultrasound findings with pathologic correlation – the crescent-in-doughnut sign. Radiology 199:688–692

del-Pozo G, Gonzalez-Spinola J, Gomez-Anson B, et al. (1996b) Intussusception: trapped peritoneal fluid detected with ultrasound – relationship to reducibility and ischaemia. Radiology 201:379–383

Demos TC, Flisak ME (1986) Coiled spring appearance of the caecum in acute appendicitis. AJR 146:45–48

DiDonato LR (1976) Pneumatosis coli secondary to acute appendicitis. Radiology 120:90

Docherty JG, Zaki A, Coutts JAP, et al. (1992) Meconium ileus: a review 1972–1990. Br J Surg 79:571–573

Dolgin SE, Beck AR, Tartter PI (1992) The risk of perforation when children with possible appendicitis are observed in the hospital. Surg Gynaecol Obstet 175:320–324

Don S, Cohen MD, Wells LJ, et al. (1992) Air reduction of an intussusception caused by a pathologic lead point in an infant. Pediatr Radiol 22:326–327

Donnelly LF (1996) CT imaging of immunocompromised children with acute abdominal symptoms. AJR 167:909–913

Doyle T, Mullany J (1986) The radiological features of Henoch-Schönlein purpura in the gastrointestinal tract. Australas Radiol 30:313–316

Drumm B, Rhoads JM, Stringer DA, et al. (1988) Peptic ulcer disease in children: aetiology, clinical findings and clinical course. Pediatrics 82:410–414

Dufour D, Delaet MH, Dassonville M, et al. (1992) Midgut malrotation, the reliability of sonographic diagnosis. Pediatr Radiol 22:21–23

Eggli KD, Potter BM, Garcia V, et al. (1986) Delayed diagnosis of oesophageal perforation by aluminium foreign bodies. Pediatr Radiol 16:511–513

Ein SH, Shandling B, Reilly BJ, et al. (1987) Bowel perforation with non-operative treatment of meconium ileus. J Pediatr Surg 22:146–147

Ein SH, Palder SB, Alton DJ, et al. (1994) Intussusception: toward less surgery? J Pediatr Surg 29:433–435

Faure C, Belarbi N, Mougenot JF, et al. (1997) Ultrasonographic assessment of inflammatory bowel disease in children: comparison with ileocolonoscopy. J Pediatr 130:147–151

Fecteau A, Flageole H, Nguyen LT, et al. (1996) Recurrent intussusception: safe use of hydrostatic enema. J Pediatr Surg 31:859–861

Fedyshin P, Kelvin FM, Rice RP (1984) Non-specificity of barium enema findings in acute appendicitis. AJR 143:99–102

Filiatrault D, Garel L (1995) Commentary: paediatric blunt abdominal trauma – to sound or not to sound? Pediatr Radiol 25:329–331

Fink AM, Alexopoulou E, Cary H (1995) Bleeding Meckel's diverticulum in infancy: unusual scintigraphic and ultrasound appearances. Pediatr Radiol 25:155–156

Finkel LI, Slovis TL (1982) Meconium peritonitis, intraperitoneal calcification and cystic fibrosis. Pediatr Radiol 12:92–93

Fleischer AC, Parker P, Kirchner SG, et al. (1983) Sonographic findings of pancreatitis in children. Radiology 146:151–155

Franken Jr. EA, Kao SCS, Smith WL, et al. (1989) Imaging of the acute abdomen in infants and children. AJR 153:921–928

Friedland JA, Siegel MJ (1997) CT appearances of acute appendicitis in childhood. AJR 168:439–442

Friedland JA, Herman TE, Siegel MJ (1995) *Escherichia coli* 0157:H7 associated haemolytic-uraemic syndrome: value of colonic colour Doppler sonography. Pediatr Radiol 25:S65–S67

Gaensler EHL, Jeffrey RB Jr., Laing FC, et al. (1989) Sonography in patients with suspected acute appendicitis: value in establishing alternative diagnoses. AJR 152:49–51

Gaines PA, Saunders AJS, Drake D (1987) Midgut malrotation diagnosed by ultrasound. Clin Radiol 38:51–53

Gaisie G, Odagiri K, Oh KS, et al. (1980) The bulbous bowel segment: a sign of congenital small bowel obstruction. Radiology 135:331–334

Gaisie G, Curnes JT, Scatliff JH, et al. (1985) Neonatal intestinal obstruction from omphalomesenteric duct remnants. AJR 144:109–112

Gaisie G, Kent C, Klein RL, et al. (1993) Radiographic changes of isolated invaginated Meckel's diverticulum. Pediatr Radiol 23:355–356

Garcia JA, Garcia-Fernandez M, Romance A, et al. (1994) Wandering spleen and gastric volvulus. Pediatr Radiol 24:535–536

Gavan DR, Hendry GMA (1994) Colonic complications of acute lymphoblastic leukaemia. Br J Radiol 67:449–452

Ghahremani GG (1986) Radiology of Meckel's diverticulum. Crit Rev Diagn Imaging 26:1–43

Glasier CM, Siegel MJ, McAlister WH, et al. (1981) Henoch-Schönlein syndrome in children: gastrointestinal manifestations. AJR 136:1081–1085

Godbole P, Sprigg A, Dickson JAS, et al. (1996) Ultrasound compared with clinical examination in infantile hypertrophic pyloric stenosis. Arch Dis Child 75:335–337

Goh DW, Brereton RJ, Spitz L (1991) Oesophageal atresia with obstructed tracheo-oesophageal fistula and gasless abdomen. J Pediatr Surg 26:160–162

Goyal MK, Bellah RD (1993) Neonatal small bowel obstruction due to Meckel diverticulitis: diagnosis by ultrasound. J Ultrasound Med 2:119–122

Grahm JM, Rokorny WJ (1980) Acute appendicitis in preschool age children. Am J Surg 139:247–250

Gross K, Desanto A, Grosfeld JL, et al. (1985) Intra-abdominal complications of cystic fibrosis. J Pediatr Surg 20:431–435

Gu L, Alton DJ, Daneman A, et al. (1988) Intussusception reduction in children by rectal insufflation of air. AJR 150:1345–1348

Guttman FN, Braun P, Grance PH (1973) Multiple atresias and a new syndrome of hereditary multiple atresias involving the gastrointestinal tract from stomach to rectum. J Pediatr Surg 8:633–640

Harned RK, Strain JD, Hay TC, et al. (1997) Oesophageal foreign bodies: safety and efficacy of Foley catheter extraction of coins. AJR 168:443–446

Hayden CK Jr. (1996) Ultrasonography of the acute pediatric abdomen. Radiol Clin North Am 34:791–806

Herman TE, McAlister WH (1991) Oesophageal diverticula in childhood associated with strictures from unsuspected foreign bodies of the oesophagus. Pediatr Radiol 21:410–412

Herman E, Siegel MJ (1991a) CT of the pancreas in children. AJR 157:375–379

Herman TE, Siegel MJ (1991b) CT of acute splenic torsion in children with wandering spleen. AJR 156:151–153

Hernanz-Schulman M, Sells LL, Ambrosino MM, et al. (1994)

Hypertrophic pyloric stenosis in the infant without a palpable olive: accuracy of sonographic diagnosis. Radiology 193:771–776

Holmes M, Murphy V, Taylor M, et al. (1991) Intussusception in cystic fibrosis. Arch Dis Child 66:726–727

Hu SC, Feeney MS, McNicholls M, et al. (1991) Ultrasonography to diagnose and exclude intussusception in Henoch-Schönlein purpura. Arch Dis Child 66:1065–1067

Hussain SM, Meradji M, Robben SGF, et al. (1991) Plain film diagnosis in meconium plug syndrome, meconium ileus and neonatal Hirschsprung disease: a scoring system. Pediatr Radiol 21:556–559

Iyer CP, Mahour GH (1995) Duplications of the alimentary tract in infants and children. J Pediatr Surg 30:1267–1270

Jackson A, Bisset R, Dickson AP (1989) Case report: malrotation and midgut volvulus presenting as malabsorption. Clin Radiol 40:536–537

Jamieson DH, Babyn PS, Pearl R (1996) Imaging gastrointestinal perforation in paediatric blunt abdominal trauma. Pediatr Radiol 26:188–194

Jewell FM, Davies A, Sandhu B, et al. (1996) Technetium-99m-HMPAO labelled leucocytes in the detection and monitoring of inflammatory bowel disease in children. Br J Radiol 69:508–514

Johns DW (1995) Disorders of the central and autonomic nervous systems as a cause for emesis in infants. Semin Pediatr Surg 4:152–156

Johnson JF (1988) Pneumatosis in the descending colon: preliminary observations on the value of prone positioning. Pediatr Radiol 19:25–27

Johnson JF, Robinson LH (1984) Localised bowel distension in the newborn: a review of the plain film analysis and differential diagnosis. Pediatrics 73:206–215

Johnson JF III, Lorenzetti RJ, Ballard ET (1993) Plain film identification of inverted Meckel diverticulum. Pediatr Radiol 23:551–552

Kangarloo H, Sample WF, Hansen G, et al. (1979) Ultrasonic evaluation of abdominal gastrointestinal tract duplication in children. Radiology 131:191–194

Kao SCS, Franken EA Jr (1995) Non-operative treatment of simple meconium ileus: a survey of the Society for Pediatric Radiology. Pediatr Radiol 25:97–100

Kao SCS, Smith WL, Abu-Yousef MM, et al. (1989) Acute appendicitis in children: sonographic findings. AJR 153:375–379

Kassner EG, Kottmeier PK (1975) Absence and retention of small bowel gas in infants with midgut volvulus: mechanisms and significance. Pediatr Radiol 4:28–30

Katz ME, Siegel MJ, Shakelford GD, et al. (1987) The position and mobility of the duodenum in children. AJR 148:947–951

Keller KS, Markle BM, Lassey PA, Chawla HS, Jacir N, Frank JL (1985) Spontaneous resolution of cholelithiasis in infants. Radiology 157:345–348

Kim OH, Chung HJ, Choi BG (1995) Imaging of the choledochal cyst. Radiographics 15:69–88

King LR, Siegel MJ, Balfe DM (1995) Acute pancreatitis in children: CT findings of intra- and extrapancreatic fluid collections. Radiology 195:196–200

Kirks DR (1992) Fluoroscopic catheter removal of blunt oesophageal foreign bodies: a pediatric radiologist's perspective. Pediatr Radiol 22:64–65

Kirks DR, Swischuk LE, Merton DF, et al. (1981) Caecal volvulus in children. AJR 136:419–422

Kirks DR, Caron KH, Bisset GS III (1992) CT of blunt abdominal trauma in children: an anatomic 'snapshot in time'. Radiology 182:631–632

Kong M-S, Wong H-F, Lin SL, et al. (1997) Factors related to detection of blood flow by colour Doppler ultrasonography in intussusception. J Ultrasound Med 16:141–144

Kunin JR, Korobkin M, Ellis JH, et al. (1993) Duodenal injuries cause by blunt abdominal trauma: value of CT in differentiating perforation from haematoma. AJR 160:1221–1223

Kurtin KR, Fitzgerald SW, Nemcek AA, et al. (1995) CT diagnosis of acute appendicitis: imaging findings. AJR 905–909

Lagalla R, Caruso G, Novara V, et al. (1994) Colour doppler ultrasonography in pediatric intussusception. J Ultrasound Med 13:171–174

Lang EV, Pinckney LE (1991) Spontaneous resolution of bile plug syndrome. AJR 156:1225–1226

Lang I, Daneman A, Cutz E, et al. (1997) Abdominal calcification in cystic fibrosis with meconium ileus: radiologic-pathologic correlation. Pediatr Radiol 27:523–527

Lee JM, Kim H, Byun JY, et al. (1994) Intussusception: characteristic radiolucencies on the abdominal radiograph. Pediatr Radiol 24:293–295

Leonidas JC, Magid N, Soberman N, et al. (1991) Midgut volvulus in infants: diagnosis with ultrasound. Radiology 179:491–493

Levin TL, Liebling MS, Ruzal-Shapiro C, et al. (1995) Midgut malfixation in patients with congenital diaphragmatic hernia: what is the risk of midgut volvulus? Pediatr Radiol 25:259–261

Lieberman JM (1994) Rotavirus and other viral causes of gastroenteritis. Pediatr Ann 23:529–535

Lim HK, Bae SH, Seo GS, et al. (1994) Assessment of reducibility of ileocolic intussusception in children: usefulness of colour Doppler sonography. Radiology 191:781–785

Lim HK, Lee WJ, Lee SJ, et al. (1996) Focal appendicitis confined to the tip: diagnosis at ultrasound. Radiology 200:799–801

Long FR, Kramer SS, Markowitz RI, et al. (1996) Radiographic patterns of intestinal malrotation in children. Radiographics 16:547–556

Lund DP, Murphy EU (1994) Management of perforated appendicitis in children: a decade of aggressive treatment. J Pediatr Surg 29:1130–1134

Macpherson RI (1993) Gastrointestinal tract duplications: clinical, pathologic, aetiologic and radiologic considerations. Radiographics 13:1063–1080

Macpherson RI, Hill JG, Otherson HB, et al. (1996) Oesophageal foreign bodies in children: diagnosis, treatment and complications. AJR 166:919–924

Macrander SJ, Lawson TL, Foley DW, et al. (1989) Periportal tracking in hepatic trauma: CT features. J Comput Assist Tomogr 13:952–957

Matsumoto T, Iida M, Sakai T, et al. (1991) Yersinia terminal ileitis: sonographic findings in eight patients. AJR 156:965–967

Maves MD, Lloyd TV, Carithers JS (1986) Radiographic identification of ingested disc batteries. Pediatr Radiol 16:154–156

McAlister WH, Kronemer KA (1996) Emergency gastrointestinal radiology of the newborn. Radiol Clin North Am 34:819–844

McDermott VG, Taylor T, Mackenzie S, et al. (1994) Pneumatic reduction of intussusception: clinical experience and factors affecting outcome. Clin Radiol 49:30–34

McNamara MJ, Chalmers AG, Morgan M, et al. (1986) Typhlitis in acute childhood leukaemia: radiological features. Clin Radiol 37:83–86

Mellor MFA, Drake DG (1994) Colonic volvulus in children: value of barium enema for diagnosis and treatment in fourteen children. AJR 162:1157–1159

Meradji M, Hussain SM, Robben SGF, et al. (1993) Plain film diagnosis in intussusception. Br J Radiol 67:147–149

Mercado-Deane MG, Burton EM, Howell CG (1995) Transverse colon volvulus in pediatric patients. Pediatr Radiol 25:111–112

Messineo A, MacMillan JH, Palder SB, et al. (1992) Clinical factors affecting mortality in children with malrotation of the intestine. J Pediatr Surg 27:1343–1345

Meyer CM III (1991) Potential hazards of oesophageal foreign body extraction. Pediatr Radiol 21:97–98

Mezoff AG, Balistreri WF (1995) Peptic ulcer disease in children. Pediatr Rev 16:257–265

Miller SF, Landes AB, Dautenhahn LW, et al. (1995) Intussusception: ability of fluoroscopic images obtained during air enemas to depict lead points and other abnormalities. Radiology 197:493–496

Moccia WA, Astacia JE, Kaude JV (1981) Ultrasonographic demonstration of gastric duplication in infancy. Pediatr Radiol 11:52

Moon D, Weeks D, Burgess B, et al. (1997) Perforated duodenal ulcer presenting with shock in a child. Am J Emerg Med 15:167–169

Moore TC (1996) Omphalomesenteric duct malformations. Semin Pediatr Surg 5:116–123

Neilson D, Hollman AS (1994) The ultrasonic diagnosis of infantile hypertrophic pyloric stenosis: technique and accuracy. Clin Radiol 49:246–247

Newman B, Bender TM (1997) Oesophageal atresia/tracheo-oesophageal fistula and associated congenital oesophageal stenosis. Pediatr Radiol 27:530–534

Newman B, Nussbaum A, Kirkpatrick JA (1987) Bowel perforation in Hirschsprung's disease. AJR 148:1195–1197

Noblett HR (1969) Treatment of uncomplicated meconium ileus by Gastrografin enema: a preliminary report. J Pediatr Surg 4:190–197

Norton KI, Luhmann KC, Dolgin SE (1993) Retrograde jejunoduodenal intussusception associated with a jejunal duplication cyst. Pediatr Radiol 23:36–361

O'Donovan AN, Habra G, Somers S, et al. (1996) Diagnosis of Hirschsprung's disease. AJR 167:517–520

O'Haller J (1991) Sonography of the biliary tract in infants and children. AJR 157:1051–1058

O'Halloran SM, Gilbert J, McKendrick OM, et al. (1986) Gastrografin in acute meconium ileus equivalent. Arch Dis Child 61:1128–1130

O'Hara SM (1996) Pediatric gastrointestinal nuclear imaging. Radiol Clin North Am 34:845–862

Pasto ME, Deiling JM, O'Hara AE, et al. (1984) Neonatal colonic atresia: ultrasound findings. Pediatr Radiol 14:346–348

Patrick LE, Ball TI, Atkinson GO, et al. (1992) Pediatric blunt abdominal trauma: periportal tracking at CT. Radiology 183:689–691

Patriquin HB, Garcier J-M, Lafortune M, et al. (1996) Appendicitis in children and young adults: Doppler sonographic-pathologic correlation. AJR 166:629–633

Peh WCG, Khong PL, Chan KL, et al. (1996) Sonographically guided hydrostatic reduction of childhood intussusception using Hartmann's solution. AJR 167:1237–1241

Perry M, Alon U, Lachter JH, et al. (1990) The value of ultrasound in Schönlein-Henoch purpura. Eur J Pediatr 150:92–94

Persliden J, Schuwert P, Mortensson W (1996) Comparison of absorbed radiation doses in barium and air enema reduction of intussusception: a phantom study. Pediatr Radiol 26:329–332

Pierro A, Donnell SC, Paraskevopoulou C, et al. (1993) Indications for laparotomy after hydrostatic reduction for intussusception. J Pediatr Surg 28:1154–1157

Pilling DW, Steiner GM (1981) The radiology of meconium ileus equivalent. Br J Radiol 54:562–565

Pollack ES (1996) Pediatric abdominal surgical emergencies. Pediatr Ann 25:448–457

Pombo F, Arnal-Monreal F, Soler-Fernandez R, et al. (1982) Multiple gastrointestinal atresias with intraluminal calcification. Br J Radiol 55:307–309

Poon TSC, Zhang AL, Cartmill T, et al. (1996) Changing patterns of diagnosis and treatment of infantile hypertrophic pyloric stenosis: a clinical audit of 303 patients. J Pediatr Surg 31:1611–1615

Potts SR, Thomas PS, Garstin WIH, et al. (1985) The duodenal triangle: a plain film sign of midgut malrotation and volvulus in the neonate. Clin Radiol 36:47–49

Powell DM, Otherson HB, Smith CD (1989) Malrotation of the intestines in children: the effect of age on presentation and therapy. J Pediatr Surg 24:777–780

Powell RW, Raffensperger JG (1982) Congenital colonic atresia. J Pediatr Surg 17:166–170

Pracos JP, Tran-Minh VA, Morin DE, et al. (1987) Acute intestinal intussusception in children: contribution of ultrasonography (145 cases). Ann Radiol 30:525–530

Pracos JP, Sann L, Genin G, et al. (1992) Ultrasound diagnosis of midgut volvulus: the "whirlpool" sign. Pediatr Radiol 22:18–20

Puylaert JBCM (1986) Acute appendicitis: ultrasound examination using graded compression. Radiology 158:355–360

Puylaert JCBM, Lalisang RI, van der Werf SDJ, et al. (1988) Campylobacter ileocolitis mimicking acute appendicitis: differentiation with graded compression ultrasound. Radiology 166:737–740

Puylaert JBCM, Vermeyden RJ, Van der Werf SDJ, et al. (1989) Incidence and sonographic diagnosis of bacterial ileocaecitis masquerading as acute appendicitis. Lancet II:84–86

Quillin SP, Siegel MJ (1992) Appendicitis in children: colour Doppler sonography. Radiology 184:745–747

Quillin SP, Siegel MJ (1993) Colour Doppler ultrasound of children with acute lower abdominal pain. Radiographics 13:1281–1293

Quillin SP, Siegel MJ (1994a) Gastrointestinal inflammation in children: colour Doppler ultrasonography. J Ultrasound Med 13:751–756

Quillin SP, Siegel MJ (1994b) Appendicitis: efficacy of colour Doppler sonography. Radiology 191:557–560

Quillin SP, Siegel MJ (1995) Diagnosis of appendiceal abscess in children with acute appendicitis: value of colour Doppler sonography. AJR 164:1251–1254

Quillin SP, Siegel MJ, Coffin CM (1992) Acute appendicitis in children: value of sonography in detecting perforation. AJR 159:1265–1268

Ratcliffe JF, Fong S, Cheong I (1992) The plain abdominal film in intussusception: the accuracy and incidence of radiographic signs. Pediatr Radiol 22:110–111

Riggs W, Parvey LS (1976) Perforated appendix presenting with disproportionate jejunal distension. Pediatr Radiol 5:47–49

Rioux M (1992) Sonographic detection of the normal and abnormal appendix. AJR 158:773–778

Robinson P (1993) The role of nuclear medicine in acute

gastrointestinal bleeding. Nucl Med Commun 14:849–855

Rohrschneider WK, Troger J (1995) Hydrostatic reduction of intussusception under ultrasound guidance. Pediatr Radiol 25:530–534

Rohrschneider W, Troger J, Betsch B (1994) The post-reduction donut sign. Pediatr Radiol 24:156–160

Ros PR, Olmsted WR, Moser RP, et al. (1987) Mesenteric and omental cysts: histologic classification with imaging correlation. Radiology 164:327–332

Rosenfield NS, Ablow RC, Markowitz RI, et al. (1984) Hirschsprung disease: accuracy of the barium examination. Radiology 150:393–400

Rothrock SG, Green SM, Hummel CB (1992) Plain abdominal radiography in the detection of major disease in children: a prospective analysis. Ann Emerg Med 21:1423–1429

Routh WD, Lawdahl RB, Lund E, et al. (1990) Meckel's diverticula: angiographic diagnosis in patients with non-acute haemorrhage and negative scintigraphy. Pediatr Radiol 20:152–156

Sargent MA, Babyn PS, Alton DJ (1994) Plain radiography in suspected intussusception: a reassessment. Pediatr Radiol 24:17–20

Saxton V, Katz M, Phelan E, et al. (1994) Intussusception: a repeat gas enema increases the non-operative reduction rate. J Pediatr Surg 29:588–589

Schey WL, Donaldson JS, Sty JR (1993) Malrotation of bowel: variable patterns with different surgical considerations. J Pediatr Surg 28:96–101

Schiavetti E, Massotti G, Torricelli M, et al. (1984) "Apple peel" syndrome. A radiological study. Pediatr Radiol 14:380–383

Schunk JE, Corneli H, Bolte R (1989) Pediatric coin ingestion: a prospective study of coin location and symptoms. Am J Dis Child 143:546–548

Seashore JH, Collins FS, Markovitz RI, et al. (1987) Familial apple peel jejunal atresia: surgical, genetic and radiographic aspects. Pediatrics 80:540–544

Sfakianakis GN, Conway JJ (1981) Detection of ectopic gastric mucosa in Meckel's diverticulum and in other aberrations by scintigraphy: 1. Pathophysiology and ten year experience. J Nucl Med 22:647–654

Shanmuganathan K, Mirvis SE, Amoroso M (1993) Periportal low density on CT in patients with blunt abdominal trauma: association with elevated venous pressure. AJR 160:279–283

Sharland MR, Chowcat NL, Quereshi SL, et al. (1989) Intestinal obstruction caused by malrotation of the gut in atrial isomerism. Arch Dis Child 64:1623–1624

Sharma V, Sharma ID (1992) Intestinal trichobezoar with perforation in a child. J Pediatr Surg 27:518–519

Shiels WE 2nd, Maves CK, Hedlung GL, et al. (1991) Air enema for reduction and diagnosis of intussusception: clinical experience and pressure correlates. Radiology 181:169–172

Shiels WE II, Kirks DA, Keller GL, et al. (1993) Colonic perforation by air and liquid enema. AJR 160:931–935

Shimanuki Y, Aihara T, Takano H, et al. (1996) Clockwise whirlpool sign at colour Doppler ultrasound: an objective and definite sign of midgut volvulus. Radiology 199:261–264

Shimkin PM (1978) Radiology of acute appendicitis - commentary. AJR 130:1001–1004

Shust N, Blane CE, Oldham KT (1993) Perforation associated with barium enema in acute appendicitis. Pediatr Radiol 23:289–290

Siegel MJ, Herman TE (1992) Periportal low attenuation at CT in childhood. Radiology 163:685–688

Siegel MJ, Shackelford GD, McAlister WH (1980) Small bowel volvulus in children: its appearance on the barium enema examination. Pediatr Radiol 10:91–93

Siegel MJ, Shackelford GD, McAlister WH (1981) Left sided congenital diaphragmatic hernia: delayed presentation. AJR 137:43–46

Siegel MJ, Martin KW, Worthington JL (1987) Normal and abnormal pancreas in children: ultrasound studies. Radiology 165:15–18

Siegler RL (1995) Haemolytic uraemic syndrome in children. Curr Opin Pediatr 7:159–163

Simonovsky V (1995) Ultrasound in the differential diagnosis of appendicitis. Clin Radiol 50:768–773

Sivit CJ (1993) Diagnosis of acute appendicitis in children: spectrum of sonographic findings. AJR 161:147–152

Sivit CJ, Kaufman RA (1995) Commentary: sonography in the evaluation of children following blunt abdominal trauma: is it to be or not to be? Pediatr Radiol 25:326–328

Sivit CJ, Eichelberger MR, Taylor GA, et al. (1992a) Blunt pancreatic trauma in children: CT diagnosis. AJR 158:1097–1100

Sivit CJ, Newman KD, Boenning DA, et al. (1992b) Appendicitis: usefulness of ultrasound in diagnosis in a paediatric population. Radiology 185:549–552

Sivit CJ, Newman KD, Chandra RS (1993a) Visualisation of enlarged mesenteric lymph nodes at ultrasound examination. Pediatr Radiol 23:471–475

Sivit CJ, Taylor GA, Eichelberger MR, et al. (1993b) Significance of periportal low-attenuation zones following blunt trauma in children. Pediatr Radiol 23:388–390

Sivit CJ, Eichelberger MR, Taylor GA (1994) CT in children with rupture of the bowel caused by blunt trauma: diagnostic efficacy and comparison with the hypoperfusion complex. AJR 163:1195–1198

Slovis TL, O'Haller J, Cohen HL, et al. (1989) Complicated appendiceal inflammatory disease in children: pyelophlebitis and liver abscess. Radiology 171:823–825

Smet MH, Marchal G, Ceulemans R, et al. (1991) The solitary hyperdynamic pulsating superior mesenteric artery: an additional dynamic sonographic feature of midgut volvulus. Pediatr Radiol 21:151–157

Smyth RL, van Velzen D, Smyth AR, et al. (1994) Strictures of the ascending colon in cystic fibrosis and high strength pancreatic enzymes. Lancet 343:85–86

Somekh E, Serrour F, Goncalves D, et al. (1996) Air enema for reduction of intussusception in children: risk of bacteraemia. Radiology 200:217–218

Spottswood SE (1994) Peristalsis in duplication cyst: a new diagnostic sonographic finding. Pediatr Radiol 24:344–345

Stein M, Alton DJ, Daneman A (1992) Pneumatic reduction of intussusception: five year experience. Radiology 183:681–684

Stone DN, Kangarloo H, Graviss ER, et al. (1980) Jejunal intussusception in children. Pediatr Radiol 9:65–68

Stringer DA (1989) Congenital and developmental anomalies of the small bowel. In: Pediatric gastrointestinal imaging. Decker, Philadelphia, pp 261–262

Stringer MD, Capps SNJ, Pablot SM (1992) Sonographic detection of the lead point in intussusception. Arch Dis Child 67:529–530

Stringer MD, Dhawan A, Davenport M, et al. (1995) Choledochal cysts: lessons from a 20 year experience. Arch Dis Child 73:528–531

Swischuk LE, Hayden CK Jr (1980) Appendicitis with perforation: the dilated transverse colon sign. AJR 135:687–689

Swischuk LE, Hayden CK Jr, Boulden T (1985) Intussusception: indications for ultrasonography and an explanation of the doughnut and pseudokidney signs. Pediatr Radiol 15:388–391

Swischuk LE, John SD, Swischuk PN (1994) Spontaneous reduction of intussusception: verification with ultrasound. Radiology 192:269–271

Taylor GA, Littlewood Teele R (1985) Chronic intestinal obstruction mimicking malrotation in children. Pediatr Radiol 15:392–394

Taylor GA, Kaufman RA, Sivit CJ (1994) Active haemorrhage in children after thoracoabdominal trauma: clinical and CT features. AJR 162:401–404

Thomason MA, Gay BB (1987) Oesophageal stenosis with oesophageal atresia. Pediatr Radiol 17:197–201

Torris JM, O'Haller J, Velcek FT (1990) Choledochal cyst and biliary atresia in the neonate: imaging findings in five cases. AJR 155:1273–1276

Towbin R, Lederman HM, Dunbar JS, et al. (1989) Oesophageal oedema as a predictor of unsuccessful balloon extraction of oesophageal foreign body. Pediatr Radiol 19:359–360

Uken P, Smith W, Franken EA, et al. (1988) Use of the barium enema in the diagnosis of necrotising enterocolitis. Pediatr Radiol 18:24–27

Vaudagna JS, McCort JJ (1975) Plain film diagnosis of retrocaecal appendicitis. Radiology 117:533–536

van der Schouw YT, van der Velden MTW, Hitge-Boetes C, et al. (1994) Diagnosis of hypertrophic pyloric stenosis: value of sonography when used in conjunction with clinical findings and laboratory data. AJR 163:905–909

Verschelden P, Filiatrault D, Garel L, et al. (1992) Intussusception in children: reliability of ultrasound diagnosis - a prospective study. Pediatr Radiol 22:741–744

Verstandig AG, Klin B, Bloom RA, et al. (1989) Small bowel phytobezoars: detection with radiography. Radiology 172:705–707

Vignault F, Filiatrault D, Brandt ML, et al. (1990) Acute appendicitis in children: evaluation with ultrasound. Radiology 176:501–504

Vinton NE (1994) Gastrointestinal bleeding in infancy and childhood. Gastroenterol Clin North Am 23:93–122

von Allmen D, Goretsky MJ, Ziegler MM (1995) Inflammatory bowel disease in children. Curr Opin Pediatr 7:547–552

Watson NA, Bisset RAL (1994) Case report: intussusception - a cause of chronic abdominal symptoms and weight loss. Clin Radiol 49:723–726

Weinberger E, Winters WD, Liddell RM, et al. (1992) Sonographic diagnosis of intestinal malrotation in infants: importance of the relative positions of the superior mesenteric vein and artery. AJR 159:825–828

Winters WD, Weinberger E, Hatch EI (1992) Atresia of the colon in neonates. AJR 159:1273–1276

Yang ST, Tsai CH, Chen JA, et al. (1995) Differential diagnosis between intussusception and gastroenteritis by plain film. Acta Paediatr Sin 36:170–175

Yeung CY, Lee HC, Huang FY, et al. (1996) Pancreatitis in children - experience with 43 cases. Eur J Pediatr 155:458–463

Yousefzadeh DK, Bickers GH, Jackson JH, et al. (1983) Tubular colonic duplication - review of 1876-1981 literature. Pediatr Radiol 13:65–71

Zerin JM, DiPietro MA (1992) Superior mesenteric vascular anatomy at ultrasound in patients with surgically proved malrotation of the midgut. Radiology 183:693–694

Zerin JM, Polley TZ Jr (1994) Malrotation in patients with duodenal atresia: a true association of an expected finding on postoperative upper gastrointestinal barium study? Pediatr Radiol 24:170–172

Ziegler MM (1994) Meconium ileus. Curr Probl Surg 31:731–777

Ziprokowski MN, Teale RL (1979) Gastric volvulus in childhood. AJR 132:921–925

4 Abdominal Pathology: Urinary Causes

N.B. Wright

CONTENTS

4.1 Introduction

The investigation of pathology related to the urinary tract forms a substantial workload for any radiology department dealing with children. The majority of conditions, either congenital or acquired, can present acutely and require urgent imaging. The object of this chapter, therefore, is to include those conditions that commonly present in the emergency setting and also to give general guidelines which can be applied to the more unusual problems, rather than cover every possible eventuality. As an illustration of

N.B. Wright, DMRD, FRCR, Consultant Paediatric Radiologist, Manchester Children's Hospital NHS Trust, Royal Manchester Children's Hospital, Hospital Road, Pendlebury, Manchester, M27 4HA, UK

the difficulties, it is worth briefly reflecting upon the commonest urinary cause for presentation to an emergency department: acute urinary tract infection (UTI). About 3% of girls and 1% of boys suffer at least one episode of UTI (Wimberg et al. 1974), but despite this the investigation remains a contentious issue, both acutely and in the long-term (Slovis 1995; Seigle and Nash 1995).

In broad terms, emergency conditions of the urinary tract in children can be separated into traumatic and non-traumatic causes. The imaging of genital tract abnormalities is reviewed elsewhere.

In non-traumatic conditions the presenting features of urinary tract pathology in infants may be non-specific; fever, feeding disorders, vomiting and diarrhoea may all be indicators, as may more localising features, such as haematuria and offensive smelling urine. On occasion overwhelming sepsis with shock and hypotension may be seen. More specific features of urinary tract pathology occur with increasing age, such as dysuria, frequency, delayed bladder control or enuresis, abdominal or loin pain and haematuria. Fever and general malaise may also be present. An abdominal mass may be palpable. Occasionally rupture of a large hydronephrosis or haemorrhage into a renal tumour may result in a shocked child requiring urgent resuscitation.

In traumatic circumstances there may be clear signs suggesting genito-urinary injury, such as evidence of penetrating injury in the loin or haematuria. Often, however (and particularly in the case of blunt abdominal trauma), specific features may be lacking and injury is only detected as a consequence of imaging the whole abdomen and pelvis.

4.2 Imaging Modalities

The full range of imaging modalities can be used to visualise the urinary tract, but in general imaging will initially include ultrasound (US) and possibly a

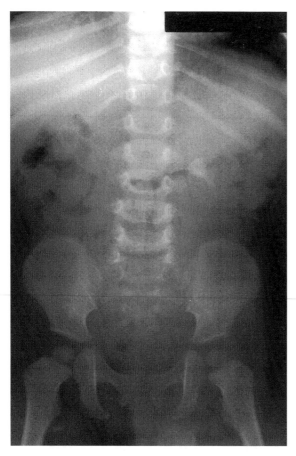

Fig. 4.1. Plain abdominal radiograph shows a left-sided staghorn calculus

plain abdominal radiograph in the non-traumatic situation, and a plain radiograph and preferably contrast-enhanced computed tomography (CT) in the trauma setting.

4.2.1
Plain Radiography

In the non-traumatic situation plain radiographs may help to identify renal or bladder calculi as a cause of abdominal pain or colic (Fig. 4.1), but more often the abdominal film is required to exclude other causes of abdominal pain, such as constipation or bowel obstruction. Gas within a perinephric collection or within the collecting system itself ("gas pyelogram") is rarely seen as a result of infection. Air may be seen in the bladder, usually as a consequence of catheterisation.

In the traumatic situation, the plain film of the abdomen or pelvis is helpful in providing sec-

ondary evidence of possible renal, bladder or urethral trauma. The presence of a lower rib fracture, fracture of the transverse process of a vertebra or loss of psoas shadow may all point to underlying renal trauma. A scoliosis may result from retroperitoneal injury. Fractures of the pelvis may suggest bladder or urethral injury, particularly if the pubic bones are affected. Occasionally the chest x-ray may be helpful, with elevation of the ipsilateral hemidiaphragm or the presence of a small pleural effusion suggesting renal injury.

4.2.2
Ultrasound

Ultrasound remains the primary imaging tool for investigating the urinary tract in the non-traumatic setting. It is non-invasive, avoids radiation, is cheap and can be performed at the bedside if necessary. All these features ensure its continued use as the first line of investigation for many acute urinary tract problems. Structural abnormalities such as focal scarring, calculi and hydronephrosis can be clearly demonstrated, as can fluid collections related to urinomas or haematomas. Where available, the use of colour Doppler and more recently power Doppler can assess renal perfusion in the trauma setting and may have a role in detecting pyelonephritis and scarring (DACHER et al. 1996). US has also been used to detect and grade vesico-ureteric reflux (VUR) using US contrast agents (see Sect. 4.3.1.2). US can be used to guide therapeutic interventional procedures such as the percutaneous drainage of a pyonephrosis or abscess.

4.2.3
Intravenous Urography

In the acute setting, intravenous urography (IVU) is now largely performed for two reasons. Firstly, in those children with suspected renal tract calculi, in whom a calculus cannot be clearly seen to lie in the urinary tract on US. Secondly, in those institutes where there is limited access to cross-sectional imaging in the trauma setting. For this purpose, 1–2 ml/kg of non-ionic, water-soluble contrast is administered intravenously. The IVU can also be used to evaluate pelvi-ureteric junction (PUJ) obstruction, in particular to exclude dilatation of the distal ureter prior to surgery, and also to confirm or exclude duplex systems.

4.2.4
Micturating Cysto-urethrography

Micturating cysto-urethrography (MCU) in the non-traumatic emergency setting is generally performed to evaluate the presence or absence of VUR and grade its severity. Cyclical voiding, that is multiple bladder fillings, may improve the sensitivity of cystography for the detection of VUR (JEQUIER and JEQUIER 1989; DITCHFIELD et al. 1994). It is generally felt appropriate to perform MCU after treatment has commenced and preferably when the urine is sterile, although some institutes will delay the MCU for 6–8 weeks. The use of antibiotics to reduce the risk of iatrogenic infection from the MCU examination has not been clearly defined. If the child has had a confirmed UTI and the *treatment* regimen has been completed (e.g. trimethoprim 4 mg/kg twice daily), most clinicians will continue with a *prophylactic* dose of antibiotic (e.g. trimethoprim 2 mg/kg at night). In these circumstances, some institutes would increase the antibiotic cover over the next 3–5 days following the MCU to *treatment* dose level to reduce the risk of ascending infection, regardless of whether VUR is identified or not. Other institutes would only increase the antibiotic dose if VUR were identified. If the child is not receiving any antibiotics, commencing a short prophylactic dose, or a treatment dose if VUR is identified, may be felt appropriate.

In the trauma setting MCU is usually restricted to evaluation of the bladder for possible perforation/rupture, although other imaging modalities, such as CT or US will often suffice.

4.2.5
Ascending Urethrography

Ascending urethrography is restricted almost exclusively to male children when there has been perineal or pelvic injury and urethral damage is suspected. A Foley catheter is introduced into the distal urethra, the balloon inflated if necessary, and water-soluble contrast injected gently to assess urethral integrity.

4.2.6
Nuclear Medicine

Nuclear medicine can be used both for physiological assessment of renal function, mainly to identify obstruction, and for the detection of acute or long-term renal damage, in the form of acute pyelonephritis and scarring. It also has a role in the detection of VUR.

There is currently much debate whether to image the kidneys in the acute stages of infection using isotope imaging or whether to delay imaging until after the acute infection has subsided. Technetium-99m (^{99}mTc)-labelled dimercaptosuccinic acid (DMSA) and ^{99}m Tc-glucoheptonate are the current radioisotopes in general use and both will detect acute pyelonephritis and renal scarring (see Sect. 4.3.1).

Diuretic renography can differentiate non-obstructive from obstructive hydronephrosis or hydroureter. ^{99}mTc-diethylene triamine penta-acetic acid (DTPA) and ^{99}mTc-mercaptoacetyltriglycine (MAG3) are the most commonly used agents. Both analogue images and time-activity curves should be obtained.

Isotope cystography by either direct (via bladder catheter injection) or indirect (via intravenous injection) methods can be used to assess VUR. Although anatomical detail is less than with radiographic cystography, especially with relation to the male urethra, some centres use isotope cystography to evaluate VUR in well-defined subgroups. Most of these groups are not directly relevant to the acute setting, but the technique is advocated by some authors as a screening tool for assessing girls with UTI (BISSETT et al. 1987).

4.2.7
Computed Tomography

Computed tomography has a major role in assessing blunt abdominal injury. It is important that the examination is enhanced with intravenous contrast and also preferably with oral contrast. Delayed images may be required, especially with the quicker spiral scanners, to detect urine extravasation from the collecting system and the bladder. CT is also useful diagnostically when assessing the extent of a renal abscess and therapeutically for guiding drainage. There may also be a limited role for contrast-enhanced CT in the assessment of acute pyelonephritis (see Sect. 4.3.1.1).

4.2.8
Magnetic Resonance Imaging

The role of MRI in genito-urinary imaging has not been fully evaluated, but there is little doubt that it can replace CT in some circumstances, especially in evaluating the extent of renal infection and tumour staging. Its usefulness in the trauma setting has not been evaluated but it seems likely that its general constraints with respect to polytraumatised patients apply (safety aspects, image acquisition time, access, etc.) and therefore its impact is likely to be small in this area.

4.2.9
Angiography

Angiography is generally indicated in the trauma setting only if renal pedicle injury is suspected or if there is gross haematuria from an unknown source. A standard percutaneous angiogram is generally performed to demonstrate the source of bleeding and assess the potential for embolisation.

4.2.10
Interventional Procedures

The commonest urinary tract interventional procedure in the emergency setting is the percutaneous drainage of a pyonephrosis or an acutely obstructed kidney. Less commonly abscesses require drainage and rarely embolisation procedures are needed in trauma patients. Most interventional procedures in children require general anaesthesia or at least assistance from anaesthetic staff.

Ultrasound is often used to guide renal puncture in pyonephrosis. A urine specimen must be obtained for culture and adequate intravenous antibiotics should be administered prophylactically during the procedure. Subsequently fluoroscopic control is used to ensure opacification of the collecting system in standard antegrade pyelogram fashion and then a pigtail catheter is inserted into the appropriate collecting system. Although the lower pole collecting system is the ideal site for the catheter, children have infected upper moieties of duplex systems more commonly than do adults and therefore may require more unorthodox catheter placement. Usually 6F or 8F catheters suffice, although the urine may be so thick with pus that larger catheters or frequent flushing with saline is required to allow free drainage. An important aspect of the procedure is the subsequent fixation of the catheter following insertion. While the catheter may seem securely placed with the child anaesthetised, young children have a habit of removing them with unnerving regularity if they

are not carefully fixed and appropriate dressings applied!

Renal abscesses may be treated in a similar fashion to pyonephrosis, although their more complex nature may require CT rather than US guidance. Less commonly urinomas, lymphocoeles and haematomas may require aspiration or drainage. There has also been recent work evaluating the use of balloon dilatation of PUJ obstruction with mixed results (WILKINSON and AZMY 1996), but this is unlikely to be performed in the acute setting.

In the trauma setting, significant haemorrhage may require embolisation, which can be performed with a number of materials such as Gelfoam, polyvinyl alcohol microspheres, coils or detachable balloons.

4.3
Non-traumatic Urinary Tract Pathology

Most renal tract abnormalities can present acutely, but the main groups of abnormalities encountered in the emergency setting are related to infection, obstruction including calculus disease, and nephrological causes resulting in haematuria or acute renal failure. Occasionally a neoplasm will present with haematuria or as an abdominal mass.

The initial radiological investigation is usually US, with subsequent imaging guided by the clinical and ultrasonic findings.

4.3.1
Infection

Infection accounts for the largest number of urinary tract presentations to the emergency department. The objective of imaging is to determine whether the infection is limited to the bladder or extends to involve the kidney, and whether there are any structural abnormalities that predispose to infection, such as VUR and obstruction. Some symptoms will help to direct imaging (Table 4.1), but unfortunately no single imaging investigation will adequately evaluate the whole urinary tract, and strategies for investigation will depend on the local availability of equipment. In general, plain abdominal radiographs are unhelpful in UTI and need be done only if calculi are suspected (KENNEY et al. 1991) or if a diagnosis outside the genito-urinary tract is being considered.

Many schemes have been proposed to evaluate UTI, but the main constraints on any proposal are

Table 4.1. Symptoms of upper and lower urinary tract infection

Lower urinary tract	Upper urinary tract
Dysuria	Pyrexia
Enuresis	Anorexia
Frequency	Loin pain
Lower abdominal pain	Malaise
	Vomiting

the availability of equipment and expertise in the local environment. Children admitted to hospital because of fever associated with UTI should undergo US shortly after their admission. This is to rule out a pyonephrosis, hydronephrosis or other secondary complication of infection, as these may need prompt intervention, such as percutaneous nephrostomy, to prevent deterioration in renal function (KANGARLOO et al. 1985). Some institutes would then perform a ^{99}mTc-DMSA renal scan to exclude acute pyelonephritis, although others would leave this for an out-patient visit after the acute infection has subsided in order to identify the presence of renal scars. In either event, there is some recent evidence to suggest that a normal ^{99}mTc-DMSA scan in a child over 4 years of age means the child can be safely discharged without the need for follow-up (VERNON et al. 1997).

After treatment has been commenced an MCU may be performed. It is not necessary to wait a prolonged period before performing the MCU although many institutes will combine MCU with a DMSA isotope renal scan and US assessment at a single attendance some 6–12 weeks after the acute infection has subsided. When deciding upon a departmental imaging strategy for the assessment of UTI, the age of the child to be investigated is a crucial factor. GLEESON and GORDON (1991) demonstrated renal scarring in 48% of children under 1 year of age with VUR. The Birmingham Reflux Study Group (1983) showed that children over 5 years of age are unlikely to develop new renal scars, although COULTHARD et al. (1997) demonstrated an equal chance of detecting scars in toddlers or teenagers with DMSA scanning after a referral for a first UTI. The British Paediatric Radiology and Imaging Group recommend MCU combined with DMSA and renal US in all children under 1 year of age with a proven UTI. Between 1 and 5 years, use of DMSA and renal US is suggested, leading to MCU if either investigation is abnormal. In the over 5's, US alone is recommended initially, with further investigation as appropriate if the US is

abnormal. This latter recommendation could be changed to include a DMSA scan as a number of studies have suggested that US alone is too insensitive for detection of renal scarring. Alternatively, it could be proposed that the DMSA examination be performed instead of US. RICKWOOD et al. (1992) concluded that US should be combined with MCU and renal scintigraphy in the young child. The older child with UTI and a normal US scan requires further investigation only if there is also evidence of systemic upset, fever and vomiting.

4.3.1.1
Acute Pyelonephritis

The most severe consequence of UTI, that is end-stage renal disease secondary to scarring, results from pyelonephritis. The object of imaging is to identify those patients with kidneys at risk of developing scars and those in whom scars have already developed and who therefore need careful monitoring. The initial investigation is usually US although it is rather insensitive (37%, TASKER et al. 1993; 39%, BJORGVINSSON et al. 1991).

In general, the grey-scale US appearances in acute pyelonephritis include a diffuse increase in renal size in the affected kidney, altered parenchymal echogenicity, loss of corticomedullary differentiation and dilatation of the pelvicalyceal system (Fig. 4.2) (MACKENZIE et al. 1994). Other features are calyceal distortion and renal pelvic and ureteric wall thickening with occasionally rounded, hypoechoic lesions present (BJORGVINSSON et al. 1991). Renal volume may increase by up to 176% in about 75% of children with acute pyelonephritis and the increase

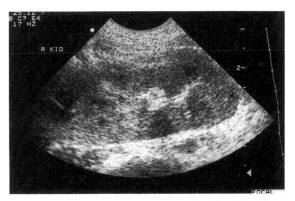

Fig. 4.2. Acute pyelonephritis. Ultrasound of the right kidney shows increased echogenicity and loss of cortico-medullary differentiation in the upper pole

is more marked in young children (DINKEL et al. 1986; JOHANSSON et al. 1988). This increase in size during the acute infection may lead to spurious readings as a baseline measure for subsequent follow-up. PICKWORTH et al. (1995) therefore recommended delaying or repeating US at least 2 weeks after the start of treatment to obtain a more accurate baseline US measure of renal length. More recently colour Doppler (EGGLI and EGGLI 1992) and power Doppler sonography (DACHER et al. 1996) have been used with some positive results. Colour Doppler may show altered (reduced or increased) perfusion to the affected portion of the kidney. On power Doppler areas of acute pyelonephritis show as triangular areas of decreased perfusion. When combined with conventional US, power Doppler increases the sensitivity of US for detecting acute pyelonephritis (89%), but it requires substantial patient co-operation and experienced operators and is time-consuming. US is also able to visualise complications of acute pyelonephritis such as renal or perirenal abscess formation. Although US is generally considered inferior to renal cortical scintigraphy in the detection of renal scarring, scrupulous attention to detail can improve its sensitivity. BARRY et al. (1998) showed that a positive predictive value of 93% and a negative predictive value of 95% could be achieved with modern real-time scanners and careful attention to technique.

There is no doubt that renal cortical scintigraphy (RCS) using ⁹⁹mTc-DMSA is effective in detecting acute pyelonephritis. Affected areas will show reduced uptake. This may be focal, multifocal or diffuse and is consistent with localised ischaemia and tubular dysfunction (MAJD and RUSHTON 1992). The presence of a preserved renal contour ("ghosting") is said to indicate acute pyelonephritis in contradistinction to focal scarring. Recent evidence has therefore suggested that RCS in the acute phase may be helpful not only in identifying acute pyelonephritis, but also more importantly in guiding treatment (MACKENZIE et al. 1994; JAKOBSSON et al. 1994; RUSHTON 1997). Others would argue that the presence of a positive scan is immaterial in the acute phase, since all children with a febrile UTI are treated as if they had acute pyelonephritis (SEIGLE and NASH 1995). Also, as parenchymal changes seen in the acute phase may completely resolve, many centres currently prefer to image the kidneys some time after the acute event (6 weeks up to 6 months). This is in order to identify permanent renal damage, since long-term prognosis is based around the presence of renal scarring (Fig. 4.3). Persisting abnormal DMSA images have been seen in 37% of children 2 years

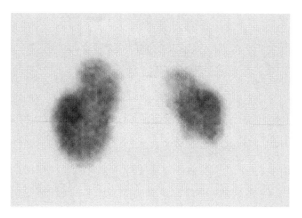

Fig. 4.3. Renal scars. DMSA renal scintigraphy shows an upper pole scar on the left and a small right kidney with multiple peripheral scars

after acute pyelonephritis (JAKOBSSON et al. 1994). The importance of identifying scarring is reflected by studies by GOONASEKERA et al. (1996) and JACOBSON et al. (1989), who found that between 10% and 23% of children with renal scarring developed hypertension in adolescence or early adulthood and that renal scarring led to end-stage kidney disease in 10%. More recently, DMSA single-photon emission computed tomography (SPECT) has been used to detect renal scars (GROSHAR et al. 1994). Presently the data available suggest it may further improve the sensitivity of the DMSA renal scan, although normal variants are known to produce "defects" in up to one-third of patients, which may increase the false-positive rate (ROSSLEIGH 1994).

The role of both contrast-enhanced CT and MRI in the diagnosis of acute pyelonephritis is also currently being evaluated. Contrast-enhanced CT will show areas of acute pyelonephritis as underperfused regions, but whether the technique is practical in a paediatric setting is debatable when DMSA scanning is relatively easy to perform and readily available in most centres. After comparing US, DMSA scans and CT in acute pyelonephritis, LAVOCAT et al. (1997) concluded that DMSA scanning is more sensitive than CT and US. They also considered CT less appropriate because of the need for sedation and the radiation exposure it involved. CT does have the added benefit over DMSA imaging, however, of better anatomical resolution and detection of perinephric disease. It may be an appropriate imaging tool in difficult cases (DACHER et al. 1993). MRI has the advantage over CT in that there is no radiation exposure and it may be potentially more sensitive. Experimental work using gadolinium-enhanced fast multiplanar inversion recovery sequences yielded a

89% sensitivity and 94% specificity in pyelonephritis induced in piglets (PENNINGTON et al. 1996). Further studies are needed for clinical validation.

4.3.1.2
Vesico-ureteric Reflux

Vesico-ureteric reflux is one of the most significant host risk factors for renal scarring and occurs in 30%–40% of those children with UTI (STRIFE et al. 1989; SMELLIE et al. 1981, 1985). In children with acute febrile UTIs, DMSA renal scans show abnormalities in 80%–90% with demonstrable VUR. There are, however, a substantial proportion (63%) of children with focal abnormalities seen on acute DMSA scanning who show no evidence of VUR even if the MCU is performed during the initial hospital admission (DITCHFIELD et al. 1994). The severity (grade) of the VUR is important, with more severe reflux, particularly intrarenal reflux, being correlated with more severe scarring. JODAL (1987) demonstrated that while 17% of children with VUR grade I or II developed scars, the figure increased to 66% with grades III–V. The grading of VUR should follow the International Classification of Vesicoureteric Reflux (International Reflux Committee 1981; LEBOWITZ et al. 1985; Table 4.2).

It is to be noted, however, that there is also more recent antenatal and neonatal evidence to suggest that some renal tracts can simulate post-infective scarring, but are actually dysplastic *ab initio*. This has been termed "foetal reflux nephropathy" and thus, children may present with end-stage renal disease with no antecedent history of UTI. The precise pathophysiological role of VUR in these children is uncertain and there is currently still much debate as to the imaging pathways which should be followed (AVNI et al. 1998).

Vesico-ureteric reflux is best demonstrated by MCU (Fig. 4.4). The MCU will also allow evaluation of the bladder and particularly the urethra, which other methods used to identify VUR, such as direct or indirect isotope cystography, are unable to image adequately. The disadvantages of MCU are its invasiveness and the need to expose the child to ionising radiation.

The role of US in the detection of VUR is controversial. Many paediatric radiologists have considered mild pelvic dilatation as a feature suggesting the presence of VUR. DAVEY et al. (1997), following a retrospective study of 455 children, found that the frequency of VUR was *no different* in kidneys with mild renal pelvic dilatation (anteroposterior diameter of the renal pelvis ≤10 mm) than in those with no distension (≤2 mm). US examinations have also shown no dilatation on the same day a child has had an MCU showing a severe grade of reflux (grade V; BLANE et al. 1993). Furthermore, US has been shown to be unreliable in the detection of renal scarring and thus needs to be combined with another imaging modality such as ^{99}mTc-DMSA renal scanning or IVU (STOKLAND et al. 1994; TASKER et al. 1993). In contradistinction to these studies, AVNI et al. (1997) found that carefully performed US in neonates detected abnormalities suggestive of reflux in 87% of kidneys subsequently found to reflux. The criteria used were renal pelvic dilatation over 7 mm, calyceal and ureteral dilatation over 3 mm, pelvic or ureteric

Table 4.2. International classification of the grade of VUR

Grade of reflux	Level of reflux and appearance
I	Ureter only
II	Ureter, pelvis, calyces No dilatation, normal fornices
III	Mild/moderate dilatation and/or tortuosity of ureter and mild/moderate dilatation of the pelvis with no/slight fornical blunting
IV	Moderate dilatation and/or tortuosity of ureter and mild dilatation of the pelvis and calyces, obliterated fornices but maintenance of papillary impressions in majority of calyces
V	Gross dilatation and tortuosity of ureter, gross dilatation of pelvis and calyces; papillary impressions lost in the majority of calyces

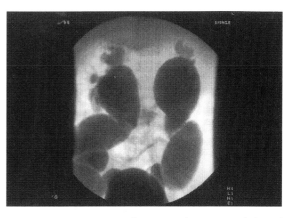

Fig. 4.4. Vesico-ureteric reflux. MCU shows severe bilateral reflux up dilated tortuous ureters into the renal pelvis and calyces (grade 5 reflux)

wall thickening greater than 2 mm, loss of corticomedullary differentiation and evidence of dysplasia. Their population was selective, however, and therefore sensitivity for these variables in the general paediatric population cannot be evaluated (POSTLETHWAITE and WILSON 1997).

In an effort to reduce radiation exposure to children, US contrast agents have been used with some success to perform micturating cystography to detect reflux (DARGE et al. 1997; BOSIO 1998). The technique requires catheterisation and then instillation of the US contrast agent in a similar fashion to a standard MCU. Real-time US of the kidneys and bladder is performed both during the infusion and during micturition to identify reflux. The results have shown good sensitivity and specificity in grading VUR. The technique is time consuming, however, and requires considerable patient cooperation. Its role in assessing the male urethra has not yet been evaluated. It is therefore currently unlikely to replace conventional x-ray MCU. Additionally, BAZOPOULOS et al. (1998) have shown that considerable reduction in radiation dose can be achieved by using digital fluoroscopic hard-copy film rather than spot films with conventional x-ray MCU, without loss in accuracy in the diagnosis and grading of VUR.

4.3.1.3
Acute Lobar Nephronia

Acute lobar nephronia, an acute focal bacterial infection, is a variant of acute pyelonephritis. It usually derives from ascending infection, often due to *E. coli*, and may entail localised infection involving either one pole of the kidney or a single moiety of a duplex system. Sonographic appearances are of an ill-defined hypo-echoic mass, lack of acoustic enhancement and reduced corticomedullary differentiation (Fig. 4.5). Occasionally a wedge-shaped echogenic area is seen consistent with a haemorrhagic form of nephritis. Doppler and colour flow imaging show reduced or absent flow in the focal abnormality. It may be difficult to distinguish it from a focal infarct or a tumour mass and therefore clinical correlation and urinalysis are crucial. DMSA renal scanning shows a photopenic area. Whereas renal abscesses appear as a thick-walled enhancing mass (see Sect. 4.3.1.4), CT of acute lobar nephronia shows a low-attenuation, ill-defined solid mass with inhomogeneous or little enhancement following intravenous contrast. Usually systemic antibiotics will suffice to

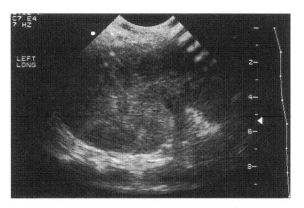

Fig. 4.5. Acute lobar nephronia. Renal ultrasound shows an enlarged upper pole of the left kidney with loss of corticomedullary differentiation in a child with pyrexia. This resolved following antibiotic treatment

obtain complete resolution although some cases will evolve into a renal abscess.

4.3.1.4
Renal Abscess

A renal abscess can result from progression of acute focal pyelonephritis or occasionally from dissemination of distant infection. The abscess can form intrarenally or within the perirenal space and is usually due to *E. coli*, or *Staphylococcus aureus* if from a distant source. Neonates are more prone to fungal abscesses. Children with diabetes mellitus, immune compromise and sickle cell anaemia are all at greater risk of developing an abscess. Initially acute pyelonephritis is often suspected clinically. On US, a mature renal abscess appears as a thick- and irregular-walled mass with hypo- or anechoic appearances centrally. In the early stages it may simulate lobar nephronia (see Sect. 4.3.1.3). Occasionally there is acoustic enhancement. Internal echoes suggest the presence of debris or possibly gas. An IVU may show localised enlargement of a renal pole or more diffuse changes and appearances may simulate a neoplasm with displacement of calyces. Localised reduction in renal function may appear as radiolucency on the IVU. This is also reflected by photopenia on DMSA renal scanning. When perinephric extension is suspected, CT is generally considered the modality of choice, although where available MRI may be substituted (Fig. 4.6). Both intrarenal and extrarenal abscesses show the typical features of a low-attenuation centre with a thick enhancing wall, possibly with septations. The extent of

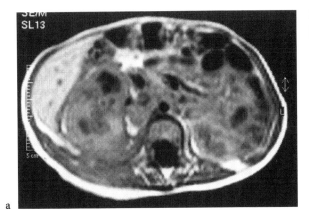

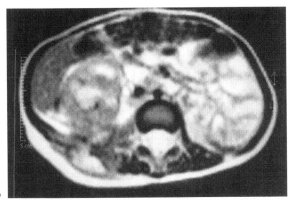

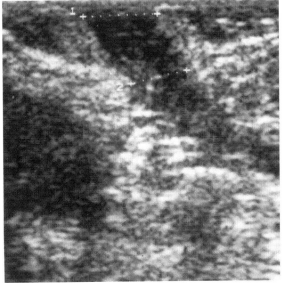

Fig. 4.6 a–c. Renal abscess. Transverse abdominal MR scan. **a** T1- and **b** T2-weighted images demonstrate an enlarged hydronephrotic right kidney with abnormal tissue extending into the posterior perirenal fascia and out into the subcutaneous region. **c** Ultrasound confirms a hypoechoic track leading subcutaneously to the skin surface

inflammatory change can be accurately assessed, with abscess potentially tracking down the psoas muscle or posteriorly through the loin. Ultimately surgical drainage may be necessary, although systemic antibiotics with percutaneous drainage of the abscess using US or CT guidance can be satisfactory.

4.3.1.5
Pyonephrosis

It is important to recognise pyonephrosis, as it requires immediate percutaneous or surgical drainage. The term refers to the presence of pus within a dilated collecting system. The dilatation is usually secondary to a congenital abnormality such as PUJ obstruction, calculus or stricture. The infective organism is often *E. coli*. If there is clinical suspicion of renal obstruction in the presence of infection, urgent US is an essential part of management. The US findings in pyonephrosis are of a dilated collecting system with internal echoes within the fluid and possibly a fluid-fluid or fluid-debris level that alters with changes in posture. When the fluid is echo-free, the diagnosis can be difficult and in such cases percutaneous aspi-

ration or drainage may be required for confirmation. The potential for significant long-term damage in an obstructed, infected kidney is high; hence the need for aggressive management. Occasionally internal echoes reflect the presence of gas-forming organisms. Severe obstruction in a non-infected kidney may result in a collecting system filled with protein and debris leading to false-positive diagnoses, but the key to the diagnosis is an overall assessment of both radiological and clinical features.

4.3.1.6
Fungal Infection

Renal candidiasis is the commonest fungal infection affecting the urinary tract. It is usually seen in premature infants and children with an impaired immune system from any cause. It would be rare for a child to present with fungal infection without a predisposing factor. Candida usually arrives in the kidney by haematogenous spread, initially affecting the parenchyma and then the collecting system, coalescing into round "fungal balls". The latter are best imaged by US and appear as echogenic masses within the collecting system or bladder, showing no acoustic shadowing or enhancement. The kidneys are usually enlarged with an echogenic parenchyma and there may be hydronephrosis and hydro-ureter secondary to PUJ and ureteric obstruction. The bladder may become thick walled and a fungal ball may become large enough to fill the entire lumen. Nephrostomy may be required to relieve obstruction and for instillation of therapeutic agents. Less commonly, aspergillosis, cryptococcosis and blastomycosis may affect the urinary tract.

4.3.1.7
Xanthogranulomatous Pyelonephritis

Xanthogranulomatous pyelonephritis (XPN) is a form of pyelonephritis probably caused by an altered response of the kidney to chronic infection. The common organisms involved are *Proteus mirabilis*, *E. coli* and *S. aureus*. XPN is usually unilateral. Children may present with a flank mass or pain, haematuria, pyuria and fever, but careful history taking often reveals a background of chronic illness, weight loss and growth retardation. There may also be a history of repeated urinary tract infections and possibly known vesico-ureteric reflux. Anaemia and leucocytosis are common findings. Initially renal malignancy is often considered in the differential diagnosis. On histological appearances, a part or the whole of the kidney may be replaced by necrotic tissue which consists of fibrogranulomatous tissue and soft yellow nodules of lipid-filled macrophages or xanthoma cells (KIERCE et al. 1985).

The diffuse type of involvement is often associated with obstruction, possibly from a staghorn calculus or related to congenital PUJ obstruction. Dilated calyces fill with purulent debris while the renal pelvis may remain relatively unchanged in calibre. The more localised form may affect a single moiety of a duplex system or simply be a focal abnormality in an otherwise normal kidney. Calyceal dilatation with pus follows infundibular calyceal obstruction, but calculi are less frequent than in the diffuse form. Children are more prone to this latter type of segmental disease.

A plain abdominal radiograph may show evidence of renal calculi, possibly a staghorn calculus, and the presence of a renal mass (Fig. 4.7). US will show renal enlargement with mixed echoes, dilated calyces containing debris and the presence of calculi. DMSA renal scanning may show a non-functioning kidney or reduced activity in the affected area. Non-function

or poor function is a frequent finding on IVU. CT demonstrates multiple, rounded masses showing patchy enhancement but generally of low attenuation and sometimes enhancement of a thickened renal fascia (COUSINS et al. 1994). CT can be substituted by MRI when the latter is available. Fine-needle biopsy has been used to confirm the diagnosis. Partial or total nephrectomy is the treatment of choice.

4.3.1.8
Cystitis

For imaging purposes cystitis can be divided into infective, non-pyogenic, haemorrhagic and the rarer pseudotumoral forms.

Repeated lower urinary tract infection in the younger child may result in a thick-walled, small-capacity bladder that is readily identified on US. The bladder may appear trabeculated. Bladder wall thickness should not exceed 3 mm with adequate distension, but obviously a child with recurrent infection may not be able to maintain an adequate volume for assessment and in these circumstances subjective evaluation is necessary. Occasionally echogenic debris can be seen within the bladder lumen. Care should be taken in evaluating children with previous surgical procedures to the bladder, particularly bladder augmentation with bowel. In these cases, the presence of echogenic debris within the bladder lumen is a common finding. The assessment of the bladder wall may also be difficult, with the bowel augmentation producing an irregular wall simulating trabeculation.

Some older children will present with recurrent symptoms of lower urinary tract infection (dysuria and frequency) but will have sterile urine, so-called non-pyogenic cystitis. This group of children will often have a normal US, but require imaging to exclude structural abnormalities.

Haemorrhagic cystitis can result from bacterial (*E. coli*), viral (adenovirus) or parasitic (*Schistosoma haematobium*) infection or can be iatrogenic, related to chemotherapy (cyclophosphamide) or radiation. Gross haematuria is the usual presenting feature, with dysuria and frequency often present. When infective in origin it usually affects 5- to 7-year-olds and is self-limiting in 2–3 weeks. Iatrogenic forms of cystitis are unusual presentations to the emergency department and the history often makes the diagnosis, with imaging simply confirming it. The presence of blood clot and bladder wall thickening can be assessed satisfactorily by US. Increased blood flow can be visualised in

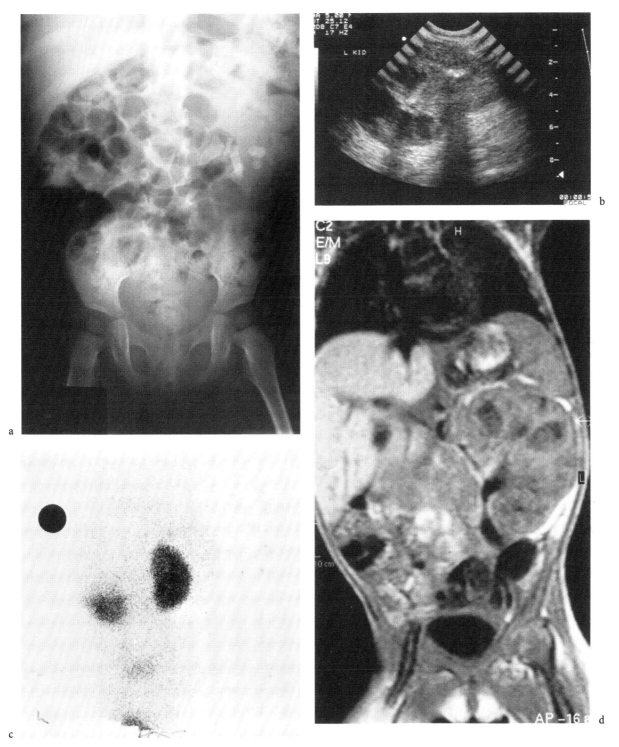

Fig. 4.7 a–d. Xanthogranulomatous pyelonephritis. **a** Plain abdominal radiograph shows numerous calculi in the left flank. **b** Ultrasound confirms the intrarenal nature of the calculi, which show significant acoustic shadowing and dilated upper pole calyces. **c** Renal DMSA scan shows reduced uptake of tracer by the left kidney. **d** Coronal T1-weighted MR image shows an enlarged left kidney with upper pole hydronephrosis and loss of lower pole cortico-medullary differentiation.

the bladder wall with colour flow US. Cystography will show a small-volume bladder with an irregular wall, although this is rarely required.

Occasionally bladder wall thickening can be focal and simulate neoplasia, so-called pseudotumoral cystitis. Again, gross haematuria and bladder irritability are the typical clinical features. In most cases the inflammatory mass is due to eosinophilic cystitis. Other causes are cystitis cystica and granulomatous cystitis. There are recognised associations with drugs, allergy and eosinophilic gastroenteritis (FRIEDMAN et al. 1993). Focal thickening of the bladder wall primarily involves the trigone, is confined to the mucosa, and is associated with generalised bladder wall thickening and unilateral or bilateral hydronephrosis. The mass is solid and broad based with a smooth or irregular outline. VUR may also be present. To the unwary, the features are easily confused with rhabdomyosarcoma of the bladder. The importance is that the condition is self-limiting, requiring only symptomatic treatment or antibiotics with a positive urine culture. Follow-up US will confirm its resolution.

4.3.1.9
Unusual Infections

Tuberculosis, schistosomiasis and hydatid disease may all affect the urinary tract, but are uncommon in children from the "developed world". These more unusual infections need to be considered in children moving into a region from endemic areas and in those returning from holiday abroad. In the emergency setting, schistosomiasis may produce gross haematuria secondary to cystitis (see Sect. 4.3.1.8). The diagnosis may be inferred when calcification of the bladder wall and ureter is seen.

4.3.2
The Urinary Tract Mass

Many of the causes for urinary tract masses in children are covered elsewhere in this chapter and include PUJ obstruction and hydro-ureteronephrosis in general, renal abscesses, and rarely renal cystic disease. Neoplasms are occasionally seen in an emergency setting, sometimes as the presenting complaint ("I can feel a lump, doctor"), or with haematuria (see Sect. 4.3.6), or rarely with a shocked child secondary to internal haemorrhage.

The initial investigation is ultrasound and a plain abdominal radiograph. In the upper abdomen, once hydronephrosis, cystic or calculus disease has been excluded and the presence of a renal or perinephric mass has been confirmed, the main differential diagnosis lies between a Wilms' tumour and neuroblastoma. It is important that other non-neoplastic causes for a mass should also be considered such as an abscess or lobar nephronia (see Sect. 4.3.1). There will often be appropriate clinical pointers to help distinguish the neoplastic from the infective cause of a mass. Once a mass is identified, some features will help to distinguish a Wilms' tumour from a neuroblastoma.

4.3.2.1
Wilms' Tumour

Wilms' tumours are the commonest renal neoplasm in childhood. They are more frequent in boys, 90% occurring under 5 years of age. They grow rapidly. Most children present with an abdominal mass discovered incidentally by a parent who will often comment that it was not there last week. Pain is due to pressure on surrounding structures or due to capsular distension, often precipitated by haemorrhage and tumour necrosis (Fig. 4.8). Haematuria may be the presenting system. Minor trauma may precipitate presentation by causing haemorrhage into the mass, the child presenting with haematuria or a palpable mass.

Wilms' tumours metastasise to the chest. Following presentation at the emergency department, the child should be referred for a plain abdominal rediograph, ultrasound of the abdomen and a chest x-ray. The mass will usually be seen on the abdominal radiograph with displacement of bowel gas around it. There may be elevation of the diaphragm with large tumours. Calcification is present in less than 10% of Wilms' tumours. The ultrasonic appearances are typical: a large intrarenal mass displacing normal cortex around it. The lesion is usually echogenic but necrosis and haemorrhage within the mass may cause a "cystic appearance". Fresh blood is echogenic. Ultrasonic assessment should include identification of breach of the tumour capsule, perirenal haematoma, patency of the renal vein and inferior vena cava or the presence of tumour thrombus within them, the presence of liver metastases (but this is rare) and normality of the contralateral kidneys. Further imaging by CT or MRI will be required to stage the tumour accurately, but this will be done following referral to oncology.

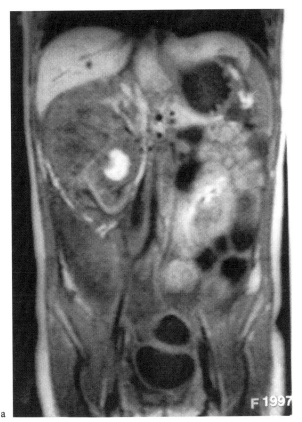

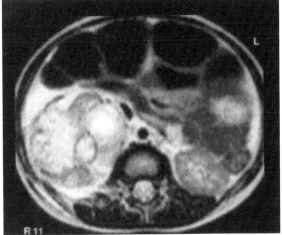

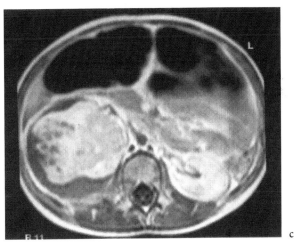

Fig. 4.8 a–c. Haemorrhagic right-sided Wilms' tumour presenting in a shocked child. **a** Coronal T1-weighted MR image shows an area of high signal in the right kidney representing haemorrhage, with inferior displacement of the kidney by a large perinephric haematoma. **b** Transverse T2-weighted sequence shows a multilobular mass replacing the right kidney in addition to a perinephric fluid collection and ascites. **c** Transverse enhanced T1-weighted sequence shows the exophytic nature of the tumour with an apparent breach of the renal capsule laterally and clear definition of the perinephric fluid component

4.3.2.2
Neuroblastoma

Neuroblastomas arise within the adrenal gland most frequently. The other sites are in the presacral region (Fig. 4.9a) or in the sympathetic chain. They occur most frequently under 5 years of age. Tumour staging is by a combination of imaging, biochemical tests and bone marrow examination. When presenting as an emergency, most children will have stage IV disease with widespread metastatic disease. Clinical presentation as an emergency is often because of abdominal distension or general debility with symptoms of bone and abdominal pain. The child looks ill, in contrast to children with Wilms' tumour. Rarer presentation is with the endocrine effects of the tumour, flushing and diarrhoea being the commonest. Orbital metastases may cause proptosis.

As for Wilms' tumour, initial imaging should be an abdominal radiograph and ultrasound. On the radiograph the mass is noted to displace bowel gas; calcification is common, the calcification often being fine (Fig. 4.9b, c). Bone destruction, commonly in the metaphysis of the upper femur, pelvic bones, or more rarely a collapsed vertebra, is not infrequent. At ultrasound examination, the presence of the adrenal mass is confirmed. Calcification is often present. Nodal disease is usually present but may be difficult to distinguish from the primary mass. If colour Doppler imaging is used, vessel encasement by tumour is evident (Fig. 4.9d), but this is easier to ap-

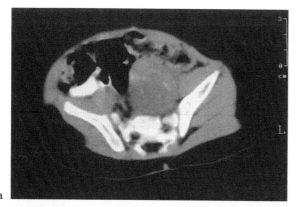

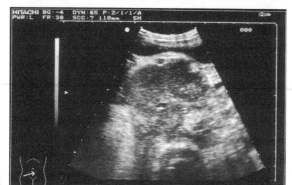

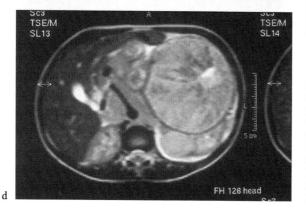

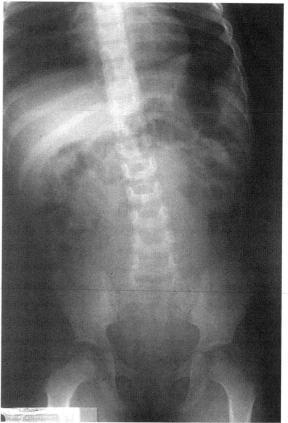

Fig. 4.9. a CT (non-enhanced) scan of child with presacral neuroblastoma in the left abdomen. The child presented with pain and a mass was found on ultrasound. **b** Large central abdominal mass containing fine calcification seen to left of spine. Note displacement of bowel gas around the mass. **c** Ultrasound shows the mainly solid mass with areas of increased echo due to calcification. **d** MRI of a different child. Note encasement of the aorta and coeliac axis by tumour nodes. The large primary tumour is seen in the left abdomen. Note breach of capsule anteromedially

preciate on MRI, as is extension into the spinal canal. Paravertebral extension of the tumour above the diaphragm may be found. A presumptive diagnosis is made by the initial imaging but subsequent imaging will include radionuclide imaging with both methylene diphosphonate (MDP) and MIBG (metaiodobenzylguanidine) and MRI, in addition to urinary collection for catecholamines and bone marrow biopsy.

Presentation of a high paravertebral or cervical neuroblastoma may be airways obstruction or a Horner's syndrome.

4.3.2.3
Other Abdominal Tumours

Retroperitoneal rhabdosarcoma is the third most frequent abdominal solid mass lesion that may present to the emergency department and may be extremely difficult to distinguish from the more frequent Wilms' tumour and neuroblastoma by imaging alone.

Abdominal lymphoma usually presents with symptoms of abdominal pain and distension. Lymphomatous infiltration of the kidneys may occur with any disseminated lymphoma. Clinically, this may present as enlarged kidneys. Ultrasonically, the kidneys are enlarged, with multiple hypoechoic mass lesions. Abdominal lymphoma may cause bilateral obstructive uropathy but this is usually discovered during ultrasonic assessment of the mass. Rarely the obstruction will be total and presents as anuria.

Rhabdomyosarcoma is the most frequent genitourinary pelvic tumour. It arises in the prostate, perineum or vagina. Symptoms are usually those of pain, haematuria, difficulty in micturition and, if bladder obstruction occurs, anuria. A lower abdominal mass is often present. This may be formed of both the tumour and the obstructed bladder. Most pelvic rhabdomyosarcomas are large solid tumours at presentation, containing little or no calcification. A botryoid form exists which on IVU appears as multiple filling defects in the bladder base. Initial imaging is an abdominal radiograph and ultrasound. On the abdominal radiograph a mass may be seen arising from the pelvis, displacing bowel gas around it. The ultrasonic appearances are those of a solid mass, displacing the bladder upwards, and there is often associated hydro-ureteronephrosis. Nodal disease may be evident in the para-aortic region but as for all other abdominal tumours, full staging requires cross-sectional imaging. A presumptive diagnosis can be made, based on the imaging and location but histological confirmation will be needed. In a few children, temporary nephrostomy drainage will be required to maintain urine output.

Presacral tumours may present with symptoms of urinary tract obstruction but more commonly present with constipation first. The main presacral lesions are presacral primitive neuroectodermal tumour, presacral neuroblastoma, sacrococcygeal teratoma and, rarely, anterior meningocele. The last-mentioned is transonic on ultrasound; the others all solid. Imaging of these lesions, once suspected, is by MRI.

4.3.3
Obstruction

4.3.3.1
Congenital Obstruction

4.3.3.1.1
THE UPPER URINARY TRACT
Pelvi-Ureteric Junction Obstruction. Abnormality at the PUJ is the commonest cause of upper urinary tract obstruction in childhood. The left kidney is affected more commonly, and the condition is bilateral in 10%–30%. Ectopic, horseshoe and malrotated kidneys are all at greater risk of PUJ obstruction, the obstruction being largely related in these cases to extrinsic compression by aberrant or multiple vessels. The contralateral kidney requires careful assessment as it may show multicystic dysplasia in 5%–10%, or may be absent or duplicated. A single moiety of a duplex kidney can be affected, and in the majority of cases it is the lower pole. Various findings have been seen at operation for PUJ: intrinsic stenosis, a focal area of dysmotility, and extrinsic compression from a band, adhesion or vessel have all been described. These all result in the same clinical and radiological features. Rarely strictures, valves and polyps may result in PUJ obstruction.

Pelvi-ureteric junction obstruction may present with abdominal distension or a palpable mass in the neonate, or with abdominal pain, haematuria, urinary tract infection or recurrent flank pain at times of increased fluid load in the older child. In a study from 1980, SNYDER et al. found that in about 55% of children the diagnosis is made before 5 years of age, and in 25% during the first year. With the more widespread use of antenatal US, it is likely that more children are now found to have a PUJ obstruction as infants. Rather than present acutely, they will be managed electively and may have surgery prior to developing any symptoms. The children who present with symptoms form a different group clinically, but recent work suggests they have a variable outcome if the degree of dilatation is not excessive: some will not require surgery and may improve spontaneously (RICKWOOD and GODIWALLA 1997).

Ultrasound is the initial diagnostic tool and shows hydronephrosis, with dilated calyces of uniform size communicating with a moderate or large renal pelvis, visible parenchyma and failure to visualise the distal ureter (Fig. 4.10). In neonates a transverse pelvic diameter greater than 10 mm is abnormal and requires investigation to exclude obstruction. Lesser degrees of dilatation (5–10 mm) may not be due to obstruction and can resolve spontaneously. Some are associated with VUR and megaureter and therefore require further imaging (DUDLEY et al. 1997). Minor degrees of dilatation may simulate an extrarenal pelvis, but the number of false-negative scans can be reduced by ensuring a well-hydrated patient. The diagnosis may be difficult in the immediate postnatal period up to about 1 week of age. At this stage the infant is relatively dehydrated and a delayed scan is indicated to reduce the false-negative rate. The renal parenchyma may be thinned and echogenic or

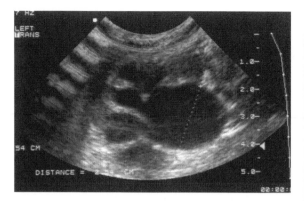

Fig. 4.10. Pelvi-ureteric junction obstruction. Transverse ultrasound image of the left kidney shows a dilated renal pelvis (25 mm) communicating with uniformly enlarged calyces distributed evenly around its periphery, typical of hydrocalycosis. No ureteric dilatation was visualised

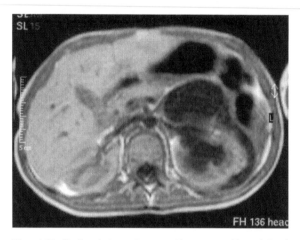

Fig. 4.11. Perinephric urinoma. Transverse T1-weighted MR scan of the upper abdomen shows a large, left-sided perinephric urinoma following rupture of a dilated pelvis secondary to PUJ obstruction

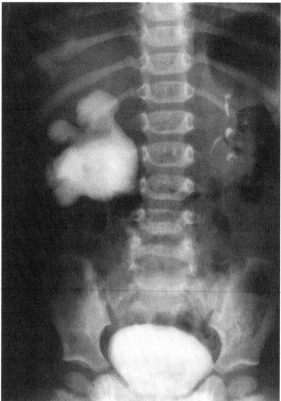

Fig. 4.12. Pelvi-ureteric junction obstruction. A single image from an IVU series confirms the dilated pelvis and calyces with no ureteric dilatation

contain small cysts consistent with areas of renal dysplasia. The degree of pelvic dilatation may be so great as to result in rupture spontaneously or following relatively minor trauma. This may lead to a perinephric urinoma (Fig. 4.11) and the spurious appearance of a non-dilated renal pelvis. Occasionally ureteric dilatation is also present as a result of concomitant VUR or distal vesico-ureteric junction (VUJ) obstruction. VUR will need to be excluded by MCU regardless of whether there is ureteric dilatation. Severe VUR with a dilated tortuous ureter may result in kinking of the PUJ and lead to obstruction that can be relieved by treatment of the reflux. The dilated ureter in this setting should be clearly evident on US and should not cause confusion.

Although the US appearances of PUJ obstruction are relatively characteristic, the degree of renal function and obstruction will need to be assessed either by isotope renography or, more traditionally, by an intravenous urogram (Fig. 4.12) (IVU). Many centres use ^{99}mTc-DTPA or ^{99}mTc-MAG3 for the isotope study with a diuretic administered either immediately prior to the injection of isotope or after a specified time interval depending on departmental policy. Progressive accumulation of tracer in the ipsilateral renal pelvis provides confirmation of obstruction and appears as gradually increasing activity on the time-activity graph (Fig. 4.13). Sometimes the obstruction is incomplete and some response to diuretic is seen. Unfortunately the appearances of the time-activity curves may bear little relationship to the mode of presentation (RICKWOOD and GODIWALLA 1997). The analogue images also require careful evaluation as these may identify unsuspected ureteric dilatation. As mentioned previously, dilatation of the ureter (megaureter) requires further investigation to exclude VUR or distal VUJ obstruction. An IVU shows similar features, with gradual

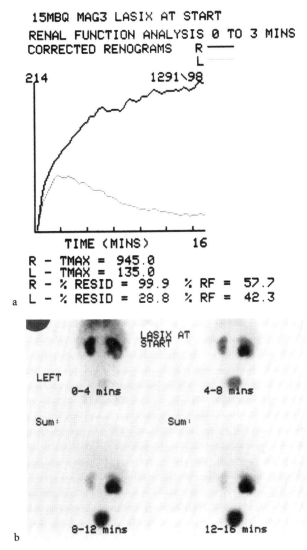

15MBQ MAG3 LASIX AT START
RENAL FUNCTION ANALYSIS 0 TO 3 MINS
CORRECTED RENOGRAMS   R ———
                        L ·······

214   1291\98

TIME (MINS)   16
R - TMAX = 945.0
L - TMAX = 135.0
R - % RESID = 99.9   % RF = 57.7
a L - % RESID = 28.8   % RF = 42.3

LASIX AT START

LEFT
0-4 mins   4-8 mins

Sum: Sum:

8-12 mins   12-16 mins

b

Fig. 4.13 a,b. Pelvi-ureteric junction obstruction. Isotope renogram shows a gradually rising right renal curve with time-activity analysis (a) and a large dilated pelvis on the analogue images (b)

accumulation of contrast within the renal pelvis necessitating the use of delayed and occasionally prone films. Early films may show a rim nephrogram when the dilatation is particularly marked and a slow, gradual filling of the calyces producing the calyceal crescent sign. Occasionally exclusion of distal VUJ obstruction is difficult, as the contrast opacification is so poor due to dilution that a dilated ureter cannot be seen. Careful US and assessment of the analogue images obtained from the isotope renogram usually resolve this problem.

Despite the use of US, isotope renography and IVU, some cases remain equivocal on clinical and

imaging grounds and therefore antegrade pyelography can be performed. This can be combined with pressure studies (Whitaker test) in the older child, although this is not done in the emergency setting.

Occasionally, PUJ obstruction is confused with renal multicystic dysplasia on US. The latter shows cysts of varying sizes that fail to communicate, the largest often lying laterally. There is also echogenic stroma between the cysts. In contradistinction, PUJ obstruction shows a large medially placed cyst (renal pelvis) communicating with smaller cysts (calyces) of uniform size distributed in an orderly fashion around it (Fig. 4.10). In difficult cases, it may be necessary to do a renal "cyst" puncture to differentiate the two conditions. Megacalicosis may also be confused with PUJ obstruction, the important distinguishing feature being the presence of numerous dilated calyces with little dilatation of the renal pelvis.

Following spontaneous rupture of a PUJ obstruction the presence of a urinoma may require evaluation by other cross-sectional imaging modalities, such as CT or MRI, to define the extent of the fluid collection (Fig. 4.11).

Megacalicosis. Infrequently, US shows numerous dilated calyces with minimal or no dilatation of the renal pelvis. There may be some thinning of the renal medulla generally, but the cortex is normal (GARCIA et al. 1987). The ureter is usually not visualised. Isotope renography shows no evidence of obstruction although some retention of tracer activity is seen within the calyces themselves. In this setting, megacalicosis is the likely diagnosis, a congenital abnormality related to hypoplasia of the renal medulla. The condition affects males more than females and is unilateral, non-familial and non-progressive. There is an association with primary megaureter; hence ureteric dilatation is occasionally seen (VARGAS and LEBOWITZ 1986). Between 20 and 25 calyces may be present, each showing a slightly short and wide infundibulum in addition to the calyceal dilatation. An IVU will show some delay in excretion of contrast into the calyces. The features may simulate reflux nephropathy or PUJ obstruction, but the usual presentation is with UTI and calculi (see Sect. 4.3.3.2). A ^{99}mTc-DMSA renal scan will confirm the presence of a normal renal cortex.

Megaureter. A megaureter is simply a dilated ureter and the majority of children with megaureter will present with UTI. There are three groups of

Table 4.3. The primary and secondary causes of megaureter

	Primary causes	Secondary causes
Refluxing megaureter	Absent intravesical ureter	Neurogenic bladder, intravesical obstruction (e.g. posterior urethral valves), ureterocoele
Obstructive megaureter	Congenital obstruction of juxtavesicular ureter by stenosis, stricture, valve or aperistaltic segment	Acquired obstruction, neurogenic bladder, ureterocoele, calculi
Non-refluxing, non-obstructive megaureter	Idiopathic, diagnosis of exclusion	Urinary infection or high urine flow (e.g. diabetes insipidus)

causes: refluxing megaureter, obstructive megaureter and non-refluxing, non-obstructive megaureter, all of which have primary and secondary causes (Table 4.3).

Ultrasound shows dilatation of the proximal or mid ureter, hyperperistalsis of the distal ureter with an adynamic narrowed segment and disproportionate dilatation of the distal ureter when compared with its ipsilateral proximal portion and the renal pelvis. Unfortunately, distinguishing the causes of megaureter cannot be based on US imaging alone. MCU will be required to exclude reflux and isotope renography to exclude obstruction. An IVU may also help to define the anatomy more clearly. A dilated ureter tapering down towards the VUJ is a typical finding (Fig. 4.14).

Miscellaneous Causes of Congenital Upper Urinary Tract Obstruction. These include obstruction related to vessels such as a retrocaval ureter, persistent left umbilical artery or right ovarian vein, or the presence of ureteric valves or diverticula either in the ureter or at the VUJ.

4.3.3.1.2
THE LOWER URINARY TRACT
Children with lower urinary tract obstruction who present acutely usually have infective symptoms such as dysuria and septicaemia. Occasionally a child may present with obstructive symptoms such as straining, dribbling or intermittent stream and rarely with acute retention. In males the commonest cause for lower urinary tract obstruction is posterior urethral valves, and in females a prolapsing ectopic ureterocoele. Other causes for obstruction are calculi, foreign bodies, blood clots, fungus balls, a bladder diverticulum, neuropathic bladder, urethral stricture, anterior urethral diverticulum, urethral polyps, prune belly syndrome, meatal stenosis and phimosis. Causes not directly attributable to the uri-

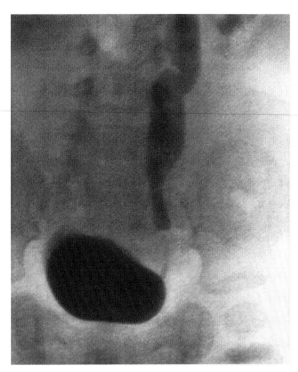

Fig. 4.14. Megaureter. Intravenous urography shows a dilated left renal pelvis and proximal ureter with tapering of the distal ureter consistent with a primary non-obstructing, non-refluxing megaureter

nary tract are usually related to pelvic masses and/or the spine, with discitis, transverse myelitis and spinal tumours sometimes presenting with dysuria or acute retention.

Features suggesting lower urinary tract obstruction are the presence of bilateral hydronephrosis with hydro-ureters in association with a thick-walled bladder. US should demonstrate these features readily and may also show the cause of the obstruction, especially if the abnormality is intravesical (calculus, ureterocoele; see Sect 4.3.4.3). US may also

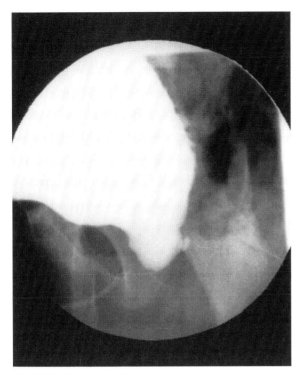

Fig. 4.15. Posterior urethral valves. MCU demonstrating dilatation of the posterior urethra and reflux of contrast into the prostatic utricle

show evidence of dilatation of the posterior urethra, suggestive of urethral valves in a male child.

Posterior Urethral Valves. Posterior urethral valves may present at any age, but generally one-third present in the first month of life, one-third in the first year and one-third thereafter (PARKHOUSE et al. 1988). The obstruction is caused by a bicuspid or unicuspid membrane arising from the posterior urethral wall at the level of the verumontanum. One-third have impaired renal function in the long-term. Deteriorating renal function is related to a number of factors: primary renal dysplasia, renal dysplasia induced by intra-uterine obstruction, intra-uterine hydronephrotic damage, UTI with or without VUR and persistent bladder dysfunction (DINNEEN and DUFFY, 1996). Paradoxically those presenting later tend to have a better prognosis. In addition to the US features suggesting lower tract obstruction described above, US may show evidence of renal dysplasia with echogenic renal parenchyma. US has also been used to assess the posterior urethra during micturition (GOOD et al. 1994). MCU is mandatory and will show a trabeculated, small bladder, possibly VUR, and a

dilated posterior urethra with little or no flow into the anterior urethra. Occasionally contrast will reflux into the utricle, prostate and urachus (Fig. 4.15). As a technical note it is essential that images are obtained with the catheter removed. Renal damage and function can be assessed by isotope studies, usually renography. Immediate treatment is usually with urethral or suprapubic catheterisation, followed by valve ablation.

4.3.3.2
Acquired Obstruction

4.3.3.2.1
CALCULUS DISEASE

Most calculi present with either UTI (55%) or haematuria (23%) or pain (20%). The causes are numerous, but most identifiable causes are related to infection, an anatomical anomaly or abnormal metabolism such as oxalosis. Thus, imaging can help in identifying the aetiology of some calculi, but certainly not the majority. Calculi can be solitary or multiple (Fig. 4.16).

The radiological investigation of choice in suspected acute obstruction secondary to calculus disease (renal colic) is IVU (WEBB 1990). If, however, there is evidence to suggest infection in the presence of obstruction, which is a common setting in children, US is the method of choice to detect dilatation of the collecting system and a possible pyonephrosis.

Ultrasound shows calculi as echogenic areas which are usually associated with acoustic shadowing if greater than 5 mm in diameter (Fig. 4.17). The overall sensitivity for detection is 96% (MIDDLETON et al. 1988). Calculi may be associated with obstruction, particularly when lying in the ureter, or may simply be lying free within the renal pelvis or bladder. When they are associated with obstruction there is often proximal dilatation of the urinary tract, although in the acute phase this may not be especially marked. A plain radiograph may demonstrate the calculus and will be required prior to an IVU. The IVU may show complete obstruction by a calculus, in which case uptake of contrast will be slow and delayed films may be required to demonstrate the level of obstruction if it is not clearly apparent. A "standing column" of contrast from the renal pelvis to the site of obstruction is a classical feature (Fig. 4.18). Occasionally a calculus may have been recently passed, leaving oedema at the VUJ with no visible

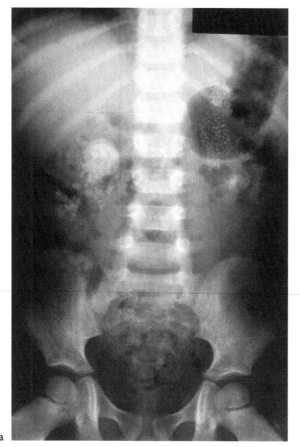

a

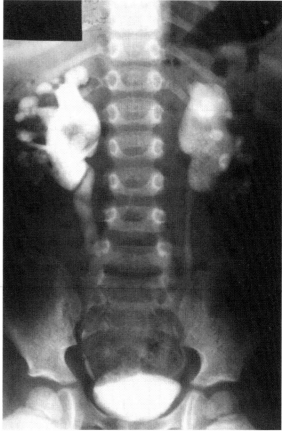

b

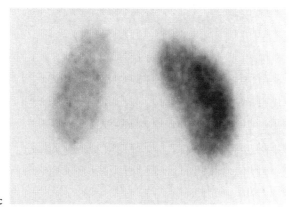

c

Fig. 4.16 a–c. Renal calculi. **a** Multiple bilateral renal calculi shown clearly on this plain abdominal film. **b** Following intravenous contrast there is dilatation of the renal pelvis and calyces bilaterally, with a dilated proximal ureter on the right. **c** A DMSA renal scan shows no focal scarring but asymmetry in tracer distribution

stone, or the calculus may be non-opaque, such as uric acid, xanthine or matrix stones. Oxalic stones are particularly dense and are often associated with nephrocalcinosis and skeletal abnormalities. Conversely, opacities may be thought to be calculi but are actually outside the urinary tract, such as an appendicolith, faecal contents or a calcified ovarian lesion. Occasionally definition of a calculus can be poor and localised CT is required for confirmation. This may be especially helpful in those children with

severe scoliosis, in whom renal position and ureteric course are difficult to define.

Bladder calculi are easily seen on US and plain films and are often freely mobile within a distended bladder (Fig. 4.19). They can also be seen on MCU, although if care is not taken, they can be obscured by contrast. They may produce intermittent bladder outlet obstruction. Rarely urethral calculi may cause acute obstruction. US of the perineum or plain films may confirm the diagnosis.

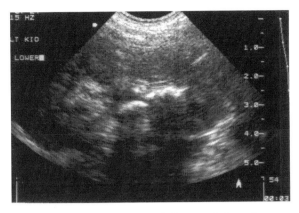

Fig. 4.17. Renal calculi. Left renal ultrasound shows the presence of linear areas of increased echogenicity in the mid and lower pole of the kidney with associated acoustic shadowing typical of calculi

4.3.3.2.2

OTHER CAUSES OF INTRINSIC OBSTRUCTION

Other miscellaneous intrinsic causes of obstruction include blood clots (see Sect. 4.3.6), localised inflammation (e.g. tuberculosis), polyps, valves and fungus balls (see Sect. 4.3.1.6).

4.3.3.2.3

EXTRINSIC CAUSES OF ACQUIRED OBSTRUCTION

Extrinsic causes of acquired obstruction include inflammatory conditions (appendicitis or Crohn's disease), retroperitoneal tumours (neuroblastoma, lymphoma) and large pelvic tumours that produce obstruction either by their mass effect or by local inflammation/infiltration. The nature and level of the obstruction will depend on the primary

a,b,c

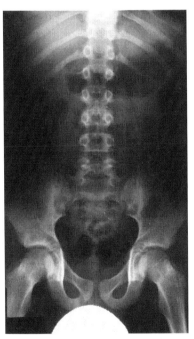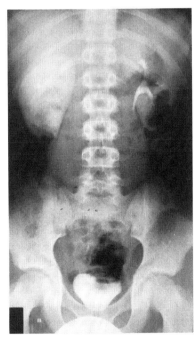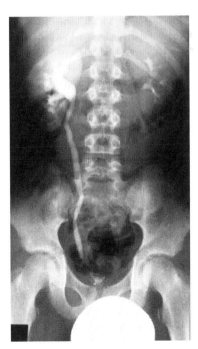

d

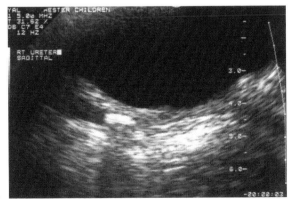

Fig. 4.18 a–d. Ureteric calculus. IVU. **a** The control film shows normal appearances. **b** Following contrast administration, there is delayed appearance of a dense right nephrogram and **c** following micturition after 1.5 h a standing column of contrast in the right ureter confirms obstruction at the VUJ. **d** Ultrasound confirms the presence of a calculus at this site

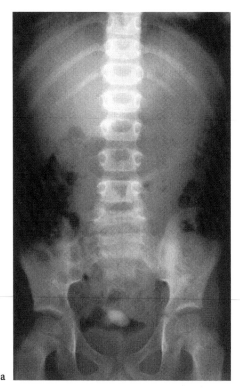

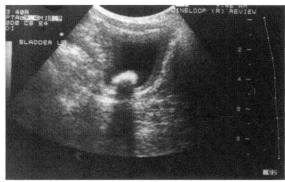

Fig. 4.19 a,b. Bladder calculus. a Abdominal radiograph shows a calcific opacity in the pelvis. b Pelvic ultrasound shows an echogenic mass in the bladder with distal acoustic shadowing consistent with a calculus

abnormality in addition to any associated lymphadenopathy. Retroperitoneal lesions tend to produce unilateral obstruction and pelvic masses, bilateral distal obstruction.

4.3.4
Duplication Anomalies and Ureterocoeles

Duplication anomalies of the renal tract are a common finding and result from abnormal ureteric budding from the wolffian duct at about 5 gestational weeks. The incidence of duplication of the ureter in the general population is about 0.8%. Duplications are twice as common in females, have an equal incidence in either kidney, are more often incomplete than complete and occur bilaterally in 20% (PRIVETT et al. 1976). Complete duplication results in each renal pelvis and its ureter draining separately into the bladder, with the upper pole (moiety) ureter entering the bladder lower and more medially than the lower pole (moiety) ureter, which usually enters in the normal site (orthotopic ureter, Weigert-Mayer law). This rule is rarely broken and the consequences are that the ureters cross in the abdomen or pelvis, and that the upper moiety ureter has a longer submucosal course. Incomplete duplication can vary from a

bifid renal pelvis to two ureters joining just prior to entering the bladder or even in its submucosa (Fig. 4.20).

4.3.4.1
Uncomplicated Duplication

An uncomplicated duplex system is one in which the presence of duplication plays no real part in or contribution to on-going pathology. Uncomplicated duplex systems are often discovered incidentally during US or IVU. On US grounds a duplex system is suspected when there is a discrepancy in renal length of greater than 1 cm and there is a split sinus echo resulting from a band of parenchyma separating the renal hilar complex. About 50% of duplex kidneys are bigger than the contralateral kidney, 40% are equal in size and 10% are smaller (PRIVETT et al. 1976). Thus the US features are inconclusive (unreliable) and an IVU may be necessary to clearly define the anatomy.

In the emergency setting, however, it is important to recognise that uncomplicated duplex systems are common and imaging should be dictated by the clinical problem to be resolved, not by the need to confirm the presence of an uncomplicated duplex

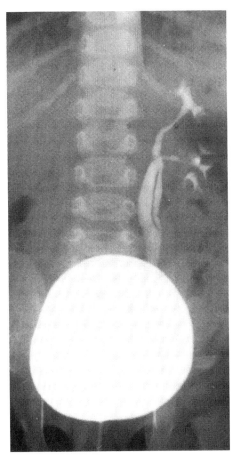

Fig. 4.20. Duplex system. MCU showing left VUR into a partially duplicated ureter and collecting system

system. In the presence of UTI, an MCU may be indicated and show reflux into the lower moiety ureter, regardless of whether there is lower pole pelvic dilatation on US.

4.3.4.2
Complicated Duplication

A complicated duplex system is one in which the presence of the duplication both contributes to and results in pathological processes, most of which become symptomatic. The usual clinical features associated with a complicated duplex system are UTI, an abdominal mass or loin pain, vaginal discharge and constant wetting. In the context of the emergency setting, it is usually UTI, loin pain and possibly the presence of a mass which initiate investigation. For the purposes of discussion, however, although incontinence and vaginal discharge rarely present

acutely, it is important to consider the origins of these symptoms with respect to duplication anomalies.

4.3.4.2.1
UPPER POLE ABNORMALITES AND URETERIC
ECTOPIA

The ureter from the upper moiety inserts medial to and below the orthotopic ureter, but it does *not* always insert into the bladder. In females it can insert alternatively into the urethra or vestibule (69%), vagina (25%), uterus and perineum. Obviously, some of these sites are outside the confines of the bladder-continence mechanism, and therefore some of the girls present with continuous wetting ("She's never been dry, doctor!"). In males the ectopic ureter may insert into the posterior urethra or utricle (57%), ejaculatory duct, vas deferens or seminal vesicle (43%). None of these sites lies distal to the external sphincter mechanism, and therefore incontinence is not a presenting symptom in males.

Urinary tract US may appear normal; otherwise there may be dilatation of the upper moiety calyces, pelvis or ureter. This is usually secondary to stenosis of the ureteric orifice. Frequently the upper moiety renal parenchyma is dysplastic and occasionally it may be difficult to visualise. The distal ureter may also be associated with a ureterocoele that may be clearly visible in the bladder. An MCU usually fails to show VUR into the upper pole, but reflux into the lower moiety may give secondary evidence of the presence of a duplex system with displacement of the ureter and the "drooping flower" appearance to its pelvis. An IVU may clearly show the presence of a duplex system (Fig. 4.21), a dilated upper moiety and ureter draining into an ectopic site, but if the function in the moiety is impaired, poor contrast definition may give misleading reassurance. It is important to analyse the images of both kidneys scrupulously for asymmetry to minimise the risk of a false-negative study. Subsequent imaging is needed to formally evaluate renal function with a DMSA renal scan and possibly an isotope renogram. In these cases not only can split renal function be calculated for each kidney, but also for each moiety (Fig. 4.22).

4.3.4.2.2
LOWER POLE ABNORMALITIES

Vesico-ureteric reflux is the commonest abnormality associated with the lower pole of a duplex system. The grade of reflux is generally more severe in duplex systems. One review (SKOOG 1992) found grade

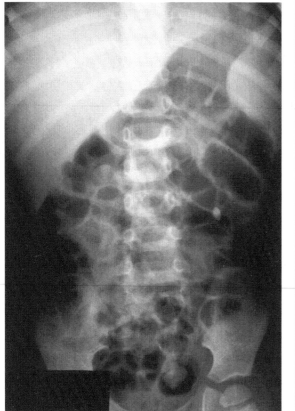

a

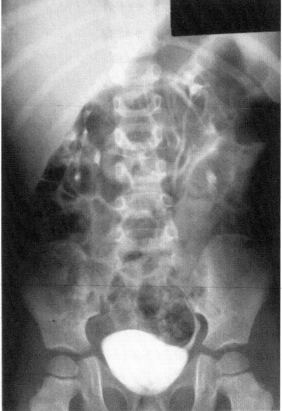

b

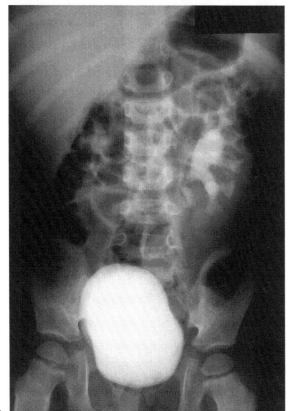

c

Fig. 4.21a–c. Duplex system with lower pole calculus. a A
control film at presentation shows a calcific opacity lateral to
the L3/4 level on the left. b Fifteen-minute film from an IVU
series shows a left duplex system with the calculi in the lower
moiety. The upper moiety is of normal calibre. c One-hour
delayed film shows contrast in a dilated lower moiety and
slightly dilated ureter. The calculus is obscured by contrast in
the lower pole calyx

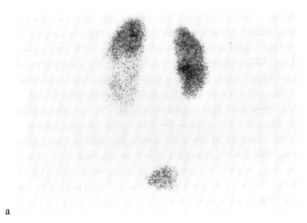

a

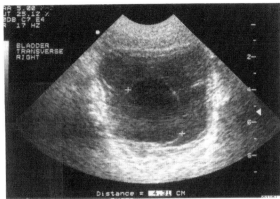

Fig. 4.23. Ureterocoele. Ultrasound shows a thin-walled ureterocoele lying in the right side of the bladder

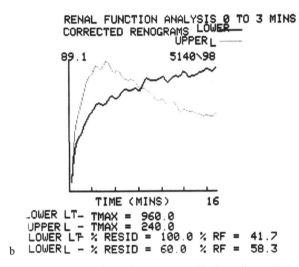

b

Fig. 4.22 a,b. Left duplex system. a Single analogue image from an isotope renogram shows clear differential uptake by the upper and lower moieties of the left kidney. The right kidney is normal. b Split renal curves from the upper and lower moieties of the left kidney alone show poor drainage of the lower moiety with a rising curve. Normal curve from the upper moiety

requires investigation along similar lines (see Sect. 4.3.3.1) (Fig. 4.22).

4.3.4.3
Ureterocoeles

Not only can the upper pole ureter insert in an abnormal site, but it is also often associated with a ureterocoele. This is a congenital cystic dilatation of the terminal submucosal or intravesical ureter. Ureterocoeles are usually associated with the upper moiety of duplex systems, but can be seen in single systems and rarely the lower moiety of duplex systems. They can be simple (stenotic, orthotopic or adult-type) or ectopic (infantile). Simple ureterocoeles are relatively unusual in children, but are slightly more common in boys and tend to be intravesical. Ectopic ureterocoeles account for about 60%–75% of ureterocoeles encountered in children and 80%–90% involve the upper moiety of a duplex system. They are more common in girls and are bilateral in 10%. Their close proximity to the bladder neck and urethra means they may present prolapsing into the introitus in girls and as acute bladder outlet obstruction in both sexes. They are usually associated with hydroureter. On US they appear as rounded, thin-walled, intravesical cysts at the base of the bladder (CREMIN 1986; Fig. 4.23). Occasionally they can fill the entire bladder with the wall of the cyst merging with the bladder wall on US appearances and leading to a false-negative scan. When sufficiently large they can also be associated with obstruction of the lower pole ureter on the ipsilateral side and the ureter(s) on the contralateral side, leading to ureteric dilatation. If the ureter associated

IV or V reflux in 27.1% of duplex and 7.6% of single systems. The lesser grades of reflux generally follow the same course as similar refluxing single systems with respect to the incidence of scarring and the resolution of reflux (BEN-AMI et al. 1989). They can therefore be treated in the same fashion. VUR is best demonstrated by MCU (see Sect. 4.3.1.2). Features on MCU or IVU that suggest the presence of a duplication include fewer calyces when compared with the normal contralateral side, lateral displacement of the kidney, an abnormal axis to the collecting system, increased distance from the upper renal contour to the opacified collecting system and a spiral course to the ureter ("Drooping flower"). PUJ obstruction may also affect the lower moiety of a duplex system and

with the ureterocoele contains debris the uretero-coele may also contain similar material, clarifying its relationship.

On MCU, the ureterocoele usually appears as a filling defect at the bladder base. Occasionally, when filling pressure is high or when the bladder is full, the ureterocoele is effaced or even inverted into its ureter to give the spurious appearance of normality or the presence of a bladder diverticulum (BELLAH et al. 1995). It is therefore always important to visualise the bladder early during the filling phase of an MCU to avoid this error. The ureterocoele may prolapse into the bladder neck or urethra during micturition. On IVU similar features may be seen, but also the ureterocoele can fill with contrast and may look like a "spring onion" or "cobra's head" (Fig. 4.24). There is often disparity between the size of the ureterocoele and the ureter. Occasionally it is difficult to determine the precise insertion point of the ureterocoele and in such cases antegrade pyelography may help to clarify the situation.

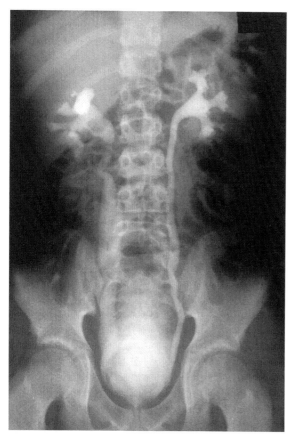

Fig. 4.24. Orthotopic ureterocoele: Single film of an IVU series shows a dilated ureter down to the bladder, where the ureterocoele is clearly seen

4.3.5
Renal Parenchymal Disease

Among the large spectrum of causes of renal parenchymal disease, those generally presenting acutely include all the causes of acute renal failure, nephrotic syndrome, thrombotic thrombocytopenic purpura and the haemolytic-uraemic syndrome. The renal parenchyma may also be involved as a result of systemic disease such as sickle cell disease, leukaemia and lymphoma.

Most nephrological causes for presentation to the emergency department do not require input from the imaging department to make the diagnosis as this is usually made biochemically. Despite this, plain abdominal films and US are often requested while the cause is being confirmed. The plain abdominal film may suggest the presence of ascites and show evidence of bowel wall thickening, but is of limited value. US frequently shows the presence of enlarged, echogenic kidneys with variable expression of corticomedullary differentiation and possibly free intraperitoneal and pleural fluid. A chest x-ray may also show pleural fluid or even consolidation in immunological causes of nephritis such as Goodpasture's syndrome. Ultimately, renal parenchymal disease may need histological analysis, necessitating renal biopsy with US or fluoroscopic guidance.

4.3.6
Haematuria

Haematuria in children can result from a number of causes, but the commonest are UTI, inflammation, trauma and calculi. Occasionally neoplasms can present solely with haematuria. The source of the blood loss logically may be from the renal parenchyma, the collecting system, the ureter, the bladder and the urethra. Occasionally the cause can be identified clinically, but frequently imaging is required. With respect to UTI, haematuria suggests direct involvement of the collecting system or lower urinary tract. Infections commonly affecting the collecting system, such as fungi, are best imaged with US.

With respect to inflammation, trauma and calculi, the reader is referred to the other relevant sections.

Neoplasms may present acutely with abdominal pain and/or haematuria. The presence of haematuria again indicates involvement of the collecting system or lower urinary tract. US should be the first imaging modality utilised, but subsequently CT or MRI will need to be performed for accurate staging. In the

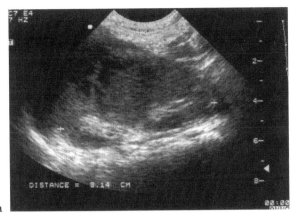

a

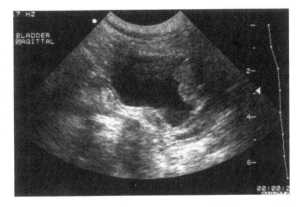

b

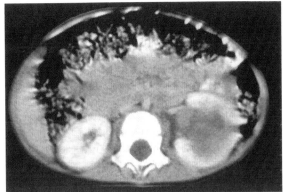

c

Fig. 4.25 a–c. Stage 1 Wilms' tumour. **a** Ultrasound shows an ill-defined iso- and hypoechoic mass in the mid-pole of the left kidney with splitting of the renal sinus echo. **b** Non-enhanced CT demonstrates the centrally placed mass which **c** following contrast fails to enhance. The normal parenchyma is displaced around the mass. No local spread or distant disease was found

upper urinary tract, Wilms' tumour usually presents with an abdominal mass but may involve the collecting system early in the disease and present with haematuria (Fig. 4.25). Renal cell carcinoma is less common. In the lower tract, rhabdomyosarcoma is the commonest malignancy and usually affects the bladder, pelvic floor or prostate (TANNOUS et al. 1989; Fig. 4.26). It commonly produces haematuria associated with straining to void or dysuria.

4.3.7
Renal Cystic Disease and Haemorrhage

The classification of renal cystic disease is complex and includes a large number of conditions that are inherited or syndromic. For the purposes of the emergency setting, children with cystic disease may present with acute pain related to associated calculi or possibly internal haemorrhage. There may be a previous history of renal cystic disease, in which case comparison with previous investigations may help to identify a specific cyst as the cause of the current problem, or the cyst(s) may be discovered de novo.

Fig. 4.26. Bladder rhabdomyosarcoma. Sagittal ultrasound of the bladder shows a lobular thickening of the bladder wall antero-inferiorly, subsequently confirmed to be neoplastic. The child presented with haematuria

Features suggesting cystic disease as a cause of the presenting complaint are a rapid increase in size of previously noted cysts or the presence of internal debris within the cyst(s) itself. Cysts are best seen using US and generally appear as well-defined, round structures associated with acoustic enhancement. When multiple cysts are present it may be difficult to define normal parenchyma, and occasionally disease is so extensive as to require numerous images to generate a "complete picture". The presence of internal echoes suggests a more proteinaceous content, possibly haemorrhage, which may be the cause of the presentation. Occasionally the cysts may rupture, leading to a perinephric collection.

It is essential that both kidneys are carefully evaluated, for the presence of bilateral cysts is more significant than a single, simple cyst. The liver, spleen and pancreas must also be scrutinised for cystic disease. IVU may suggest the presence of a mass lesion with calyceal splaying or distortion and a DMSA scan may show a cyst as a photopenic area. Rarely a Wilms' tumour may present with a multicystic mass. In the neonate, an abdominal mass may be the presenting feature of polycystic disease, with ultrasound showing large echogenic kidneys occasionally with macrocysts. Multicystic dysplasia may also present as a renal mass in the infant.

4.3.8
Urachal Anomalies

The urachus is a normal embryological structure that joins the urogenital sinus with the allantois. It generally undergoes a process of involution that commences during the 4th to 5th month of gestation and continues on into the first few months of life. Involution is usually complete by 6 months of age. The process of involution has been recently visualised using US (ZIEGER et al. 1998) and generally causes no problems. Abnormal regression of the urachus, however, can result in a number of abnormalities: patent urachus, urachal diverticulum, urachal sinus and urachal cyst. The usual presenting feature is one of a discharging umbilicus or sinus, or of a palpable mass. In either event the initial examination is US, preferably utilising a high-resolution probe. Cystic abnormalities associated with the urachus are easily demonstrated, although MCU or fistulography may be necessary (NAGASAKI et al. 1991).

4.4
Traumatic Urinary Tract Pathology

Trauma to the genitourinary tract in children is usually as a result of blunt abdominal injury and occurs in about 10% of cases. Penetrating injuries are more unusual. In either case, the overwhelming priority of the initial management of the child is to obtain haemodynamic and cardiorespiratory stabilisation.

While this is occurring, some basic but essential plain radiography is mandatory. A child presenting with blunt abdominal injury requires a radiograph of the pelvis and a chest x-ray. A lateral cervical spine film is also advisable, but this should be guided by the clinical history and examination. A formal abdominal film including the pelvis may be preferred to the pelvic x-ray alone as it may help to confirm the position of a nasogastric tube, the bowel gas pattern, the presence of a pneumoperitoneum and any abnormal soft tissue masses suggesting the presence of a haematoma or urinoma. Depending on the availability, the next investigation, regardless of whether there is suspected urinary tract injury, should be a contrast-enhanced abdominal CT examination. Both oral (1%–2%) and intravenous contrast (1–2 ml/kg) should be administered and there should be a low threshold for repeating the scans after a short delay (5 min) to enhance the detection of urine/contrast extravasation from a ruptured urinary tract. This is particularly so when using spiral/helical scanning techniques. Alternatively intravenous urography and US can be used to assess the urinary tract although they do have some limitations.

In the trauma setting, much emphasis is often placed on the presence of haematuria as a marker of urinary tract injury. The need to image the genitourinary tract in paediatric trauma should, however, be based as much upon the clinical evaluation of the patient as on the presence of haematuria, since major injuries may not even produce microscopic haematuria (ABOU-JAOUDE et al. 1996). Blunt abdominal trauma can result in gross or microscopic haematuria and predicts the presence, but not the severity of urinary tract injury (KARP et al. 1986; STEIN et al. 1994). Despite this, a child with a normal blood pressure and microscopic haematuria (less than 50 red blood cells per high-power field) is unlikely to have sustained significant renal injury (STALKER HP et al. 1990).

Although blunt injury following a road traffic accident is the commonest mode of presentation to the emergency department and penetrating injuries do occur intermittently, non-accidental injury, including sexual abuse, should always be considered if the history or setting seems inappropriate.

4.4.1
Renal Injury

Renal injury following blunt abdominal trauma is more frequently seen in children than adults and

Table 4.4. Classification of renal injury

Grade 1	Contusions and small haematoma, capsule intact
Grade 2	Lacerations limited to the cortex
Grade 3	Deep lacerations/fractures extending into the collecting system
Grade 4A	Segmental infarcts
Grade 4B	Vascular pedicle injury

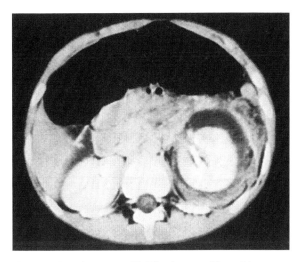

Fig. 4.27. Renal trauma. CT following a traffic accident confirms the presence of a left-sided perinephric collection of low attenuation consistent with a perinephric urinoma. Free fluid is also present in the right subhepatic space

occurs in 1.2%–15% of cases. The kidneys are comparatively larger than in adults, and are less well protected, having less perinephric fat and thinner abdominal musculature. The left kidney is more susceptible to injury and the presence of pre-existing renal tract anomalies, such as a pelvic or horseshoe kidney or hydronephrosis, which occurs in about 5% of children, increases the likelihood of damage.

The general objective of imaging is not only to establish the degree of damage to the injured kidney, but also to demonstrate normal function of the contralateral kidney before any surgery is contemplated. There are a number of proposed systems for classifying renal injury, but any system should be practical and relevant to management issues. Accordingly, the Hessel and Smith (YALE-LOEHR et al. 1989) system is easy to use in the emergency setting (Table 4.4).

Contrast-enhanced CT is the imaging modality of choice, but if CT is unavailable, US can be performed. In general, however, it underestimates the extent of renal damage. Fresh haemorrhage usually appears echogenic, with reduction in echogenicity with time. MAYOR et al. (1995) suggested that microscopic haematuria following blunt abdominal injury in an otherwise asymptomatic patient requires only US evaluation and a series of subsequent urinalyses; in the acute phase, however, US could miss renal contusions, which would be evident 24–48h later. Mayor et al. commented that parenchymal bleeding could be echogenic or echo-poor and reported that intravenous pyelography (IVP) was more accurate in detecting all types of renal injury (80.8% vs 40.1%), but their study did not involve the use of Doppler techniques. A normal IVP excluded severe renal injury. IVP was unhelpful in children following blunt trauma with asymptomatic microscopic haematuria, but IVP and US complemented each other in the setting of gross haematuria or if isolated renal injury was suspected (loin pain, ecchymosis, haematoma). US was useful in identifying perinephric and retroperitoneal abnormalities as well as associated injuries.

As indicated above, contrast-enhanced CT is the examination of choice when renal injury is suspected

in a multiply injured, but haemodynamically stable child. It is quick and non-invasive and is able to assess a number of organ systems simultaneously. This is important as most renal damage (82%) is associated with other injuries (MCALEER et al. 1993). In a review of 4000 children presenting to a US Trauma Centre, MCALEER et al. found that isolated renal damage occurs rarely, in about 0.22% of admissions. ABDALATI et al. (1994) reported that 5% of children sustaining blunt abdominal injury had CT evidence of renal injury. The outcome of these injuries depended on the initial CT grade of renal injury: contusions, small haematomas and lacerations healed without significant complications (grades 1 and 2). Segmental infarcts resulted in tissue loss proportional to the degree of vessel occlusion, the volume of tissue lost being related to the extent of hypo-attenuation seen on the CT examination. Vascular pedicle injury resulted in complete loss of renal function, but the highest complication rate (30%) was associated with deep lacerations and fractured kidneys. KUHN and BERGER (1981) and SIEGEL and BALFE (1989) found these to be the commonest renal injury, with fractures or lacerations extending through the renal capsule. These often resulted in either a perirenal haematoma or a urinoma (Fig. 4.27) if the collecting system was involved.

On CT, a renal fracture appears as an irregular, frequently wedge-shaped, low-attenuation defect, which is optimally seen following contrast enhancement (Fig. 4.28). Recent fresh haemorrhage shows a greater density than non-enhanced renal paren-

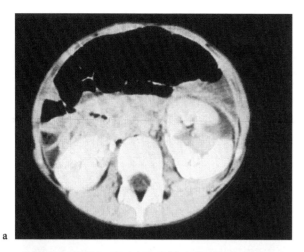

a

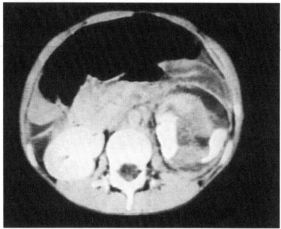

b

Fig. 4.28 a,b. Fractured kidney. **a** CT shows a fractured kidney on the left, extending from the parenchymal surface into the renal pelvis. **b** Contrast leakage confirms rupture of the renal collecting system

chyma, whereas urinomas appear as lower density. Despite this, it may be difficult to distinguish haematoma from urinoma on CT and occasionally delayed imaging may help clarify the situation, with contrast-opacified urine entering the collection in a urinoma (Fig. 4.28b). Once a urinoma has been identified, monitoring of its progress is generally best performed by ultrasound. Occasionally percutaneous drainage is required if the urinoma fails to resolve or becomes symptomatic. Subcapsular haematomas appear as lentiform or occasionally oval collections and may be associated with mass effect, distorting the renal contour. Perirenal fluid collections are often larger, are confined by Gerota's fascia and may completely surround the kidney. The presence of large quantities of retroperitoneal fluid in the interfascial or anterior pararenal space or psoas

muscle is associated with more severe injury, but its absence does not exclude significant renal trauma (SIEGEL and BALFE 1989).

Severely shattered kidneys are well demonstrated by contrast-enhanced CT, with the vascular integrity of the remaining parenchyma clearly visualised. Despite the obvious extensive abnormality these cases may be treated conservatively with little long-term scarring. Occasionally partial or complete nephrectomy may be required, but it is essential that the function of the contralateral kidney be assessed beforehand. Renal pedicle damage is clearly identified on CT, with failure of any renal enhancement indicating pedicle damage requiring prompt surgery. The follow-up of renal injury is generally best performed by nuclear medicine techniques to assess residual function.

4.4.2
Ureteric Injury

Ureteric injuries are unusual in children and often go undetected initially. The typical site for damage is the proximal ureter and around the PUJ, where compression of the ureter against the ribs or transverse processes of the upper lumbar vertebrae results in transection or partial rupture. The diagnosis may be made on CT (SIEGEL and BALFE 1989) or IVU if the radiologist remains alert to the possibility and identifies perinephric, perihilar or retroperitoneal extravasation of contrast. With CT this may require delayed images. Features that suggest PUJ disruption include an intact renal parenchyma, no perirenal haematoma, contrast seen almost entirely in the medial perirenal area and no opacification of the ureter distal to the disruption (KENNEY et al. 1987). Other features may include loss of the psoas shadow and the presence of a focal mass or fluid collection. In the long term, stricture and fistula formation and retroperitoneal fibrosis may occur.

4.4.3
Bladder Injury

Both intra- and extraperitoneal bladder rupture can occur rarely following blunt abdominal injury. SIVIT et al. (1995) found seven bladder ruptures (four intraperitoneal and three extraperitoneal) in a series of 1500 children sustaining blunt abdominal trauma over a 10-year period. Rupture may be suspected clinically if there is gross macroscopic haematuria or spurious anuria resulting from free intraperitoneal leakage of urine. The diagnosis is usually made by retrograde cystography, US or contrast-enhanced CT. Cystography is generally considered the best technique but is invasive and may be difficult to perform in the presence of pelvic fractures. Bladder rupture can be missed by contrast-enhanced CT although delayed imaging of the pelvis following intravenous contrast injection appears to improve the sensitivity (SIVIT et al. 1995).

Extraperitoneal rupture is more common and is often associated with fracture of the superior pubic ramus. Cystography and CT will show evidence of localised perivesical leakage of contrast. Secondary signs of perivesical haematoma or fluid collection may be seen with US or CT, although with an empty bladder US assessment will be difficult. The treatment is generally conservative with transurethral or suprapubic catheterisation.

Intraperitoneal rupture can have more serious consequences with peritonitis and metabolic disturbances. If there is free leakage of urine into the peritoneum, the bladder may appear small and underfilled with urine ascites present in the abdomen. US will clearly show the presence of free intraperitoneal fluid, although it may not be immediately apparent that it is urine and not a haemoperitoneum. The wall defect is difficult to identify in the contracted bladder and may only be demonstrated when the bladder is distended or during attempted micturition. Extravasated contrast spills into the peritoneum, filling the paracolic gutters and outlining bowel loops. When leakage of contrast occurs superiorly, it may be difficult to distinguish intraperitoneal from extraperitoneal rupture. If extraperitoneal, contrast may track superiorly and anteriorly to the umbilicus in the prevesical space, and inferiorly and laterally around the rectum. If intraperitoneal, it will lie in a more lateral position and will usually communicate with the lateral paracolic gutters (SIVIT et al. 1995).

4.4.4
Urethral and Perineal Trauma

Injury to the perineum from straddle trauma and pelvic fractures may result in urethral damage, particularly in males. Gross haematuria in the presence of a pelvic fracture is strongly suggestive of urethral injury. The child may still be able to void if the tear is incomplete. In blunt abdominal injury and pelvic fracture, it is the posterior urethra at the level of the

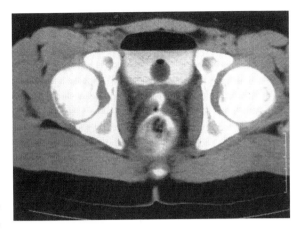

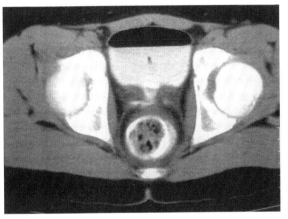

Fig. 4.29 a,b. Traumatic vesicocolic fistula. CT cystogram images (a,b) show a vesicocolic fistula in this male child who sustained a penetrating injury to the perineum. No oral or rectal contrast was administered

urogenital diaphragm that is usually damaged, with straddle-type injuries more likely to result in anterior urethral damage. Ascending urethrography is the investigation of choice and may demonstrate peri-urethral extravasation of contrast. The presence of bladder filling suggests an incomplete tear. If urethral damage is present, suprapubic catheterisation is the initial treatment. Although unusual, traumatic rupture of the urethra can occur in girls and usually occurs at the level of the urogenital diaphragm (PATIL et al. 1982). These injuries are difficult to visualise radiographically, but they may be demonstrated using a modified urethrography technique. The close proximity of the urethra to the vagina with the urethrovaginal septum intervening means that urethral and vaginal injuries often occur concurrently. OKUR et al. (1996) reviewed 38 girls sustaining lower genitourinary tract injuries, most of which followed a fall or motor vehicle accident. The most frequent injuries were to the vulva (63%)

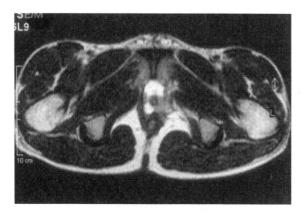

Fig. 4.30. Penetrating perineal injury. Transverse T1-weighted MR scan of the pelvis shows asymmetry of the levator ani group of muscles in the left side of the perineum following a penetrating injury

and vagina (53%), with 6 girls having rupture of the urethra.

Examination under anaesthetic and primary repair is the optimum treatment, with radiology having a minimal contribution apart from assessment of associated abdomino-pelvic injury. Penetrating injuries, labial contusion and introital laceration all suggest child abuse if the history is inappropriate.

Penetrating injuries of the perineum may produce bladder injury generating fistulous tracks to the skin surface or between body cavities. These cases generally require cystography, sinography or a contrast enema for accurate delineation. Occasionally CT may be helpful in conjunction with the contrast study to define the extent of the track (Fig. 4.29). Perineal injury can also result in extensive disruption of the perineal muscles, resulting in urinary or faecal incontinence. In these circumstances MRI may be helpful in delineating the structural damage prior to reconstruction (Fig. 4.30).

References

Abdalati H, Bulas DI, Sivit CJ, Majd M, Rushton HG, Eichelberger MR (1994) Blunt renal trauma in children: healing of renal injuries and recommendations for imaging follow-up. Pediatr Radiol 24:573–576

Abou-Jaoude WA, Sugarman JM, Fallat ME, Casale AJ (1996) Indicators of genitourinary tract injury or anomaly in cases of pediatric blunt trauma. J Pediatr Surg 31:86–90

Avni EF, Ayadi K, Rypens F, et al. (1997) Can careful US examination of the urinary tract exclude vesicoureteric reflux in the neonate? BJR 70:977–982

Avni EF, Hall M, Schulman CC (1998) Congenital uro-nephropathies: is routine voiding cystourethrography always warranted? Clin Radiol 53:247–250

Barry BP, Hall N, Cornford E, et al. (1998) Improved ultrasound detection of renal scarring in children following urinary tract infection. Clin Radiol 53:747–751

Bazopoulos EV, Prassopoulos PK, Damilakis JE, et al. (1998) A comparison between digital fluoroscopic hard copies and 105-mm spot films in evaluating vesicoureteric reflux in children. Paediatr Radiol 28:162–166

Bellah RD, Long FR, Canning DA (1995) Ureterocele eversion with vesicoureteric reflux in duplex kidneys: findings at voiding cystourethrography. Am J Roentgenol 165:409–413

Ben-Ami T, Gayer G, Hertz M, et al. (1989) The natural history of reflux in the lower pole of duplicated collecting systems: a controlled study. Pediatr Radiol 19:308–310

Birmingham Reflux Study Group (1983) Prospective trial of operative versus non-operative treatment of severe vesicoureteric reflux in children: two years' observation in 96 children. BMJ 287:171–174

Bissett III GS, Strife JL, Dunbar JS (1987) Urography and voiding cystourethrography: findings in girls with urinary tract infection. Am J Roentgenol 148:479–482

Bjorgvisson E, Madj M, Eggli KD (1991) Diagnosis of acute pyelonephritis in children: comparison of sonography and 99mTc-DMSA scintigraphy. Am J Roentgenol 157:539–543

Blane HH, Di Pietro MA, Zerin JM, et al. (1993) Renal sonography is not a reliable screening examination for vesicoureteric reflux. J Urol 150:752–755

Bosio M (1998) Cystosonography with echocontrast:a new imaging modality to detect vesicoureteric reflux in children. Pediatr Radiol 28:250–255

Coulthard MG, Lambert HJ, Keir MJ (1997) Occurrence of renal scars in children after their first referral for urinary tract infection. BMJ 315:918–919

Cousins C, Somers J, Broderick N, et al. (1994) Xanthogranulomatous pyelonephritis in childhood: ultrasound and CT diagnosis. Pediatr Radiol 24:210–212

Cremin BJ (1986) A review of the ultrasonic appearances of posterior urethral valve and ureterocoeles. Pediatr Radiol 16:357–364

Dacher J-N, Boillot B, Eurin D, et al. (1993) Rational use of CT in acute pyelonephritis: findings and relationships with reflux. Pediatr Radiol 23:281–285

Dacher J-N, Pfister C, Monroc M, et al. (1996) Power Doppler sonographic pattern of acute pyelonephritis in children: comparison with CT. Am J Roentgenol 166:1451–1455

Darge K, Troeger J, Rohrschneider W, et al. (1997) Contrast sonography for the detection of vesicoureteric reflux in children. Abstracts of 34th Congress of ESPR, p 72

Davey MS, Zerin JM, Reilly C, Ambrosius WT (1997) Mild renal pelvic dilatation is not predictive of vesicoureteral reflux in children. Pediatr Radiol 27:908–911

Dinkel E, Orth S, Dittrich M, Schulte-Wisermann H (1986) Renal sonography in the differentiation of upper from lower urinary tract infection. Am J Roentgenol 146:755–780

Dinneen MD, Duffy PG (1996) Posterior urethral valves. Br J Urol 78:275–281

Ditchfield MR, de Campo JF, Nolan TM, et al. (1994) Risk factors in the development of early renal cortical defects in children with urinary tract infection. Am J Roentgenol 162:1393–1397

Dudley JA, Haworth JM, McGraw ME, et al. (1997) Clinical relevance and implications of antenatal hydronephrosis. Arch Dis Child 76:F31–34

Eggli KD, Eggli D (1992) Color Doppler sonography in pyelonephritis. Pediatr Radiol 22:422–425

Friedman EP, de Bruyn R, Mather S (1993) Pseudotumoral cystitis in children: a review of the US features in four cases. Br J Radiol 66:605–608

Garcia CJ, Taylor KJW, Weill RM (1987) Congenital megacalyces: US appearance. J US Med 6:163–165

Gleeson FV, Gordon I (1991) Imaging in urinary tract infection. Arch Dis Child 66:1282–1283

Good CD, Vinnicombe SJ, Dicks-Mireaux C, Mather S, King A (1994) Voiding urethrosonography in the diagnosis of posterior urethral valves in male infants. Royal College of Radiologists annual scientific meeting, programme and abstracts, p 40, Norwich, Sept 1994

Goonasekara CDA, Shah V, Wade AM, Barrat TM, Dillon MJ (1996) 15-year follow-up of renin and blood pressure in reflux nephropathy. Lancet 347:640–643

Groshar D, Moskovitz B, Gorenberg M, et al. (1994) Quantitative SPECT of technetium-99m-DMSA uptake in the kidneys of normal children and in kidneys with vesicoureteric reflux: detection of unilateral kidney disease. J Nucl Med 35:445–449

International Reflux Committee (1981) Medical versus surgical treatment of primary vesicoureteric reflux. Paediatrics 67:392–400

Jacobson SH, Eklof O, Eriksson CG, et al. (1989) Development of hypertension and uraemia after pyelonephritis in childhood. BMJ 299:703–706

Jakobsson B, Berg U, Svensson L (1994) Renal scarring after acute pyelonephritis. Arch Dis Child 70:111–115

Jequier S, Jequier J-C (1989) Reliability of voiding cystourethrography to detect reflux. Am J Roentgenol 157:807–810

Jodal U (1987) The natural history of bacteriuria in childhood. Infect Dis Clin North Am 1:713–719

Johansson B, Troell S, Berg U (1988) Renal parenchymal volume during and after acute pyelonephritis measured by ultrasonography. Arch Dis Child 63:1309–1314

Kangarloo H, Gold RH, Fine RN, et al. (1985) Urinary tract infection in infants and children evaluated by US. Radiology 154:367–373

Karp MP, Jewett TC, Kuhn JP, Allen JE, Dokler ML, Cooney DR (1986) The impact of CT scanning on the child with renal trauma. J Pediatr Surg 21:617–623

Kenney PJ, Panicek DM, Witanowski LS (1987) CT of ureteral disruption. J Comput Assist Tomogr 11:480–484

Kenney IJ, Arthur RJ, Sweeney LE, et al. (1991) Initial investigation of childhood urinary tract infection: does the plain abdominal x-ray still have a role? Br J Radiol 64:1007–1009

Kierce F, Carroll R, Guiney EJ (1985) Xanthrogranulomatous pyelonephritis in childhood. Br J Urol 57:261–264

Kuhn JP, Berger PE (1981) CT in the evaluation of blunt abdominal trauma in children. Radiol Clin North Am 19:503–513

Lavocat MP, Granjon D, Allard D, Gay C, Freycon MT, Dubois F (1997) Imaging of pyelonephritis. Pediatr Radiol 27:159–165

Lebowitz RL, Olbing H, Parkkulaien KV, Smellie JM, Tammuren-Mobius TE (1985) International system of radiographic grading of VUR. Pediatr Radiol 15:105–109

MacKenzie JR, Fowler K, Hollman AS, et al. (1994) The value of US in the child with an acute urinary tract infection. Br J Urol 74:24–244

Majd M, Rushton HG (1992) Renal cortical scintigraphy in the diagnosis of acute pyelonephritis. Semin Nucl Med 22:98–111

Mayor B, Gudinchet F, Wicky S, Reinberg O, Schnyder P (1995) Imaging evaluation of blunt renal trauma in children: diagnostic accuracy of intravenous pyelography and ultrasonography. Pediatr Radiol 25:214–218

McAleer IM, Kaplan GW, Scherz HC, Packer MG, Lynch FP (1993) Genitourinary trauma in the pediatric patient. Urology 42:563–568

Middleton WD, Dodds WJ, Lawson TL, Foley WD (1988) Renal calculi: sensitivity for detection with US. Radiology 167:239–244

Nagasaki A, Handa N, Kawanami T (1991) Diagnosis of urachal anomalies in infancy and childhood by contrast fistulography, ultrasound and CT. Pediatr Radiol 21:321–323

Okur H, Kucukaydin M, Kazez A, et al. (1996) Genitourinary tract injuries in girls. Brit J Urol 78:446–449

Parkhouse HF, Barratt TM, Dillon MJ, et al. (1988) Long-term outcome of boys with posterior urethral valves. Br J Urol 62:59–62

Patil V, Nesbitt R, Meyer R (1982) Genitourinary tract injuries of the pelvis in females: sequelae and their management. Br J Urol 54:32–38

Pennington DJ, Lonergan GJ, Flacic CE, et al. (1996) Experimental pyelonephritis in piglets: diagnosis with MR imaging. Radiology 201:199–205

Pickworth FE, Carlin JB, Ditchfield MR, et al. (1995) Sonographic measurement of renal enlargement in children with acute pyelonephritis and time needed for resolution: implications for renal growth assessment. Am J Roentgenol 165:405–408

Postlethwaite RJ, Wilson B (1997) Ultrasonography vs cystourethrography to exclude vesicoureteric reflux in babies. Lancet 350:1567–1568

Privett JTJ, Jeans WD, Roylance J (1976) The incidence and importance of renal duplication. Clin Radiol 27:521–530

Rickwood AMK, Godiwalla SY (1997) The natural history of pelvi-ureteric junction obstruction in children presenting clinically with the complaint. Br J Urol 80:793–796

Rickwood AMK, Carty HM, McKendrick T, et al. (1992) Current imaging of childhood urinary infections: prospective survey. BMJ 304:663–665

Rossleigh MA (1994) The interrenicular septum: a normal anatomical variant seen on DMSA SPECT. Clin Nucl Med 19:953–955

Rushton HG (1997) The evaluation of acute pyelonephritis and renal scarring with technitium 99m-dimercaptosuccinic acid renal scintigraphy: evolving concepts and future directions. Pediatr Nephrol 11:108–120

Siegel MJ, Balfe DM (1989) Blunt renal and ureteral trauma in childhood: CT patterns of fluid collections. Am J Roentgenol 152:1043–1047

Seigle R, Nash M (1995) Is there a role for renal scintigraphy in the routine initial evaluation of a child with urinary tract infection? Pediatr Radiol 25:S52–S53

Sivit CJ, Cutting JP, Eichelberger MR (1995) CT diagnosis and localisation of rupture of the bladder in children with blunt abdominal trauma: significance of contrast material extravasation in the pelvis. AJR 164:1243–1246

Skoog SJ (1992) Spontaneous resolution of vesicoureteric reflux in the duplicated system: a comparison with single system VUR. In: Patil V (ed) Dialogues in pediatric urology: a new look at duplication of ureters. Miller, New York, pp 7–8

Slovis TL (1995) Is there a single most appropriate imaging workup of a child with an acute febrile urinary tract infection? Paediatr Radiol 25:S46–S49

Smellie JM, Normand ICS, Katz G (1981) Children with urinary infection: a comparison of those with and those without vesicoureteric reflux. Kidney Int 20:717–722

Smellie JM, Ransley PG, Normand ICS, Prescod N, Edwards D (1985) Development of new renal scars: a collaborative study. BMJ 290:1957–1960

Snyder HN, Lebowitz Rl, Colodny AH, Bauer SB, Retik AB (1980) Ureteropelvic junction obstruction in children. Urol Clin North Am 7:273–290

Stalker HP, Kaufman RA, Stedje K (1990) The significance of hematuria in children after blunt abdominal trauma. Am J Roentgenol 154:569–571

Stein JP, Kaji DM, Eastham J, et al. (1994) Blunt renal trauma in the pediatric population: indications for radiographic evaluation. Urology 44:406–410

Stokland E, Hellstrom M, Hansson S, et al. (1994) Reliability of ultrasonography in identification of reflux nephropathy in children. BMJ 309:235–239

Strife JL, Bisset GS, Kirks DR, et al. (1989) Nuclear cystography and renal sonography: findings in girls with urinary tract infection. Am J Roentgenol 153:115–119

Tannous WN, Azous EM, Homsy YL, et al. (1989) CT and US imaging of pelvic rhabdomyosarcomas in children: a review of 56 patients. Pediatr Radiol 19:530–534

Tasker AD, Lindsell DRM, Moncrieff M (1993) Can US reliably detect renal scarring in children with urinary tract infection? Clin Radiol 47:177–179

Vargas B, Lebowitz RL (1986) The coexistance of congenital megacalyces and primary megaureter. Am J Roentgenol 147:313–316

Vernon SJ, Coulthard MG, Lambert HJ, et al. (1997) New renal scarring in children who at age 3 and 4 years had had normal scans with dimercaptosuccinic acid: follow up study. BMJ 315:905–908

Webb JAW (1990) Ultrasonography in the diagnosis of renal obstruction. BMJ 301:944–946

Wilkinson AG, Azmy A (1996) Balloon dilatation of the pelviureteric junction in children: early experience and pitfalls. Pediatr Radiol 26:882–886

Wimberg J, Anderson HJ, Bergstrom T, et al. (1974) Epidemiology of symptomatic UTI in childhood. Acta Paediatr Scand 63 [Suppl 252]:1–20

Yale-Loehr AJ, Kramer SS, Quinlan DM, LaFrance ND, Mitchell SE, Gearhart JP (1989) CT of severe renal trauma in children: evaluation and course of healing with conservative therapy. AJR 152:109–113

Zieger B, Sokol B, Rohrschneider WK, et al. (1998) Sonomorphology and involution of the normal urachus in asymptomatic newborns. Pediatr Radiol 28:156–161

5 Genital Emergencies

A.S. HOLLMAN and S. MACDONALD

CONTENTS

5.1
Introduction

Genital emergencies are infrequent compared with other acute paediatric emergencies but the potential for such adverse outcomes as testicular wastage and infertility, with their associated psychological problems, necessitates rapid diagnosis and optimum management.

5.2
Genital Emergencies in Boys

5.2.1
Problems in Clinical Assessment

Acute genital pathology in boys comprises acute scrotal and acute penile disorders. Penile emergencies are, on the whole, clinically evident and include

A.S. HOLLMAN, MD, Consultant Paediatric Radiologist, Department of Paediatric Radiology, Royal Hospital for Sick Children, Yorkhill, Glasgow G3 8SJ, UK
S. MACDONALD, MD, Consultant Paediatric Radiologist, Department of Paediatric Radiology, Royal Hospital for Sick Children, Yorkhill, Glasgow G3 8SJ, UK

phimosis, paraphimosis, meatal ulceration and priapism. Imaging is not usually required for diagnosis or management.

The term "acute scrotum" describes the scrotum with acute pain, swelling and other signs of inflammation (FLANIGAN et al. 1981). Prompt and accurate diagnosis is required to avoid testicular damage and to ensure timely surgery is not withheld in appropriate cases (NOSEWORTHY 1993). The diagnostic accuracy of clinical assessment of acute scrotal pathology has been shown to be incorrect in up to 50% of cases (RILEY et al. 1976). Clinical symptoms and signs are non-specific, variable and commonly misleading because of the marked tenderness and swelling; some clinicians have therefore advocated that such cases warrant surgical exploration (STEINHARDT et al. 1993).

5.2.2
Role of Imaging

The diagnosis of acute scrotal pathology is based on combined clinical and imaging evaluation. Ultrasound is the mainstay for imaging of the scrotum and has a high sensitivity in determining the location and nature of the pathology and in differentiating cystic from solid lesions and testicular from paratesticular pathology (HAMM 1997). Sonography in isolation is non-specific, and the clinical features are also required for diagnostic specificity (FOURNIER et al. 1985).

Nuclear scintigraphy, using technetium-99 m sodium pertechnetate, was considered to be the gold standard imaging modality to diagnose testicular torsion. It has an overall sensitivity of 95% in the paediatric population (BABCOCK 1995). The disadvantages of this investigation include the radiation burden (estimated at 0.0032 Gy to the testes) (STEIN et al. 1980), and the difficulty in arranging an immediate "out of hours" service, which results in delay in surgery. The inability to differentiate complicated epididymo-orchitis from missed torsion is also a major drawback (BARLOON and WEISSMAN 1996; INGRAM and HOLLMAN 1994).

Early Doppler studies were disappointing in evaluating the acute scrotum. Continuous wave Doppler without the facility to accurately localise flow proved unreliable (RODRIGUEZ et al. 1981; LEE et al. 1983; BRERETON 1981; NASRALLAH et al. 1977). Conventional duplex Doppler does not significantly increase the accuracy of evaluation because of the difficulty in detecting flow in small testicular vessels in children. Colour Doppler imaging represents a significant technical advance and provides colour flow data from vessels within the entire field of imaging while providing simultaneous and detailed anatomical information. There are a few caveats in its use in the acute scrotum. Perfusion is usually absent in complete torsion but observable in partial torsion or between episodes of intermittent torsion. In addition, blood flow may be increased due to reactive hyperaemia following spontaneous detorsion (INGRAM et al. 1993; RALLS et al. 1991). Operator experience and the sensitivity of the colour Doppler equipment used are likely to influence diagnostic accuracy, and a child with a single testis precludes comparison of the findings with those of the contralateral asymptomatic side (PRYOR et al. 1994). Lastly, the small size of the paediatric testicular vasculature leads to additional difficulty as flow in the normal testis in very young children may be difficult to demonstrate (INGRAM and HOLLMAN 1994).

Power Doppler imaging is a technique reported to increase the sensitivity and the detection of blood flow by a factor of 3–4 (BABCOCK et al. 1996). Coded on the basis of total energy (amplitude) of the Doppler signal, it relates more to the number of scatterers than to speed or direction of flow. Power Doppler imaging is only minimally angle dependent and conveys no directional or velocity information. The gain may be substantially increased without incurring noise artefact. Recent work has shown that power Doppler imaging is more sensitive than colour Doppler imaging in detecting intratesticular flow and that testicular flow in healthy children is symmetrical, underscoring the fact that asymmetry of flow between the two sides is an important parameter (BAETH and SHORTLIFFE 1997).

5.2.3
Scrotal Ultrasound: Technique

High-resolution linear array transducers (7, 10 or 15 MHz) are utilised and afford excellent near-field spatial resolution. The sensitivity is adjusted to detect low flow rates, i.e. 2–3 cm/s. Overall colour gain is increased until there is "speckle" artefact within the testis. It is then reduced to eliminate this artefact. The power setting is minimised. The ultrasound room is kept warm and the older child should be afforded privacy by excluding unnecessary personnel. Whilst a towel is used to give scrotal support in the older child, the scrotum is usually too small in the infant to warrant this. The penis is reflected onto the anterior abdominal wall and restrained by an overlying paper towel. A generous layer of pre-warmed gel is administered to act as a stand-off and to limit the cremasteric reflex, which can cause retraction of the testis into the inguinal canal. Direct contact scanning commences on the asymptomatic side, with measurement of testicular length, breadth and height. The scrotal wall thickness is assessed and the echogenicity of testis and epididymis are evaluated. Compared with the testis in adults, the testis in infants and children is hypoechoic and only attains the adult pattern at puberty (HAMM and FOBBE 1995). The testicular artery, which courses with the spermatic cord, provides the primary blood supply to the testicle. It gives rise to prominent capsular and intratesticular arteries which course bidirectionally within the testicular parenchyma. However, identification of this pattern may prove difficult in the pre-pubertal testis in which flow is often evidenced by pulsatile foci of intratesticular colour flow patterns. Where colour flow is demonstrated a spectral Doppler arterial wave form is recorded. Detectable flow is not expected in the normal epididymis. Care is taken not to misinterpret scrotal hyperaemia as capsular flow. Vessels demonstrated at the testicular surface might originate from the pudendal artery supplying the parietal tunica vaginalis or dartos muscle and may simulate the testicular artery. Unlike in adults, in whom a low resistive arterial pattern is described (MIDDLETON et al. 1989), a high resistive pattern can be normal in children and should not be mistaken for pathology (BARTH and SHORTLIFFE 1997). The spermatic cord is then imaged along its length to ensure there is normal parallel flow of the testicular vessels (BARD et al. 1995). The procedure is then repeated on the symptomatic side and the results compared.

The testis is approximately 1 cm in diameter at birth. The length remains relatively static during the first decade and rapidly increases under the hormonal drive of puberty, to attain 3–4 cm in length at 15 years. The testicular volume can be calculated from the formula for a prolate ellipse (depth ×

Table 5.1. Conditions presenting predominantly with testicular pain and swelling

Acute testicular torsion
Torsion of testicular appendages or epididymis
Inflammatory conditions including orchitis, epididymitis and epididymo-orchitis
Acute scrotal oedema (including idiopathic scrotal oedema and vasculitis in Henoch-Schönlein purpura)
Incarcerated inguinal hernia
Traumatic conditions including testicular rupture, haematoma and haematocele
Symptomatic spermatocele and varicocele
Haemorrhage into scrotal tumour
Scrotal gangrene
Acute scrotal swelling resulting from remote intra-abdominal pathology

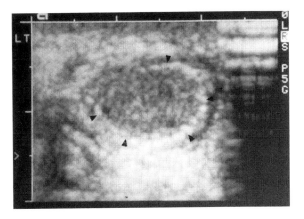

Fig. 5.1. Neonatal torsion of the testis. A 2-day-old infant was noted to have a discoloured scrotum which was firm to palpation. Longitudinal scan shows a normal sized testis with a peripheral echogenic rim (*arrowheads*). Colour Doppler assessment showed no intratesticular blood flow. An orchidectomy was performed, removing a necrotic testis

breadth × length × 0.5). It has, however, been suggested that a formula of length × breadth × height × 0.65 is more accurate (RIFKIN 1990).

5.2.4
Causes of the Acute Scrotum

The causes of the acute paediatric scrotum are given in Table 5.1. Differentiation must be made between an inflammatory condition warranting expectant therapy and acute testicular torsion which threatens testicular viability and demands prompt surgical intervention. The window of opportunity may be tragically narrow. Achieving a balance in management may be fraught with difficulty. A blanket policy of mandatory scrotal exploration in all cases of acute scrotum would subject large numbers of children to unnecessary surgery. Prompt accurate diagnosis with colour Doppler and power Doppler imaging may limit testicular loss.

5.2.4.1
Torsion of the Testis

Torsion of the testis has a biphasic age incidence with the first peak in the neonatal period and the second in adolescence. Torsion occurs when the testicle is abnormally mobile and twists on its vascular pedicle.

5.2.4.1.1
NEONATAL (EXTRAVAGINAL) TORSION
In neonates, the loose attachment of the cord and testis to surrounding structures predisposes to torsion of the entire suprascrotal cord (extravaginal torsion). The event may occur in utero (LEACH and MASIH 1983). Complete infarction is usually the rule but detorsion has rarely led to recovery of the testis. Orchidopexy of the contralateral gonad is indicated to safeguard its future (LYON 1961). Neonatal torsion is thought to account for the "vanishing testis" syndrome which presents later in life as unilateral cryptorchidism (STEPHENS 1982).

Torsion results in haemorrhagic infarction with necrosis of the testis with subsequent fibrosis and occasional calcification. The testicular parenchyma appears inhomogeneous on ultrasound. The presence of an echogenic rim marginating the testis suggests infarction (Fig. 5.1). The appearance may be due to oedema or fibrosis of the tunica albuginea. Alternatively, it may be due to a relative increase in echogenicity of the coverings of the infarcted testis as it undergoes necrosis (ZERIN et al. 1990).

5.2.4.1.2
INTRAVAGINAL TORSION
The second peak in incidence is during the testosterone drive of puberty when there is a four- or fivefold increase in testicular volume. This can precipitate torsion in those with an anatomical predisposition. The tunica vaginalis may insert high on the cord, leading to the "bell clapper deformity", which allows the testicle to twist on its vascular pedicle within the tunica vaginalis and results in intravaginal torsion (PARKER and ROBINSON 1971). This anomaly is commonly bilateral.

Table 5.2. Testicular torsion: ultrasound findings and outcome

Duration of symptoms	Grey-scale/colour Doppler findings	Testis salvage rate
<4 h	No change on grey scale Absent or reduced flow Spiral twist of spermatic cord vessels	85%–97%
4–6 h	Testicular enlargement, hypoechoic Absent or reduced flow Spiral twist of cord vessels	85%–97%
>12 h	Mixed echogenicity, hydrocele, scrotal wall thickening	20%–80%

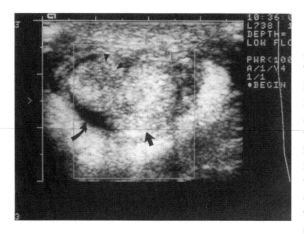

Fig. 5.2. Torsion of testis. This 4-year-old boy presented with sudden onset of severe pain in the scrotum. Longitudinal scan demonstrates an enlarged heterogeneous testis (*arrow*), a swollen epididymis (*arrowheads*) and a small hydrocele (*curved arrow*). Colour Doppler imaging showed no flow in the testis. An infarcted torted testis was removed at surgery

The cardinal symptom of testicular torsion is sudden scrotal pain, commonly at night, followed by swelling occurring in an otherwise completely healthy boy. There may be nausea, anorexia, pyrexia (in 25%) and pyuria (in 30%). These features cause diagnostic difficulty in discrimination from inflammatory aetiologies. The event is painless in 10% (HORSTMAN and MIDDLETON 1994; CASS et al. 1980).

The role of imaging is to provide an accurate diagnosis, thus maximising testicular salvage rates. Intra- and extravaginal torsion may not be distinguishable sonographically. Grey-scale sonographic findings are non-specific and indeed may be entirely normal (MIDDLETON et al. 1990). However, a testis with definite hyperechogenicity is usually unsalvageable (Fig. 2) (BARLOON and WEISSMAN (1996). The findings on grey scale relate to the duration of torsion (BIRD et al. 1983) (Table 2).

The sensitivity of colour Doppler imaging is currently comparable with that of scintigraphy. The most frequent finding is absent flow in the intratesticular vessels. Less commonly there may be markedly decreased testicular flow in true torsion. If symptoms have been present for more than 12 h there may be an associated increased peritesticular flow. In incomplete torsion, there may be reduced flow and in this situation, comparison with the contralateral testis is crucial (MEZA et al. 1992). If flow on the symptomatic side is reduced, surgical intervention is indicated as there may be incomplete torsion (LUKER and SIEGEL 1994). BARD et al. (1995) have elegantly demonstrated the spiral twist of the spermatic cord immediately above the testis. The role of power Doppler imaging in evaluating intratesticular flow has been discussed (BARTH and SHORTLIFFE 1997).

Testicular torsion is a surgical emergency because complete torsion with occlusion of the testicular artery for approximately 6 h results in subsequent necrosis (KAPLAN and KING 1970; LEEPAGE 1986). Testicular viability is influenced not only by the duration but also by the degree of torsion, with at least a 360° turn being required to cause infarction (BUICKS et al. 1990; LERNER et al. 1990). Surgical treatment comprises derotation and repositioning of the testicle with bilateral orchidopexy commonly employing four quadrant non-absorbable sutures (LEWIS et al. 1995).

Detorsion may be attempted manually using ultrasound guidance as an initial procedure aimed at immediately restoring blood flow (FRAZIER and BUCY 1975; BLOOM et al. 1992). Torted testes usually turn inward or medially so manual detorsion rotates the testis in an outward direction. Detorsion of the spermatic cord is evidenced by cessation of pain with reperfusion, and can be documented by colour Doppler imaging (DIZA-BALL et al. 1990; FITZGERALD et al. 1992). Manual detorsion may al-

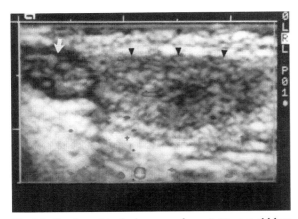

Fig. 5.3. Torsion of testicular appendage. A 10-year-old boy presented with acute scrotal pain. Longitudinal scan shows an echogenic mass (*arrow*) above the normal testis (*arrowheads*). Surgery performed for persistent pain at 10 days confirmed torsion of the appendix testis

low for less urgent surgical intervention and an improved chance of testicular salvage.

5.2.4.2
Torsion of the Appendices of the Testis and the Epididymis

The testicular appendage (or hydatid) is present in about 90% of males. It varies between 1 and 10 mm in diameter and is the most frequently twisted (90% of cases) of the four appendages. The other appendices are the appendix epididymis (vestige of the wolffian tubule), the paradidymis, the vas aberrans and the organ of Giraldés (or the appendix of the cord). The peak incidence for appendage torsion is between 7 and 12 years. Boys with a twisted testicular or epididymal appendage rarely have systemic symptoms such as nausea and vomiting and are usually much more comfortable than those with testicular torsion. Scrotal swelling, which is commonly due to an acute hydrocele, and erythema are usually manifest. Approximately 25% have a history of antecedent trauma or vigorous activity. Maximal tenderness is often at the upper pole of the testis, with the pathognomonic feature of the tender blue nodule (the "blue dot sign") (DRESNER 1973).

Grey-scale sonography demonstrates a normal testis, an enlarged epididymis and a reactive hydrocele. The torted appendage may be seen as an echogenic or hypoechoic mass in 30% of cases (Fig. 5.3). On colour flow imaging there is markedly increased epididymal flow, normal or slightly increased testicular flow and absent flow in the torted appendage. The condition may be confused with an acute epididymitis. However, this is not clinically relevant as both conditions are treated conservatively.

5.2.4.3
Epididymo-orchitis

The epididymis is more commonly affected by infection than the testis. Traditional teaching was that epididymitis is uncommon in pre-pubertal boys. However, recent work suggests that it is commoner than previously thought (SIEGEL et al. 1987; PATRIQUIN et al. 1993). Epididymitis may develop as a consequence of urethral instrumentation, the presence of an indwelling urethral catheter, underlying genito-urinary anomalies including reflux of sterile urine, dysfunctional voiding and recent scrotal trauma (NOSEWORTHY 1993; LIKIT et al. 1987). Orchitis may be associated with epididymitis, presumably representing a direct extension of the inflammation. Isolated orchitis is unusual and is generally of viral origin; the infections implicated include mumps, coxsackie, echovirus and adenovirus. The presentation is of gradual onset of scrotal pain and swelling over several days. Dysuria is a frequent symptom and there may be associated lower abdominal or loin pain.

Ultrasonic imaging in epididymitis reveals enlargement of the epididymis and an associated hydrocele, but the testis is frequently normal on grey-scale sonography (Fig. 5.4). The homogenicity of the testicular texture is usually preserved in orchitis. On colour Doppler imaging, the normal paediatric epididymis shows no flow, so that the presence of any epididymal vascularity represents inflammation (LUKER and SIEGEL 1994). There may be focal or diffuse hypervascularity within the testis in orchitis (SUBRAMANYAM et al. 1985). Pulsed Doppler waveforms show abnormally increased diastolic flow but are not necessary to secure the diagnosis of acute inflammation. Management is expectant although full work-up of the urinary tract is indicated.

Complications of epididymo-orchitis are often well demonstrated on sonography and include pyocele, abscess formation (which may appear as a complex testicular fluid collection) and testicular ischaemia. This may occur when the inflamed epid-

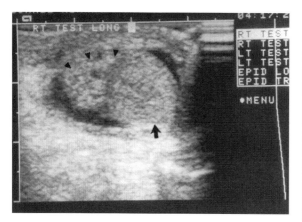

Fig. 5.4. Epididymitis. This 2-year-old boy presented with a 4-day history of scrotal pain and swelling. Ultrasound, shows an enlarged epididymis (*arrowheads*), a normal testis (*arrow*) and a small hydrocele. Doppler imaging showed marked increased flow in the testis and epididymis and parallel flow in spermatic cord vessels

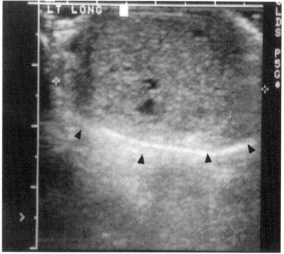

Fig. 5.5. Yolk sac testicular tumour. This 3-year-old boy presented as an emergency when his mother noted a swollen left hemiscrotum. Longitudinal scan demonstrates a moderately large echogenic mass replacing the normal left testis (*arrowheads*)

idymis produces increased pressure within the tough tunica albuginea and venous outflow from the testis is impaired. Pulsed Doppler waveforms are useful to establish the diagnosis. Testicular atrophy may develop after severe orchitis or a protracted course.

5.2.4.4
Tumours

The most common presentation of a testicular tumour is a lump or painless scrotal swelling. However, 25% of patients complain of pain, which is usually dull or heavy, and 10% experience acute pain caused by haemorrhage into or infarction of the tumour. Most testicular tumours in boys are malignant, germ cell tumours such as teratomas accounting for approximately 80% and non-germ cell tumours (Sertoli or Leydig cell) for the remaining 20%.

Metastatic testicular deposits from solid tumours such as neuroblastoma are rare, but acute scrotal pain may result from infiltration of the testis or cord by leukaemic deposits (STOFFER et al. 1975). Although the diagnosis is normally made clinically, ultrasound confirms the diagnosis and demonstrates testicular enlargement with areas of altered echogenicity (Fig. 5.5). There may be calcification or cystic areas. The homogeneous echo texture of the normal testicular parenchyma represents an excellent background for the detection of intratesticular lesions. Impalpable lesions as small as 3–5 mm in diameter are reliably detected. Recent work has

shown that in cases of testicular tumour, colour Doppler imaging may demonstrate a hypervascular mass in the face of normal grey-scale sonography in paediatric practice, contrary to the adult experience (LUKER and SIEGEL 1994).

5.2.4.5
Trauma

Scrotal haematoma, haematocele, testicular laceration or fracture can result from trauma (RABINOWITZ and HULTERT 1995). Fracture results from a direct blow to the testicle when it is caught between the symphysis pubis or thigh and the crushing object. The sonographic findings have a decisive influence on clinical management. If left untreated, serious complications such as ischaemic atrophy leading to impaired spermatogenesis or subsequent infection may occur (HAMM 1997). The prognosis for testicular salvage improves with early surgery and repair, especially if performed within 72 h of injury (SCHAFFER 1985).

Ultrasound examination is sensitive for detection of injury but has poor specificity for delineating the pathology. Haematocele is a collection of blood between the tunica albuginea and tunica vaginalis and appears as a "hydrocele-like" collection with numerous small internal echoes (Fig. 5.6). An intratesticular haematoma appears as a hyper-

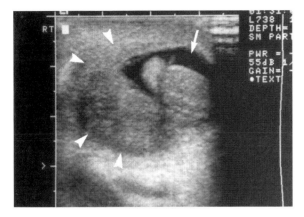

Fig. 5.6. Scrotal haematoma and haematocele. This 2-year-old boy fell astride a fence, sustaining marked scrotal bruising. A large scrotal haematoma (*arrowheads*), haematocele (*arrow*) and a normal intact testis were demonstrated on ultrasound, leading to conservative management

or hypoechoic avascular mass with displacement of peripheral vessels on colour Doppler imaging. Sonographic findings in fracture are non-specific. Discrete fracture planes are seen in only 17% of cases (CORRALES et al. 1993) and extruded parenchyma or testicular fragmentation, whilst pathognomonic, are rarely seen. Colour Doppler imaging enhances accuracy by determining the pattern of testicular perfusion. However, recent work suggests that sonography will not reliably differentiate between intratesticular haematoma without rupture and testicular rupture (CASS and LUXENBERG 1991).

Thus, in cases of low suspicion of serious testicular injury (low force, minimal swelling or ecchymosis of the scrotum) the role of sonography may be to show an intact testis and the absence of haematocele, thereby circumventing operative intervention.

An additional consequence of trauma, constituting a genital emergency, is rupture of the bulbous portion of the urethra with involvement of the deep fascia of the penis. This results in extravasation of urine into the scrotum. It may be difficult to distinguish sonographically from hydrocele or haematocele. However, if there is a dissection along soft tissue planes, a characteristic onion-peel appearance of the area may result.

5.2.4.6
Acute Tense Hydrocele

Hydrocele is one of the most common causes of scrotal swelling in boys and is associated with a patent processus vaginalis. Occasionally the presentation is acute and is associated with acute increases in intra-abdominal pressures caused by coughing or straining at stool. The swelling is not usually tender and is usually diagnosed clinically. However, if the hydrocele is tense and the surrounding tissue indurated, transillumination may not be possible. In these circumstances sonography demonstrates an echo-free zone with good sound transmission; the underlying testis may be displaced posteriorly but is well visualised. The fluid envelops the testis except posteriorly, where the testis is attached to the epididymis. The sonographic examination should be extended to include the inguinal canal to see whether the processus vaginalis is patent or not. Secondary hydrocele may be associated with epididymo-orchitis, missed torsion or scrotal trauma. Chronic hydrocele or that secondary to underlying inflammation may show scrotal wall thickening and is frequently septate.

5.2.4.7
Scrotal Hernia

Scrotal hernia in a child is due either to a persistent processus vaginalis or to a congenital sac. Although it is usually an obvious clinical diagnosis, confusion may occur with acute tense hydrocele or torsion of an ectopic testicle. Grey-scale sonography will demonstrate loops of bowel and occasionally omental fat descending through the inguinal canal into the scrotum. Colour Doppler imaging may alter the clinical management in an incarcerated hernia when the intestine and the testis are at risk of infarction (RABINOWITZ and HULTERT 1995). Ischaemic necrosis of the testis may occur due to compression of spermatic vessels between the incarcerated contents of the inguinal hernia and the fibrous sheath of the cord. This complication is thought to occur almost exclusively during the first few months of life. The testis may appear hypoechoic with reduced colour flow. Spectral Doppler may demonstrate reduced or absent diastolic flow in the affected testis on comparison with the contralateral testis. Prompt surgical intervention safeguards testicular viability.

5.2.4.8
Symptomatic Varicocele

Varicocele, dilatation of the pampiniform venous plexus, occurs in 15% of males, with an onset in early adolescence. Eighty-five percent of cases are left sided. The majority are idiopathic but in young boys obstruction to venous flow may be secondary to a renal tumour with left renal vein or intracaval tumour extension. The lesion is most commonly encountered towards the lower pole of the testis. Although readily evident clinically, grey-scale sonography may establish the diagnosis if the vessels of the pampiniform plexus are greater than 2–3 mm in diameter. Colour Doppler imaging shows dilated tubular structures with low flow best demonstrated with venous flow augmentation following pressure on the cord or during a Valsalva manoeuvre. Formal abdominopelvic sonography for evidence of neoplasia may be prudent. The outcome in childhood varicocele can include interference with testicular development and possible subfertility later in life.

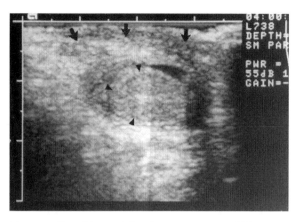

Fig. 5.7. Idiopathic scrotal oedema. A 10-year-old boy presented with a short history of marked scrotal swelling. Longitudinal scan shows scrotal wall thickening (*arrows*) with a normal testis (*arrowheads*) and epididymis. The clinical features resolved within 36 h

5.2.4.9
Acute Scrotal Oedema

Acute scrotal oedema is the result of an inflammatory process and causes a painful scrotum in young children in whom the normal scrotal skin is less than 3 mm thick and has no detectable blood flow. Thickening of the scrotal skin may be seen in cellulitis, trauma, Henoch-Schönlein purpura and idiopathic scrotal oedema. Idiopathic scrotal oedema is thought to be due to perineal infection or a localised form of angioneurotic oedema as peripheral eosinophilia is often an associated finding. Grey-scale sonography will demonstrate thickened scrotal skin, normal testis and epididymis and in some cases a small hydrocele (Fig. 5.7). Colour Doppler imaging shows increased flow in the scrotal wall and a slight increase in testicular and epididymal flow.

Scrotal involvement in Henoch-Schönlein purpura is not uncommon as 15%–38% of affected males suffer scrotal wall involvement (Laor et al. 1992). This small vessel vasculitis generally affects children between 2 and 10 years old. The vasculitis may infrequently involve the testis and epididymis. In this case, clinical differentiation from testicular torsion may prove difficult (Ross et al. 1987). In uncomplicated cases, however, the imaging characteristics are as seen in idiopathic scrotal oedema and obviate the need for surgical exploration. Conservative management is indicated.

5.2.4.10
Unusual Causes of Acute Scrotum

There are a handful of rare causes of the acute scrotum in boys but the majority do not constitute a diagnostic problem clinically. Imaging is rarely necessary, for example, in cases of Fournier's gangrene or insect bites. There are some imaging issues nevertheless. Acute scrotal pathology may reflect intra-abdominal pathology. Blood may track down a patent processus vaginalis from a ruptured abdominal organ, from tumour or from neonatal adrenal haemorrhage, or may be secondary to iatrogenic causes such as transfemoral cardiac catheterisation or renal biopsy. Ascitic fluid may similarly track into the scrotum, as may cerebrospinal fluid in patients with ventriculoperitoneal shunt, or pus from perforated appendicitis.

5.2.5
Summary

The ultimate goal of management of the acute scrotum in childhood is avoidance of testicular loss. This requires a high degree of diagnostic accuracy and prompt surgical intervention in cases of torsion. In acute scrotal conditions, overlap of history and clinical features of the possible aetiology occasionally makes a definitive diagnosis difficult. Colour Doppler imaging and lately power Doppler imaging add useful information regarding perfusion and aid in the diagnosis of testicular and scrotal disorders. An optimal diagnostic service requires close clinical and radiological collaboration and adequate expertise. This allows management decisions to be made on the basis of combined clinical and ultrasound findings.

5.3
Genital Emergencies in Girls

5.3.1
Imaging of the Normal Female Paediatric Pelvis

5.3.1.1
Pelvic Ultrasound: Technique

Pelvic ultrasound in girls provides a near-ideal imaging modality to exclude suspected pelvic pathology. It often provides the only imaging necessary for the diagnosis of many pelvic conditions, with computed tomography (CT) and magnetic resonance imaging (MRI) being required for more complex cases. The examination is performed without sedation or anaesthesia. A full bladder is essential to scan the female reproductive tract. This can be difficult to achieve in infants and young children due to their lack of bladder control (COHEN and HALLER 1989). If the bladder is not adequately full, then having given the baby or child a drink, it is worth repeating the examination every 15 min until optimum imaging is achieved. This requires time and patience.

A 7-MHz probe is ideal for an infant or young child, a 5-MHz probe being used for older children and adolescents. A 3-MHz probe is only needed for very large or obese older children. A midline sagittal scan and transverse scan is made of the uterus, recording the uterine length, the antero-posterior (AP) diameters of the fundus and cervix, and whether an endometrial echo is present or not. The ovaries are measured for length on a longitudinal scan, and for width and depth on transverse views. Ovarian volume is determined using the formula for a prolate ellipsoid (length × width × depth × 0.5). The kidneys and adrenal glands should also be included in the study for completeness.

5.3.1.2
Pelvic Ultrasound: Normal Anatomy

The neonatal uterus is pear shaped and is larger in size than in the early childhood years, measuring approximately 3.5 cm in length. An echogenic endometrial echo is seen in 97%, a myometrial "halo" in 29% and a small amount of fluid in the uterine cavity in 23% of neonates (NUSSBAUM et al. 1986).

With the withdrawal of maternal oestrogen, there is a gradual reduction in size over the first few months of life, until the uterine shape changes to the prepubertal shape in which the length is 2.6–2.8 cm, the cervix is twice as long as the body of the uterus, and the endometrial echo disappears. There is then little change in the uterine size or shape until the onset of puberty, when the uterus rapidly increases in size and initially becomes tubular in shape. The AP diameters of the cervix and the fundus are similar at this stage. After puberty, the uterus has a pear-shaped appearance, is 5–8 cm in length, and has a fundus to cervix ratio of 3 : 1.

At least one ovary can be visualised by an experienced operator in 80% of children under 5 years and in 90% of children over 5 years. The ovaries are relatively high in position in the pelvis in infants and young children, but can be found anywhere between the lower border of the kidney and the broad ligament (SIEGEL 1991). Each ovary is typically 1.5 cm in length, 0.4 cm wide and 0.3 cm in depth, with a volume of less than 1 cc under the age of 2 years. Small cysts under 5 mm are often present and represent unstimulated follicles. At puberty, the ovarian size rapidly increases, and the mean ovarian volume after puberty is 5.2 cc, length 3 cm, width 1 cm and breadth 1.2 cm. The number and size of follicles similarly increase at this time.

5.3.1.3
Transvaginal Ultrasound

Transvaginal scanning requires the insertion of a high-frequency narrow endocavity probe into the vagina, and therefore is unsuitable for young children or virginal adolescents. Although transvaginal scanning has been slow to be adopted for use in children, sexually active teenagers find the procedure acceptable and excellent detail of the uterus, adnexa and cul-de-sac can be obtained. It is of particular value in girls who are obese, have surgical dressings obscuring the abdominal wall, or lack a urinary bladder.

5.3.2
Vaginal Discharge

5.3.2.1
Introduction

Vaginal discharge is a common complaint in girls (COHEN and HALLER 1989). A vaginal foreign body and infection should be considered, and if the discharge is bloody then vaginal tumours and precocious puberty should also be excluded (PHELAN

1994). Visual and digital inspection of the child's vagina may be problematic, and a pelvic ultrasound examination may be an easier alternative.

5.3.2.2
Vaginal Foreign Body

The history of a foreign body inserted into the vagina is rarely obtained from the child but usually there is a history of a persisting foul smelling and even bloody discharge. Foreign bodies are various and include toilet paper, toys, beads and food. Plain radiographs are rarely of diagnostic value as foreign bodies are not usually radio-opaque.

On pelvic ultrasonography, a vaginal foreign body is suspected if there is a discrete area of echogenicity with acoustic shadowing in the vagina. This may be difficult to elicit because of the proximity of the vagina to the rectum, which in itself produces acoustic shadowing from faeces and gas. The echogenicity is variable depending on the nature of the foreign body (Fig. 5.8). A more recent report (CASPI et al. 1995) indicated that careful attention should be given to another sign of a vaginal foreign body, that of focal indentation of the posterior bladder wall disrupting the normal smooth bladder contour. CT and MRI have rarely been reported to be of value, and if there is strong clinical suspicion of a foreign body then an examination under general anaesthesia should be performed.

5.3.3
Vaginal Bleeding

5.3.3.1
Introduction

Vaginal bleeding in early childhood (i.e. in prepubertal girls) causes a great deal of parental concern. In the newborn period, vaginal bleeding may occasionally occur, and is secondary to withdrawal of maternal oestrogen.

After the neonatal period and before the age of 10 years, vaginal bleeding should be taken seriously and meticulously evaluated. Vaginal bleeding may originate from vulvar, vaginal or uterine causes. Local vulvar lesions include infection (vulvo-vaginitis), urethral prolapse, trauma or skin conditions such as lichen sclerosis. Vaginal causes that should be considered include vaginal tumours and foreign bodies. Bleeding that arises from the endometrium is usually

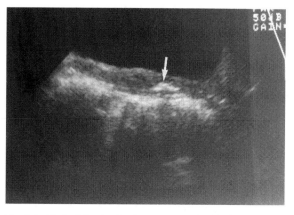

Fig. 5.8. Vaginal foreign body. A 20-month-old girl presented with purulent vaginal discharge. A discrete echogenic lesion with posterior acoustic shadowing (*arrow*) is shown on this sagittal scan of the uterus and vagina. A toy bead was removed

associated with sexual precocity (precocious puberty), but occasionally the bleeding may be isolated with no other features of puberty and is termed premature menarche. In a recent large series of girls with premenarchal bleeding (IMAI et al. 1995), 74% resulted from a local lesion in the vagina, 61% had vulvo-vaginitis, 13% urethral prolapse, 13% trauma, 7% foreign bodies and 7% vaginal tumours. The remaining 26% of patients bled as a result of precocious puberty. In another review in girls under the age of 10 years with vaginal bleeding the findings were that 54% had a local vulvar lesion, 21% had a malignant genital tumour, 21% had precocious puberty and in 25% no cause could be found (HILL 1989).

5.3.3.2
Vaginal Tumour

Rhabdomyosarcoma is the most common malignant tumour of the genital tract in young girls, usually under the age of 4 years. The clinical presentation is commonly with vaginal bleeding, associated with a palpable abdominal mass. There may also be a polypoid mass protruding from the vagina or urethra. Typical ultrasonic features are of a mixed echogenic soft tissue mass in the vagina. The tumour may extend out into the pelvis and may obstruct the proximal vagina and cervix, resulting in fluid accumulating in the uterus. Lymph node metastases are difficult to assess ultrasonically, and CT and MRI staging is appropriate for accurate tumour evaluation (Fig. 5.9). Chemotherapy, surgery and radio-

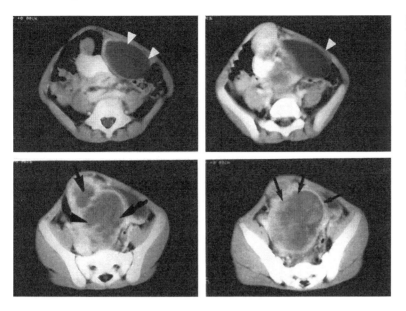

Fig. 5.9. Vaginal rhabdomyosarcoma. This 3-year-old girl presented with a pelvic mass, pain and inability to micturate. CT scan demonstrates a large irregular mixed attenuation vaginal tumour (*arrows*) causing bladder outlet obstruction (*arrowheads*)

therapy can result in survival approaching 90% (ESTROFF 1997).

Primary adenocarcinoma of the vagina and cervix is rare. Vaginal clear cell adenocarcinoma is associated with maternal diethylstilboestrol exposure. This tumour affects girls over the age of 7 years and survival rates of more than 90% are reported for localised tumours. Features found on various imaging modalities are similar to those of vaginal rhabdomyosarcoma.

5.3.3.3
Precocious Puberty

Sexual precocity or precocious puberty is the development of secondary sexual characteristics before the age of 8 years or the onset of menses before the age of 9 years. There are two main forms: central precocious puberty due to precocious activation of the hypothalamic-pituitary-gonadal axis, and precocious pseudo-puberty, with increased levels of sex steroids from other causes, such as ovarian or adrenal tumour (KORNREICH et al. 1995).

The role of ultrasound in this situation is twofold. Firstly to confirm, along with a positive luteinising hormone-releasing hormone (LHRH) test, that the child has precocious puberty. The uterus is inappropriately enlarged for the child's age, is typically pear shaped and has a midline endometrial echo. The ovaries are symmetrically enlarged, the volume frequently exceeds 3 cc, and they are megalocystic with six follicles greater than 3 cm in size in each ovary.

The second role of ultrasound is as a screening examination to rule out an ovarian or adrenal tumour (HALLER et al. 1978). An ovarian tumour should be considered if there is asymmetrical enlargement of one ovary (COHEN and HALLER 1989).

Premature menarche is a rare entity in which young girls present with recurrent vaginal bleeding in the absence of other signs of puberty. These girls have normal pelvic anatomy on ultrasound, with uterine and ovarian sizes appropriate for their age. Premature menarche is a benign self-limiting condition, and provided the hormonal profile and pelvic sonographic examination are normal, then parental reassurance is appropriate (MURAM et al. 1983).

5.3.4
Acute Pelvic Pain

5.3.4.1
Introduction

Acute pelvic pain in girls may be secondary to a wide range of gynaecological pathology and non-gynaecological causes (GIDWANI and KAY 1994). Gynaecological conditions that should be considered include congenital malformations, pelvic inflammatory disease, tumours, ovarian torsion and, in older children, complications of pregnancy. Non-gynaecological causes are more common, including appendicitis, gastroenteritis, urinary tract infection, bone and joint infection and trauma. Whilst the history is of invaluable help to the clinician, the clinical examination is often difficult in children. Pelvic ultrasound has therefore become a simple and reliable diagnostic tool to aid precise diagnosis. CT and MRI have been used only as secondary complementary imaging modalities (STONE 1992).

5.3.4.2
Congenital Uterovaginal Anomalies

Approximately 1%–5% of females have an anomaly of the genital tract, and as the female reproductive tract partly derives from the mesonephric duct, associated renal anomalies are common. Girls with these uncommon uterovaginal anomalies may present as an emergency because of vaginal obstruction resulting in abdominal or pelvic pain and an abdominal mass (Fig. 5.10). The vaginal obstruction may be caused by an imperforate hymen, complete vaginal membrane, vaginal stenosis or distal vaginal atresia.

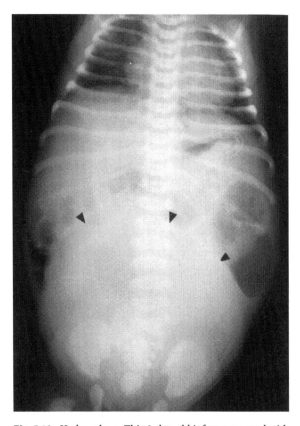

Fig. 5.10. Hydrocolpos. This 2-day-old infant presented with a large abdominopelvic mass. Plain film of the abdomen shows a large soft tissue mass arising from the pelvis (*arrowheads*). Ultrasonic assessment confirmed a huge hydrocolpos. An imperforate hymen was identified and treated

These conditions are usually encountered either in the neonatal period or in adolescence at the time of the menarche. The clinical diagnosis of these anomalies is notoriously inaccurate: hence the importance of the radiological evaluation to identify and define these malformations.

Ultrasound represents the initial imaging modality of choice. A hydrocolpos, a distended fluid-filled vagina, is demonstrated as a tubular cystic midline mass between the bladder and rectum. The uterus may also be fluid filled (hydrometrocolpos) in which case the vagina is 5–9 times more dilated than the uterus. If there has been bleeding into the fluid (haematometrocolpos) there may be echoes within the mass. In vaginal atresia, the dilated proximal vaginal segment is evident, whilst the distal collapsed vagina cannot be well defined (Fig. 5.11) (SHATZKES et al. 1991).

In imperforate hymen, the vagina is dilated throughout its length. The fallopian tube may also be dilated in these congenital anomalies, and if the pelvic mass is large enough an obstructive uropathy may result from distal ureteric compression. Complex anomalies are best further defined with MRI, as the multiplanar scanning and excellent anatomical detail best depict the extent of the lesion, facilitating the planning of further surgical intervention.

5.3.4.3
Ovarian Torsion

Torsion of an ovary and fallopian tube can occur at any age; most commonly, however, it occurs in the first two decades of life, and it is rare in infancy. Torsion may result from the ovary being abnormal (cyst, tumour), or it may be that the adnexae are normal but hypermobile in young people. In the early stages of torsion, there is impaired venous and lymphatic drainage resulting in vascular congestion and ovarian stromal oedema. If the torsion detorts the ovary may return to normal. If the torsion is unremitting then haemorrhagic infarction ensues. In infants the torsion is often extrapelvic in location, in older girls the mass is adnexal in position (SCHMAHMANN and HALLER 1997). The torted ovary may become detached from auto-amputation and obtain a collateral blood supply from elsewhere in the abdomen (COHEN and HALLER 1989).

Children present with lower abdominal pain and vomiting and have a leucocytosis. They may have had similar episodes of pain previously. The symp-

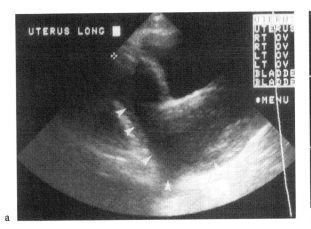

a

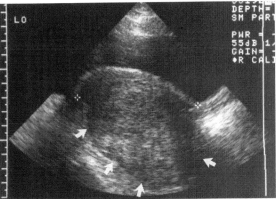

Fig. 5.12. Torted ovarian cyst. This 12-year-old girl presented with sudden onset of pelvic pain. Longitudinal ultrasound scan of the pelvis shows an echogenic midline mass in the pouch of Douglas (*arrows*). Colour Doppler imaging showed the mass to be avascular. An infarcted torted ovarian cyst was removed

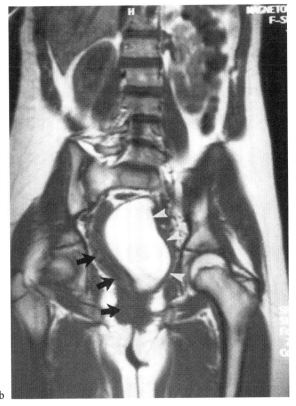

b

Fig. 5.11 a,b. Uterine didelphus with vaginal obstruction. This 13-year-old girl presented with acute pelvic pain and normal menses. Longitudinal ultrasound scan (a) and MRI of the pelvis (b) shows a haematometrocolpos (*arrowheads*) of the left uterus and vagina which was due to distal vaginal atresia. The non-obstructed right-sided uterus and vagina can also be seen (*arrows*)

toms may mimic appendicitis if the torsion is right sided. Fifty percent of patients have a palpable abdominal mass.

Ultrasound imaging demonstrates an abdomino-pelvic mass, often in a midline location (SIEGEL 1991). The mass is usually echogenic, but may be cystic or cystic with septations (Fig. 5.12). There is often fluid in the pouch of Douglas. The only specific sign is said to be the presence of multiple small peripherally located cysts (8–12 mm), resulting from vascular congestion with fluid transudation into follicles. MRI or CT can be confirmatory of the mass but ultrasound usually suffices for planning the surgical approach.

5.3.4.4
Pelvic Inflammatory Disease

Although rare in young children, the incidence of pelvic inflammatory disease amongst teenagers continues to rise (THORPE and MURAM 1994) owing to girls becoming sexually active at a younger age. Infection spreads in an ascending fashion from the vagina, through the cervix into the endometrium and the fallopian tubes. Girls may present with acute pelvic pain, vaginal discharge or dyspareunia, and on examination often exhibit pain on movement of the cervix or adnexa.

Transvaginal ultrasound has been shown to provide superior anatomical detail and more abnormalities than transabdominal ultrasound (BULAS et al. 1992). In mild cases ultrasound findings may be normal. In more severe cases, the uterine cavity may contain a little fluid and the uterine outline may be indistinct due to inflammation. If a hydrosalpinx or pyosalpinx is present, then there is a dilated tubular cystic adnexal structure. Tubo-ovarian abscesses may be unilateral or bilateral, and can be cystic or echogenic in appearance. Fluid in the pouch of Douglas may be evident.

Magnetic resonance imaging has also been used to define the complications of pelvic inflammatory disease but its accuracy is very similar to that of transvaginal ultrasound (FEDELE et al. 1990). Laparoscopy, however, can demonstrate the precise extent of the disease, and immediate treatment can be implemented by drainage of abscesses and sampling of fluid to plan appropriate antimicrobial therapy (CANDIANI et al. 1997).

5.3.4.5
Pregnancy

Adolescent pregnancy is not uncommon, and a complication of pregnancy should always be suspected in a post-pubertal sexually active adolescent who presents with acute pelvic pain. A recent period of amenorrhoea is usual, but the diagnosis of pregnancy should not be rejected if this is not the case. The index of suspicion is particularly high if the pelvic pain is accompanied by vaginal bleeding and/or a pelvic mass.

The diagnosis of pregnancy is made most accurately and rapidly with a pregnancy test. If the pregnancy test is positive, transabdominal ultrasound is performed first, but if this is non-diagnostic, transvaginal ultrasound may be acceptable to the patient.

If the patient has acute pelvic pain, then ectopic pregnancy or threatened abortion must be considered. It is important to determine whether the pregnancy is intrauterine and whether the fetus is viable or not. If the serum human chorionic gonadotrophin (hCG) level is >2500 mIU/ml, a gestational sac should be identified within the uterus with a transvaginal probe. If no sac is seen with this hCG level, then the patient should be assumed to have an ectopic pregnancy. If the hCG level is >5000 mIU/ml, a fetal pole should also be demonstrable (ESTROFF 1997). Most ectopic pregnancies develop in the fallopian tube but they can occur in other locations, including the cervical canal and other sites in the abdomen or pelvis. Actual ultrasonic demonstration of an ectopic pregnancy is difficult due to its tubal location, and only rarely is a fetal heart identified in a sac in an adnexal mass. Free fluid in the pouch of Douglas suggests that the ectopic pregnancy is leaking (SIEGEL 1991). If a gestational sac is not demonstrated in the uterus (and with serial measurements

the hCG level falls), then it can be assumed that the pregnancy has failed and a spontaneous abortion has occurred.

Laparoscopy is becoming an increasingly useful diagnostic test in paediatrics to localise unexplained pelvic pain and is of great value in ruling out early ectopic pregnancy if ultrasound has been non-confirmatory. Modern treatment of ectopic pregnancy is with either systemic chemotherapy using methotrexate or by laparoscopic salpingotomy and aspiration.

5.3.5
Genital Trauma

The incidence of genital trauma is unknown, as studies are often drawn from biased populations such as those reported by authors who have an interest in child sexual abuse. Accidental injury to the external genitalia occurs typically from blunt trauma arising from a straddle injury (for example over a bicycle crossbar or over a fence), or a direct kick to the pelvic region or from road traffic injuries. Haematomas and lacerations occur in the perineal, vaginal and vulvar area, and these injuries rarely require surgical repair.

Imaging is only necessary if associated internal injuries are suspected and must be tailored to the child's clinical condition (SCLAFANI et al. 1985). A penetrating vaginal tear can result in a large retroperitoneal haematoma. Perineal injuries can extend into the anus and rectum, and road traffic injuries to the pelvis may be associated with fractures of the bony pelvis and bladder and bowel rupture. Ultrasound, CT and contrast studies of the bladder and colon may then be necessary (RIMZA 1994).

5.3.6
Summary

Invasive diagnostic investigations such as hysterosalpingography are now rarely necessary to assess the paediatric female pelvis. Pelvic ultrasound provides immediate imaging of pelvic structures, and is often the only investigation necessary to assess the child with pelvic pain or a pelvic mass. MRI can be reserved for more complex situations such as complex congenital abnormalities and large pelvic masses.

References

Babcock DS (1995) Which is the most sensitive study for testicular torsion in children: doppler sonography or testicular nuclear scan (letter)? AJR 165:224

Babcock DS, Patriquin H, La Fortune M, Dauzat M (1996) Power Doppler sonography: basic principles and clinical applications in children. Pediatr Radiol 26:109–115

Bard C, Verac C, Couture A, Ferran JL (1995) Spiral twist in testicular torsion. 52nd Congress, European Society of Paediatric Radiology, Utrecht 1995. Book of Abstracts, p 36

Barloon TJ, Weissman AM (1996) Diagnostic imaging of patients with an acute scrotal pain. Am Fam Physician 53:1730–1739

Barth RA, Shortliffe LD (1997) Normal paediatric testis: comparison of the power Doppler and colour Doppler ultrasound in the detection of blood flow. Radiology 204:389–393

Bird K, Rosenfield AT, Taylor KJW (1983) Ultrasonography in testicular torsion. Radiology 147:527–534

Bloom DA, Wan J, Key DW (1992) Disorders of the male external genitalia and inguinal canal. In: Kelelis PP, King LR, Belman AB (eds) Clinical paediatric urology, vol 2. W.B. Saunders, Philadelphia, p 1033

Brereton RJ (1981) Limitation of the Doppler flow meter in the diagnosis of the acute scrotum in boys. Br J Urol 53:380–383

Buicks DD, Markell BJ, Birkhert TK, Balsard ZW, Haluszka MM, Canning DA (1990) Suspected testicular torsion and ischaemia: evaluation with colour Doppler sonography. Radiology 175:815–821

Bulas DI, Ahlstrom PA, Sivit CJ, Blask AR, O'Donnell RM (1992) Pelvic inflammatory disease in the adolescent: comparison of transabdominal and transvaginal sonographic evaluation. Radiology 183:435–439

Candiani M, Canis M, Giambelli E, et al. (1997) Laparoscopic management of pelvic pain and adnexal masses in adolescents and paediatric patients. Ital J Gynecol Obstet 9:82–86

Caspi B, Zalel Y, Katz Z, Appelman Z, Insler V (1995) The role of sonography in the detection of vaginal foreign bodies in young girls: the bladder indentation sign. Pediatr Radiol 25:560–561

Cass A, Luxenberg M (1991) Testicular injuries. Urology 37:528–530

Cass AS, Cass BB, Veraragharan K (1980) Immediate exploration of the unilateral acute scrotum in young male subjects. J Urol 124:829–832

Cohen HL, Haller JO (1989) Pediatric and adolescent genital abnormalities. Clin Diagn Ultrasound 24:187–215

Corrales JG, Corbel L, Cipoolla B (1993) Accuracy of ultrasound diagnosis after blunt testicular trauma. J Urol 150:1834–1836

Diaz-Ball FL, Moreno AG, Toney MAO, et al. (1990) One dose technetium-99m pertechnenate imaging in acute testicular torsion followed by manual detorsion. Clin Nucl Med 15:76–79

Dresner ML (1973) Torsed appendage: diagnosis and Management: blue dot sign. Urology 1:623–626

Estroff JA (1997) Emergency obstetric and gynecologic ultrasound. Radiol Clin North Am 35:921–957

Fedele L, Dorta M, Brioschi D (1990) Magnetic resonance evaluation of gynecologic masses in adolescents. Adolesc Pediatr Gynecol 3:83–88

Fitzgerald SW, Erickson S, Dewire DM, et al. (1992) Colour Doppler sonography in the evaulation of the adult acute scrotum. J Ultrasound Med 1:543–548

Flanigan RC, Dekernien JB, Persky L (1981) Acute scrotal pain and swelling in children: a surgical emergency. Urology 17:51–53

Fournier GR, Faye JR, Laing C, Brooke Jeffrey R, McAninch JW (1985) High resolution scrotal ultrasonography: highly sensitive but non-specific diagnostic techniques. J Urol 134:490–493

Frazier WJ, Bucy JG (1975) Manipulation of torsion of the testicle. J Urol 114:410

Gidwani GP, Kay M (1994) Dysmenorrhoea and pelvic pain. In: Sanfippo JS, Muram D, Lee PA, Dewhurst J (eds) Pediatric and adolescent gynecology. W.B. Saunders, Philadelphia, pp 233–249

Haller JO, Kassner G, Staiano S, Schneider M (1978) Ultrasonic diagnosis of gynecologic disorders in children. Pediatrics 62:339–342

Hamm JR (1997) Differential diagnosis of scrotal mass by ultrasound. Eur Radiol 7:668–679

Hamm B, Fobbe F (1995) Maturation of the testis: ultrasound evaluation. Ultrasound Med Biol 21:143–147

Hill NCW (1989) The aetiology of vaginal bleeding in children. A 20 year review. Br J Obstet Gynaecol 96:467–470

Horstman WG, Middleton WD (1994) Testicular and scrotal imaging. In: A categorical course in genitourinary radiology. Radiological Society of North America, pp 159–173

Imai A, Horibe S, Tamaya T (1995) Genital bleeding in premenarchal children. Int J Gynecol Obstet 49:41–45

Ingram S, Hollman AS (1994) Colour Doppler sonography of a normal paediatric testes. Clin Radiol 49:266–267

Ingram S, Hollman AS, Azmy A (1993) Testicular torsion: missed diagnosis on colour Doppler sonography. Pediatr Radiol 23:483–484

Kaplan GW, King LR (1970) Acute scrotal swelling in children. J Urol 104:219–223

Kornreich L, Horev G, Blaser S, Daneman D, Kauli R, Grunebaum M (1995) Central precocious puberty: evaluation by neuroimaging. Pediatr Radiol 25:7–11

Laor T, Atala A, Teele RL (1992) Scrotal ultrasonograaphy in Henoch-Schönlein sndrome. Pediatr Radiol 22:505–506

Leach G, Masih BK (1983) Neonatal torsion of testicle. Urology 16:604–605

Lee LM, Wright JE, McLaughlin MG (1983) Testicular torsion in the adult. J Urol 130:93–94

Leepage LI (1986) Torsion of the testis. In: Welch KJ, Randolph JG, Raritch MM, et al. (eds) Paediatric surgery. Year Book Medical, Chicago, pp 1330–1334

Lerner RM, Mevorach RA, Hulbert WC, Rabinowitz R (1990) Colour Doppler ultrasound in the evaluation of acute scrotal disease. Radiology 176:355–358

Lewis AG, Bukowski PDJ, Wacksmans J, Sheldon CA (1995) Evaluation of acute scrotum in the ER. J Pediatr Surg 30:272–282

Likitnukul S, McCracken GH, Nelson JD (1987) Epididymitis in children in adolescents. A 20 year retrospective study. Am J Dis Child 141:41–44

Luker GD, Siegel MJ (1994) Colour Doppler sonography of the scrotum in children. AJR 163:649–655

Lyon RP (1961) Torsion of the testis in childhood: a painless emergency requiring contralateral orchidopexy. JAMA 178:702–705

Meza MP, Amundson GM, Aquilina JW, Reitalman C (1992) Colour flow imaging in children with clinically suspected testicular torsion. Pediatr Radiol 22:370–373

Middleton WD, Throne DA, Melson GL (1989) Colour Doppler ultrasound of the normal testis. AJR 152:293–297

Middleton WD, Siegel BA, Melson GL, Yates CK, Androle GI (1990) Acute scrotal disorders: prospective comparison of colour Doppler ultrasound and testicular scintigraphy. Radiology 177:177–181

Muram D, Dewhurst J, Grant JB (1983) Premature menarche: a follow up study. Arch Dis Child 58:142

Nasrallah PF, Manzone D, King LR (1977) Falsely negative Doppler examinations in testicular torsion. J Urol 118:194–195

Noseworthy J (1993) Testicular torsion. In: Ashcraft KW, Holder TM (eds) Paediatric surgery, 2nd edn. Saunders, Philadelphia, pp 595–601

Nussbaum AR, Sanders RC, Jones MD (1986) Neonatal uterine morphology as seen on real time US. Radiology 160:641–643

Parker RM, Robinson JR (1971) Anatomy and diagnosis of torsion of the testicle. J Urol 106:243–247

Patriquin HB, Yazbeck S, Trinn B (1993) Testicular torsion in infants and children: diagnosis with Doppler sonography. Radiology 188:781–785

Phelan E (1994) Gynecology and intersex. In: Carty H, Shaw D, Brunelle F, Kendall B (eds) Imaging children. Churchill Livingstone, Edinburgh, pp 755–784

Pryor JL, Watson LR, Day DL, Abbit PL, Howards SS, Gonzalet RJ, Reinberg U (1994) Scretal ultrasound for evaluation. J Urol 151:693–697

Rabinowitz R, Hultert WC (1995) Acute scrotal swelling. Common problems in paediatric urology. Urol Clin North Am 22:101–105

Ralls PW, Larsen D, Johnston MB, Lee KP (1991) Colour Doppler sonography of this scrotum. Semin Ultrasound CT MR 12:109–114

Rifkin MD (1990) Measurement of scrotal contents. In: Goldberg BB, Kurtz AB (eds) Atlas of ultrasound measurements. Year Book Medical Publishers, Chicago, pp 180–186

Riley TW, Mosbaugh PG, Colls JL, Newman DM, Vanhove ED, Heck LL (1976) Use of radioisotope scan in evaluation of intrascrotal lesions. J Urol 116:472–474

Rimza ME (1994) Genital trauma. In: Sanfilippo JS (ed) Pediatric and adolescent gynecology. W.B. Saunders, Philadelphia, pp 528–534

Rodriguez DD, Rodriguez WC, Rivera JJ, Rodriguez S, Otero AA (1981) Doppler ultrasound versus testicular scanning in the evaluation of the acute scrotum. J Urol 125:343–346.

Ross WS, Davis LMR, Reynolds JR (1987) Epididymal involvement in H.S.P. mimicking testicular torsion. J R Coll Surg Edinb 32:247

Schaffer R (1985) Ultrasonography of scrotal trauma. Urol Radiol 7:245

Schmahmann S, Haller JO (1997) Neonatal ovarian cysts: pathogenesis, diagnosis and management. Pediatr Radiol 27:101–105

Sclafani SJA, Becker JA, Shaftan GW (1985) Strategies for the radiologic management of genitourianry trauma. Urol Radiol 7:231–244

Shatzkes DR, Haller JO, Velcek FT (1991) Imaging of uterovaginal anomalies in the pediatric patient. Urol Radiol 13:58–66

Siegel MJ (1991) Female pelvis. In: Siegel MJ (ed) Pediatric sonography. Raven Press, New York, pp 311–344

Siegel A, Snyder H, Duckett J (1987) Epididymitis in infants and boys: underlying urogenital anomalies and efficacy or imaging modalities. J Urol 138:1100–1103

Stein BS, Kendall AR, Harke HT, Naiman JL, Karafin L (1980) Scrotal imaging in the Henoch-Schönlein syndrome. J Urol 124:568–569

Steinhardt GF, Boyarsky S, MacKey R (1993) Testicular torsion: pitfalls of colour Doppler sonography. J Urol 150:461–462

Stephens FD (1982) Embryopathy of malformations (guest editorial). J Urol 127:13

Stoffer TJ, Nesbit MT, Levitt STI (1975) Extramedullary involvement of the testes in childhood leukaemia. Cancer 35:1203–1211

Stone SC (1992) Pelvic pain in children and adolescents. In: Carpenter SFK, Rock JA (eds) Pediatric and Adolescent gynecology. Raven Press, New York, pp 267–278

Subramanyam BR, Honi SC, Hitton S (1985) Diffuse testicular disease: sonographic features and significance. Am J Roentgenol. 145:1221–1224

Thorpe EM, Muram D (1994) Sexually transmitted diseases in adolescence. In: Sanfilippo JS, Muram D, Lee PA, Dewhurst J (eds) Pediatric and adolescent gynecology. W.B. Saunders, Philadelphia, pp 310–335

Zerin JM, Di Pietro MA, Grignon A, Shea D (1990) Testicular infarction in the newborn. Ultrasound findings. Pediatr Radiol 20:329–330

6 Emergency Room Neurological Presentation

L.J. ABERNETHY and R. E. APPLETON

CONTENTS

6.1
Introduction: Investigation and Management of Acute Neurological Conditions in Childhood

When a child presents with an acute neurological illness, the first priority is to determine whether immediate supportive treatment is necessary to maintain respiration and circulation. Whatever the underlying condition, prevention of secondary neurological injury from hypoxia, ischaemia or meta-

L.J. ABERNETHY, MB, ChB, Consultant Paediatric Radiologist, Royal Liverpool Children's NHS Trust, Alder Hey Children's Hospital, Eaton Road, Liverpool L12 2AP, UK
R. E. APPLETON, MB, BS, Consultant Paediatric Neurologist, Royal Liverpool Children's NHS Trust, Alder Hey Children's Hospital, Eaton Road, Liverpool L12 2AP, UK

bolic upset is crucial. After basic life support measures have been instituted as necessary, a good history and clinical examination are essential. Complex investigations, including imaging of the brain and spine, may then be appropriate. It must be stressed that it can be extremely dangerous to commence radiological investigations before the general condition of the child has been stabilised.

Computed tomography (CT) and magnetic resonance imaging (MRI) may both be used appropriately in acute neurological conditions of childhood. CT is usually more accessible, and permits rapid brain imaging. CT has real advantages over MRI in acute head injury and subarachnoid haemorrhage. Acute haemorrhage and supratentorial space-occupying lesions (conditions requiring immediate active management) are demonstrated accurately. MRI has greater sensitivity for posterior fossa tumours and more subtle brain abnormalities, but this must be balanced against the longer imaging times and the difficulties in monitoring a sick child within the MRI environment. MRI has a unique role in the investigation of suspected acute spinal cord lesions, and should be considered the investigation of choice for acute paraplegia.

6.2
Trauma

Head injury in children is a common problem and may present considerable clinical difficulty. A child with a significant head injury may not lose consciousness immediately, and neurological signs of intracranial haemorrhage may evolve slowly. In young children, the skull is much less rigid than in an adult, and the presence or absence of a skull vault fracture is not a reliable indicator of intracranial haemorrhage or brain injury (HARWOOD-NASH et al. 1971; LLOYD et al. 1997). Skull radiographs tend to be over-used in children with closed head injuries; they are of limited value, except in special situations such as suspected child abuse, when the presence of fractures must be documented, or when there are clinical signs of a depressed or compound fracture.

Close clinical observation is the key to good management of closed head injuries, with early brain imaging if the mechanism of injury or clinical signs give any indication of intracranial damage. CT is usually the most appropriate modality for rapid brain imaging in a child who requires close observation and monitoring. A child with a head injury may be too restless or agitated to obtain a satisfactory scan, and in this situation general anaesthesia is necessary; sedation without protection of the airway is contra-indicated.

The possibility of non-accidental injury must always be considered when signs of intracranial haemorrhage or brain injury are found in a young infant. The specific features of non-accidental injury are discussed in Chap. 10.

6.2.1
Extradural and Subdural Haematoma

Children with an extradural or subdural haematoma may present with a range of clinical signs, including irritability, drowsiness, a declining conscious level and focal neurological deficits (with or without headache). These features may develop soon after the injury, or sometimes after a 'lucid interval' of 24–72 h. In this situation urgent CT is indicated; early neurosurgical intervention is required to prevent secondary neurological damage, and is potentially life-saving in preventing cerebral herniation and brainstem compression.

On CT, acute extradural haematoma shows a characteristic pattern of a biconvex, well-defined collection of uniformly high attenuation, lying between the surface of the brain and the inner table of the skull, which does not cross the line of cranial sutures (Fig. 6.1). However, an acute subdural haematoma may sometimes simulate these appearances. In an actively bleeding extradural haematoma, areas of low attenuation may be present.

Small extradural haematomas in the middle or posterior cranial fossa, or near the skull vertex, may be missed on axial CT scans. MRI can demonstrate these lesions more accurately, using coronal T1-weighted images. Acute haematomas show uniform high signal, although in the hyperacute situation, blood may be almost iso-intense with the underlying brain parenchyma.

Acute subdural haematomas typically appear on CT as crescentic, high-attenuation collections, but some may contain both high and low attenuation

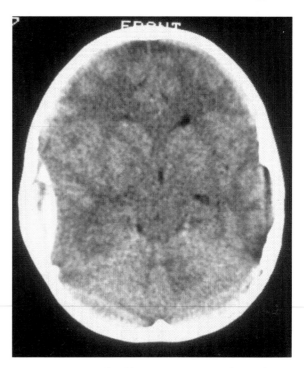

Fig. 6.1. Acute extradural haematoma. CT scan shows a lense-shaped, high-attenuation collection on the right side between the skull vault and the surface of the brain

(Fig. 6.2). Large collections produce mass effect, with inward buckling of the cerebral cortex, compression of the lateral ventricle and midline shift. Subdural haematomas may track along the falx cerebri and over the tentorium; MRI is more sensitive than CT in demonstrating small collections in these locations.

On CT, extra-axial haematomas gradually decrease in density with time, becoming isodense with brain at about 2 weeks. Chronic subdural haematomas have a density equal to cerebrospinal fluid (CSF). The signal characteristics of extra-axial haematomas on MRI scans also change with time; this is a complex process related to lysis of red cells, conversion of haemoglobin to deoxyhaemoglobin, and then breakdown, first to methaemoglobin and then to haemosiderin. In the first few hours after injury, a haematoma may be isointense with brain on T1-weighted images and hypointense on T2-weighted images. A haematoma then develops a characteristic hyperintensity, firstly on T1-weighted images and then on T2-weighted images, which makes even small collections conspicuous. This process commences at the edges of the collection and progresses towards the centre. Then, as blood breakdown products are absorbed, the hyperintensity on T1 gradually diminishes until the collection has identical signal characteristics to CSF.

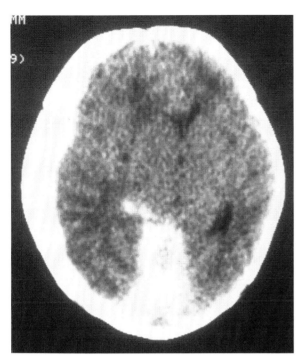

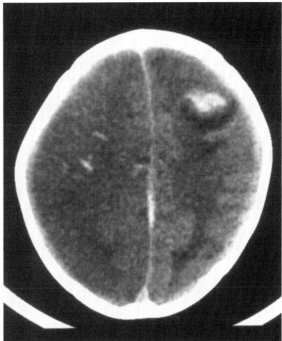

Fig. 6.2. Acute subdural haematoma. CT shows a crescentic, high-attenuation collection over the convexity of the right cerebral hemisphere and above the tentorium

Fig. 6.3. Cerebral contusion. CT shows a high-density lesion with surrounding oedema in the left frontal lobe. There is diffuse oedema in the right cerebral hemisphere, which contains some small focal haemorrhages consistent with shearing injury

6.2.2
Cerebral Contusion

Cerebral contusions are frequently found following moderate or, more commonly, severe head trauma. They may be single or multiple and are more commonly seen in the frontal, occipital and anterior temporal regions. In infants and young children, contre-coup cerebral contusions (opposite the site of direct injury) should raise the possibility of non-accidental injury. Contusions comprise both haemorrhage and brain necrosis and may be followed by the development of oedema, resulting in further neurological deterioration.

Computed tomography reveals cerebral contusions as areas of irregular high density with surrounding oedema; large lesions may produce mass effect with ventricular compression and midline shift (Fig. 6.3).

6.2.3
Diffuse Axonal Injury/Cerebral Oedema

Diffuse axonal injury/cerebral oedema is a feature of more severe closed head injury and pathologically causes extensive disruption of axons and synapses

and multiple, small areas of shearing-induced haemorrhage throughout the brain, particularly within the corpus callosum and frontal lobes. Clinically, this results in varying periods of unconsciousness, deep coma or death; focal neurological signs and seizures rarely occur. CT performed acutely shows diffuse cerebral oedema, but may not show the multiple haemorrhagic lesions. Severe cerebral oedema produces loss of differentiation between grey and white matter, diffuse low density throughout the brain, and compression of the ventricular system and basal cisterns (Fig. 6.4). Focal oedema may produce mass effect and midline shift. In children who survive the acute episode, MRI, particularly with gradient-echo sequences, may show evidence of multifocal haemorrhage within the cerebral substance, visible as areas of signal inhomogeneity due to the presence of blood breakdown products.

6.2.4
Cervical Spine Injury

Children with severe head injuries, particularly if associated with loss of consciousness, should be managed as if they have sustained an injury to the cervical spine until proven otherwise. Young chil-

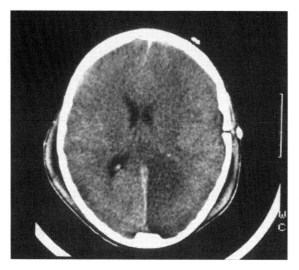

Fig. 6.4. CT scan shows severe, diffuse cerebral oedema following trauma. There is a left occipital infarct, probably due to transtentorial cerebral herniation with compression of the left posterior cerebral artery

dren are particularly vulnerable to cervical spinal cord injury. Immobilisation of the neck should be instituted promptly and maintained until radiological investigation has been completed; however, even if there is no evidence of an unstable cervical spine injury, the possibility of spinal cord injury without radiological abnormality (SCIWORA) must be considered, particularly if the mechanism of injury suggests that a forced flexion or extension of the neck has occurred. The flexibility of the spine in young children allows significant spinal cord injury to occur in the absence of radiographic signs of fracture or dislocation (OSENBACH and MENEZES 1989; PANG and WILBERGER 1982).

In children who are conscious, symptoms and signs suggesting cervical cord damage include:

- Neck pain
- Paraesthesia/loss of sensation from the neck downwards
- Loss or weakness of voluntary movement in upper or lower limbs, or both
- Priapism (persistent penile erection – implies complete spinal cord injury)
- Bladder/anal dysfunction
- Hypotension and bradycardia (frequently develop following complete cord injury)

Most cervical cord damage is sustained at the time of the initial injury; however, between 5% and 10% of patients will develop a neurological deficit later following further displacement of an unstable neck in-

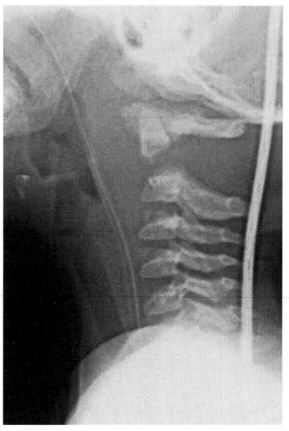

Fig. 6.5. Lateral radiograph of the cervical spine. Fracture of the C2 vertebra caused by flexion injury. Anterior displacement of the upper fragment disrupts the anterior and posterior vertebral lines

jury or cervical disc herniation. Primary cord damage cannot be reversed; it is these secondary injuries which are potentially preventable, which emphasises the importance of early immobilisation and thorough radiological assessment. If the mechanism of injury suggests that cord injury is possible, immobilisation of the cervical spine should be maintained until full neurological assessment can be performed, if necessary waiting until the child regains consciousness.

Radiological assessment of the cervical spine begins with carefully performed plain radiographs; a single lateral film taken in the emergency room is a useful starting point to demonstrate a major fracture or gross instability, but it should not be assumed that a normal lateral film excludes a significant injury. The lateral film must be scrutinised carefully for signs of vertebral fracture or discontinuity in the anterior and posterior vertebral lines and the laminar line which indicate an unstable flexion or extension injury (Fig. 6.5). Antero-posterior (AP) and lateral radiographs may be supplemented by fine-section CT to detect an occult fracture (Fig. 6.6). In a conscious, cooperative child with local pain and tenderness but no neurological signs, careful flexion and extension views with close medical supervision are appropriate to exclude instability. An unstable cervical spine injury requires halo traction or vertebral fusion to protect the spinal cord.

If there are clinical signs of cord injury, MRI is the investigation of choice. MRI is the most sensitive means of demonstrating surgically remediable abnormalities such as extradural haematoma or ruptured intervertebral discs; MRI may also demonstrate oedema or haemorrhage within the spinal cord, and injury to spinal ligaments and vertebral growth plates. (Fig. 6.7).

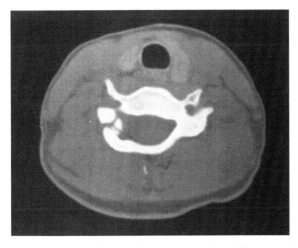

Fig. 6.6. CT scan of cervical spine. Comminuted fracture of the lamina of the C5 vertebra, not visible on conventional radiograph

6.3
Subarachnoid and Cerebral Haemorrhage

Bleeding into the subarachnoid space may follow trauma (particularly in the neonate) or a spontaneous rupture of an aneurysm or an arteriovenous malformation (AVM), or rarely in association with a cerebral tumour. Up to a third of all cases of subarachnoid haemorrhage may be idiopathic, although it is likely that a high proportion of these may have

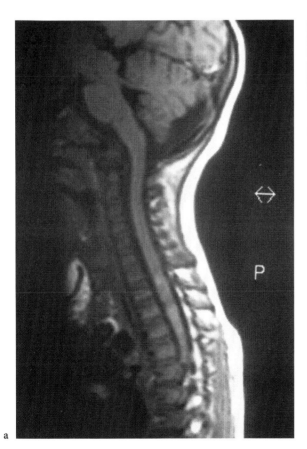

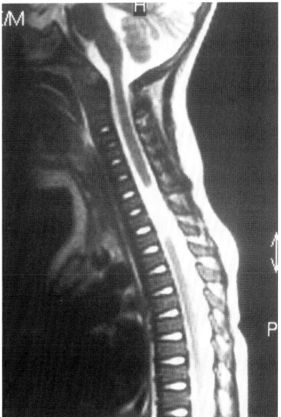

a   b

Fig. 6.7 a,b. MRI of cervical spinal cord. Cord contusion at C7–T2 due to flexion injury, without radiographic evidence of fracture or dislocation. **a** Sagittal T1-weighted spin-echo image. **b** Sagittal T2-weighted turbo spin-echo image

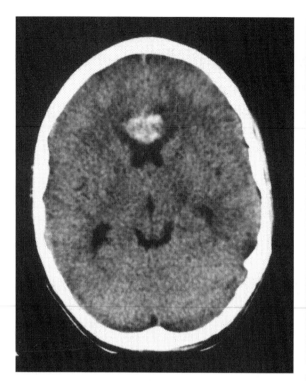

Fig. 6.8. Cerebral haemorrhage from an arteriovenous malformation in a 15-year-old boy. CT without contrast shows a haematoma in the anterior interhemispheric fissure

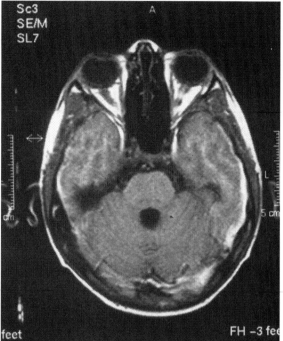

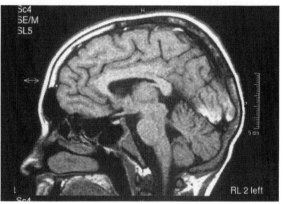

Fig. 6.9 a,b. Subarachnoid haemorrhage visible on T1-weighted MR images in a child with thrombocytopenia due to leukaemia. **a** Axial image showing high-signal blood in the CSF spaces around both temporal lobes: **b** Sagittal image showing blood around the occipital pole

been caused by bleeding from a cryptic AVM. The clinical features of a subarachnoid haemorrhage vary, depending upon its severity, from an acute onset of headache with back pain or stiffness, meningism, focal or generalised seizures (a common presentation in the neonatal period), hemiplegia, coma or death. The onset of symptoms is usually sudden and may occur either at rest or during exercise, coughing or a forced Valsalva manoeuvre. In infants and young children this acute presentation may occur on the background of an increasing head circumference, heart failure and a cranial bruit if the cause of the haemorrhage has been a large AVM or a vein of Galen aneurysm.

Computed tomography without intravenous contrast is the initial radiological investigation of choice; subarachnoid blood is manifest as high-attenuation fluid filling the basal cisterns and the cortical sulci and fissures. Blood may be present within the ventricles and there may be an intracerebral haematoma, visible as a space-occupying lesion of high attenuation (Fig. 6.8). CT is more sensitive than MRI in the detection of acute haemorrhage, particularly within the basal cisterns, and is also sensitive for

complications of haemorrhage, such as ischaemic infarction and hydrocephalus. However, CT is sensitive to the presence of subarachnoid blood only in the first few days after acute haemorrhage; in the subacute situation, blood-containing CSF loses its high density on CT, but becomes conspicuous on T1-weighted MR images (Fig. 6.9).

A large vascular malformation or vein of Galen aneurysm will be visible on CT, particularly after contrast enhancement, but in many cases subse-

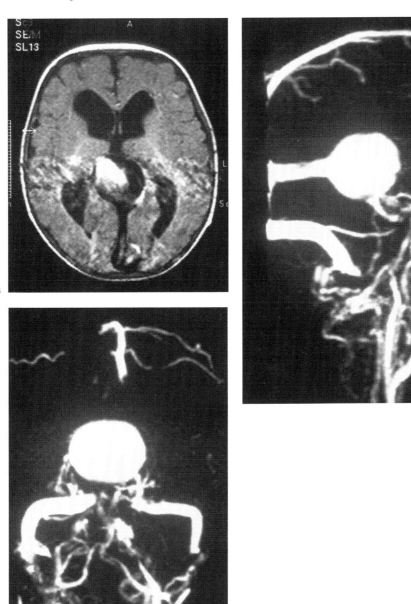

Fig. 6.10 a–c. Vein of Galen malformation in a 5-month-old child. **a** Axial T1-weighted spin-echo images show artifact from rapid, turbulent blood flow within the midline malformation. There is dilatation of the lateral ventricles. **b** Sagittal and **c** coronal reconstructions of phase-contrast MR angiography

quent MRI and MR angiography will be helpful to demonstrate a vascular malformation (Fig. 6.10). However, the presence of acute haemorrhage makes it difficult to obtain a satisfactory MR angiogram. Conventional cerebral angiography is still necessary in many cases, but this is usually performed electively, after the child's condition has been stabilised.

6.4
Acute Confusional States/Behavioural Disorders

Delirium or acute confusional state is the generally accepted term for an acute, transient, global organic disorder of higher central nervous system function resulting in impaired consciousness and attention. It may arise as a consequence of a primary brain lesion (e.g. trauma, migraine, raised intracranial pressure, encephalitis/meningitis, ictal or post-ictal epileptic state, subarachnoid haemorrhage) or cerebral involvement secondary to a systemic illness (e.g. any infection, cardiac failure, hypo/hyperglycaemia, Addisonian crisis, hepatic disease) or intoxication (e.g. prescribed or illicit drugs, poisons, alcohol). In children, infectious, toxic or metabolic causes are most common. A detailed history and careful physical examination should provide important clues to the aetiology and therefore help to guide the most urgent and appropriate investigations. Blood and urine analyses are the most important initial investigations; electroencephalography (EEG) may also be required, depending on the clinical features. Neuroimaging is indicated in most cases, but particularly if there is no obvious toxic or metabolic cause. CT is usually appropriate; if the child is restless or agitated, general anaesthesia may be necessary to enable satisfactory completion of the scan.

6.5
Acute Asphyxia

Children who have suffered an acute episode of asphyxia or cardiorespiratory arrest (for example, near drowning or post cardiac bypass surgery) may show signs of profound neurological impairment at presentation. After the clinical condition has been stabilised, brain imaging is often indicated to assess the degree of irreversible brain injury. CT may show no abnormality for the first 24h; non-specific signs of cerebral oedema may be the earliest abnormality. Between 1 and 3 days following the original injury, scans may show diffuse loss of cerebral grey–white matter differentiation and decreased density within the grey matter of the basal ganglia and cortex (Fig. 6.11). Haemorrhage in the basal ganglia and cortex may occur between 4 and 6 days.

The acute reversal sign refers to a CT finding of diffusely decreased density of cerebral grey and white matter; in severe cases there is reversal of the densities of grey and white matter, the cortex becoming less dense than the underlying white matter. The interface between grey and white matter becomes indistinct or is lost completely. There is typically sparing of the basal ganglia, thalami and cerebellum, which show relatively increased density (Fig. 6.12). Prognosis for neurological recovery is very poor once this sign has developed (HAN et al. 1989).

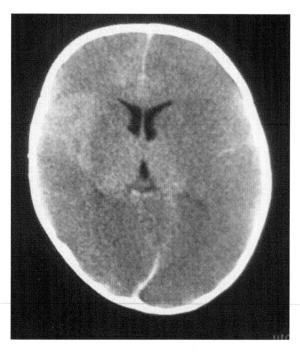

Fig. 6.11. Acute asphyxia. CT shows diffuse cerebral oedema with loss of grey-white matter differentiation 24h after an episode of near drowning. There is relative sparing of the thalami and the cortex around the right sylvian fissure

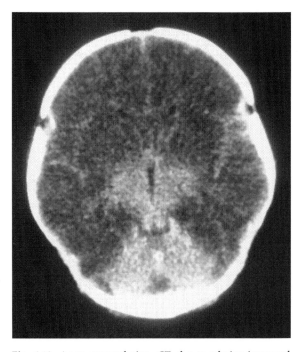

Fig. 6.12. Acute reversal sign. CT shows relative increased density of basal ganglia and cerebellum, 48h after an episode of acute asphyxia

Magnetic resonance scans show only subtle abnormalities in the first 1–3 days, consisting of T1 and T2 prolongation in the basal ganglia and insular cortex. Blurring of the junction between the cortex and the subcortical white matter on T1-weighted images and a line of T2 prolongation at this site together represent an early sign of significant cortical damage (Barkovich 1995). Diffusion-weighted imaging has shown promise in showing acute hypoxic-ischaemic damage with greater sensitivity.

After 7 days, both CT and MRI show progressive changes of cerebral atrophy when irreversible cerebral damage has occurred. It should be noted that scans performed around 7 days after an episode of asphyxia are particularly likely to be misleading, as the acute changes of oedema may have resolved, while the atrophic changes have not yet become apparent. Imaging at 14 days is more likely to give a reliable guide to long-term prognosis.

6.6
Acute Metabolic Encephalopathies

There are a number of inborn errors of metabolism which may cause progressive or relapsing encephalopathy in childhood. In some cases, a metabolic disorder may have an acute onset in a child whose development has been normal. Examples of this type of disorder are Leigh syndrome and glutaric aciduria type 1. Early diagnosis of these conditions is of great importance for genetic counselling.

6.6.1
Leigh Syndrome

Leigh Syndrome refers to a group of inherited neurodegenerative disorders with a characteristic complex of clinical manifestations and imaging features. A number of different biochemical or genetic defects, related to pyruvate metabolism, have been identified. Leigh syndrome has an episodic or chronic progressive clinical course, but its onset may be acute. Affected children may present in the first few years of life with hypotonia and psychomotor deterioration, or acutely during an intercurrent illness or infection or even during, or in recovery from, a surgical procedure. There may be a systemic lactic acidosis during an acute episode, or peripheral blood lactate may be normal while CSF lactate is increased. CT and MRI show characteristic bilateral, sym-

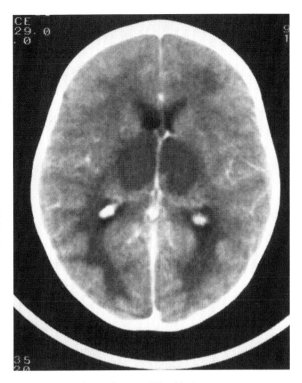

Fig. 6.13. Leigh syndrome. CT with intravenous contrast shows symmetrical low attenuation within the basal ganglia and thalami

metrical abnormalities localised to the putamen and globus pallidus. On CT the affected areas show abnormally low attenuation (Fig. 6.13); MRI is more sensitive, affected areas showing prolonged T1 and T2. In more severe cases, the caudate nuclei, periaqueductal grey matter, dorsal pons, cortical grey matter and cerebral white matter may be affected (Fig. 6.14).

6.6.2
Glutaric Aciduria Type 1

Glutaric aciduria type 1 may present during infancy or early childhood as an acute encephalopathy, although it more frequently causes slowly progressive neurological deterioration, including developmental plateau or regression and the appearance of involuntary movements (choreoathetosis and dystonia). Macrocephaly is a frequent finding. Glutaric aciduria type 1 is an autosomal recessive condition which results from deficiency of the mitochondrial enzyme glutaryl-CoA dehydrogenase. Neuroimaging shows a bilateral, symmetrical pattern of basal ganglia abnormality, manifest as low attenuation on CT and

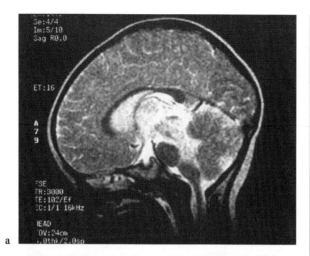

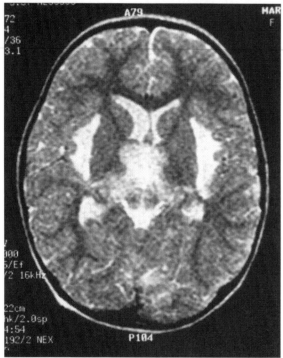

Fig. 6.14 a,b. Leigh syndrome. MRI: T2-weighted turbo spin-echo images (a sagittal; b axial) show high signal in the basal ganglia (particularly in the putamen), thalami and dorsal brainstem

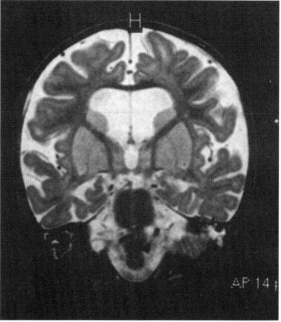

Fig. 6.15. Glutaric aciduria type 1. MR image (T2-weighted coronal turbo spin-echo) shows bilateral, symmetrical high signal within the basal ganglia

6.7
Acute Disseminated Encephalomyelitis

Acute disseminated encephalomyelitis (ADEM) usually follows a viral infection or immunisation with a latent period of a few days to several weeks, and tends to affect younger children (less than 10 years of age). It is believed to represent an autoimmune reaction to infection, causing a vasculitis. Affected chidren may present with headaches, fever, hemiplegia or other focal deficits, seizures, or acutely disturbed consciousness, including coma. Mortality is estimated at 10%–20%; survivors may recover completely, but some are left with neurological deficits.

Computed tomography may show multifocal or diffuse white matter damage, but may be normal early in the course of the disease, and may sometimes remain normal throughout. MRI shows multiple, bilateral focal lesions with an asymmetrical pattern of distribution (Fig. 6.16) (ATLAS et al. 1986). The lesions are predominantly within the cerebral white matter, but may extend into adjacent cortical grey matter or into the basal ganglia (BAUM et al. 1994). There is usually no mass effect. Occasionally, MRI may show predominantly grey matter lesions. There is a variant of this condition, acute

prolonged T1 and T2 on MRI (Fig. 6.15). There may also be global retardation of white matter myelination and atrophy of the frontal and temporal lobes. Similar abnormalities may be seen in other inborn errors of metabolism such as methylmalonic aciduria and proprionic aciduria, which may present as an acute encephalopathy associated with lactic acidosis.

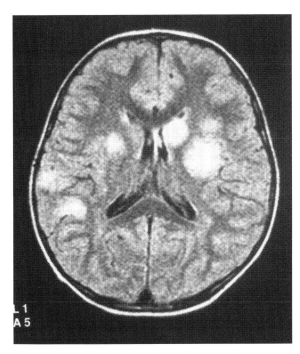

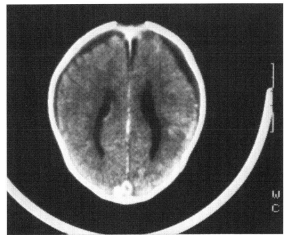

Fig. 6.17. Complicated bacterial meningitis. Contrast-enhanced CT scan shows meningeal enhancement, subdural effusions and signs of sagittal sinus thrombosis

Fig. 6.16. Acute disseminated encephalomyelitis in a 6-year-old boy. MRI (axial T2-weighted turbo spin-echo) shows multiple, bilateral, asymmetrical white matter lesions

haemorrhagic encephalomyelitis, in which the lesions show evidence of haemorrhage on CT or MRI, and tend to show oedema or mass effect.

6.8
Acute Cerebral Infection

6.8.1
Bacterial Meningitis

The symptoms and signs of meningitis may differ depending on the age of the child. In young infants the presentation may be acute and non-specific including fever, irritability, vomiting, lethargy, neck stiffness, a bulging anterior fontanelle and seizures. In older children, headache, vomiting and neck stiffness are more prominent; if seizures occur they may be focal or generalised and are difficult to control, frequently progressing to status epilepticus. The onset of seizures is frequently followed by a rapid decline in consciousness, resulting in coma.

Children suspected of having acute bacterial meningitis require immediate treatment with intravenous antibiotics. The diagnosis may be confirmed by lumbar puncture and examination of CSF, but treatment must not wait for investigations to be per-

formed. Lumbar puncture must be avoided if consciousness is impaired or if there are clinical signs of raised intracranial pressure, as it may precipitate herniation of the brain, or coning. Herniation of the brain is a common post-mortem finding in children who die from meningitis, and may occur without lumbar puncture. Rapid deterioration in conscious level or the development of focal neurological signs suggest coning. Herniation of the cerebellar tonsils and medulla through the foramen magnum leads to respiratory abnormalities, decerebrate posturing and flaccidity; transtentorial herniation of the uncus of the temporal lobe may be manifest as a unilateral fixed dilated pupil and a contralateral hemiparesis.

Brain imaging is of no value in the immediate diagnosis of bacterial meningitis (CABRAL et al. 1987). It is an insensitive method for the detection of raised intracranial pressure, and is unhelpful in determining whether lumbar puncture is safe (RENNICK et al. 1993). It has also been shown that CT is unhelpful in children with acute bacterial meningitis who have stable focal neurological signs, convulsions, or prolonged fever (HEYDERMAN et al. 1992). The role of brain imaging is in the identification of complications of meningitis (hydrocephalus, subdural empyema, cerebral abscess, sinus thrombosis, infarction) or the exclusion of focal brain pathology simulating meningitis clinically (Fig. 6.17). Cerebral abscess and subdural empyema are uncommon complications which usually occur more than 7 days after the onset of symptoms. CT or MRI is therefore indicated if there are progressive focal neurological signs, prolonged decreased level of consciousness, prolonged or focal seizures, increasing head circumference, evidence of continuing infection or recurrence of symptoms. However, brain imaging should not be undertaken until after initiation of antibiotic treatment, control of raised intracranial pressure and, if necessary, intubation and ventilation.

6.8.2
Herpes Simplex Encephalitis

The herpes simplex viruses are widely prevalent and commonly cause subclinical or minor infections, but can cause encephalitis with rapidly progressive, devastating neurological damage. Type 1 herpes simplex virus, a common cause of orofacial infections, is the cause of herpes simplex encephalitis in most patients over the age of 6 months. Type 2 herpes simplex virus is usually associated with genital infections but may cause congenital or neonatal encephalitis.

The challenge of management of herpes simplex encephalitis is to institute antiviral therapy rapidly in order to limit the long-term sequelae. In typical cases of type 1 herpes simplex encephalitis, there are non-specific prodromal symptoms of viral infection; neurological symptoms such as depressed conscious level, seizures and hemiparesis then develop and progress rapidly. Unfortunately, CT and MRI are not sensitive in the early stages of the disease. CT usually shows no abnormality before the fifth day, when signs of focal oedema or haemorrhage may become apparent in the temporal or frontal lobes. MRI is more sensitive and specific, showing prolongation of T1 and T2 in inferior frontal or medial temporal lobe structures (Fig. 6.18) (SCHROTH et al. 1987).

6.8.3
Cerebral Abscess

Cerebral abscesses are uncommon in childhood; most occur in children with predisposing conditions such as congenital heart disease or pulmonary arteriovenous malformations (which permit paradoxical embolism), infective endocarditis, cystic fibrosis or immunosuppression. Direct extension may occur from paranasal sinus or middle ear infection. Affected children present with fever, headaches, confusion, altered consciousness, seizures or focal neurological signs. Abscesses begin as areas of cerebritis; central necrosis then occurs and a capsule forms

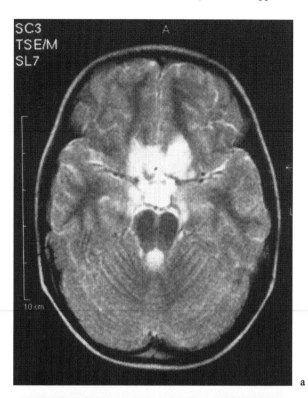

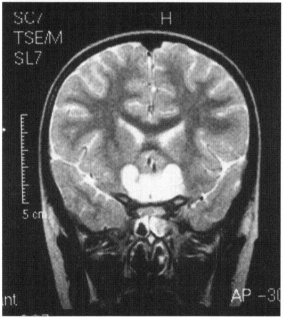

Fig. 6.18 a,b. Herpes simplex encephalitis. MRI (T2-weighted turbo spin-echo) shows cortical oedema in the inferior frontal lobes. **a** Axial and **b** coronal images

around the lesion; this process usually evolves over a period of 7–14 days. However, children may present acutely with a fully developed, capsulated abscess. On CT, cerebral abscesses appear as low-density

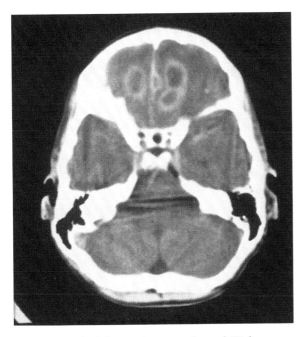

Fig. 6.19. Cerebral abscess. Contrast-enhanced CT shows cystic frontal lobe lesions with marked ring enhancement

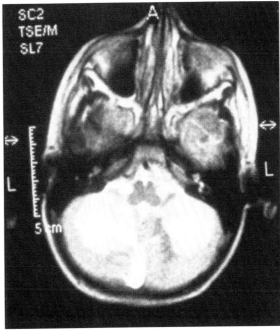

Fig. 6.20. Post-viral cerebellitis. MRI (axial T2-weighted turbo spin-echo) shows bilateral, symmetrical areas of high signal within the cerebellar hemispheres

lesions with well-defined margins of higher density; following intravenous contrast, the abscess wall usually enhances vividly (Fig. 6.19). On MRI, cerebritis and early abscesses show low signal on T1- and high signal on T2-weighted images; as the abscess wall appears it is initially hyperintense on both T1- and T2-weighted images, but subsequently becomes isointense on T1- and hypointense on T2-weighted images. Following intravenous gadolinium, the abscess wall shows marked enhancement on T1-weighted images (HAIMES et al. 1989).

6.9
Acute Ataxia

Acute ataxias are most often caused by intoxication (particularly drugs and alcohol), infections (e.g. mumps and other enteroviruses) or post/para-infectious disorders (e.g. varicella cerebellitis). Ataxia accompanied by headache, vomiting and irritability may be post-traumatic in origin or caused by a brain tumour; in this situation CT or MRI must be undertaken to exclude a posterior fossa haematoma or tumour. Rarely, children with an underlying metabolic or progressive degenerative condition (e.g. mitochondrial cytopathies, Leigh syndrome, maple syrup urine disease) may present during an

intercurrent infection or illness with acute ataxia; again, neuroimaging is usually indicated to exclude a structural lesion.

Neuroimaging in acute, viral-induced ataxia is often normal and is probably unjustified in clinically typical cases. T2-weighted MR images may show bilateral, symmetrical areas of high signal in the cerebellar hemispheres (Fig. 6.20), but these appearances are not specific; lead poisoning, multiple sclerosis or vasculitis may produce identical appearances. Acute onset ataxia which develops days or weeks after a viral infection (usually, but not invariably, in association with other neurological signs) may represent acute disseminated encephalitis and MRI may demonstrate the characteristic lesions seen in this condition.

Rarely, acute ataxia occurring in the absence of any additional neurological symptoms or signs may represent an episode of demyelination (e.g. multiple sclerosis); MRI may demonstrate signs of plaques within the brainstem and cerebellum, and asymptomatic cerebral lesions may also be present, particularly in the periventricular white matter and corpus callosum. The lesions of multiple sclerosis are typically multiple and confluent and show high signal on T2-weighted images. However, solitary lesions with mass effect may occur at the onset of multiple sclerosis, especially in children and adolescents (OSBORN et al. 1990). Demyelinating disease usually has a more insidious onset, and neuroimaging need not necessarily be undertaken as an emergency investigation.

6.10
Headache/Suspected Tumour

A detailed history and examination of children with acute headache will identify the underlying cause in most cases. It must be emphasised that a brain tumour may present either acutely or more gradually over a period of days, weeks or months. In addition, the headache may be either intermittent or steadily progressive, whether presenting acutely or more gradually. In children between the ages of 4 and 10 years, the most common site of a brain tumour is in the posterior fossa; in younger children, supratentorial tumours are more common. When a tumour is associated with an acute headache, this is often associated with haemorrhage within the tumour and is commonly accompanied by seizures, focal neurological signs and some alteration in consciousness. When the headache is more chronic in duration, additional clues from both the history and the examination which tend to suggest the diagnosis include:

- Greater severity of the headache in the early hours of the morning/on awakening, with some improvement during the course of the day
- Vomiting (which may be effortless and frequent) either accompanying or preceding the headache
- A plateau or regression in the child's development
- A head circumference larger than either parent
- Head tilt
- Papilloedema or optic atrophy

In these situations, and importantly *whenever* a brain tumour is suspected clinically, neuroimaging is indicated using either CT or MRI initially (Fig. 6.21); skull radiographs are unnecessary, inappropriate and may be unjustifiably reassuring. If a tumour of the brainstem is suspected, and if cough, micturition or defecation significantly exacerbates the headache, then MRI rather than CT is the preferred imaging technique.

Migraine is not uncommonly diagnosed initially in children who are subsequently found to have a brain tumour. In migraine, the headache symptoms are usually characteristic: the headache is always paroxysmal, and never persistent or steadily pro-

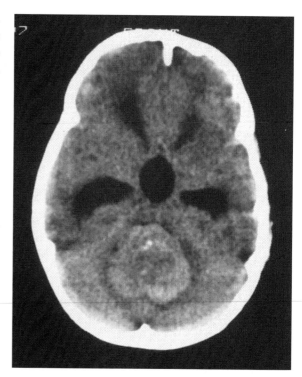

Fig. 6.21. Medulloblastoma presenting with symptoms of raised intracranial pressure in a 21-month-old child. CT with contrast enhancement shows an enhancing mass in the midline of the cerebellum with secondary hydrocephalus and periventricular oedema

gressive and, ideally, there should be a family history of migraine (in the child's parents or first-degree relatives); in addition the vomiting in migraine commonly follows (rather than precedes) the onset of headache by many minutes to hours. Children presenting with a first episode of hemiplegic migraine, particularly in the absence of a positive family history, should undergo neuroimaging with either CT (initially) or MRI. If the attacks of hemiplegia are always on the same side, are followed by residual neurological signs or are accompanied by additional symptoms or signs, then further investigations may be indicated, including angiography, echocardiography, and haematological and metabolic studies (see Sect. 6.12).

6.11
Seizure Disorders

There is universal concern among both parents and clinicians that a child presenting with a first epileptic seizure (including a febrile convulsion), whether brief or prolonged (status epilepticus), has an underlying brain tumour. In reality, this is most uncommon; brain tumours are the cause of seizures in only 1%–2% of children with epilepsy. However, it is important to classify the type of epileptic seizure. In primary generalised seizures, tumours will be found in less than 1% of affected children. In partial or focal seizures (in which only one part of the face or body or both are affected), with or without secondary generalisation, tumours may be identified in 4%–6% of children.

Skull radiography has no role in the imaging of children with epilepsy or febrile convulsions. CT is an appropriate initial scanning technique for the exclusion of a brain tumour; however, in a number of children who have an initial normal scan, later scans (particularly MRI) may reveal a slow-growing lesion only after months or years. MRI is the preferred initial imaging technique for children with complex partial seizures and infantile spasms.

The following groups of children with epilepsy require a brain scan:

- Children who have a neurological deficit or asymmetry (e.g. hemiparesis)
- Children who have evidence of a neurocutaneous syndrome (e.g. neurofibromatosis and tuberous sclerosis)
- Children with simple or complex partial seizures
- Children with infantile spasms or myoclonic seizures (presenting in the first year of life)
- Children under the age of 12–18 months who present with a complicated febrile seizure (i.e. focal or prolonged or followed by residual neurological signs)
- Children whose seizure control deteriorates for no obvious reason following an initial period of good control
- Children whose first epileptic seizure is prolonged (lasting more than 20–30 min)

The majority of these groups of children do not require neuroimaging as an emergency investigation. Exceptions include those who present with a prolonged convulsion or a complicated febrile seizure. CT is a satisfactory emergency scanning technique in these situations to detect a space-occupying lesion or signs of hypoxic-ischaemic brain injury. MRI may be required subsequently as it is more sensitive in identifying lesions within the temporal lobes and subtle areas of cerebral dysgenesis (e.g. focal cortical dysplasia and grey matter heterotopia).

Children who present with absence seizures, benign partial epilepsy or a simple febrile seizure (i.e. one that occurs in children between 18 months and 4 years of age, is generalised in nature, lasts less than 5 min and is not followed by any neurological signs) do not need brain imaging.

6.12
Stroke

Acute stroke must be considered when a child suddenly develops a hemiparesis or other focal neurological disturbance. Stroke is uncommon in children and in most cases is not permanent or irreversible, but is related to a transient and predominantly unilateral disturbance of cerebral function, usually in association with a prolonged seizure (when it is termed Todd's paresis), migraine or infection. Congenital malformations or tumours of the brain may occasionally present in this way, without any previous history of weakness. The predominant features of a haemorrhagic stroke (including a spontaneous bleed of an arteriovenous malformation) are impairment or loss of consciousness and seizures, as well as hemiparesis. Rare but well-recognised causes of stroke in childhood include hypertensive encephalopathy, congenital or acquired cardiac or vascular lesions and a number of haematological, biochemical or metabolic disorders such as sickle cell disease, homocystinuria, coagulopathies and mitochondrial cytopathies, specifically MELAS (mitochondrial encephalopathy, lactic acidosis and stroke). Trauma to the neck or pharynx, which may have been apparently trivial or even overlooked, may cause a stroke as a result of a dissecting aneurysm of the carotid or vertebral artery. No cause is found in up to 25% of children who have had a stroke, although it is very likely that this figure will decline with further improvements in neuroimaging and laboratory investigations.

Neuroimaging is indicated in all children who present with a stroke or stroke-like episode; CT is a useful initial technique, particularly for determining whether the stroke is haemorrhagic or ischaemic. Acute haemorrhage is visible as a focal area of increased density. Non-haemorrhagic infarction is visible as a well-defined, often wedge-shaped area of low density involving both grey and white matter with loss of grey-white differentiation. MRI may give a better indication of the extent of ischaemic lesions (Fig. 6.22), revealing cortical high signal intensity on T1-weighted images; in neonates and young infants, the changes may be extremely subtle as the ischaemic cortex may become isointense with the

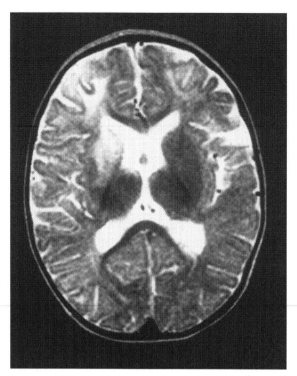

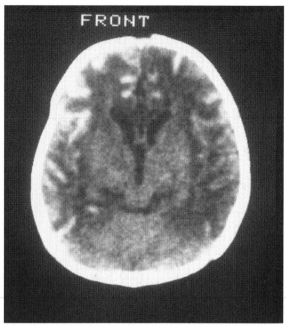

Fig. 6.23. Sagittal sinus thrombosis. CT scan shows bilateral haemorrhagic venous infarcts

Fig. 6.22. Multiple embolic cerebral infarcts in a child with congenital heart disease. MRI (axial T2-weighted turbo spin-echo) shows multiple foci of high signal involving both grey and white matter

underlying white matter. MRI may also reveal an occult vascular malformation or show direct evidence of vascular occlusion; for example, a dissecting aneurysm of the carotid artery may be visible on T1-weighted images as a crescent of high signal intensity narrowing the flow void within the lumen of the vessel.

Magnetic resonance angiography is a useful noninvasive method for the evaluation of the major cerebral vessels. However, the resolution of MR angiography is significantly inferior to that of conventional cerebral angiography, which may be required depending upon the clinical situation and results of initial investigations.

Chest radiography and echocardiography are indicated to demonstrate or exclude a cardiac source of embolisation, even in those children not previously known to have a cardiac abnormality.

The timing of neuroimaging is important; scanning undertaken soon after the onset of stroke may demonstrate no abnormality. CT performed as an emergency is usually unhelpful in distinguishing between an embolic or thrombotic stroke although

clearly multiple infarcts suggest an embolic or vasculitic aetiology. However, early CT will identify haemorrhage reliably.

6.13
Sinus Thrombosis

Sinus thrombosis may occur as a complication of middle ear infection, meningitis, dehydration, septicaemia or jugular vein thrombosis caused by a central venous line. Clinical diagnosis is difficult; signs include irritability, alteration of consciousness and seizures.

Sinus thrombosis causes venous infarction, visible on CT as zones of oedema, infarction and haemorrhage, typically involving the convexities of both cerebral hemispheres (Fig. 6.23). Hydrocephalus occurs when sagittal sinus thrombosis interferes with reabsorption of CSF.

Magnetic resonance imaging and MR venography are valuable in confirmation of sinus thrombosis without the need for cerebral angiography (Fig. 6.24). Sagittal and axial T1-weighted images may show lack of flow void and high-intensity thrombus within the superior sagittal sinus. MR venography (phase contrast MR angiography, velocity 20 cm/s)

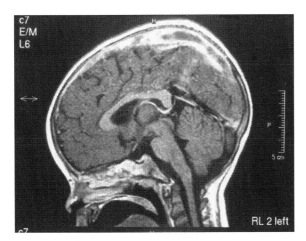

Fig. 6.24. Sagittal sinus thrombosis. Thrombus is visible in the superior sagittal sinus on a sagittal T1-weighted MR image

demonstrates absence of flow in the involved segments of the venous sinuses.

6.14
Facial Palsy

Acute isolated facial palsy is most commonly idiopathic in origin, when it is termed Bell's palsy; although a cause is rarely found, it is believed to be immune mediated, following a preceding respiratory viral infection. The weakness, which is usually sudden in onset and maximal within a few hours, may be preceded by pain or paraesthesia in the ear canal ipsilateral to the facial weakness. The weakness is lower motor neurone in type and there is frequently accompanying hyperacusis and impaired lacrimation, salivation and taste. Other causes of ipsilateral facial weakness (hypertension, middle ear infection, trauma or tumour) should be excluded before accepting a diagnosis of idiopathic facial palsy. Neuroimaging is not indicated for every child with an acute, isolated facial palsy; however, if other cranial nerve palsies or other neurological deficits develop, or if the facial palsy has shown no improvement after a month, then imaging is indicated, preferably with MRI. Detailed MRI of the posterior fossa, internal auditory meatus and petrous temporal bones will help to exclude a tumour such as an acoustic neuroma or the rare facial neuroma, and complications of middle ear or mastoid infection. In idiopathic Bell's palsy, MRI may show thickening and abnormal enhancement of the facial nerve in its course through the facial canal (Tien et al. 1990).

6.15
Acute Visual Failure

Children rarely experience acute visual loss; when it occurs the loss is usually episodic or recurrent, usually in association with epileptic seizures or migraine, rather than being isolated and persistent. Unilateral loss due to orbital disease is associated with eye pain, redness and proptosis, and is usually caused by post-septal orbital cellulitis, orbital tumour or haemangioma. CT or MRI of the orbits is indicated to confirm or exclude these aetiologies.

Visual loss with a relative afferent pupillary defect (abnormal pupillary response to a light shone in one or both eyes) suggests damage to the optic nerve; causes include optic neuritis, optic nerve glioma, trauma, leukaemic/lymphomatous infiltration of the optic nerve head and demyelination (e.g. multiple sclerosis). Visual loss with retained pupillary responses is more suggestive of a lesion involving the optic chiasm, tract or radiation, when usually there will be an accompanying visual field defect. When there is visual loss without clinical signs of orbital disease, urgent MRI is appropriate as this is the most appropriate modality to demonstrate intrinsic optic nerve lesions or mass lesions such as a craniopharyngioma causing optic chiasm compression (Fig. 6.25). Craniopharyngiomas typically appear as multicystic suprasellar masses; the cyst contents may show high signal on T1-weighted images, which is characteristic, but in other cases the fluid shows low signal. The solid portions of the tumour show marked enhancement following intravenous gadolinium.

6.16
Acute Paraplegia

Acute onset of paraplegia is a neurological emergency requiring immediate investigation. MRI is the imaging modality of choice, as sagittal and coronal images can display the whole length of the spinal cord. The primary role of imaging is to exclude an extrinsic lesion causing cord compression, including vertebral tumours such as aneurysmal bone cyst, giant cell tumour and Ewing sarcoma (Fig. 6.26), paraspinal tumours (neuroblastoma, ganglioneuroblastoma, ganglioneuroma), leukaemia, lymphoma, metastases (Fig. 6.27) and Langerhans cell granulomatosis. Epidural abscess is an uncommon cause

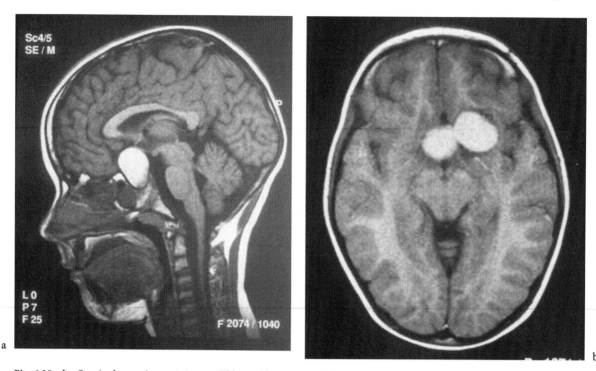

a   b

Fig. 6.25 a,b. Craniopharyngioma. A 9-year-old boy with acute visual failure. MR shows a cystic suprasellar lesion containing fluid with short T1. **a** Sagittal and **b** axial T1-weighted spin-echo images

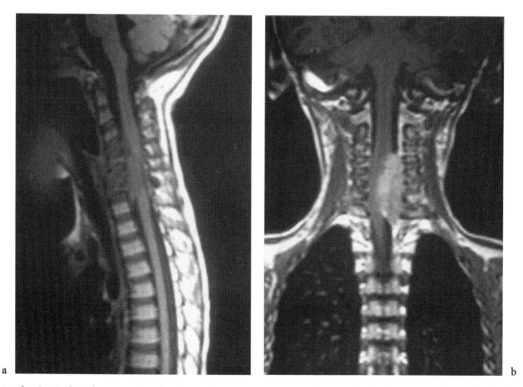

a   b

Fig. 6.26 a,b. Cervical cord compression due to vertebral Ewing's tumour. MRI: **a** sagittal and **b** coronal T1-weighted spin-echo images

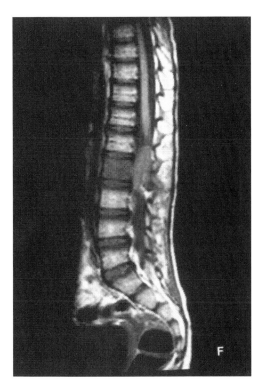

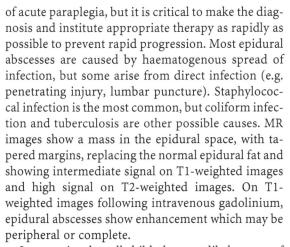

Fig. 6.27. Metastatic disease from a Wilm's tumour within the lumbar spinal canal MRI: sagittal T1-weighted spin-echo image shows replacement of the normal marrow signal within the L2 vertebra, with an adjacent mass within the spinal canal just below the conus of the spinal cord

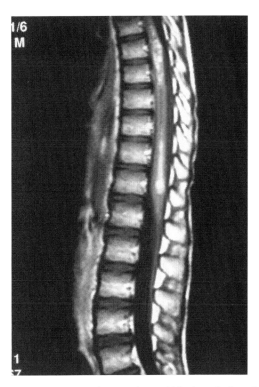

Fig. 6.28. Spontaneous haemorrhage within the spinal cord in a 7-year-old. MRI: sagittal T1-weighted spin-echo image shows expansion of the lower part of the spinal cord. The acute haematoma shows short T1 (high signal)

of acute paraplegia, but it is critical to make the diagnosis and institute appropriate therapy as rapidly as possible to prevent rapid progression. Most epidural abscesses are caused by haematogenous spread of infection, but some arise from direct infection (e.g. penetrating injury, lumbar puncture). Staphylococcal infection is the most common, but coliform infection and tuberculosis are other possible causes. MR images show a mass in the epidural space, with tapered margins, replacing the normal epidural fat and showing intermediate signal on T1-weighted images and high signal on T2-weighted images. On T1-weighted images following intravenous gadolinium, epidural abscesses show enhancement which may be peripheral or complete.

In a previously well child, the most likely cause of acute paraplegia is an intrinsic, self-limiting inflammatory process in the spinal cord, such as transverse myelitis or a rapidly evolving Guillain-Barré syndrome. Back pain and sphincter disturbance are more common in transverse myelitis. In transverse myelitis, MRI scans may show no abnormality, but there may be a focal area of T1 and T2 prolongation

within the cord; sensitivity appears to be increased by intravenous gadolinium, as the affected segments of the cord may show enhancement (AL DEEB et al. 1997; PARDATSHER et al. 1992).

Spinal cord tumours (astrocytomas and ependymomas) usually present with insidious onset of symptoms, but occasionally present with acute paraplegia, often with sphincter disturbance, usually as a result of haemorrhage. Haemorrhage into the spinal cord may also be due to an arteriovenous malformation, and in some cases no underlying cause is found (Fig. 6.28).

References

Al Deeb SM, Yaqub BA, Bruyn GW, Biary NM (1997) Acute transverse myelitis. A localized form of postinfectious encephalomyelitis. Brain 120:1115–1122

Atlas SW, Grossman RI, Goldberg HI, Hackney DB, Bilaniuk LT, Zimmerman RA (1986) MR diagnosis of acute disseminated encephalomyelitis. J Comput Assist Tomogr 10:798–801

Barkovich AJ (1995) Pediatric neuroimaging, 2nd edn. Raven Press, New York

Baum PA, Barkovich AJ, Koch TK, Berg BO (1994) Deep gray matter involvement in children with acute disseminated encephalomyelitis. Am J Neuroradiol 15:1275–1283

Cabral DA, Flodmark O, Farrell K, Speert DP (1987) Prospective study of computed tomography in acute bacterial meningitis. J Paediatr 111:201–205

Fenichel GM (1997) Altered states of consciousness. In: Fenichel GM (ed) Clinical paediatric neurology – a signs and symptoms approach, 3rd edn. W.B. Saunders, New York, pp 47–76

Haimes AB, Zimmerman RD, Mrogello S, et al. (1989) MR imaging of brain abscesses. Am J Neuroradiol 10:279–291

Han BK, Towbin RB, De Courten-Myers G, McLaurin RL, Ball WS (1989) Reversal sign on CT: effect of anoxic/ischemic cerebral injury in children. Am J Neuroradiol 10:1191–1198

Harwood-Nash DC, Hendrick EB, Hudson AR (1971) The significance of skull fracture in children. A study of 1187 patients. Radiology 101:151–160

Heckmann JM, Eastman R, Handler L, Wright M, Owen P (1993) Leigh disease (subacute necrotizing encephalomyelopathy): MR documentation of the evolution of an acute attack. Am J Neuroradiol 14:1157–1159

Heyderman RS, Robb SA, Kendall BE, Levin M (1992) Does computed tomography have a role in the evaluation of complicated acute bacterial meningitis in childhood? Dev Med Child Neurol 34:870–875

Lloyd DA, Carty H, Patterson M, Butcher CK, Roe D (1997) Predictive value of skull radiography for intracranial injury in children with blunt head injury. Lancet 349:821–824

Osborn AG, Harnsberger HR, Smoker WRK, Boyer RS (1990) Multiple sclerosis in adolescents: CT and MR findings. Am J Neuroradiol 11:489–494

Osenbach RK, Menezes AH (1989) Spinal cord injury without radiographic abnormality in children. Pediatr Neurosci 15:168–175

Pang D, Wilberger JE Jr (1982) Spinal cord injury without radiographic abnormalities in children. J Neurosurg 57:114–129

Pardatsher K, Fiore DL, Lavano A (1992) MR imaging of transverse myelitis using GD-DTPA. J Neuroradiol 19:63–67

Rennick G, Shann F, de Campo J (1993) Cerebral herniation during bacterial meningitis in children. Brit Med J 306:953–955

Schroth G, Gawehn J, Thron A, Vallbracht A, Voigt K (1987) Early diagnosis of herpes simplex encephalitis by MRI. Neurology 37:179–183

Tien RD, Dillon WP, Jackler RK (1990) Contrast enhanced MR imaging of the facial nerve in 11 patients with Bell's palsy. Am J Neuroradiol 11:735–741

7 Back Pain and Spinal Trauma

K.E. Halliday and J.M. Somers

CONTENTS

7.1
Introduction

Back pain is a surprisingly common problem amongst the young, with between 30% and 74% of schoolchildren reporting having suffered from it (Salminen et al. 1992; Balague et al. 1988, 1994, 1995; Olson et al. 1992; Bodner et al. 1988). Most episodes are due to soft tissue injury and will resolve spontaneously within a few weeks (Afshani and Kuhn 1997). Chronic muscular low back pain occurs far less frequently in children than in adults (Gerbino and Micheli 1995). Self-limiting back pain is more common in girls, sedentary children and those who play competitive sport (Balague et al. 1994; Brattberg and Wickmann 1992; Salminen et al. 1993).

K.E. Halliday, FRCR, MD, Consultant Paediatric Radiologist, Queen's Medical Centre, Nottingham NG7 2UH, UK
J.M. Somers, FRCR, MD, Consultant Paediatric Radiologist, Nottingham City Hospital, Hucknall Rd, Nottingham NG5 1PB, UK

Children with persistent or severe pain are seen infrequently, accounting for only 2% of non-trauma referrals to an orthopaedic clinic (Turner et al. 1989). These children must, however, be taken seriously since of those who do present to a specialist, up to 90% have objective problems and around 50% have serious spinal disease (Turner et al. 1989; Hensinger 1995).

While it is vital that those children with persistent and severe pain are identified and investigated thoroughly, it is equally important that children are not irradiated unnecessarily. It should be appreciated that radiographs of the lumbar spine constitute a relatively high-dose investigation. Overall, in the British population, lumbar spine films contribute the second highest medical radiation dose after computed tomography (CT) (Nrpb 1992). It is important to avoid exposing the young to unnecessary investigation for episodes of short-lived pain but a balance must be struck between this and not missing lesions requiring treatment.

In this chapter we will review the possible causes of persistent back pain and suggest suitable imaging strategies. In addition spinal trauma in children will be discussed.

7.2
Trauma

Injuries to the spine may result from either accidental or, more rarely, non-accidental trauma. Most spinal injuries occur in motor vehicle pedestrian or cycling accidents, but falls play an increasing role as the child grows older. The greater flexibility of the juvenile spine produces different patterns of injury to those found in adults. Repetitive micro-trauma is a common cause of low back pain in young athletes (Gerbino and Micheli 1995), with some sports having a particularly strong association. In one study the incidence of degenerative changes in the spine on magnetic resonance imaging (MRI) was found to be 9%, 43% and 63% in pre-elite, elite and

Olympic gymnasts respectively (GOLDSTEIN et al. 1991). Spondylolysis and Scheuermann's disease are both thought to be caused by repetitive microtrauma.

7.2.1
Spinal Trauma

The initial radiographic survey in children admitted with a history of trauma is a lateral cervical spine to try and include a view of the C7/T1 disc, a chest x-ray and an abdomen x-ray, to include the pelvis. The cervical collar is not removed until the x-ray is declared normal and the neurological evaluation is also normal. In less violent trauma, anteroposterior (AP) and lateral views of the region of the trauma are taken.

7.2.1.1
Lumbar Spine

Lumbar spine injuries are usually hyperflexion/extension injuries. Lateral flexion may result in avulsion of a transverse process. The simplest injury is a stable compression wedge fracture. With increasing levels of trauma, fracture dislocation and burst fractures occur, and with these there is a high incidence of associated organ injury. The spinal cord ends at the lower border of T12; the cord itself therefore usually escapes injury but there may be damage to the cauda equina or filum terminale. The initial radiographs in suspected lumbar spine trauma should be an AP and lateral view. Review of the radiographs should include noting normal height of vertebral bodies and disc spaces, normal facetal and spinous process alignment and intact transverse processes. A fragment of bone projected over the spinal canal on the lateral view is indicative of a posterior limbus fracture, an injury that usually occurs following sudden exertion.

Simple wedge fractures are infrequently associated with other organ injury. They often occur from falls from heights. Plain radiographs may underestimate the number of vertebrae involved. MRI or scintigraphy will often reveal more but does not alter clinical management.

All other fractures should be assessed by CT, with MRI added if there is suspicion of cauda equina or filum terminale damage. CT should be tailored to show the spine. A general abdominal survey is inadequate to delineate spinal fractures properly (GLASS et al. 1994). Long-term orthopaedic complications of

lumbar spine injury include kyphosis and growth failure secondary to vertebral endplate damage.

Young passengers secured with lap belts have an increased risk of lumbar spine injury than those in three point diagonal belts. These injuries are often accompanied by severe abdominal injury and may be associated with paraplegia. Lap belts are designed to be strapped over the pelvis. In adults, they are prevented from rising up by the anterior superior iliac spine and abrupt deceleration forces are dissipated by rotation at the hip joint and absorbed by the belt and the pelvis. In children, however, the belt often lies over the abdomen at the waist unless the child is raised up on a booster seat. Even if the belt and passenger are correctly positioned, the small juvenile anterior superior iliac spine means that the belt slips up on impact and the child "submarines" below the belt. With sudden deceleration the abdomen absorbs the force and there is hyperflexion of the lumbar spine. The relatively heavy heads of children exacerbate this situation (JOHNSON and FALCI 1990).

Injury typically occurs at L1 and L2 and involves a transverse fracture with or without dislocation of the posterior spinal elements. (Fig. 7.1). Chance fracture is a transverse fracture through the spinous process while a Smith's fracture is through the posterior part of the vertebral body. Posterior distraction may or may not be accompanied by an anterior compression fracture. These fractures may be visible on AP and lateral radiographs, but thin-section CT with sagittal and coronal reconstruction allows a more accurate assessment of the injury. In particular bony fragments within the spinal canal are identified more reliably.

Spondylolysis. Acute spondylolysis (fracture of the pars interarticularis) can occur as a result of a single episode of violent hyperextension (GERBINO and MICHEL 1995; vide infra).

7.2.1.2
Thoracic Spine

Wedge fractures of the thoracic spine may occur after falls from a height and are the most frequent thoracic spine injury (Fig. 7.2). Long-term sequelae are few, but there may be a resultant kyphosis. Radiographs may show displacement of the paraspinal lines due to haematoma on the AP view. Some wedging of thoracic vertebrae is a normal finding in children aged 6 years and above and may cause confusion in the context of trauma. If there is diagnostic

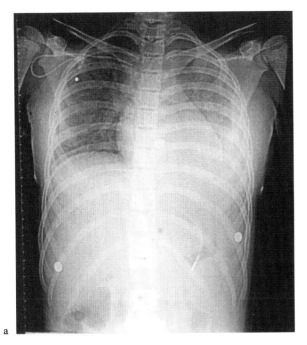

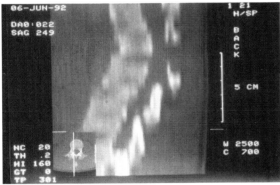

Fig. 7.1. a Fifteen-year-old girl with fracture subluxation at L1/2. Note the widened disc space. b Sagittal CT reconstruction showing disruption of the spinous processes, angular kyphosis and subluxing vertebrae

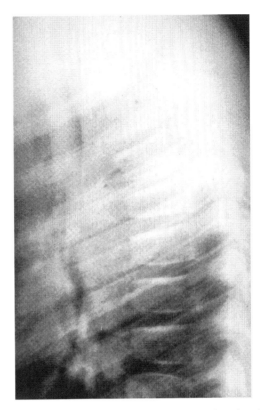

Fig. 7.2. Lateral radiograph of the thoracic spine showing multiple vertebral compression fractures

7.2.1.3
Cervical Spine

The cervical spine in children differs from that in adults in that it is much more flexible and facets are more horizontal. The fulcrum below the age of 8 years lies at C2/3. Most movement occurs at C2/3 and C3/4 rather than at C5/6, as it does in the adult. These features affect the frequency and pattern of injury as well as the appearance of normal films. Loss of cervical lordosis is quite normal in children. Forward displacement of C2 on C3 and less commonly C3 on C4 with flexion (pseudosubluxation) is also normal and can be differentiated from significant injury because the spinolaminar line remains intact and the facets retain their normal relationship (Figs. 7.3, 7.4). Increased flexibility also allows a greater atlanto-dental interval in children, which may be up to 5 mm.

A further pitfall in children is widening of the prevertebral space if the neck is x-rayed in flexion, which may simulate prevertebral bleeding. A repeat radiograph with the head in extension eliminates this.

The normal ring apophysis in the immature vertebra must not be mistaken for an avulsion fracture.

doubt a bone scan will identify acute fractures. CT will show the full extent of the lesion and MRI may be required to identify the extent of cord damage. Dislocations of the thoracic spine are very unusual because of the splinting effect of the ribs. Similarly, burst fractures are uncommon as the normal thoracic kyphosis prevents vertical compression. Injury at the upper thoracic level is serious, resulting in neurological damage, and may be associated with injury to the great vessels.

Spinal cord injury without radiological abnormality (SCIWORA) may occur in the upper thoracic region; this is discussed in more depth in the section on the cervical spine.

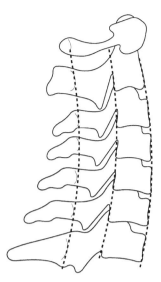

Fig. 7.3. Diagram of normal lateral cervical spine radiograph. A continuous smooth line can be drawn along the anterior and posterior borders of the vertebral bodies and along the spinolaminar junction

Cervical spine fractures are very uncommon in children, accounting for only 2% of all spinal injuries (EVANS and BETHEM 1989; RENTON 1994b). In a recent audit of over 250 cervical spine examinations in children under 10 years old presenting to the Accident and Emergency Department with a history of trauma in Nottingham, no significant injury was identified. In addition 33% of lateral films and 34% of peg views were technically inadequate or had to be repeated, reflecting how difficult it is to obtain these radiographs in agitated youngsters. It is not necessary to image the cervical spine in children unless there is a history of severe trauma and in this setting a lateral view alone will suffice. These patients often have other serious injuries, particularly head injuries. If it is difficult to obtain a good lateral view of the cervical spine by conventional means it may be possible to perform a lateral scanogram of the neck during the course of a cranial CT. If abnormalities are identified on the lateral view, accurate delineation of the injured area should be undertaken with axial CT.

Anteroposterior views are useful in the lower cervical spine in older children when jumped facets become more frequent. Most serious injuries at the lower cervical and upper thoracic spine are visible on the AP view, when loss of alignment of the facets or spinous processes is visible. Open mouth views of the odontoid peg are difficult and are not routinely indicated.

When fractures do occur, they are mainly in the atlas and axis, which are uncommon sites for adult injury. Atlanto-occipital dislocation is usually fatal and in most cases is associated with severe brain injury. There is usually massive widening of the prevertebral soft tissues, and displacement forward of nasogastric tube if one is in place. With this injury, children usually have a cardiorespiratory arrest at the accident site. An injury exclusive to children is the odontoid synchondrotic slip, which occurs at the synchondrosis between the ossification centre for the body of C2 and that for the odontoid peg (CONNOLLY et al. 1995) (Fig. 7.5). This injury is frequently fatal and usually accompanied by other very severe injuries, but conversely, due to the width of the canal at this level some children escape without neurological deficit.

The extreme flexibility of the spine can sometimes allow the spinal cord to be damaged without bony injury, the so-called spinal cord injury without radiographic abnormality (SCIWORA) (Fig. 7.6), which is said to account for up to 5% of paraplegia in childhood (OSENBACH and MENEZES 1982). SCIWORA by definition has normal radiographs and MRI is required to demonstrate the cord injury (OENBACH and MENEZES 1982; PANG and WILBERGER 1982). The presence of a SCIWORA lesion is clinically suspected because of paraplegia but this can be missed initially in an unconscious child.

The paediatric cervical spine matures at around 8 years of age, after which it responds to trauma in a more adult fashion, with an increased incidence of fractures in the lower cervical vertebrae. These include flexion and extension fractures, with compression injury, and as the child approaches adulthood, facetal dislocations. The principles of stable and unstable injuries that apply in adult practice now apply.

Torticollis. Children frequently present to Accident and Emergency with torticollis. Usually this is due to muscular strain and resolves within a week with conservative management. Other causes of acquired torticollis include inflammatory or neoplastic neck masses, paroxysmal torticollis of infancy, gastro-oesophageal reflux and posterior fossa tumours (TOM et al. 1991; BRATT and MENELAUS 1992; MAHESHWARAN et al. 1995). Most frequently, however, it is due to minor trauma. Plain radiographs are difficult to interpret because of rotation. Horizontal beam, shoot through and lateral radiographs with tube angulation to overcome the rotation are sometimes helpful, but unless there is a history of serious trauma, or positive neurology, they are not indicated. CT is preferable to multiple poor radiographs. Most post-traumatic torticollis resolves within a

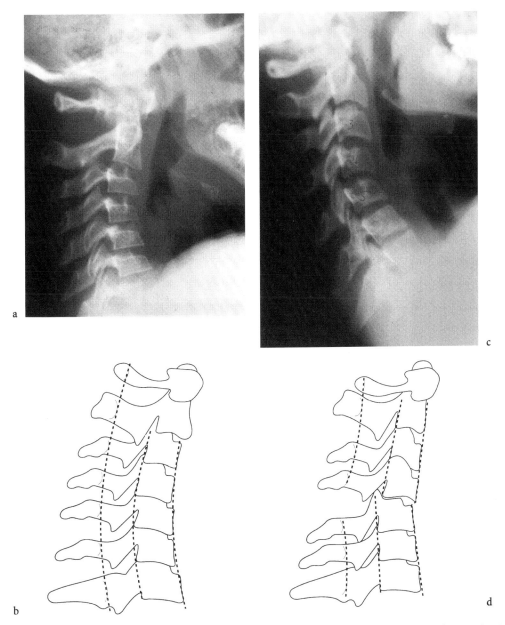

Fig. 7.4. a Pseudosubluxation seen on a lateral view taken in flexion **b** Diagram of pseudosubluxation, the spinolaminar line remains intact. **c** Dislocation at C4/5; all lines are broken and the interspinous distance is increased. **d** Diagram of **c**

week with conservative management. If the condition persists, a diagnosis of rotary subluxation should be considered.

Atlanto-axial Rotary Fixation. Rotary subluxation or fixation of the atlanto-axial joint also presents with torticollis. This may be traumatic or due to local inflammation following infection or surgery (Grisel's syndrome); it may also be the first presentation of juvenile chronic arthritis. Atlanto-axial rotary fixation has been classified into five types according

to the degree and direction of displacement of the atlas. The exact aetiology is unknown, but it may be related to a capsular tear at the atlanto-axial joint. Very rarely it may be associated with occipital-atlanto rotary fixation. It is commoner in children than adults (MAHESHWARAN et al. 1995). The condition may be difficult to diagnose with plain radiography, particularly in those cases without displacement of the atlas in the antero-posterior plane. An open mouth peg view will show displacement of the odontoid peg relative to the lateral masses of C2

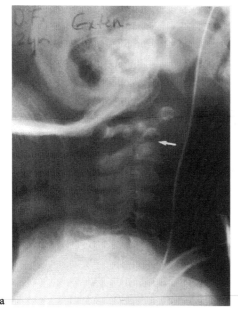
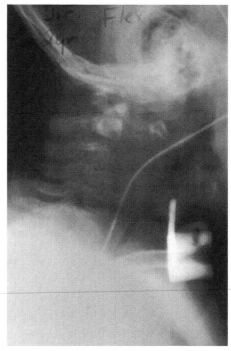

Fig. 7.5. a Lateral view of the cervical spine in this 2-year-old shows a fracture through the odontoid synchondrosis (*arrow*). Note that the child has a tracheostomy due to associated neurological injury. **b** Flexion view shows marked anterior subluxation of the atlas

but it may be difficult to obtain. CT or MRI is therefore the investigation of choice. MRI has the advantage of demonstrating associated injury to the transverse and alar ligaments and compression of the thecal sac, but may be difficult in young children (Tom et al. 1991; Maheshwaran et al. 1995). Scans should be performed with the head rotated in either direction; if the abnormal relationship between the atlas and the axis is maintained, the diagnosis is confirmed (Fig. 7.7). This condition requires more aggressive treatment than transient post-traumatic torticollis, and orthopaedic referral is indicated.

7.2.2
Non-Accidental Injury

Compression fractures of the vertebral bodies of the lower thoracic and upper lumbar spine are not uncommon in victims of child abuse. Avulsion fractures of the spinous processes are highly specific for child abuse but are rare. Cervical spine fractures have also been described (Rooks et al. 1998). Such fractures result from hyperflexion and hyperextension associated with violent shaking (Nimkin and Kleinman 1997). There may be associated rib and

metaphyseal fractures or intracranial injury. In cases where there is doubt, delayed films and scintigraphy may be helpful.

7.2.3
Fatigue Fractures

Fatigue fractures, also known as stress fractures, occur through normal bone and are the result of repetitive micro-trauma. They are not unusual in the spines of young people. The lumbar spine is commonly affected but fractures may also occur in the sacrum (Haasbeek and Green 1994). Spondylolysis is the name given to a fatigue fracture of the pars interarticularis. If bilateral, anterior subluxation of the vertebral body on the vertebra below (spondylolisthesis) may occur. A genetic predisposition is recognised, a family history being associated with an increased risk of developing the condition. It is three times more frequent in Caucasians than Afro-Caribbeans and occurs in up to 50% of Inuit (Stewart 1953). The condition occurs most frequently in boys and it may occur in children with normal spinal anatomy. Congenital spinal anomalies, such as asymmetric development of the facets

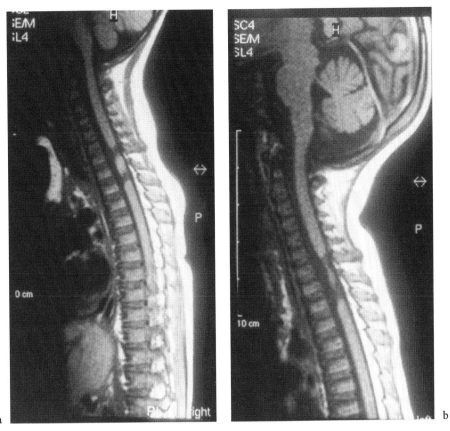

Fig. 7.6. a,b. SCIWORA injury: The radiographs were normal but the child, aged 2 years, was paraplegic. T1-weighted MR images **a** 1 month after injury and **b** 6 months later. Note cord disruption at two levels and subsequent atrophy

and transitional vertebrae (GERBINO and MICHELI 1995; PAYNE and OGILVIE 1996), may increase susceptibility to spondylolysis . Typically spondylolysis involves the fifth lumbar vertebra, but may also occur at the fourth and rarely higher levels.

Spondylolysis is rare before the age of 5 years and then gradually increases in frequency to the age of 20, when it reaches adult prevalence (5%) (HENSINGER 1995). The lesion is thought to be due to repetitive hyperextension of the immature spine. The pars interarticularis is the weakest part of the vertebra and is relatively thin in young people (HENSINGER 1995). Repeated hyperextension, such as occurs during fast bowling or "back walk-overs" in gymnastics, results in a shearing stress across the pars which can result in stress fracturing. In support of this theory, the incidence of the condition is highest amongst gymnasts, cricketers, ballet dancers, figure skaters, tennis and volley-ball players (GERBINO and MICHELI 1995; HENSINGER 1995).

Spondylolysis and spondylolisthesis are often asymptomatic, but if pain does develop, it usually oc-

curs during the adolescent growth spurt and typically radiates to the back of the thighs.

Plain films demonstrate lucency within the pars interarticularis on an AP view. Acute lesions are, in general, narrow with irregular edges, whereas smooth rounded edges to the defect suggest chronicity (HENSINGER 1995; PAYNE and OGILVIE 1996). Spondylolisthesis is best demonstrated on the lateral view and is graded 1–4 according to the degree of slippage (Fig. 7.8). Oblique views demonstrate up to 20% more defects than can be seen on the AP film but are not necessary if the lesion is visible on the standard frontal and lateral views. In these circumstances oblique views do not add further information. Therefore, in a suspected case of spondylolysis oblique films should only be requested following review of the AP and lateral films by a radiologist or orthopaedic surgeon. The high radiation dose and relatively insensitivity of these views should preclude their routine use in children with back pain. Similarly, coned views of the lumbar-sacral junction increase patient dose without an improvement in the diagnostic yield and should not be performed rou-

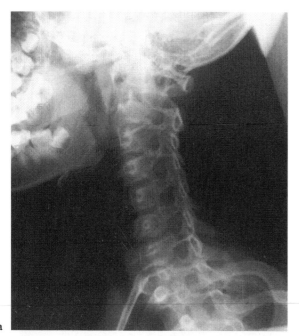

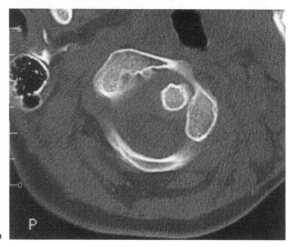

Fig. 7.7. a Atlanto-axial rotary subluxation. On this oblique view of the cervical spine the atlas is seen to lie in a true lateral position while the other cervical vertebrae are oblique. This is due to rotation at the atlanto-axial joint. **b** CT confirms the rotation. The relationship of C1 and C2 was maintained with the head rotated in both directions

tinely. Both plain films and planar bone scans are insensitive to unilateral spondylolysis, which occurs in 20%–25% of cases (HENSINGER 1995). Single-photon emission tomography (SPET) detects significantly more lesions than planar scintigraphy (GERBINO and MICHELI 1995; HENSINGER 1995; MANDELL and HARCKE 1993; BELLAH et al. 1991; COLLIER et al. 1985; READ 1994; KRISS; et al. 1996) and is now the investigation of choice following plain radiography when spondylolysis is suspected, par-

ticularly if the duration of symptoms is less than 1 year (HARVEY et al. 1998) (Fig. 7.9).

Computed tomography defines spondylolysis and provides more accurate anatomical information than MRI (HELMS 1995) (Fig. 7.9). SPET is also of value since it demonstrates osteoblastic activity in the pars region. This helps to differentiate between an actively healing lesion and a chronic non-union of the pars, which may be of assistance when choosing between operative and non-operative therapy. Furthermore, SPET can be used to assess the response to treatment (HENSINGER 1995). Pre-spondylotic stress reactions in the pars may be seen with SPET and MRI; on the later the pars appears hypo-intense on T1-weighted images (YAMANE et al. 1993).

7.2.4
Disc Degeneration and Herniation

Magnetic resonance imaging evidence of disc degeneration is not uncommon in late adolescence but symptomatic disc degeneration is less frequent. Degenerative changes, as evidenced by reduced disc hydration, are seen on MRI in almost 40% of 15 year olds with low back pain and more than 25% of asymptomatic controls. Disc herniation is less common than in adults, but 1%–4% of disc herniations occur in adolescents and may be seen in children as young as 12 years (Fig. 7.10). Disc herniation is very rare before puberty (AFSHANI and KUHN 1991; HENSINGER 1995; PAYNE and OGILVIE 1996). There may be a familial predisposition (VARLOTTA et al. 1997), but repetitive micro-trauma from intense sporting activity is usually the cause of disc disease. Gymnasts are at the greatest risk of disc degeneration, whilst those playing contact sports are at increased risk of herniation (GERBINO and MICHELI 1995). Herniation of the nucleus pulposus tends to be larger than in adults (AFSHANI and KUHN 1991). In spite of this, the usual clinical presentation is with back pain without radiation. Sciatica and sensory and deep tendon reflex changes are uncommon (SALMINEN et al. 1992; AFSHANI and KUHN 1991; HENSINGER 1995; PAYNE and OGILVIE 1996). Disc herniation is important to identify, since the results of surgery are good (DELUCA et al. 1994; EBERSOLD et al. 1987; SHILLITO 1996). AP and lateral radiographs are usually normal and MRI is the investigation of choice.

Disc disease may be associated with lesions of the vertebral endplate, both anteriorly and posteriorly, and displacement of small bony fragments into the spinal canal. These changes may occasionally be

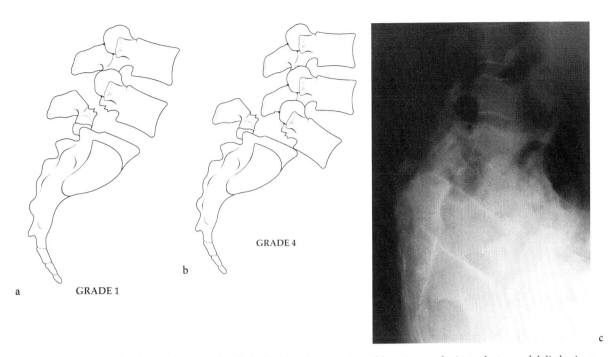

Fig. 7.8. a Diagram showing grade 1 spondylolisthesis. **b** Further anterior subluxation results in grade 4 spondylolisthesis. **c** Radiograph of grade 4 spondylolisthesis

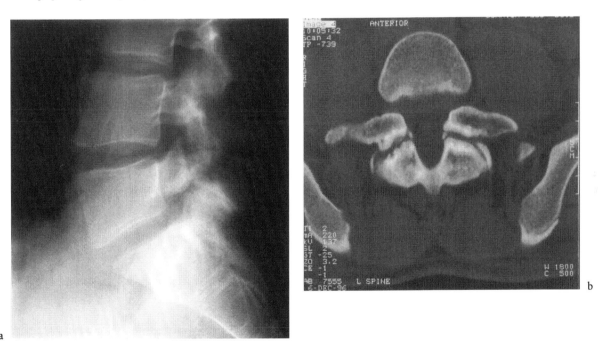

Fig. 7.9. a There is a defect in the pars interarticularis of L5. **b** CT confirms that the defect is bilateral. **c** SPET in another patient shows unilateral increased uptake due to an active lesion in the right pars interarticularis

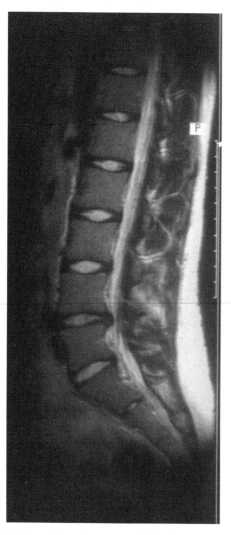

Fig. 7.10. Acute disc prolapse at L4/5. Plain films were normal

seen on lateral radiographs, CT and MRI and typically occur at the inferior margin of L4. There has been dispute as to the origin of this lesion, which appears to be associated with repetitive strain and may represent slipping of the vertebral apophysis, herniation of the nucleus pulposus into the inferior margin of the vertebra or an osteochondritis of the endplate (HENSINGER 1995; IKATA et al. 1995). Acute herniation of the nucleus pulposus may occur rarely in young athletes (GERBINO and MICHELI 1995).

7.2.5
Scheuermann's Disease

Scheuermann's disease is a radiographic diagnosis which results from underlying disc degeneration but is often described as an independent entity. This is a

common condition affecting 31% of male patients and 21% of female patients with back pain (AFSHANI and KUHN 1991). Two forms are described. The commoner thoracic form is not usually associated with pain but results in kyphosis. The diagnosis may be made incidentally on thoracic spine radiographs, for example in an Accident and Emergency Department, in which case the disease may not be the cause of back pain. The diagnosis is made on the lateral radiographs and is defined as a thoracic kyphosis greater than 45° where at least three consecutive thoracic vertebrae are wedged by 5° or more. Associated Schmorl's nodes (herniation of the intervertebral disc into the vertebral end plate, giving rise to a small central well-defined defect) and disc space narrowing occur frequently and are demonstrated well on radiographs. A degree of vertebral wedging may also be seen normally in children. These features, in the absence of kyphosis, are not diagnostic (HENSINGER 1995). Standing films are preferable because they accentuate the kyphotic deformity. The less common lumbar form may be associated with pain. The radiographic findings are similar, but it occurs at the thoraco-lumbar junction and involves fewer vertebrae.

Scheuermann's disease is believed to be caused by excessive and repetitive loading on the immature spine such as occurs in young weight-lifters or gymnasts. Individuals with "straighter" spines, i.e. those with lumbar hypolordosis and thoracic hypokyphosis, are at increased risk (GERBINO and MICHELI 1995).

Once the diagnosis of Scheuermann's disease has been made and is deemed the cause of pain, further investigation is seldom necessary. Bone scintigraphy, performed to eliminate other causes of back pain, may show increased uptake on delayed images and SPET may show subtle, diffuse, accumulations of tracer. Uptake is much less marked than in infection or trauma (MANDELL and HARCKE 1993). Scheuermann's disease is also well demonstrated on MRI, with reduced disc height and hydration. Other changes such as Schmorl's nodes are also seen on MRI. The condition is usually self-limiting and vertebral changes heal slowly during the remaining growth period. However, Schmorl's nodes and disc space narrowing may persist (HENSINGER 1995).

An increased incidence of spondylolysis (up to 50%) has been reported in patients with Scheuermann's disease (HENSINGER 1995; PAYNE and OGILVIE 1996). This may be due to kyphosis causing a compensatory increase in lumbar lordosis, resulting in hyperextension strain at the pars interarticularis.

7.3
Inflammatory Lesions

7.3.1
Discitis

Childhood discitis is a low-grade infective condition generally agreed to be due to staphylococcal infection (CRAWFORD et al. 1991; RENTON 1994). The incidence is highest in infants and young children between the ages of 6 months and 4 years. A second peak occurs between 10 and 14 years. Many patients have a history of a recent febrile illness and in the older age group up to 20% give a history of recent trauma (RENTON 1994). Back pain is the presenting feature in older children. In young children postural alteration and difficulty weight bearing (CRAWFORD et al. 1991) may be presenting features. Symptoms are often poorly localised and clinical diagnosis is difficult. Children frequently undergo multiple investigations for hip irritability and abdominal pain. Systemic evidence of infection may be minimal. The erythrocyte sedimentation rate (ESR) is usually raised but the white cell count and temperature are often normal. Cultures of blood and aspirated material are often negative (HENSINGER 1995).

Plain film changes occur relatively late in the course of the condition, with the earliest signs of disc space narrowing and endplate irregularity occurring 2–4 weeks after the onset of symptoms (Fig. 7.11). This is most easily seen on the lateral films. However, when a supine abdominal radiograph is performed to investigate abdominal pain, the disc spaces should be routinely scrutinised. Scintigraphic abnormality occurs several weeks before radiographic abnormality, with increased uptake in the whole vertebral body rather than just the endplate. Planar bone scans may be normal in as many as 25% of cases (CRAWFORD et al. 1991). SPET may be positive in these cases and this, combined with the pinhole collimation technique, can be useful in determining the exact distribution of activity (BELLAH et al. 1991). MRI is sensitive and accurately defines the site of the lesion. There is loss of disc height with increased signal in the adjacent vertebral bodies on T2-weighted images (Fig. 7.11). Gadolinium

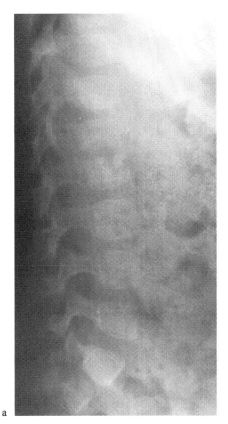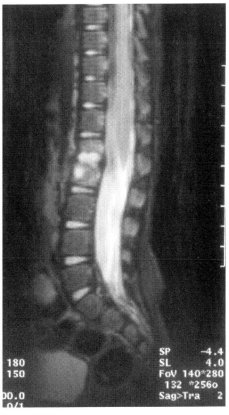

a   d

Fig. 7.11 a,b. Discitis. **a** There is erosion of adjacent endplates at L1/2 and loss of disc height. **b** Sagittal T2-weighted spin-echo sequence demonstrates high signal within the L1/2 disc space extending into the adjacent vertebral bodies. There is no epidural extension

enhancement may demonstrate discrete abscess formation. Increased signal within the disc itself, which is characteristic of adult discitis, is not always seen in children (CRAWFORD et al. 1991; SZALAY et al. 1987).

During the healing phase, sclerosis of endplates is seen radiographically. The disc space narrowing frequently persists and occasionally there is adjacent vertebral enlargement (CRAWFORD et al. 1991).

Juvenile calcific discitis is a rare condition seen most commonly in the cervical spine, though it can occur in the thoracic and lumbar regions. It is commoner in boys, usually occurring around the age of 7 years. There may be fever and raised ESR (HENSINGER 1995). It is a self-limiting inflammatory condition in which calcification occurs in the intervertebral disc without any metabolic abnormality (RENTON 1994a). Plain films show calcification confined to the nucleus pulposus that resolves spontaneously (HENSINGER 1986).

7.3.2
Connective Tissue Disorders

Juvenile rheumatoid arthritis (JRA) and ankylosing spondylitis (AS) may present with back pain. Both conditions may be associated with uveitis, and sacro-iliitis may be seen in AS. The sacro-iliac joints appear very irregular on radiographs before skeletal maturity and the diagnosis of sacro-iliitis depends on other modalities. CT shows subchondral sclerosis, loss of joint space, osseous erosions and ankylosis. Nevertheless, currently MRI is the modality of choice for the diagnosis of sacro-iliitis: it is more sensitive than CT, does not involve ionising radiation and allows images to be obtained in the coronal plane. Cartilage loss and erosions are well shown on T1-weighted images. T2-weighted images show areas of increased signal intensity in the synovial compartment of the joint (MURPHY et al. 1991). Scintigraphy is rarely indicated since it is difficult to interpret owing to the normally increased uptake in this region in young people.

In many cases the diagnosis of JRA and AS rests on clinical features and serology. Rheumatoid factor is less commonly positive in JRA than in adult rheumatoid arthritis, but anti-nuclear factor is positive in 50% of cases. The HLA B27 gene marker is found in 94% of those with AS (GERBINO and MICHELI 1995).

7.3.3
Osteomyelitis

Osteomyelitis is seen predominantly in the first decade. Children present with pain and stiffness and there may be tenderness over the spine. Infection of the vertebra initially involves the disc and early radiographic and scintigraphic findings are similar to discitis. Only one vertebra is usually involved, unlike in discitis, where adjacent endplates are affected (MANDELL and HARCKE 1993; RENTON 1994a). The lesion is best seen on CT, where it appears as a central destructive focus in the vertebral body. The earliest plain film features are a lucent defect above the growth plate. Paravertebral abscess formation is uncommon except in tuberculosis. It is important to distinguish between discitis and osteomyelitis because the course of the former is usually benign, with complete resolution of pain whatever the treatment (CRAWFORD et al. 1991), whilst osteomyelitis is far more destructive. Spinal deformity (most commonly kyphosis) may result. Ankylosis also occurs and can be followed by hypoplasia of the vertebrae. Premature degeneration is seen in adult life (RENTON 1994a). MRI is particularly useful to assess spinal cord involvement. Epidural and extradural abscess formation is well seen with gadolinium enhancement.

The incidence of tuberculosis (TB) is once again increasing worldwide (STOKER 1994) and is an important diagnosis to consider, particularly in patients from TB endemic areas. Tuberculous disease may involve several levels (RENTON 1994a); the disc is normally spared and a soft tissue mass is frequently present (Fig. 7.12). Late effects of childhood infection include bony fusion and a progressive kyphosis or gibus deformity; these may result in respiratory compromise or paraplegia (RENTON 1994a).

7.4
Neoplasms

7.4.1
Intraspinal Lesions

Intraspinal lesions should be considered in children less than 4 years old. Children may present with pain, gait abnormalities or bladder dysfunction. Ependymoma is the commonest intramedullary tumour (AFSHANI and KUHN 1991). It usually occurs distally in the region of the conus, filum terminale or cauda equina (AFSHANI and KUHN 1991). Malignant astrocytomas also occur. Benign tumours such

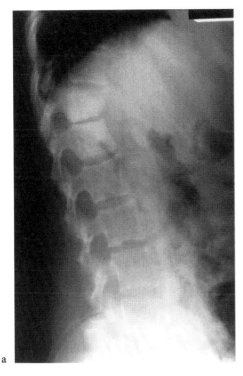

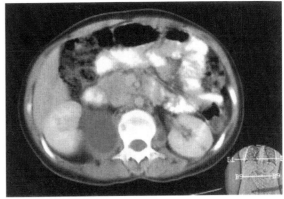

Fig. 7.12 a,b. Tuberculous osteomyelitis. a There is sclerosis in the vertebral bodies of T12 and L1 with erosion of the endplates and a developing kyphosis. b CT through L1 shows sclerosis of the vertebral body and bilateral paravertebral tuberculous abscesses

as dermoids and neurofibromata may give rise to pain and non-neoplastic lesions such as diastematomyelia and syringomyelia should be considered. Neurological signs are usually present and often precede the onset of pain.

Plain films may show interpedicular widening, pedicle erosion or a bony spur. On the lateral film there may be scalloping of the posterior aspect of the vertebral bodies. In infants, where the posterior spinal elements are not yet ossified, ultrasound can be very useful to examine spinal contents and can be used to identify tethering of the cord, spinal dysraphism and intraspinal tumours. Following laminectomy, ultrasound may also be used for follow-up of spinal tumours in older children (SEIGEL and MCALISTER 1995). MRI is, however, the investigation of choice in the older child with a suspected intraspinal lesion.

7.4.2
Neoplasms of Bone

7.4.2.1
Benign Neoplasms

Osteoid osteoma is a benign tumour of bone arising between the ages of 5 and 24 years; 10% occur in the spine, usually in the pedicles or posterior elements. It comprises a central area of highly vascular osteoid tissue (the nidus), with surrounding bony sclerosis. The lesion classically presents with a painful scoliosis. The pain typically occurs at night and may be dramatically relieved by aspirin; however, since this drug is no longer used in children this feature is not often noted.

If visible at all on plain films, osteoid osteomas present as a well-defined sclerotic region in the vertebral appendages. The lucent nidus may be visible (Fig. 7.13). The whole lesion is usually less than a centimetre in diameter. If the diagnosis is suspected, a bone scintigram should be performed, which will be strongly positive due to intense osteoblastic activity. SPET is not usually necessary. Thin-slice CT, at high resolution, provides the definitive diagnosis, demonstrating a sclerotic area surrounding a small nidus (Figs. 7.13, 7.14). Scintigraphy can be used intra-operatively to identify the lesion and limit resection (MANDELL and HARCKE 1993).

Osteoblastoma has a similar presentation and histology to osteoid osteoma but is larger (2–10 cm in diameter) and more aggressive. In addition it is not usually as painful as osteoid osteoma (AFSHANI and KUHN 1991). The spine is involved in 30%–50% of cases (GITELIS and SCHAJOWICZ 1989; COPLEY and DORMANS 1996). These tumours occur between the

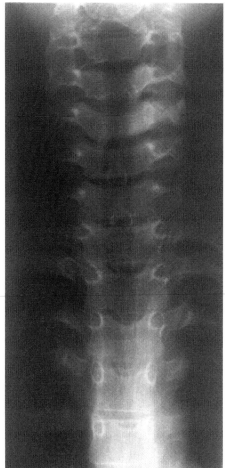

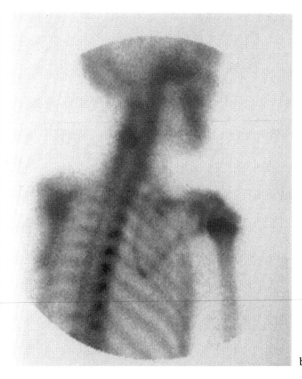

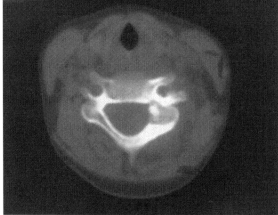

Fig. 7.13. a AP view of the cervical spine shows ill-defined sclerosis in the region of the pedicle and transverse process of C5. b Bone scintigram shows a well-defined area of increased activity corresponding to the area of abnormality on the radiograph. c CT shows a well-defined lucency in the pedicle with a central sclerotic nidus. These features are typical of an osteoid osteoma

ages of 10 and 35 years and, as with osteoid osteoma, there is a male preponderance. Osteoblastoma may rarely metastasise and in the cervical or thoracic regions can give rise to spinal cord compression.

Radiographically these are well-circumscribed lytic lesions, which may be expansile (GITELIS and SCHAJOWICZ 1989). Surrounding sclerosis is much less marked than in osteoid osteoma (COPLEY and DORMANS 1996). CT is useful to delineate bone expansion or destruction but MRI is superior in assessing spinal cord involvement.

Aneurysmal bone cyst occurs in the spine. It is commoner in thoracic or lumbar vertebral bodies or in the sacrum but can occur in the posterior

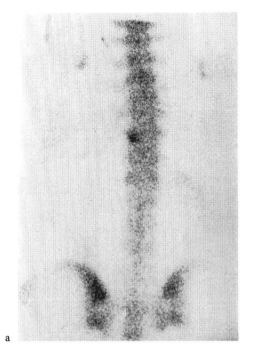

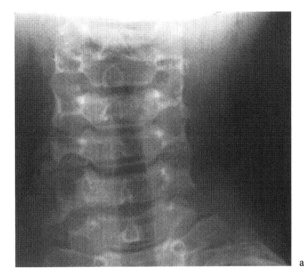

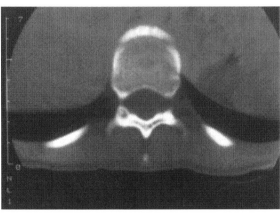

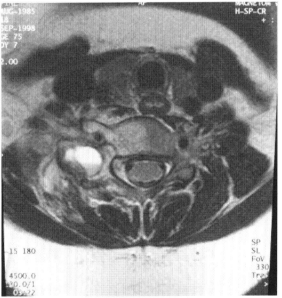

Fig. 7.14. **a** Bone scintigram performed on a teenager with painful scoliosis, in whom plain films were normal. There is a discrete area of increased uptake in the region of the pedicle of T11. **b** CT scan shows a well-defined lucent lesion less than 1 cm with a central sclerotic nidus – an osteoid osteoma

Fig. 7.15. **a** Aneurysmal bone cyst. AP view of the cervical spine shows expansion of the transverse process of C6. **b** MRI of the lesion shows a fluid-fluid level within it. This feature is typical of aneurysmal bone cyst but is not pathognomonic

elements. The tumour may be present for a long time without causing symptoms and often presents with pathological fracture. Radiographs show an eccentrically placed lytic lesion and there may be some collapse, or frank vertebra plana. Typically aneurysmal bone cyst is seen as a doughnut lesion of increased uptake on a bone scan, but this appearance is not specific. The lesions are well demonstrated on CT and MRI and fluid-fluid levels may be seen (AFSHANI and KUHN 1991; TSAI et al. 1990) (Fig. 7.15). Aneurysmal bone cysts recur in 10%–

20% of patients following treatment (BELLAH et al. 1991).

Eosinophilic granulomata involve the spine in 10% of lesions. They are commonest in the thoracic spine and found least frequently in the cervical region. Plain films are more sensitive than bone scans and classically show vertebra plana (Fig. 7.16). In the earlier phase, prior to collapse, there is asymmetrical or minimal loss of height and even vertebral expansion. Bone scintigraphy is positive before the vertebral body collapses but lacks specificity. However,

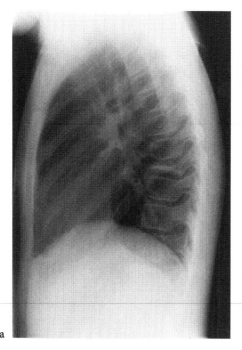
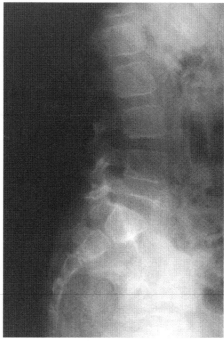

a   b

Fig. 7.16. Vertebra plana at T8 (**a**) and L5 (**b**); both cases are secondary to eosinophilic granuloma

for complete identification of multiple lesions radiographic and scintigraphic skeletal surveys are necessary (MANDELL and HARCKE 1993).

Rare tumour-like conditions that affect the spine include haemangioma and lymphangioma. Most are asymptomatic and solitary but occasionally they may cause pain and cord compression. These conditions have typical plain film findings with expansion of the affected vertebral body or bodies, osteopenia and coarsening with striation or honeycombing of the trabecular pattern. Several adjacent vertebrae may be affected, particularly with lymphangioma, as may the ribs in thoracic lesions. CT demonstrates these plain film findings elegantly and may define a soft tissue or intraspinal element. MRI demonstrates very high signal on T2 and short tau inversion recovery (STIR) sequences and best demonstrates cord involvement (ROSS et al. 1987; LAREDO et al. 1986).

7.4.2.2
Malignant Neoplasms

Primary malignant neoplasms are rare in the spine, the commonest being Ewing's sarcoma (Fig. 7.17), which usually presents between the ages of 5 and 20 years with pain and a mild leucocytosis (GHELMAN

1989). Plain films may demonstrate bone destruction or abnormal bone texture and there may be a soft tissue mass. MRI more accurately demonstrates the extent of the lesion, including marrow involvement. The differential diagnosis includes osteosarcoma (Fig. 7.18) but this tumour occurs more commonly in long bones than the spine (AFSHANI and KUHN 1991).

Leukaemia may present with generalised osteoporosis and multiple collapsed vertebrae. (Fig. 7.19). MRI shows decreased signal on T1-weighted images due to leukaemic infiltration of fatty bone marrow. This is more difficult to appreciate in younger children, who normally have red marrow which has a lower signal than fat. Patchy decrease in marrow signal may persist for many years after successful treatment, which may make follow-up difficult (OJALA et al. 1998).

Primary lymphoma of bone is the third most common primary bone tumour of childhood (AFSHANI and KUHN 1991), and it can involve the spine. Disseminated lymphoma may also be seen in bone. Lesions are lytic or sclerotic. MRI demonstrates bone, bone marrow and soft tissue involvement.

The commonest metastatic bone tumours are neuroblastoma and rhabdomyosarcoma. Up to 70% of patients with neuroblastoma have bony metastases at some time and the spine is the com-

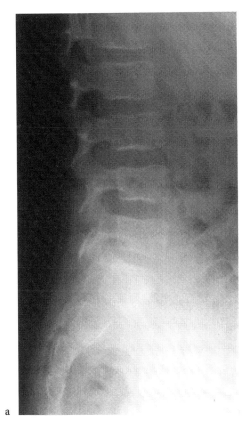

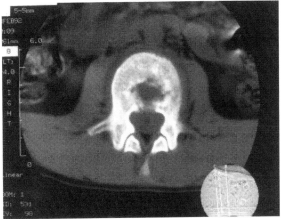

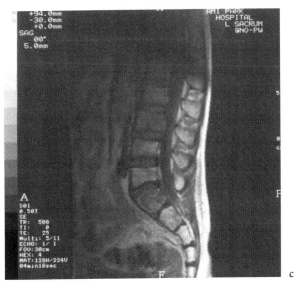

Fig. 7.17. a There is expansion and diffuse sclerosis of the S1 vertebral body. **b** CT shows destruction and sclerosis of the vertebral body with a small soft tissue mass. **c** Sagittal T1-weighted MR scan shows abnormally low signal in the S1 vertebral body. Biopsy revealed Ewing's sarcoma

monest site. Lesions typically resemble those found in the metaphyses, with permeative bone destruction and a variable amount of periosteal reaction. Cortical lesions are detected with technetium-99 m methylene diphosphonate scintigraphy and marrow metastases with iodine-123 metaiodobenzylguanidine (MIBG) scintigraphy. Either or both may be positive in an individual patient and both techniques are recommended for staging. MRI with contrast enhancement is also sensitive for the detection of marrow metastases in the axial skeleton and may occasionally be positive when MIBG scintigraphy is negative.

Between 30% and 70% of children with rhabdomyosarcoma have skeletal metastases. Bone-metastasising renal tumour of childhood, retinoblas-toma and teratocarcinoma are rarer causes of spinal metastases.

7.5
Scoliosis

Scoliosis rarely presents as an emergency but it may be discovered in a child who presents with pain. Back pain from idiopathic or structural scoliosis is rare but may occur after surgery (Gerbino and Micheli 1995; Fabry et al. 1989). Plain radiographs are excellent for assessing the degree of scoliosis and these should be performed standing (Hensinger 1995; Payne and Ogilvie 1996). The typical pattern of an idiopathic scoliosis is a right thoracic left lumbar

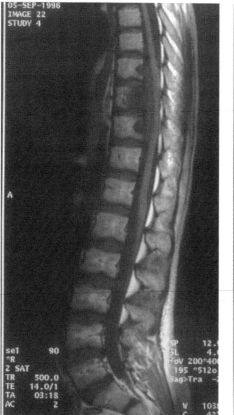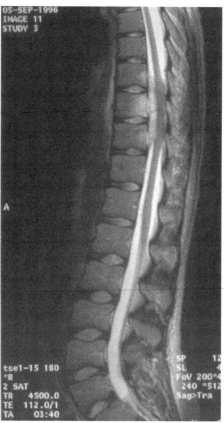

a   b

Fig. 7.18 a,b. A teenager undergoing treatment for osteosarcoma developed back pain. Bone scintigraphy was negative. **a** T1 and **b** T2-weighted sagittal MRI demonstrates metastases within the vertebral bodies of T8–T10 with epidural extension

curve. If there is a different pattern or scoliosis is painful or rapidly progressive, particularly in a boy, then a non-idiopathic aetiology should be sought (HENSINGER 1995). A bone scan is the initial investigation of choice to exclude an occult bony neoplasm. MRI is an alternative or first-line investigation and may be required to assess the spinal cord.

7.6
Extrinsic Lesions

Pain may be referred to the back from other parts of the skeleton such as the hips or sacro-iliac joints. Other extrinsic causes of back pain include renal infection, vesico-ureteric reflux or pelvi-ureteric junction obstruction, retroperitoneal infection, tumour (Fig. 7.20) and pleural disease. Back pain may complicate systemic disease such as sickle cell disease, where pain is due to bone infarction. Children with cystic fibrosis also report an increased

incidence of back pain, which may be due to a chronic flexed posture and kyphosis associated with cough, lung hyperinflation and dyspnoea (ROSE et al. 1987).

7.7
Miscellaneous Conditions

7.7.1
Congential Skeletal Abnormalities

A transitional vertebra forming a pseudarthrosis with the iliac wing or sacrum is uncommon in children but can result in painful degenerative arthritis (GERBINO and MICHELI 1995). These congenital malformations are usually an incidental finding on plain films but in cases where they are thought to be the cause of pain, scintigraphy may be helpful to assess the activity in the area. Localised congenital spinal fusion may also give rise to pain. Spinal stenosis may present with back pain in children or

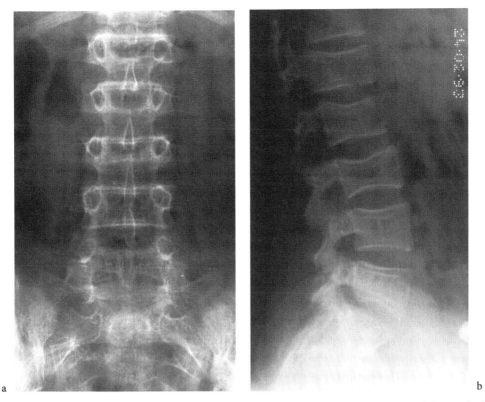

Fig.7.19. a These is generalised osteopenia with coarsening of the trabecular pattern. **b** Loss of height of the vertebral bodies is seen, with biconcavity of the endplates. This patient had leukaemia

give rise to focal neurology from cord compression. Achondroplastic children are particularly prone to spinal canal stenosis.

7.7.2
Osteoporosis

Painful insufficiency fractures are seen in the thoracic and lumbar spine in patients with osteoporosis secondary to treatment with steroids. Patients with idiopathic juvenile osteoporosis often have profound spinal involvement (DIMAR et al. 1995). Further radiological investigation beyond plain radiographs is not usually necessary.

7.7.3
Congenital Torticollis

Pseudotumour of infancy, also known as fibromatosis colli, presents in infants between 2 and 4 weeks of age with a firm, painless mass in the distal sternomastoid muscle. The children are brought to the Accident and

Emergency Department because of parental concern that pain is preventing the baby from turning its head and it is for this reason that it is discussed here. This lesion is also discussed in chap. 11. If untreated, it progresses to fibrosis and congenital muscular torticollis in 20%. This in turn may result in scoliosis, craniofacial asymmetry and occasionally ocular and vestibular abnormalities. Early treatment with physiotherapy has good results, being effective in more than 80% of cases (DAVIDS et al. 1993; CHENG and AU 1994). Torticollis is the third most common congenital musculoskeletal abnormality after congenital dislocation of the hip (CDH) and talipes and is associated with CDH, talipes and breech delivery (PORTER and BLOUT 1995; WHYTE et al. 1989). The condition is more common in boys and on the right side (CHAN et al. 1992). The aetiology is unclear. Causative theories include: venous outflow obstruction (CHAN et al. 1992), ischaemia, muscle rupture with haematoma formation and a perinatal compartment syndrome (DAVIDS et al. 1993). The diagnosis may be confirmed with ultrasound, which demonstrates a focal or diffuse enlargement of the sternomastoid, more commonly in the lower third (CHAN et al. 1992). The

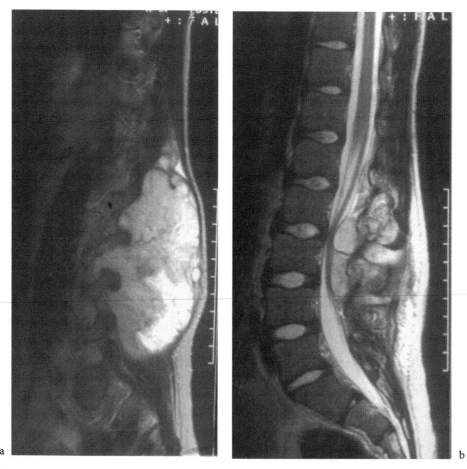

Fig. 7.20 a,b. Primitive neuro-ectodermal tumour arising in the posterior spinal muscles and invading the spinal canal

mass may be homogeneous or heterogeneous, and iso-, hypo-, or hyperechoic relative to normal muscle; it may contain foci of calcification (CHAN et al. 1992) (Fig. 7.21). MRI of established torticollis is not usually indicated but demonstrates low signal on T1- and T2-weighted images, confirming fibrosis (WHYTE et al. 1989).

7.8
Conclusions

Persistent back pain in children is uncommon and has a high likelihood of being associated with a treatable or serious underlying condition. Standing AP and lateral radiographs are the initial films. Coned lumbosacral junction and oblique views are rarely indicated. If pain continues, or there are suspicious features such as pain at night, increasing pain, weight loss, neurological signs, fever or raised

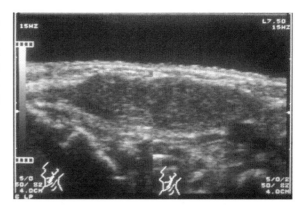

Fig. 7.21. A longitudinal sonogram of the left sternomastoid demonstrates a fusiform swelling of the mid and lower part of the muscle; the swelling is of homogeneous echogenicity. The appearances are typical of a sternomastoid tumour

ESR, further investigation is indicated. The most useful investigations are bone scintigraphy, including SPET scanning, MRI and CT; these should be carefully tailored to answer the clinical question.

References

Afshani E, Kuhn JP (1991) Common causes of low back pain in children. Radiographics 11:269–291

Balague F, Nordin M, Skovron ML, Dutoit G, Yee A, Waldburger M (1994) Non-specific back pain among school children: a field survey analysis of some associated factors. J Spinal Disord 7:374–379

Balague F, Skovron ML, Nordin M, Dutoit G, Waldburger M (1995) Low back pain in schoolchildren. a study of familial and psychological factors. Spine 20:1265–1270

Balague F, Dutoit G, Waldburger M (1988) Low back pain in schoolchildren. An epidemiological study. Scand J Rehabil Med 20:175–179

Bellah RD, Summerville DA, Treves ST, Micheli LJ (1991) Low back pain in adolescent athletes: detection of stress injury to the pars interarticularis with SPECT. Radiology 180:503–507

Bodner RJ, Heyman S, Drummond DS, Gregg JR (1988) The use of single photon emission computed tomography (SPECT) in the diagnosis of low back pain in young patients. Spine 13:1155–1160

Bratt HD, Menelaus MB (1992) Benign paroxysmal torticollis of Infancy. J Bone Joint Surg Br 74:449–451

Brattberg G, Wickman V (1992) Prevalence of back pain and headache in Swedish schoolchildren: a questionnaire survey. Pain Clin 5:211–220

Chan YL, Cheng JCY, Metreweli C (1992) Ultrasonography of congenital muscular torticollis. Pediatr Radiol 22:356–360

Cheng JCY, Au AWY (1994) Infantile torticollis: a review of 624 cases. J Pediatr Orthop 14:802–808

Collier BD, Johnson RP, Carrera GF, et al. (1985) Painful spondylolysis or spondylolisthesis studied by radiography and single-photon emission computed tomography. Radiology 154:207–211

Connolly B, Emery D, Armstrong D (1995) The odontoid synchondrotic slip: an injury unique to young children. Pediatr Radiol 25:s129–s133

Copley L, Dormans JP (1996) Benign pediatric bone tumours. Pediatr Clin North Am 43:949–966

Crawford AH, Kucharzyk DW, Ruda R, Smitherman HC (1991) Diskitis in children. Clin Orthop 266:70–79

Davids JR, Wenger DR, Mubarak SJ (1993) Congenital muscular torticollis: sequela of intrauterine or perinatal compartment syndrome. J Pediatr Orthop 13:141–147

Deluca PF, Mason DE, Weiand R, Howard R, Bassett GS (1994) Excision of herniated nucleus pulposus in children and adolescents. J Pediatr Orthop 14:318–322

Dimar JR, Campbell M, Glassman SD, Puno RM, Johnson JR (1995) Idiopathic juvenile osteoporosis. An unusual cause of back pain in an adolescent. Am J Orthop 24:865–869

Ebersold MJ, Lynn MD, Quast M, Bianco AJ (1987) Results of lumbar discectomy in the pediatric patient. J Neurosurg 67:643–647

Evans DL, Bethem D (1989) Cervical spine injuries in children. J Pediatr Orthop 9:563–568

Fabry G, Van Melkbeek J, Bockx E (1989) Back pain after Harrington rod instrumentation for idiopathic scoliosis. Spine 14:620

Gerbino PG, Micheli LJ (1995) Back injuries in the young athlete. Clin Sports Med 14:571–590

Ghelman B (1989) Radiology of bone tumours. Orthop Clin North Am 20:287–312

Gitelis S, Schajowicz F (1989) Osteoid osteoma and osteoblastoma. Orthop Clin North Am 20:313–325

Glass RBJ, Sivit CJ, Sturm PF, Bulas DI, Eichelberger MR (1994) Lumbar spine injury in a pediatric population: difficulties with computed tomographic diagnosis. J Trauma 37:815–819

Goldstein JD, Berger PE, Windler GE, Jackson DW (1991) Spine injuries in gymnasts and swimmers. An epidemiologic investigation. Am J Sports Med 19:463–468

Haasbeek JF, Green NE (1994) Adolescent stress fractures of the sacrum: two case reports. J Pediatr Orthop 14:336–338

Harvey CJ, Richenberg JL, Saifuddin A, Wolman RL (1998) Pictorial review: the radiological investigation of lumbar spondylolysis. Clin Radiol 53:723–728

Helms CA (1995) Fundamentals of skeletal radiology. Saunders, Philadelphia, p 211

Hensinger RN (1986) Orthopedic problems of the shoulder and neck. Pediatr Clin North Am 33:1495–1509

Hensinger RN (1995) Acute back pain in children. Instr Course Lect 44:111–126

Ikata T, Morita T, Katoh S, Tachibana K, Maoka H (1995) Lesions of the lumbar posterior endplate in children and adolescents an MRI study. J Bone Joint Surg Br 77:951–955

Johnson DL, Falci S (1990) The diagnosis and treatment of pediatric lumbar spine injuries caused by rear seat lap belts. Neurosurgery 26:434–441

Kriss VM, Elgazzar AH, Gelfand MJ, Golsch GJ (1996) High-resolution multi-detector SPET imaging of the pediatric spine. Nucl Med Commun 17:119–124

Laredo JD, Reizine D, Bard M, Merland JJ (1986) Vertebral hemangiomas: radiologic evaluation. Radiology 161:183–189

Maheshwaran S, Sgouros S, Jeyapalan K, Chapman S, Chandy J, Flint G (1995) Imaging of childhood torticollis due to atlanto-axial rotary fixation. Childs Nerv Syst 11:667–671

Mandell GA, Harcke T (1993) Scintigraphy of spinal disorders in adolescents. Skeletal Radiol 22:393–401

Murphy MD, Wetzel LH, Bramble JM, Levine, E, Simpson KM, Lindsley HB (1991) Sacroiliitis: MR imaging findings. Radiology 180:239–244

Nimkin K, Kleinman PK (1997) Imaging of child abuse. Pediatr Clin North Am 44:615–635

NRPB (1992) Protection of the patient in X-ray and computed tomography. London. HMSO

Ojala AE, Paakko E, Lanning FP, Harila-Saari AH, Lanning BM (1998) Bone marrow changes on MRI in children with acute lymphoblastic leukaemia 5 years after treatment. Clin Radiol 53:131–136

Olsen TL, Anderson RL, Dearwater SR, Kriska AM, Cauley JA, Aaron DJ, Laporte RE (1992) The epidemiology of low back pain in an adolescent population. Am J Public Health 82:606–608

Osenbach RK, Menezes AH (1982) Spinal cord injury without radiographic abnormality in children. Pediatr Neurosci 15:168–174

Pang D, Wilberger JE Jr (1982) Spinal cord injury without radiographic abnormalities in children. J Neurosurg 57:114–129

Payne WK, Ogilvie JW (1996) Back pain in children and adolescents. Pediatr Clin North Am 43:899–917

Porter SB, Blount BW (1995) Pseudotumour of infancy and congenital muscular torticollis. Am Fam Phys 52:1731–1736

Read MTF (1994) Single photon emission computed tomography (SPECT) scanning for adolescent back pain. A sine qua non? Br J Sports Med 28:56–57

Renton P (1994a) Infections of bones and joints. In: Carty H, Shaw D, Brunelle F, Kendall B (eds) Imaging children. Churchill Livingstone, London, pp 1203–1259

Renton P (1994b) The musculoskeletal system: trauma. In: Carty H, Shaw D, Brunelle F, Kendall B (eds) Imaging children, 1st edn. Churchill Livingstone, London, pp 1073–1187

Rooks VJ, Sisler C, Burton B (1998) Cervical spine injury in child abuse: report of two cases. Pediatr Radiol 28:193–195

Rose J, Gamble G, Schultz A, Lewiston N (1987) Back pain and spinal deformity in cystic fibrosis. Am J Dis Child 141:1313–1316

Ross JS, Masaryk TJ, Modie MT, Carter JR, Mapstone T, Dengel FH (1987) Vertebral hemangiomas: MR imaging. Radiology 165:165–169

Salminen JJ, Pentti J, Terho P (1992) Low back pain and disability in 14-year-old school children. Acta Paediatr 81:1035–1039

Salminen JJ, Osanken A, Maki P, Pentti J, Kujala UM (1993) Leisure time and physical activity in the young. Int J Sports Med 14:406–410

Seigel MJ, McAlister WH (1995) Musculoskeletal system and spine. In: Seigel MJ (ed) Pediatric sonography, 2nd edn. Raven, New York, pp 513–551

Shillito J (1996) Pediatric lumbar disc surgery: 20 patients under 15 years of age. Surg Neurol 46:14–18

Stewart TD (1953) The age incidence of neural-arch defects in Alaskan natives, considered from the standpoint of etiology. J Bone Joint Surg Am 35:937–950

Stoker N (1994) Tuberculosis in a changing world. BMJ 309:1178–1179

Szalay EA, Green NE, Heller RM, Horev G, Irchner SG (1987) Magnetic resonance imaging in the diagnosis of childhood discitis. J Pediatr Orthop 7:164–167

Tom LWC, Rossiter JL, Sutton LN, Davidson RS, Potsic WP (1991) Torticollis in children. Otolaryngol Head Neck Surg 105:1–5

Tsai JC, Delinka M, Fallon MD, Zlatkin MB, Kressel HY (1990) Fluid-fluid level: a nonspecific finding in tumours of bone and soft tissue. Radiology 175:779–782

Turner PG, Green JH, Galasko CSB (1989) Back pain in childhood. Spine 14:812–814

Varlotta GP, Brown MD, Kelsey JL, Golden AL (1991) Familial predisposition for herniation of a lumbar disc in patients who are less than twenty-one years old. J Bone Joint Surg Am 73:124–128

Whyte AM, Lufkin RB, Bredenkamp J, Hoover L (1989) Sternocleidomastoid fibrosis in congenital muscular torticollis: MR appearance. J Comput Assist Tomogr 13:163–166

Yamane T, Yoshida T, Imatsu K (1993) Early diagnosis of lumbar spondylolysis by MRI. J Bone Joint Surg Br 75:764–768

8 The Child with a Limp

R.E.R. Wright and C.W. Majury

CONTENTS

R.E.R. Wright, FRCR, FFRRCSI, Consultant Radiologist, Ulster Hospital, Upper Newtownards Road, Dundonald, Belfast BT 16 ORH, UK
C. Majury, FRCR, FFRRCSI, Consultant Radiologist, Ulster Hospital, Upper Newtownards Road, Dundonald, Belfast BT16 ORH, UK

8.1 Introduction

Children frequently present to the Accident and Emergency Department unable to weight bear or with a limp. For most the radiological investigation is straightforward, involving plain film radiography of the abnormal area. However, because of the increasing availability of new imaging modalities, the desire to reduce unnecessary radiation exposure and the better understanding of disease processes, there are an increasing number of possible pathways where utilisation of other techniques is appropriate. This chapter seeks to outline the common disease processes which may produce a limp and to draw attention to the rarer but clinically important conditions to look out for. Our preferred diagnostic pathways are given together with a brief explanation of the strengths and limitations of each technique. Attention is drawn to common radiological "traps" which may befall the unwary accident and emergency physician.

Any abnormal gait may be referred to as a limp. Pain may produce a limp, as may structural abnormalities such as limb length discrepancy and angular limb deformity. Good clinical history taking can often identify the cause of the limp such as direct trauma to a localised area or factors suggesting systemic onset, such as fever (RENSHAW 1995). It is important to record the time period over which the limp developed, whether the limp is painful, whether the limp is worse at the beginning of the day (as in juvenile arthritis) or at the end of the day (as with muscle weakness) or whether it is constant (as might be the case with a tumour). One should ask whether the patient or parents can localise the pain. A past history of developmental delay or deterioration in walking should be ascertained (e.g. spinal cord tumour).

The child should be examined in minimal clothing below the waist and should be observed barefoot. The gait is best assessed in an open area rather than a small examination cubicle. The child should be asked to run, hop and walk on toes or heels, which will help to identify less obvious weakness and co-ordination problems. The child's shoe should be inspected for unusual wear patterns. Spinal deformity and pelvic asymmetry should be noted. The site of pain should be localised by palpation initially or by observing the patient's gait in order to select the most appropriate radiographic projections or imaging modality. With a painful limp arising from pathology in the hip, the patient will place the affected limb on the ground and will lean laterally over the hip. This places the hip into abduction, thereby centralising the body's centre of gravity directly over the femoral head and shaft of the femur and distributing the weight in a more diffuse fashion along the entire limb. Characteristically, the child will lean over the hip to take the weight off the limb as quickly as possible (DABNEY and LIPTON 1995).

In a painful limb arising from pathology in the knee, the knee is typically bent, the body leans away from the affected limb, the foot is planted on the ground quickly and weight bearing occurs instantly on and off, shifting the trunk weight onto the normal limb. If the limp is due to foot or ankle pathology, the patient leans the body towards the contralateral extremity, touching the foot and ankle down just briefly, with the weight shifting immediately onto the opposite side.

A working knowledge of the likely pathologies expected within given age groups is important (Table 8.1). Without doubt the most important aetiological factor for limp in children and adolescents is trauma. Between the ages of 1 and 3 years a frequent fracture is through the base of the first metatarsal and less frequently through the necks of the second to fifth metatarsals. Both are easily missed by junior, inexperienced casualty doctors. Fractures of the tibia occur with minimal trauma in this age group and are usually spiral fractures of the tibial shaft or compression fractures of the distal tibia. Limping secondary to non-accidental injury must always enter the differential diagnosis (Fig. 8.1). Osteomyelitis is also less common but must be remembered, especially if there are local signs of heat, tenderness and swelling.

Table 8.1. Common differential diagnoses of limp by age

Toddler (1–3 years)
Developmental dysplasia
Discitis
Genu varum or genu valgum
Congenital leg length discrepancy
Toddler's fracture
Foreign body

Child (4–10 years)
Transient synovitis
Septic arthritis
Legg-Calvé-Perthes disease
Blount disease
Acquired leg length discrepancy (secondary to trauma)

Adolescent
Slipped capital femoral epiphysis
Patellofemoral disorders
Stress fracture
Tarsal coalition
Septic arthritis

Conditions affecting all ages
Osteomyelitis
Tumour

Between the ages of 3 and 10 years, trauma is still the most common cause of limp (Fig. 8.2). Painful limps of hip origin are more commonly seen with transient synovitis of the hip or with Legg-Calve-Perthes disease (Fig. 8.3). Juvenile chronic rheumatoid arthritis is seen in this age group as well as osteomyelitis and occasionally septic arthritis.

After 10 years of age until skeletal maturity is reached, trauma, again, is the most likely cause; however, a host of pain syndromes of adolescence occur, the most important of which is slipped capital femoral epiphysis. Back pain may radiate into the lower extremities with accompanying limp. A good history and clinical examination should localise the abnormality in more than 90% of cases prior to radiography.

There are potentially hundreds of possible causes of limp and many different approaches have been taken in an attempt to classify them. A reasonably comprehensive classification is given in Table 8.2. In practice, however, a classification such as this is cumbersome to the emergency physician faced with a distressed child and probably equally distressed parents. We believe a more pragmatic approach is to classify limp by the likely cause in a given anatomical area. Whilst not quite as comprehensive, in practice this will allow the clinician to focus rapidly onto the site and cause of the presenting symptoms.

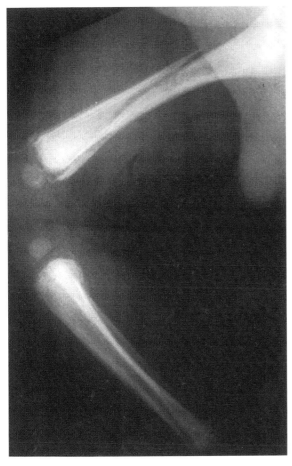

Fig. 8.1. Spiral femoral fracture and metaphyseal fractures due to non-accidental injury

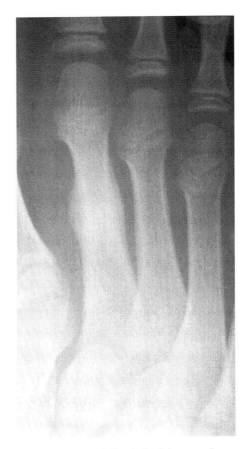

Fig. 8.2. Fracture through the shaft of the second metatarsal demonstrating periosteal reaction

8.2
Imaging Modalities

8.2.1
Plain Film Radiography

Plain film radiography remains the mainstay of radiological investigation and will often be sufficient (BLUMHAGEN 1994). To minimise radiation doses to the patient, care must be taken to select the most appropriate projections; however, radiation dose must be kept in perspective. Carefully taken radiographs using minimal doses compatible with diagnostic images do not constitute a hazard. The radiation risk/benefit ratio must be considered. In our view the advantages of a positive or negative study in confirming or excluding a lesion clearly outweigh any potential hazard associated with radiation.

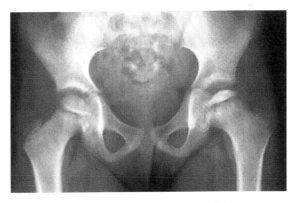

Fig. 8.3. Legg-Calvé-Perthes disease of the left hip

An attempt should be made by the medical officer to localise the most likely site of pain. In this situation a diagram is often worth a thousand words in helping the radiographer to select the most appropriate projection. If there is a history of trauma and a fracture is suspected, the radiograph should cover the whole of the affected bone to ensure that a syn-

Table 8.2. Causes of limp

Painful causes of limp	Non-Painful Causes of limp
A. Trauma	A. Neurological disorders
1. Local superficial lesions	1. Flaccid paralysis
2. Ligamentous strains and sprains	2. Spastic paralysis
3. Tendon disorders	3. Ataxia
4. Muscle bruising	B. Muscle disorders
5. Fractures	1. Muscular dystrophy
6. Non-accidental Injury	2. Arthrogryphosis
7. Patellar subluxation	C. Joint disorders
B. Inflammatory conditions	1. Stiffness or contractures
1. Transient synovitis	2. Instability
2. Acute rheumatic fever	D. Bony disorders
3. Juvenile rheumatoid arthritis	1. Leg length discrepency
4. Systemic lupus erythematosus	2. Slipped capital femoral epiphysis
5. Polyarteritis nodosa	3. Coxa vara
6. Dermatomyositis	4. Blount's disease
7. Henoch-Schönlein purpura	5. Epiphyseal dysplasias
8. Serum sickness	E. Functional states
9. Ulcerative colitis	1. Hysteria
C. Infections	2. Mimicry
1. Osteomyelitis	
2. Septic arthritis	
3. Discitis	
4. Epidural infection	
5. Acute appendicitis	
6. Retroperitoneal masses	
7. Acute iliac adenitis	
8. Mesenteric lymphadenitis	
D. Aseptic necrosis and osteochondritis	
1. Legg-Calvé-Perthes disease	
2. Osgood-Schlatter's disease	
3. Freiberg's disease	
4. Köhler's disease	
5. Sever's disease	
6. Osteochondritis dissecans	
7. Chondromalacia patellae	
8. Sinding-Larsen disease	
E. Neoplasms	
1. Leukemia	
2. Malignant bone tumours	
3. Benign bone tumours	
F. Non-malignant haematological disorders	
1. Haemophilia	
2. Sickle-cell anaemia	
3. Scurvy	
4. Phlebitis	

chronous further fracture or dislocation is not present. Two projections preferably at 90° to each other are always recommended in trauma cases as subtle fractures are often missed on one view alone. It may also be necessary to obtain comparison views of the opposite limb as epiphyseal lines or accessory ossification centres may mimic a fracture. If these are deemed necessary, they must be taken in the same position as the affected limb to enable direct comparison. In order to avoid unnecessary radiation, in the first instance an immediate report should be sought from a radiologist or senior clinician. The practice of requesting radiographs prior to examination is to be deprecated.

Correct positioning of the patient is particularly important to show the soft tissue planes around joints. The radiographic signs of inflammation and joint effusion are subtle and on hip radiographs can only be interpreted when both the pelvis and femora are positioned without rotation. The three fat planes around the hip (psoas, obturator and gluteal) are bowed away from the joint with an effusion but these

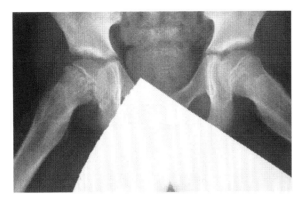

Fig. 8.4. Frog-leg lateral projection demonstrating slipped capital femoral epiphysis. (Note the gonadal radiation protection device)

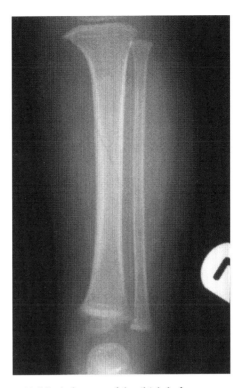

Fig. 8.5. Toddler's fracture of the tibial shaft

fat planes lie outside the muscles and an effusion needs to be very large to displace them (MAJOR and HELMS 1996). The most frequent cause for apparent displacement is a rotated position of the leg or pelvis. Ultrasound of the hip is the most sensitive way to detect an effusion. Frog-leg lateral views of the hip are required when Legg-Calvé-Perthes disease or a slipped capital femoral epiphysis is suspected to show the early changes in outline or the position of the epiphysis (HARCKE and GRISSON 1990; HOWARD et al. 1993; Fig. 8.4).

Radiographs of the spine are obtained if spine pathology is suspected. Special views, such as obliques to show a spondylolysis, may be necessary but should be performed only after discussion with the radiologist. It should be remembered that because of the spine's close proximity to the reproductive organs and its deep location within the body, a good radiograph requires a relatively high radiation dose. The radiation burden must always be remembered but unnecessary fear must not restrict the appropriate use of radiographs. The benefit/risk ratio is overwhelmingly in favour of the x-ray.

Radiographs should ideally be assessed in a darkened room with a proper viewing box and "bright light" with extraneous light covered off. Studying radiographs in a well-lit examination cubicle with many distractions increases the chances of missing abnormalities.

A useful aide memoire is the AABCS system for interpreting images:

A = Adequacy
A = Alignment
B = Bones
C = Cartilage and joints
S = Soft tissues

The radiographic exposure is important. Too great an exposure leads to dark radiographs where the soft tissues are difficult to see. Too pale and bony detail may be lost. As a general rule, the soft tissues should be easily defined without the use of a bright light (Fig. 8.5).

In our opinion it is undesirable to routinely request comparison views of normal limbs. Good texts are available illustrating normal and developmental variants and should be located in the emergency department. Most radiologists are happy to be consulted where difficulty remains. That is what we are here for!

Many departments operate a "red dot" system in which the radiographer flags up a suspected abnormality. The success of the system requires a clear understanding of its purpose. The red dot does not constitute a report but is only meant to direct the attention of the emergency practitioner to a possible abnormality. The absence of a red dot does not remove the medical officer's responsibility to critically examine the radiograph. In our experience up to 95% of abnormalities may be accurately detected with an over-call rate of approximately 20%, mostly related to normal variants and normal growth features. There is, however, a great variation between radiographers' ability to identify abnormalities. The careful implementation of such a system can reduce the unnecessary "call backs" for missed fractures, in particular during out-of-hours periods when expert interpretation may not be freely available.

It is important that the emergency physician has a reliable fail-safe mechanism to minimise the impact of mistakes in interpretation. Mechanisms should be in place for a correlation of the official radiological report and the initial assessment by the A&E practitioner or physician so that discrepancies are swiftly identified and appropriate action taken. All x-rays should ideally be reported within 24 h but due to working practices this may not be achievable, especially at weekends. Each individual department must have appropriate arrangements to identify those films in which delayed reporting takes place to minimise missed lesions.

8.2.2
Ultrasonography

Ultrasonography uses high-frequency sound waves which are transmitted into the tissues, an image being built-up from the reflected signals.

Ultrasonic imaging or ultrasonography has been described as the perfect imaging modality for assessing children when used appropriately. The examination is non-traumatic. An ultrasound examination can yield a wealth of information regarding cartilage, tendons, muscles and fluid, all areas difficult to interpret on plain radiography. A large amount of work has been done on the biological effects of diagnostic ultrasound but to date no adverse effects have been detected in humans using pulsed ultrasound at diagnostic intensities. The relatively low cost of examinations and the wide availability of equipment often render it the next line of investigation after plain radiography.

Ultrasound has a number of drawbacks, however. It cannot image bone well although it provides good detail of surrounding soft tissues, cartilage, tendons and muscles. It is operator dependent and so operators should have paediatric and musculoskeletal ultrasound experience. The examination requires the co-operation of the patient and in very painful regions the examination may be limited. The equipment should be of modern, high specification with suitable transducers and probes. For musculoskeletal work this means a high-frequency 10-mHz linear array probe in addition to sector and curvilinear

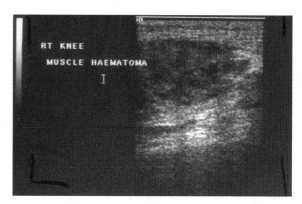

Fig. 8.6. Right calf muscle haematoma demonstrated by ultrasound

probes. Applications include the assessment of hip structure and stability in infants, the recognition of hip joint effusion, the demonstration of fluid and oedema adjacent to bone, periosteal oedema and subperiosteal abscess in osteomyelitis, the evaluation of muscle haematomas or other masses, and the demonstration of injuries to tendons (Fig. 8.6). Ultrasound is the imaging modality of choice when assessing the testis. When assessing the pelvis, a full bladder is required to assess potential pathologies such as appendicitis, abscess or pelvic haematoma which may present with hip pain.

Doppler interrogation can now usefully assess blood flow to areas of abnormality, which may be increased with inflammation or reduced with ischaemia. This is a rapidly expanding area in which changes in practice occur from month to month as equipment improves and experience grows.

8.2.3
Scintigraphy

Scintigraphy involves the labelling of a bone-seeking pharmaceutical substance which is actively incorporated into the musculoskeletal system with a radioactive isotope. It is introduced via an intravenous injection. The most commonly used isotope is technetium-99m methylene diphosphonate (MDP), which is taken up in areas of new bone formation. Hence in areas of increased bony activity such as fracture, infection or tumour the isotope is concentrated and its level can be measured using a gamma camera. Skeletal scintigraphy has a high sensitivity for the detection of lesions, but a low specificity (CARTY et al. 1984). As obtaining the image requires the patient to lie still for several minutes, some children may need to be sedated for the procedure.

The growing metaphyses are metabolically highly active in children, necessitating the use of high-resolution techniques such as pin-hole collimation to resolve subtle abnormalities. When bones or joints are assessed individually, care must be taken to image the contralateral bones or joints at exactly the same distance from the collimator face. A full bladder precludes images of the pelvis and in certain circumstances catheterisation of a sedated child may be necessary.

The appearance of the normal growth zone on scintigraphic images varies with the patient's age. After 2 years of age the growth zone is represented by a transverse linear band of increased activity which usually lies flat or slightly convex in the direction of the diaphysis. Moderate or marked convexity of this margin is abnormal. In children of 18 months or younger, the growth zone has an ovoid or elliptical form, which may be caused in part by flexion of the adjacent joint. At all ages, the demarcation of intense growth zone activity from the diaphysis is sharp; blurring of this sharp margin is due to either motion or an abnormality. With good-quality images paediatric skeletal scintigraphy is a reliable and accurate method for the detection of osteomyelitis, fracture and primary or metastatic bone neoplasms (Fig. 8.7). A two-phase scan (images taken immediately after injection of the radiotracer and late images taken 2h later) is required in the appendicular skeleton. In the axial skeleton, a late phase is often all that is needed. If it is possible to acquire images during injection this is very helpful in the assessment of vascular flow and hyperaemia, i.e. a three-phase scan. Interpretation of the scintigram should always be done in conjunction with interpretation of the plain radiographs.

8.2.4
Computed Tomography

Computed tomography (CT) is a cross-sectional imaging technique where an x-ray beam and detector rotate around the patient's body producing a two-dimensional image of the section or slice in the x-ray field. Modern CT equipment can image slices from 1 to 10mm in thickness, with most slices taking 3s or less to complete. Spiral or helical CT may produce images in an even shorter time. High-definition CT is regarded as the most accurate means of assessing

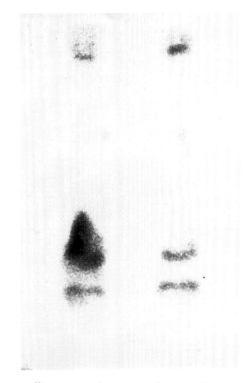

Fig. 8.7. ^{99m}Tc isotope bone scan of osteogenic sarcoma in distal femur

bony anatomy. Three-dimensional reconstruction is of value in trauma. There is a relatively high radiation dose to the patient when compared with plain film radiography. Sedation for patients between 6 months and 6 years may be necessary but depends on the skill of the technician as well as the child's behaviour. Children less than 6 months old will often lie still after a bottle feed and normal children older than 6 years will respond to a clear explanation. It is essential that whatever sedation is utilised, a clear protocol is adhered to and that adequate resuscitation equipment and appropriately trained personnel are at hand. To reduce the radiation dose to a minimum it is often possible to select relatively low-dose scanning parameters, adjusting the kilovoltage (kV) and current (mAs) to levels much lower than would be required for adult scanning.

The advantages of CT include excellent contrast between soft tissues of different density (Fig. 8.8). Bony detail is excellent, especially when sharp mathematical algorithms are applied. Multiplanar reconstructions are invaluable in assessing complex fractures such as are found in the acetabulum. Specific areas where CT is of particular use include the assessment of pelvic fracture, tumours, os-

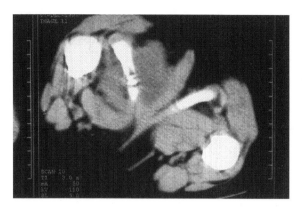

Fig. 8.8. CT demonstrating soft tissue abscess around ischial tuberosity

teomyelitis including pyogenic sacro-iliitis, femoral anteversion, spondylolysis and tarsal coalition. Imaging in suspected infection should be done following intravenous contrast administration.

8.2.5
Magnetic Resonance Imaging

Magnetic resonance imaging (MRI) utilises high-strength magnetic fields and associated radio-frequency changes to produce images. Images are obtainable in multiple planes. There is excellent soft tissue differentiation. MRI has become the method of choice for imaging many cartilage and soft tissue lesions. There is no ionising radiation. Scanning times tend to be longer than with CT and access to the patient during the procedure more limited. Hence sedation or general anaesthesia is more often required. Image sequences should include T1/T2 and fat suppression techniques (LAUR et al. 1996).

Image planes should be individually assessed. Axial images are always indicated but coronal and sagittal images are required to supplement these. The choice depends on the area of investigation. Cost and availability remain disadvantages. Intravenous gadolinium enhancement is required in suspected inflammatory or neoplastic lesions.

Magnetic resonance imaging has provided a new non-invasive and more accurate approach to the diagnosis and evaluation of several conditions, including osteonecrosis in Legg-Calvé-Perthes disease, osteochondral fractures, meniscal tears and knee anomalies, soft tissue masses, and primary or secondary neoplasms of bone. MR images should be interpreted together with plain films and not viewed in isolation.

8.3
Spinal Lesions

Standard radiographs: AP and lateral
Supplementary projections: Obliques
Most appropriate further imaging: MRI, CT and scintigraphy

Children with spinal lesions present with focal back pain, a limp due to referred pain or alteration in gait that is often interpreted as a limp.

8.3.1
Spondylolysis/Spondylolisthesis

Spondylolysis is a stress fracture of the pars inter-articularis portion of the posterior vertebral arch that is most commonly seen at L5, less commonly at L4 and rarely above that level. Less than 50% of the children who have spondylolysis will develop spondylolisthesis (the forward displacement of the vertebral column through the disc space directly below the vertebra with the spondylolytic lesions). Both lesions are rarely seen below the age of 5 years and occur most commonly between 10 and 15 years. They usually present with low back pain often associated with unilateral or bilateral buttock or posterior thigh pain but with no radiation. A limp is not uncommon.

Eighty percent of the lesions are seen on the lateral view and most of the rest on the oblique projection, which should only be acquired if the lesion is not visible on the lateral view. When imaging the pars obliquely, the vertebral body and processes have an appearance resembling a "Scotty dog", the lucency of the pars defect forming the dog's collar around its neck. Although not often necessary, a technetium bone scan will display increased activity at the defect when plain films fail to do so. CT scanning will also visualise the lesion. If one is looking specifically for spondylolysis the normal scanning angle of the CT gantry may be reversed to cause apparent elongation of the "pars" and elegant demonstration of the lesion. Spondylolisthesis is best detected on the lateral projection.

Scintigraphic planar imaging and single-photon emission computerised tomography (SPECT) may prove useful in identifying lesions. Initially a planar imaging sequence is carried out but if required, SPECT may be utilised as a second sequence in highly selected cases.

Most patients may be managed conservatively but up to 40% will require surgical stabilisation of the involved level.

8.3.2
Herniated Nucleus Pulposus

Herniated nucleus pulposus is rare in young children but its frequency increases in adolescents. The presentation is much the same way as in adults, with back pain, unilateral sciatic pain and a limp. Plain radiographs are frequently entirely normal, but in a large disc protrusion there may be loss of disc space height. Remember that compared with its higher counterparts the normal L5/S1 disc space is normally smaller in height by up to 50%. Confusion may arise where there is a transitional lumbosacral junction with partial sacralisation of the lumbar spine, in which case additional or vestigial disc spaces may be seen. Nomenclature of disc spaces can be confusing when describing such lesions, so it is best to label the spaces clearly with a chinagraph pencil directly on the radiograph to avoid confusion.

Computed tomography scanning will demonstrate most lumbar disc lesions of significance but, as already mentioned, requires a relatively large radiation dose. Scans are routinely performed aligned contiguously to each of the lower three lumbar disc spaces and images presented to demonstrate bony and soft tissue abnormalities. This allows two-dimensional reconstruction, a technique particularly useful when looking for sequestrated disc fragments.

Magnetic resonance imaging, where readily available, is the imaging method of choice for assessing disc lesions. The entire lumbar spine can be assessed without ionising radiation, tissue differentiation is better, and sagittal and coronal images can be produced without reconstruction artefact.

The majority of paediatric patients respond to such conservative measures as limited activity or bed rest and analgesia. The indications for surgery are progressive neurological deficit, cauda equina involvement or failure to improve after adequate conservative treatment.

After surgery, the cause of recurrent pain is difficult to assess radiologically as fibrotic change may be indistinguishable from disc recurrence. Contrast-enhanced CT and MRI both have a role in this difficult area.

Following lumbar vertebral fracture, disc herniation may occur when a segment of the vertebral end-plate is avulsed by its annular attachment together with a portion of the disc. The avulsed fragment may be seen as a calcified opacity over the spinal canal. Once it is suspected, CT or MRI will demonstrate the full extent of the lesion.

Anterior juvenile discitis is due to degeneration and anterior disc herniation into the vertebral endplate, most frequently superiorly but in some cases inferiorly. A bridging syndesmophyte may develop. The lesion is most frequent in athletic children. The radiographic appearances are often mistaken for infection, especially at a single level. The children may present with back pain and a limp. In general no further imaging is required.

8.3.3
Spinal Neoplasms

Neoplasms of the bony spine, spinal cord or other neural structures can produce extremity pain, weakness and limping. Presentation is usually insidious. Most benign and all malignant spinal tumours will require biopsy and/or definitive surgical treatment. AP radiography may rarely show bony thinning and erosion with widening of the interpedicular distance, or alteration in vertebral body texture, but is usually normal. MRI is the imaging method of choice and the child should then be referred to a specialist centre rather than subjecting the child to CT or CT myelography. Myelography in children is only rarely required since MRI scanning has become available, the main residual value being CT myelography in the demonstration of cervical root avulsion not shown by MRI.

8.3.4
Discitis and Vertebral Infection

Regardless of whether an acute spinal infection is confined to the disc space, involves the adjacent vertebral body end-plate or involves both the disc space and the vertebral body, the patient will present with severe back pain, often asymmetric leg pain, muscle spasm and limping. In young infants and toddlers, the presentation may be with abdominal symptoms – crying, constipation, colic or drawing the legs up to the tummy. Alteration in behaviour or posture is a clue. The child may refuse to stand-up or bend, etc. Staphylococcal bacterial infection is the most widely accepted aetiology of discitis, although other mechanisms such as trauma have been proposed.

Early radiographs may be normal for up to 2 weeks after presentation. The earliest sign is loss of disc space height (Fig. 8.9). In evaluating disc space narrowing, note that the discs normally become

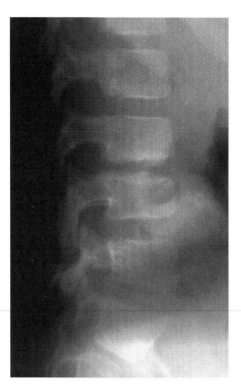

Fig. 8.9. Discitis at L2/L3

Table 8.3. Types of spinal dysphraphism

Open spinal dysraphism
Meningomyelocoele
Meningocoele

Closed spinal dysraphism
Lipomeningocoele
Diastematomyelia
Split notochord syndrome
Dermal sinus
Thickened or tight filum terminale
Anterior sacral meningocoeles
Lateral meningocoele
Caudal regression syndrome
Sacrococcygeal teratoma

nous gadolinium will help to highlight a related epidural abscess with MRI. Treatment is often conservative with appropriate antibiotics (Du Lac et al. 1990).

8.3.5
Spinal Dysraphism

Malformations of the neural tube or of the musculoskeletal structures of the spine may occur as isolated abnormalities or be associated with more widespread disease.

Plain radiographs may show associated segmentation of the vertebrae or fusion anomalies or there may be widening of the spinal canal indicative of a spinal mass or diastematomyelia (Fig. 8.10).

Ultrasound is an excellent way to demonstrate the level of the conus, a tethered cord or syrinx up to about 6 months but is of only limited value in the older child. If a lesion is found, MRI will be required to supplement ultrasound and image the whole cord fully.

For clinical purposes dysraphism is divided into open and closed types (Table 8.3). In closed spinal dysraphism there is absence of a cystic mass or presence of unbroken skin over the abnormality and is the type most likely to present with a limp. In many cases there is usually a skin blemish, hairy patch, subcutaneous lipoma or sinus associated. The child presenting with a discharging sinus or neurocutaneous mark and a limp should be urgently investigated with MRI to exclude a sinus track into the spinal canal. These children have a high risk of developing meningitis. MRI may show thickening or tethering of the spinal cord.

slightly wider at each segment proceeding from the lower thoracic region caudally to L5. Even a subtle loss of height or lack of the normal increase is suggestive in the appropriate setting. The L5/S1 space is normally narrower than L4/L5; thus at this level direct bone changes are more helpful. After a few weeks the vertebral end-plate usually becomes indistinct or destroyed. During healing areas of sclerosis may develop.

Scintigraphy demonstrates increased radiotracer deposition in the vertebral end-plate adjacent to the affected disc. The findings are generally shown well on parallel-hole collimator images, but pin-hole collimation improves image quality. If the abnormally intense area of activity is not in the end-plate but is in the pedicle or another part of the posterior arch, other possibilities such as fracture or osteoid osteoma should be considered. The MRI appearances are variable depending upon the patient's age and the stage of the disease. Because the findings change very little during the healing phase in spite of a good clinical response, MRI is not useful for monitoring this phase, except for identifying complications such as neural impingement from the protruding disc or paravertebral abscess. Enhancement with intrave-

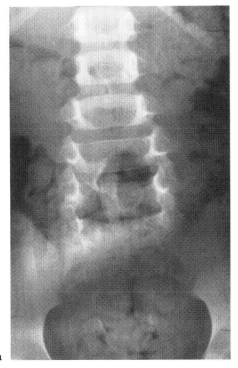

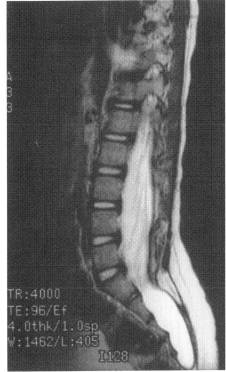

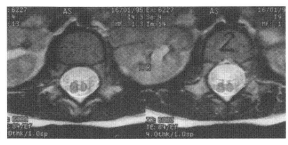

Fig. 8.10. a Widened interpedicular distance (courtesy of Dr. K. Bell). **b** MRI axial image showing split cord. **c** Same patient as in **b**. MRI sagittal section demonstrating lipoma

8.4
Bony Pelvis and Hips

Standard radiographic projections:
    AP or frog-leg lateral
Supplementary:
    Frog-leg lateral
    Judet's view for suspected acetabular fractures or,
        preferably, CT

In general only one projection is required. If the suspected diagnosis is slipped capital femoral epiphysis then the frog-leg lateral projection is the preferred baseline projection; otherwise, the AP is preferred (Fig. 8.11).

In 94% of cases a correct diagnosis of pelvic trauma can be made from only an AP radiograph. Major trauma is usually self-evident and unlikely to present with simply a limp, but there are a number of subtle pelvic injuries which can be difficult to identify. Epiphyseal lines may be misinterpreted as fractures because the apophyses of the ischial tuberosity, lesser trochanter and iliac crest do not unite until the end of the late teens. The Y-shaped (tri-radiate) cartilage separating the pubis, ischium and ilium in the acetabular floor does not fuse until puberty. The commonest fracture of the acetabulum is in the posterior rim after a posterior dislocation of the hip.

Avulsion fractures at the sites of muscle insertions into apophyses are a frequent cause of pain in athletic children. The lesions are easily overlooked. Acute injuries are usually identified. Chronic repetitive microtrauma may produce very irregular bone regeneration which may lead to erroneous diagnosis of tumour. An awareness of the problems should prevent unnecessary further investigation. Most of

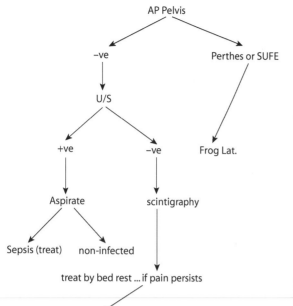

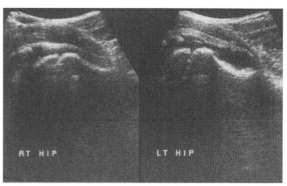

Fig. 8.12. Hip ultrasound showing normal right side and a large effusion on the left

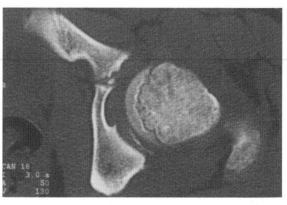

Fig. 8.13. CT of acetabular fracture sustained after a schoolboy rugby tackle

CT or MRI if required to resolve a doubtful lesion

Fig. 8.11. Pathway for investigating hip pain. U/S, Ultrasound; Perthes, Legg-Calvé-Perthes disease, SUFE, slipped upper femoral epiphysis

the lesions are visible on the plain radiographs. Ultrasound at the site of the muscle insertion will also show disruption of the normal muscle fibres.

At initial presentation of a suspected hip or pelvic disorder a single radiograph only is required. The initial radiograph should be performed without gonad protection in order not to obscure the pelvic ring; however, if subsequent projections or follow-up radiographs are required, gonadal protection in the form of lead shielding should be applied. Correct positioning of such shields require a full range of shield sizes to be readily available and much skill on the part of the radiographer!

The frog-leg lateral projections are useful in cases of suspected subtle slipped capital femoral epiphysis or in Perthes' disease.

Ultrasound is now proving invaluable in the assessment of the non-traumatic painful hip (DORR et al. 1988; GOPAKUMAR et al. 1992; HARCKE and GRISSON 1990; HOWARD et al. 1993; MIRRALES et al. 1989; TRAN-MINH et al. 1993). A high-frequency linear probe is utilised with the patient lying supine and the hip imaged in the sagittal plane. The right and left hips are compared and must be examined in the same position. Good practice is to leave the painful limb in a comfortable position and place the non-painful limb into the same position. Fluid can easily be visualised within the joint. A depth of fluid be-

tween the femur and joint capsule of greater than 4 mm is considered significant, as is a discrepancy in depth of more than 2 mm between the painful and non-painful side (Fig. 8.12).

Computed tomography is invaluable where subtle or complex pelvic trauma is suspected and is preferable to multiple radiographic projections. Narrow section imaging through the acetabulum in particular is useful in assessing fractures in this region, especially if surgical reconstruction of the acetabulum is considered (Fig. 8.13). Three-dimensional reconstructions are found useful by the orthopaedic surgeons in planning the correct surgical procedure.

The various hip lesions that cause limping are listed in Table 8.4.

8.4.1
Transient Synovitis

Transient synovitis is the most common non-traumatic cause of an acute limp in a child. The diag-

Table 8.4. Hip lesions that cause limping

Transient synovitis
Septic arthritis
Legg-Calvé-Perthes disease
Slipped capital femoral epiphysis
Developmental dysplasia
Arthritides

nosis is one of exclusion of more serious pathology such as arthritis or Legg-Calvé-Perthes disease.

The cause is unclear, but may be related to a non-specific inflammatory response to viral or streptococcal infection (MARCHAL et al. 1987). The interferon system appears to be activated by the process, acting as a mediator of inflammation (TOLAT et al. 1993).

Typically, the patient presents with a limp associated with pain in the hip, thigh or knee. Males are more commonly affected than girls in a ratio of 2:1, and the typical age of presentation is between 3 and 10 years. There may be a history of fever or suspicion of recent viral infection in up to half the patients. The child is not systematically unwell but there is limitation of joint movement. The white cell count is usually normal. Sepsis is often considered as idiopathic synovitis often develops at the time of an intercurrent respiratory illness, this being the cause of mild increases in C-reactive protein (CRP), erythrocyte sedimentation rate (ESR), and white cell count.

Joint aspiration in older children is essential in cases of suspected sepsis although in these cases open arthrotomy is often still preferred (BERMAN et al. 1995).

Complete bed rest is the appropriate therapy and may require hospital admission, depending on home circumstances. Full recovery is often within 4–6 days but may take up to 2 weeks. Recovery is accelerated by aspiration of an effusion which decompresses the joint. The frequency of long-term sequelae is thought to be very low but occasionally avascular necrosis has been documented. The relationship between Legg-Calvé-Perthes disease and transient synovitis is unclear. Recurrence rates vary between 18% and 29% and usually occur within 1 year. There are no features which will reliably predict recurrence.

Radiographic assessment is carried out to exclude other pathology such as Legg-Calvé-Perthes disease, neoplasm or osteomyelitis. Occasionally radiographic signs of joint effusion are noted as evidenced by displacement of the normal pelvic fat lines (MAJOR and HELMS 1996; ROSENBORG and

MORTENSSON 1986). Reliance should not be placed upon such signs, which are usually absent, and where synovitis is suspected, ultrasound examination is indicated. This reliably demonstrates the presence of a hip effusion and is a quick, safe and painless procedure in experienced hands. Even so, up to 40% of clinically suspicious irritable hips will have a normal scan. Scintigraphy is useful for exclusion of early Legg-Calvé-Perthes disease and osteomyelitis but in our experience is required only in a small proportion of patients, mainly those with persistent pain (CARTY et al. 1984; SPENCE et al. 1994). Scintigraphy does not reliably distinguish transient synovitis from other causes of acute synovitis, but in the appropriate clinical setting may support the diagnosis. The scintigram is either normal or shows generalized uptake around a joint without evidence of focal pathology. Full views of the spine and pelvis together with pin-hole views of the hips are required.

8.4.2
Septic Arthritis

In children, septic arthritis affects the knee in 40% of cases, the hip in 23% and the ankle in 13% (BARTON et al. 1987). Septic arthritis should be regarded as an emergency as the consequences of delayed treatment are severe and include arthritis, ankylosis, osteonecrosis and growth disturbance.

The enzymatic products of pyogenic bacterial inflammation are potent chondrolytic agents which account for the rapid development of joint damage. Raised intracapsular pressure can produce ischaemia of the femoral head.

At presentation, the patient is usually systematically unwell and has a fever. The age distribution is lower than for transient synovitis, with about half the patients being less than 2 years old; the male:female incidence is equal. Occasionally, limp and pain are the only clinical findings, with the diagnosis being made by joint aspiration. Localising signs are poor, presentation being with pyrexia of unknown origin and limitation of active limb movement. This is particularly true if hip sepsis is secondary to retroperitoneal or psoas infection. *Haemophilus influenza* and *Staphylococcus aureus* are the most common organisms but other frequent pathogens include Streptococci, *Neisseria gonorrhoeae* and *N. meningitidis*. Tuberculosis is well known to affect joints but seldom presents acutely in Western Europe. In endemic areas it may present as a cold abscess.

The clinical and laboratory data usually clinch the diagnosis. Plain radiographs are required to exclude associated metaphyseal osteomyelitis and to establish a baseline for the assessment of delayed complications.

Ultrasound examination of the hip is useful for identifying and measuring the size of effusion, which is larger than in most cases of transient synovitis. Increased echogenicity of the effusion and marked synovial hypertrophy are more suggestive of sepsis than of transient synovitis. Aspiration is always required where the diagnosis is suspected and this may be done under ultrasound guidance with a co-operative child. Distressed children require a general anaesthetic and in these circumstances arthrotomy with joint washout is preferable.

Scintigraphy with technetium-99m-labelled phosphates yields abnormalities within 3 days of onset but is non-specific (SPENCE et al. 1994). A focus of uptake in the metaphysis indicates metaphyseal osteomyelitis. Septic arthritis without osteomyelitis appears as diffuse increased uptake around the joint. Rarely a totally photopenic femoral head is seen. This is due to avascular necrosis secondary to tamponade of the blood supply and carries a poor prognosis. In children with suspected bone infection the spine and sacro-iliac joints must also be imaged as hip pain may be referred. Septic arthritis of the sacro-iliac joint differs from that in most other joints, as bone involvement occurs early in the course of disease (ABBOTT and CARTY 1993). Scintigraphy is therefore appropriately positive at an early stage.

Computed tomography will show bony changes of secondary osteomyelitis earlier than plain films. Either CT or MRI will be useful in assessing abscess formation within the pelvis, which may present clinically with an apparent septic arthritis but have a normal appearance on hip ultrasonography.

8.4.3
Legg-Calvé-Perthes Disease

Legg-Calvé-Perthes disease is an avascular necrosis of the capital femoral epiphyses occurring in young children, most commonly between the ages of 4 and 8 years. The aetiology is unclear (THOMPSON and SALTER 1987). There is evidence that the vascular anatomy of the proximal femur is in a transitional stage of development between the ages of 4 and 7 years, rendering the blood supply to the femoral head especially vulnerable during this period. Clini-

cally the child usually presents with a limp with an insidious onset. There is a strong male preponderance. Pain is usually in the groin area, but may be referred to the thigh or knee. On physical examination, there is often a limited range of hip movement, especially abduction and internal rotation. The hip abductors may be weak with a positive Trendelenburg test. Leg length inequality may be present in the more severe cases (WEINER 1993).

Legg-Calvé-Perthes disease is bilateral in 5%–20% of patients but the onset of infarction is seldom simultaneous. When a child presents with bilateral simultaneous infarction, primary causes of avascular necrosis such as sickle-cell disease or Gaucher's disease, then steroid therapy, should be considered.

Treatment objectives include minimising stress on the femoral head, limiting lateral subluxation of the femoral head and optimising congruity between the femoral head and acetabulum. Bed rest, abduction bracing, innominate osteotomy and varus derotational osteotomy are some of the options.

At presentation the clinical and radiological issue is to distinguish between Legg-Calvé-Perthes disease and idiopathic synovitis before radiographic changes occur.

The earliest radiographic feature on the AP and frog-leg views of both hips is widening of the joint space (KANIKLIDES et al. 1996). This is a non-specific sign which may also be seen in transient synovitis. Ultrasonic demonstration of an effusion is unusual, being more common earlier in the disease than later, but high-resolution ultrasound may show changes in the femoral head. Early bone changes include fissuring of the femoral capital epiphysis, which represents a subchondral fracture and is often seen only in the frog-leg lateral view, slight increase in the density of the epiphysis and slight irregularity in its outline. As the disease progresses the femoral head becomes increasingly fragmented, flattened and sclerotic (Fig. 8.14) and is displaced laterally within the joint. Lucent defects may develop in the metaphysis and broadening of the femoral neck and metaphysis may occur. In severe cases there may also be secondary acetabular change (Figs. 8.15, 8.16).

A simple classification is to have only two groups depending on whether less than or more than half of the femoral head is affected. This can be judged from the length of the fissure fracture on the plain film or the findings on scintigraphy. The first group has a good long-term prognosis. The early changes are shown on scintigraphy before there are any radiographic changes. The avascular area appears as a defect, the size of which is a good indicator of

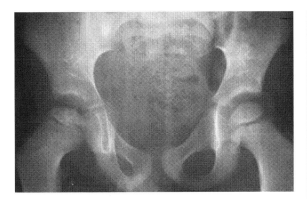

Fig. 8.14. Right-sided Legg-Calvé-Perthes disease

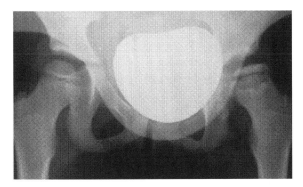

Fig. 8.15. More pronounced left-sided Legg-Calvé-Perthes disease (note female gonadal protection)

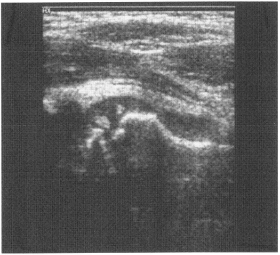

Fig. 8.16. Ultrasound of hip in a case of Legg-Calvé-Perthes disease, showing epiphyseal fragmentation and an effusion

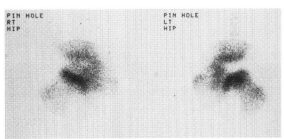

Fig. 8.17. Scintigram using pin-hole collimation. Note photopenic affected left hip

prognosis. With pin-hole collimator magnification views, the anatomy of the infarct within the femoral head can be clearly seen as a region of photopenic activity (KANIKLIDES et al. 1996; SPENCE et al. 1994; Fig. 8.17).

Magnetic resonance imaging is more accurate than scintigraphy in detecting osteonecrosis in adults. Comparison of the two modalities in Legg-Calvé-Perthes disease depends to a large extent on the technical aspects of the procedures (HENDERSON et al. 1990; RANNER et al. 1989). On MRI, the earliest appearance of the avascular region is as a well-demarcated area of low signal intensity on T1-weighted spin-echo images. The lesion is usually isointense on T2-weighted images early on. Decreased signal on T1-weighted images may persist for many years despite apparent radiographic healing (Fig. 8.18).

Patients younger than 6 years of age have a good result in 70% of cases regardless of treatment (IPPOLITO et al. 1987). Treatment includes home traction, a range of motion exercises, non-weight

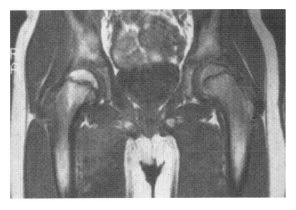

Fig. 8.18. MRI of Legg-Calvé-Perthes disease (T1-weighted image) demonstrating loss of marrow signal on the affected left hip

bearing and the administration of non-steroidal anti-inflammatory drugs. In patients 6–8 years of age, treatment depends on the height of the lateral pillar (outer width) of the physis. If it is less than half that of the opposite hip, the condition can be managed with containment treatment (brace or osteotomy). Range-of-movement exercises are performed and adductor tenotomy considered if a fixed adduction contracture exists. Patients who are older than 9 years of age are the most difficult to treat and have the worst prognosis. The need for surgical containment of the femoral head is most common in this age group. Muscle release is sometimes also necessary to regain hip motion.

8.4.4
Slipped Capital Femoral Epiphysis

Slipped capital femoral epiphysis (SCFE) is a hip disorder of adolescence. Most cases are idiopathic but some children have an associated endocrine disease such as hypothyroidism which may be subclinical. This should be excluded in all children presenting with SCFE. The SCFE lesion is a chronic lesion and technically is a Salter type fracture through the growth plate. The patient usually presents with hip pain or referred knee or thigh pain medially, the pain having been present for some time. The child walks with a Trendelenburg limp with the leg externally rotated. The pain may be referred to the knee. The typical body habitus is that of an overweight teenager, more frequently a girl. Prognosis is dependent on the duration, stability and degree of slippage. Acute slippages with less than 2 weeks of symptoms tend to be unstable and have a worse prognosis. Cartilage necrolysis (chondrolysis) and avascular necrosis of the femoral head are the two most common complications. Between 25% and 40% will be bilateral but most bilateral cases do not present concurrently.

Because a slipped epiphysis is at risk of further slippage, and the risk of avascular necrosis of the femoral head increases with the degree of slip, this problem should be dealt with urgently. The patient should be maintained in bed rest with traction until definitive surgical management with internal fixation of the hip has been accomplished.

The majority of slipped epiphyses are treated by percutaneous or limited exposure in situ pin fixation with one or two pins: the patients are then mobilised rapidly on crutches and discharged pain-free within 1–2 days. With unilateral slips, prophylactic pin fixation of the normal side is a matter of debate (BUSCH and MORRISEY 1987).

Antero-posterior and frog-leg lateral projections of the pelvis are essential for detection of subtle minimal posterior slippage and both views should be

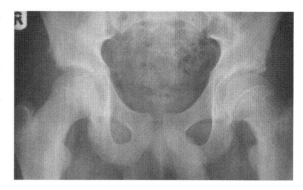

Fig. 8.19. Subtle left-sided SCFE

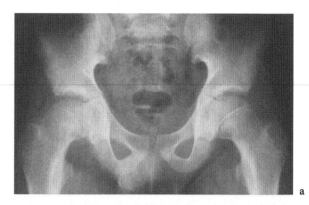

a

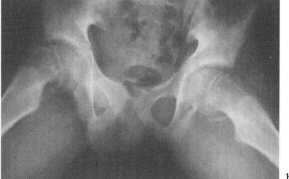

b

Fig. 8.20. a Bilateral SCFE. b Frog-leg lateral projection. The slip is easier to see on this projection

performed in a child in the appropriate age group (Figs. 8.19, 8.20).

In the earliest stage (preslip) the only change on the radiograph may be apparent widening of the epiphyseal plate with associated osteopenia.

With mild slippage (defined as up to 1 cm displacement) the AP view in neutral position may appear deceptively normal. The epiphysis will be widened with slightly irregular margins and failure of the lateral corner of the epiphysis to extend lateral to the lateral femoral neck if a line is drawn along the neck. The frog-leg position view makes the findings much easier to detect because the femoral head displacement is perpendicular to the x-ray beam. In a moderate slip, the head is displaced more than 1 cm but less than two-thirds of the width of the femoral neck. Displacement of greater than two-thirds of the width of the femoral neck is described as severe slip. Avascular necrosis of the femoral head is uncommon except in moderate or severe slips, particularly after open reduction (JONES et al. 1990). This complication is identified most effectively with skeletal scintigraphy or MRI. When viewing the images, the contralateral hip must always be closely reviewed so that bilateral disease is not missed – an easy error when the disease is symmetrical.

8.4.5
Pelvic Tumours

Children with tumours within the pelvis or of the bony pelvis may present with a history of insidious onset of a painful limp. Bony tumours most frequently found in the child's pelvis include Ewing's sarcoma, eosinophilic granuloma, aneurysmal bone cyst, osteoblastoma of the sacrum and rarely haemophilic pseudotumour. Presacral tumours are more likely to present with back pain. Due to the presence of bowel gas overlying the bones these lesions are often difficult to detect, especially as the attention is mainly on the hip joint itself. Ewing's sarcoma, in particular, may be associated with a large, soft tissue mass.

Most tumours show bone destruction. Features seen in appendicular skeleton tumours, such as cortical disruption and periosteal new bone, are more difficult to appreciate. The radiological features of the individual lesions are well described in standard texts.

Tumours of the pelvic organs may present with a limp due to pressure effects or bone erosion. Plain film clues on a pelvic radiograph include the presence of a soft tissue mass, displacement of bowel gas or calcification. Once a pelvic tumour is suspected, pelvic ultrasound should be performed.

8.5
Soft Tissue Pelvis and Scrotum

Standard radiographs:
    AP, pelvis
Most appropriate further imaging:
    Ultrasound
    MRI

There is usually clinical evidence that suggests this location of the pathology, but in cases of persistent obscure hip or groin pain pelvic ultrasound and, if this is negative, further imaging with MRI may reveal the pathology. Hip and groin pain may be the clinical presentation of intraperitoneal pathology such as a pelvic abscess or inflammatory lymph nodes in the groin or retroperitoneal pathology such as a psoas abscess.

In order to visualise soft tissue structures within the pelvis the patient must have a reasonably full bladder. The bladder presents a natural acoustic window which enhances the ultrasonic signal and displaces gas-filled bowel loops out of the field of view. A medium-frequency probe is preferred, allowing visualisation of ovaries and uterus in the female and deep pelvic tissues in the male, but bowel ultrasound requires a high-frequency linear array probe.

Abscess and tumour are the two most important pathologies which can present with an abnormal gait due either to psoas spasm or voluntary guarding. When abscess is present, the clinical history often suggests this as there is fever and localised pain. A recently formed abscess will appear as an echo-poor collection similar in echogenicity to bladder contents. Gas may be identified within it. After a few days the abscess begins to organise and appears a more inhomogeneous collection with septations. Care must be taken not to mistake mirror artefact derived from the bladder for a deep retrovesical abscess; in addition it should be noted that constipation with a large stationary solid faecal mass containing no air can be mistaken for a solid tumour. The right iliac fossa should be regarded as "tiger terrain" for ultrasound, with a high degree of skill required to elicit useful information. The aim of the examination is to confirm or exclude appendicitis in the case of pain (Figs. 8.21–8.23). A technique of graded compression is used to gently displace overlying bowel loops until the appendix is visualised. With experience this can be done in most cases.

The appendix may appear swollen and fail to compress in the normal manner. An appendicolith may be visualised within its lumen. A localised fluid collection may be present around it, as may localised ileus. Recent studies suggest that Doppler analysis of blood flow within the appendix may prove useful in identifying areas of hyperaemia due to inflammation within the appendix. Perhaps the greatest value of ultrasound examination is in ruling out other possible pathologies such as ovarian cyst rupture or mesenteric adenitis. CT has a role in confirming appendicitis in difficult cases. If ultrasonic evaluation is not conclusive, MRI is the preferred means of assess-

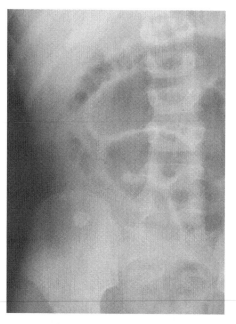

Fig. 8.21. Plain abdominal radiograph demonstrating a calcified appendicolith and localised ileus with appendicitis

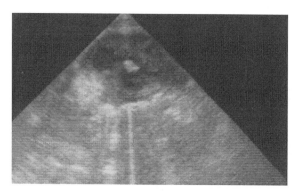

Fig. 8.22. Calcified appendicolith and adjacent soft tissue swelling on ultrasound

ing the pelvis. The directly acquired coronal and sagittal images that MRI can produce are more appropriate for imaging anatomy of pelvic organs than axially acquired CT images.

Testicular pain or swelling may present with a limp although clinical history and examination usually identify the problem. Pain can be referred to the testis from other parts of the genito-urinary tract: a trap for the unwary! If imaging is required, ultrasound is the preferred modality. A high-frequency (10-MHz) linear probe is essential to produce good near-field resolution. Abnormalities such as torsion, epididymitis or tumour are readily identified in most cases. The use of colour flow imaging has enhanced

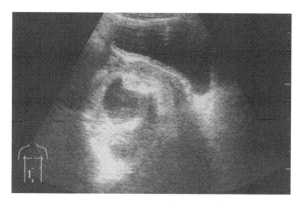

Fig. 8.23. Retrovesical appendix abscess visualised with ultrasound

the ability of the sonographer to differentiate between these two entities. These lesions are discussed in detail in Chaps. 3 and 5.

8.6
The Knee

Routine radiographic projections:
    AP
    Lateral
Additional projections:
    Skyline patella – for patellar-femoral joint
    Tunnel views – for loose body
Other imaging modalities
    MRI for meniscal lesions and radiographically negative pain

Most children presenting at the emergency department with knee pain have suffered acute trauma or a penetrating injury. Fractures around the knee are discussed in Chap. 9 and full investigation of suspected foreign bodies in Chap. 11. The other main presentation is with acute exacerbation of chronic knee pain or with chronic knee pain which the child no longer tolerates. This may arise from pathology in the ligaments, ligamentous attachments, the joint, and the muscles. Anterior knee pain is a common clinical presentation in girls. The likely cause of knee pain varies with age and activity. For example, a meniscal cyst is more frequent in young children and meniscal tears almost unknown. Patellar tendinitis and Osgood-Schlatter's lesions are more common in athletic children.

Most knee injuries are confined to the soft tissues and are invisible on plain radiographs. Nevertheless, an AP and a lateral film should still be the starting

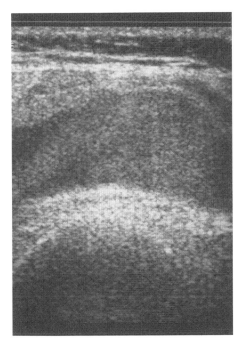

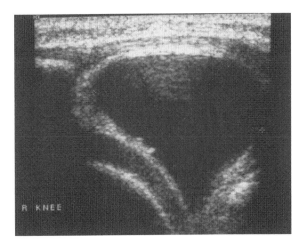

Fig. 8.25. Baker's cyst of the right knee as shown by ultrasound

Fig. 8.24. Traumatic bursitis as demonstrated by blood within bursa on ultrasound

point of radiographic investigation. There is a complex arrangement of ligaments around the knee. These include the medial, lateral and cruciate ligaments. Injury to any of these complexes may cause instability. The anterior cruciate ligament is attached to the medial tibial spine. Tibial spine fractures are more frequent than torn cruciate ligaments, so avulsion fractures of this spine or of the base of the intercondylar eminence are important. In children there is a greater elasticity of ligaments and tendons than in adults. In children both acute and chronic knee injuries are more frequently apophyseal avulsions at the site of muscle and tendon insertion, whereas adults are more likely to tear a ligament or tendon. The menisci help in smooth movement, including rotation of the joint, and are not normally visible on plain films. Occasionally a soft tissue mass is seen if there is a meniscal cyst or popliteal cyst. There are several bursae around the knee, not all of which communicate with the joint cavity. Fluid in these may cause pain (Figs. 8.24, 8.25). Radiographs are usually normal but the lesions are well seen on MRI. A lipohaemarthrosis is identified as a fat-fluid level on a decubitus film in some cases of acute trauma. Effusions are commonly seen in the suprapatellar bursa behind the quadriceps tendon when there is trauma or arthritis.

8.6.1
Patellar Anomalies

The patella starts to ossify between the ages of 3 and 6 years. Several ossification centres may fail to fuse, simulating fractures. A pseudarthrosis may be present between these and lead to pain in active children. Fractures of the patella will tend to have sharp margins and will be associated with soft tissue swelling and a clear history of injury. The fabella is a small accessory ossicle lying in the lateral head of the gastrocnemius posterolateral to the knee and should not be mistaken for an avulsed fragment. An ununited accessory ossification centre of the fibular head will have a smooth corticated margin, unlike a fracture.

8.6.2
Pellegrini-Stieda Lesion

A thin line of ossification may also be seen in the medial collateral ligament next to the insertion point of the medial femoral condyle. This is caused by an old avulsion injury of this ligament with subsequent calcification within the subperiosteal haematoma (Pellegrini-Stieda disease) and should not be confused with a recent injury.

8.6.3
Fibrous Cortical Defect

Fibrous cortical defects are the most commonly seen benign lesion of long bones and are usually identified incidentally on radiographs. They are often located

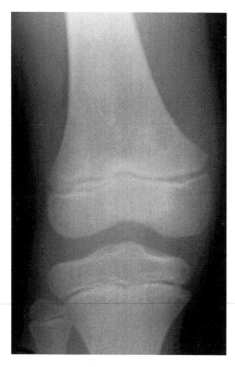

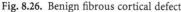

Fig. 8.26. Benign fibrous cortical defect

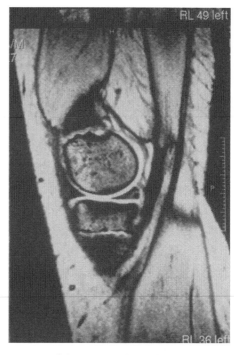

Fig. 8.27. Tear of the posterior horn of the meniscus

in the distal metaphysis of the femur posteriorly. The defect is limited to the cortex (Fig. 8.26). The lesion is well corticated with sclerotic margins and is usually asymptomatic. Pain only occurs when there is a fracture through it. This is often impossible to detect on plain radiography but may be identified with MRI. Fibrous cortical defects are hot on scintigraphy. Irregular ossification of the distal femur may occur and can be confused with trauma or tumour. These, however, are not locally painful and will have no associated soft tissue change.

8.6.4
Meniscal Lesions

Cartilaginous and ligamentous damage is almost impossible to assess on plain film radiography. On the lateral projection, however, with a good soft tissue exposure, an ovoid or sausage-shaped swelling may be identified beneath the suprapatellar ligament, indicative of an effusion. Ultrasound has some limited use in specific soft tissue injuries but MRI is the imaging method of choice for identifying cartilage and cruciate ligament injury and should be requested if meniscal or ligament injury is suspected once an acute haemarthrosis has been aspirated. On

MRI the normal menisci are seen as structures of uniformly low signal intensity. A meniscal tear is identified by the presence of an increased intrameniscal signal that extends to the surface of the structure (Fig. 8.27). This may be associated with bone oedema or a bone bruise (Fig. 8.28). Tears of the medial meniscus are more common than lateral tears. This has been attributed to the greater degree of mobility of the lateral meniscus because of its rather loose attachment to the synovium. Lateral meniscal tears, however, may accompany a developmental anomaly, the discoid meniscus, which may be related to an abnormal attachment of its posterior horn to the tibial plateau and repetitive abnormal movements, with subsequent enlargement and thickening of meniscal tissue. The discoid meniscus may be suggested clinically by a loud clicking sound on flexion and extension of the knee and radiographically on the plain film AP view by an abnormally wide lateral joint compartment (LAUR et al. 1996). On MRI the discoid meniscus is thick and lacks the central thinning typical of the normal meniscus. Increased signal due to degenerative change is common (Fig. 8.29). A discoid medial meniscus may also be seen but is rare compared with the lateral lesion. A meniscal cyst may be identified as a soft tissue mass lateral to the joint (Fig. 8.30).

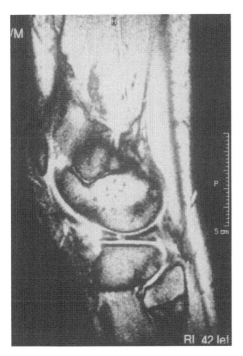

Fig. 8.28. Tear of the posterior horn of the lateral meniscus. Note extensive signal alteration in distal femoral condyle due to bone bruising

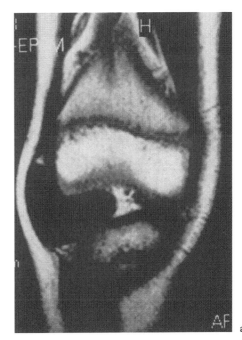

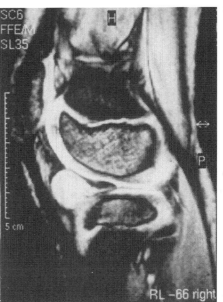

Fig. 8.30. a T1-weighted and b T2-weighted images of a medial meniscal cyst

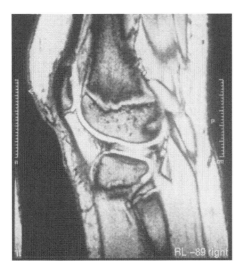

Fig. 8.29. Discoid lateral meniscus. Note high signal throughout the meniscus due to degenerative change

8.6.5
Osgood-Schlatter's Disease

Osgood-Schlatter's disease results from repeated micro- traction injuries to the patellar tendon. It is not a true osteochondrosis of the anterior tibial tuberosity. The tibial tubercle, however, frequently ossifies irregularly and a useful distinguishing feature between normal variant and the osteochondritis of Osgood-Schlatter is the lack of soft tissue swelling. Ultrasound examination may demonstrate the distal part of the patellar tendon to be thickened and hypoechoic, and it can contain fragments from the anterior tibial tuberosity. With Osgood-Schlatter's disease there is always overlying tenderness.

In the quadricipital patellar bicipital tendons, knee tendinitis may be demonstrated with ultrasound. Calcifications are rare but pathognomonic of the chronic stage. Ultrasound is the most easily accessible method for showing tendon fibres. In contrast to MRI, ultrasound is able to show micro-rupture, owing to its high resolution. MRI is indicated if ultrasound is negative and has the advantage of being able to demonstrate all the knee structures.

Sinding-Larsen disease is a condition similar to Osgood-Schlatter's disease but in this instance the lower pole of the patella is affected. Radiologically, a sleeve of bone is present at the lower pole of the patella.

8.6.6
Osteochondritis Dissecans

Osteochondritis dissecans is a marginal stress fracture generally accepted as an impaction injury. A subchondral fragment separates and may form a loose body within a joint (DE SMET et al. 1990). This may be unossified cartilage or subchondral bone. The condition is more common in males between the ages of 4 and 15 years. It is more frequent on the medial side of the joint and typically occurs on the convex surface of the distal femoral condyles (Fig. 8.31). Other common sites are the capitellum and the superior aspect of talus (Fig. 8.32). Tunnel views may be required to visualize the loose particle of osteochondritis dissecans but if this is cartilaginous it may not be seen. CT and MRI may both elegantly demonstrate these lesions and have a complementary role (Fig. 8.31). It is easier to see ossified loose bodies with CT. The coronal and sagittal imaging display of MRI is most appropriate. MRI will demonstrate the bony fragment separated from the main bony structure (usually the medial femoral condyle) by a low-intensity line (Fig. 8.31). The relationship of the bony defect to the overlying cartilage is clearly visualized in a manner which is difficult with other modalities. Osteochondritis dissecans is often accompanied by bone bruising and oedema which may be identified with MRI while being undetectable with other imaging techniques (KEARNEY and CARTY 1997). Bone oedema appears as an area of low signal in the bone on T1-weighted and as a high-signal area on STIR imaging.

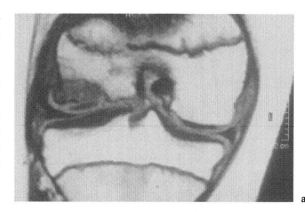

a

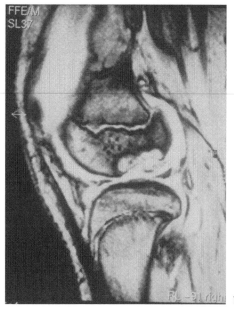

b

Fig. 8.31. a T1-weighted image. Note large osteochondral defect on the femoral condyle. b T2-weighted image. Different child. High signal within the osteochondral defect is seen on this image contiguous with the joint, indicating communication with the joint and lack of articular coverage. Note fluid in the suprapatellar bursa

tion most commonly affects adolescent girls. The abnormality is only rarely visible on plain knee radiography and appears as a defect on the femoral surface of the patella, sometimes associated with a loose fragment (Fig. 8.33). MRI is the imaging method of choice but CT may show some lesions.

8.6.7
Chondromalacia Patella

In chondromalacia patella the articular cartilage of the patella becomes softened and pitted. The condi-

8.6.8
Blount's Disease

Blount's disease is unusual disorder in which there is a growth abnormality of the medial aspects of the

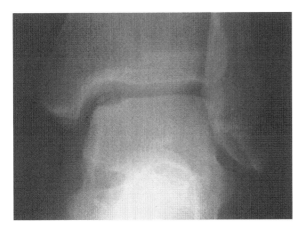

Fig. 8.32. Osteochondritis dissecans

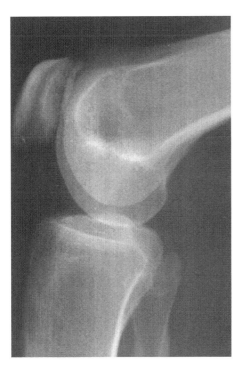

Fig. 8.33. Chondromalacia patella demonstrated by irregularity of the articular surface of the patella

tibial epiphyseal ossification centre, growth plate and metaphysis at the knee, resulting in bowing of the tibia, which in contrast to the normal physiological bowing of infancy has its apex in the proximal rather than the middle third of the tibial shaft. Plain films usually reveal adequate diagnostic information. Blount's disease does not usually present as an emergency but may present as an incidental finding in children who complain of knee pain from other causes.

8.6.9
Patellar Subluxation

Normal patellar stability depends on the shape and integrity of the articular surfaces of the patello-femoral joint and off the local muscles and tendons. If the patello-femoral groove is shallow, the lateral femoral condyle hypoplastic or the local muscles abnormal, the natural tendency to lateral subluxation may be potentiated by trauma. Plain film evaluation will show the dislocation but CT may be required to demonstrate the associated osteochondral fractures. Typically the patella subluxes laterally and in so doing an osteochondral fragment may become detached from the medial border of the patella.

8.7
The Lower Leg and Ankle

Standard radiographs:
   Tibia and fibula – AP and lateral
   Ankle – AP and lateral
Supplementary views:
   Strained inversion
Most appropriate further imaging pathway:
   CT for bony injury
   Ultrasound for soft tissue injury
   Scintigraphy

There are numerous centres of ossification around the ankle which may be confused with trauma. The os trigonum is present in about a quarter of the population. It arises adjacent to the posterior tubercle of the talus. It is a normal variant and does not cause pain except on occasion in small children when movement occurs at the junction with normal bone. This is confirmed by scintigraphy. In the os trigonum syndrome, a focal hot spot is identified. Other accessory ossification centres that may cause confusion are accessory epiphyses at the malleoli and an accessory epiphysis of the navicular bone. This often may be painful with excess activity. With normal variants localised soft tissue swelling is absent and the detached fragment is fully corticated and has a smooth contour. Injury to a developing physis may result in premature closure of all or part of a physis with consequent deformity or limp. Physeal and epiphyseal injuries are more frequent in children than the ligamentous tears more typical of adult injury. The current Royal College of Radiologist guidelines for ankle radiography state that a radiograph is unlikely to show a fracture if the patient is able to continue to weight bear with moderate ease, has no swelling or joint tenderness over the bones and has no swelling over the anterior talofibular ligament. In many injuries to the ankle a radiograph may not be required at all.

Commonly with an X-ray request in ankle injury the physician may ask for both an ankle and foot radiograph. Both examinations are often unnecessary, especially if there is careful clinical demonstration of point tenderness.

8.7.1
Toddler's Fracture

"Toddler's" fracture is a term used to describe an undisplaced spiral fracture of the distal tibial shaft in patients between the ages of 9 months and 3 years when weight bearing is just beginning (MELLICK and REESOR 1990; SHRAVAT and HARROP 1996) (Fig. 8.34). More recently, calcaneal fractures have also been identified as part of the toddler's fracture spec-

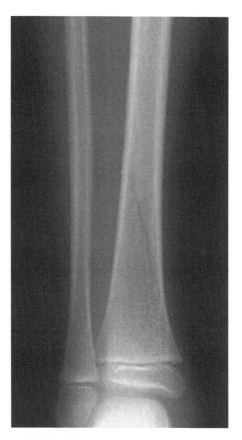

Fig. 8.34. Toddler's fracture

trum (LALIOTES et al. 1993). The relatively trivial mechanism of injury is deceptive in these patients. The child presents with a limp or pseudoparesis without a clear-cut history of trauma. The physical signs are subtle and the initial radiograph may be normal in up to a third of patients. A good-quality radiograph may show a faint hair-line fracture. This may have the typical single helix or spiral staircase configuration. The fracture is usually stable. Scintigraphy will demonstrate the fracture and its location usually before it is evident on radiography. Increased activity is shown in the diaphysis of the tibia. Scintigraphy allows a positive diagnosis to be made quickly. Management of a suspected toddler's fracture is to encourage non-weight bearing either by rest or immobilisation in plaster until the pain settles and to repeat the radiograph after 10 days to 2 weeks, by which time the radiograph is positive. The fracture may be seen due to resorption of bone along the fracture line and periosteal new bone is visible.

It is important to be aware that the vast majority of toddler's fractures result from accidental injury if this is the only bony lesion. Child abuse is unlikely, unlike in children with spiral long bone fractures found elsewhere. If there is no history of even minor trauma the main differential diagnosis is early osteomyelitis and the differentiation is often difficult. In osteomyelitis the increased uptake is often more focal in the metaphysis. Further differentiation is by correlation with the clinical findings, history and symptomatic progression. In difficult cases MRI may be of help.

8.7.2
Stress Fracture

A further cause of limp is a stress fracture of the tibia, fibula or metatarsal. Stress fractures are more frequent in athletic children but fibular stress fractures are not infrequent in toddlers. There is no history of injury. Radiographic appearances will depend on the degree of repair and location. In the tibia, the fracture is seen as a transverse fracture posteriorly but may extend across the width of the bone (Fig. 8.35). In the fibula there is often longitudinal reaction (Fig 8.36). On MRI, these fractures are associated with extensive marrow oedema and often periosteal oedema, and may be mistaken for more sinister lesions. Correlation with the plain radiographs will help to avoid mistakes.

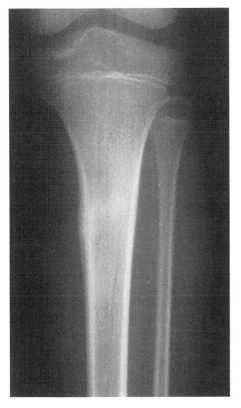

Fig. 8.35. Stress fracture of the tibia

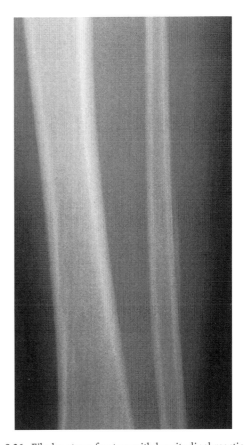

Fig. 8.36. Fibular stress fracture with longitudinal reaction

8.7.3
Shin Splints

Three causes of lower limb pain in athletic children are recognised: stress fractures (discussed in Chap. 9), shin splints and compartment syndrome. Shin splints are due to a fascial thickening at the anchoring points of the muscular compartments on the lateral and medial borders of the tibia. Such thickening is related to excessive exercise of the foot flexors. Ultrasound shows fascial thickening and oedema but scintigraphy is probably the most sensitive way of demonstrating the lesion, which appears as longitudinal areas of increased uptake along the tibial cortex. There are usually no plain film changes. The condition is found in athletic children.

8.7.4
Achilles Tendinitis

Achilles tendinitis and rupture are easily assessed by ultrasound. The tendon may appear swollen

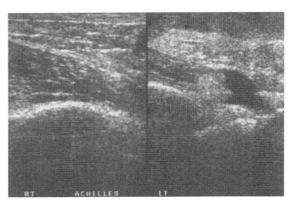

Fig. 8.37. Ultrasound of torn left Achilles tendon

and is sometimes hypoechoic. If it is ruptured, a haematoma may be visible together with the retracted and disorderly arranged muscle fibres. As with all ultrasound it is important that the normal side is compared with the affected side. Achilles rupture is found in older teenage athletic children and not in young children (Fig. 8.37).

8.7.5
Reflex Sympathetic Dystrophy Syndrome

Sometimes known as post-traumatic painful osteoporosis or Sudeck's atrophy, reflex sympathetic dystrophy syndrome is a severe form of osteoporosis that may occur after a fracture or even after relatively mild injury. The patient presents with a painful tender extremity with hyperaesthesia, diffuse soft tissue swelling, joint stiffness, vasomotor instability and dystrophic skin changes. On the radiograph the appearance is characterized by soft tissue swelling and severe patchy osteoporosis which progresses rapidly. Scintigraphy demonstrates increased uptake in the affected areas, particularly around the joints, without focal pathology. In children disuse of a limb for whatever reason will result in relatively rapid development of osteopenia, which can easily be confused with true reflex sympathetic dystrophy syndrome.

8.8
The Foot

Standard radiographic views:
  Foot – AP
  – Oblique

Supplementary views:
  Lateral soft tissue (for foreign body)
  Lateral and axial os calcis projection
Most appropriate further imaging:
  CT for complex fracture
  Scintigraphy
  MRI
  Ultrasound for foreign body

8.8.1
Trauma

Trauma around the foot which results in fractures is usually easily recognised on acute radiographs. Foot pain and limp may result from chronic stress injury, unrecognised fractures, congenital abnormalities and soft tissue and tendon injuries. Acute fractures are discussed in detail in Chap. 9. Fractures of the base of the fifth metatarsal result from inversion of the foot which produces tension on the peroneus brevis attached to the base of the fifth metatarsal (NICHOLSON and O'KEEFE 1995) (Fig. 8.38). Metatarsal fractures are common and readily seen unless they are "stress" fractures due to repeated subcortical trauma to a normal bone, usually the second metatarsal (MICHELI and FEHLANDT 1994) (Fig. 8.2).

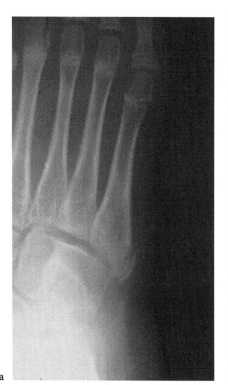 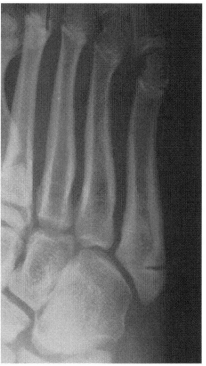

a   b

Fig. 8.38. a Normal unfused epiphysis at base of 5th metatarsal. **b** Fracture of 5th metatarsal base

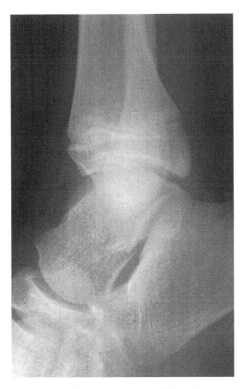

Fig. 8.39. Fracture through the waist of the talus

The child presents with a limp. This type of fracture is due to repetitive micro-trauma on normal bone and is typically seen in young dancers and military recruits subjected to sudden unaccustomed exercise. Delayed radiographs (2–3 weeks after injury) will usually show reparative periosteal new bone; however, scintigraphy will show the characteristic focal areas of increased uptake after 24–48 h.

Most crush calcaneal fractures cause depression of the posterior facet of the calcaneus, which reduces Bohler's angle, best assessed on the lateral radiograph. A missed calcaneal fracture can lead to pain. A pseudocyst of the calcaneus is a relatively frequently seen normal variant. The radiological appearances are characteristic – a well-defined lucent lesion with absent trabeculation. Micro-fractures may occur through this area of weakness and cause pain. Isolated fractures of the tarsal bones other than the calcaneus are uncommon but may be subtle, missed initially and cause the child to present with a limp (Fig. 8.39). This is especially true of the navicular bone, where stress fractures occur in athletic children. As with occult fractures at the wrist, if the radiograph is persistently negative with continuing pain then scintigraphy and possibly CT may be diagnostic.

8.8.2
Avascular Necrosis

The foot is a relatively common site to be affected by variants of avascular necrosis. Freiberg's infarction typically involves the head of the second metatarsal and may heal with resultant flattening of the second metatarsal head. It is most common in 12- to 15-year-old girls and is related to repetitive stress. Early signs are subtle or easily overlooked. Mild flattening of the metatarsal head is an early sign. Pain frequently precedes radiographic changes. Kohler's disease of the tarsal navicular bone is typically seen in boys aged 3–6 years. Calcaneal apophysitis, known as Sever's disease and resulting in pain on heel palpation, is seen primarily in boys aged 8–12 years. A dense and irregular calcaneal apophysis is usually a normal variant and is only of significance where there is localised pain and asymmetry. Both this and Kohler's disease are clinical diagnoses. The normal variant of an irregular tarsal navicular must not be confused with avascular necrosis.

Ossification centres, particularly at the base of the fifth metatarsal may cause confusion, but the line of this centre runs parallel to the long axis of the foot whereas most fractures are horizontal (Fig. 8.38).

Accessory ossification centres are usually bilateral and have a smooth rounded contour with intact cortical margins. Sesamoid bones of the great toe arise from two or more centres that fail to unite and may resemble an epiphyseal fracture. A cyst in the calcaneus caused by overlapping normal trabecular arches is normal and should not be misinterpreted as indicating disease.

8.8.3
Tarsal Coalition

Congenital foot deformity may present with a limp either in isolation or as part of a more complex neurovascular developmental disorder (FIXEN 1998). Tarsal coalition though a congenital lesion will not usually present until adolescence. The child presents with subtalar pain and has a rigid joint. A plain oblique radiograph may show a calcaneonavicular bar. This may also be shown on the lateral projection where the elongated anterior process of the calcaneum is said to resemble an "ant-eater" (OESTREICH et al. 1987). Talo-calcaneal coalition is less common and cannot be identified on plain radiography. Where there is strong clinical evidence of tarsal coalition but the plain films are unclear or

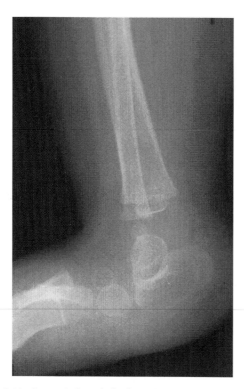

Fig. 8.40. Congenital vertical talus

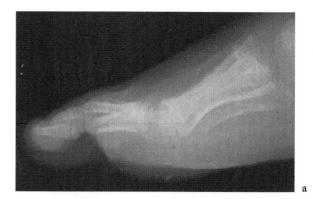

a

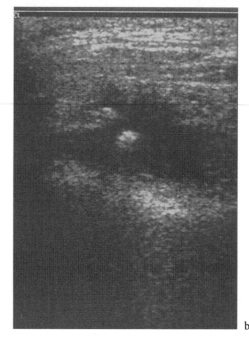

b

Fig. 8.41. a Foreign body in soft tissues of sole. **b** Same patient: ultrasound identifies the foreign body

indeterminate then either CT imaging or MRI will elegantly demonstrate the anatomy. The CT should be done with 4-mm slices at 3-mm intervals to avoid confusion due to unossified cartilage. Both feet should be examined in both the transverse and long axis of the foot. MRI is particularly useful for demonstrating cartilaginous bars where no bony component is apparent; however, the diagnosis is nevertheless usually suggested on CT as there is an irregular edge at the site of the pseudarthrosis.

Congenital vertical talus, otherwise known as " rocker bottom foot", is a rare disorder and often associated with other major syndromes. The Eyre-Brook view is most useful. The disorder occasionally presents as a limp due to abnormal stresses on the associated muscles (Fig. 8.40).

Ultrasonic assessment of the foot may identify non-opaque foreign bodies and should be the next investigation in the case a suspected foreign body with negative radiography (Fig. 8.41). Morton's neuroma is commonly a problem of adults, but it is occasionally seen in the older teenager. It is a thickening of the digital nerve between the heads of the metatarsals. It may best be diagnosed by ultrasound or MRI.

8.8.4
Arthropathy

The most frequent arthropathy in childhood is juvenile chronic arthritis (JCA). When it presents in the polyarticular form, the diagnosis is relatively easy. Monoarticular forms are more difficult. The affected joint is painful and often warm, leading to the clinical suspicion of infected arthritis. The pain in JCA is usually worse in the morning. Typically in the early stages, radiographs are normal and do not show periarticular osteopoenia or erosion. Mild soft tissue swelling may be evident. Ultrasound may show an effusion. The diagnosis is essentially clinical. Other arthropathies that may present to the emergency

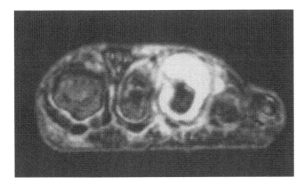

Fig. 8.42. MRI of pigmented villonodular synovitis of metatarsal phalangeal joint

room because of pain or focal inflammation include septic arthritis, discussed later in this chapter, post-traumatic arthritis, Lyme disease and pigmented villonodular synovitis (Cotton et al. 1995). The last-mentioned may involve the joint or first the tendon sheath. The radiological appearances of joint involvement are those of monoarticular erosive arthropathy with associated soft tissue swelling. Tendon sheath involvement presents as a mass, raising concern that there is a neoplasm. Investigation is ideally done with gadolinium-enhanced MRI but the diagnosis ultimately depends on biopsy (Fig. 8.42).

Investigation of these cases is not appropriate for an emergency room attendance. The primary role is to exclude infection, palliate pain and then ensure early referral to an appropriate rheumatological clinic for further investigation.

8.8.5
Foreign Body

The child who presents with a clear history of penetrating foot wound and a known foreign body penetration seldom presents a clinical problem. If the foreign body is radiopaque then a plain radiograph should be carried out to confirm removal. Initial radiographs should be taken in two planes, the entry point being identified with a metallic marker. Non-opaque foreign bodies such as wood fragments are not visible and radiographs are unhelpful. A foreign body granuloma may form, the child then presenting with a limp and palpable thickening around the lesion. This may present some months after the initial injury, which is often forgotten, and thus there is clinical concern that there is a more sinister lesion such as tumour or fibromatosis. The first investigation should be ultrasound performed using a linear

array, high-resolution probe in scan planes at right angles to each other. The foreign body is seen as an echogenic area within the lower density granuloma.

8.9
Osteomyelitis

Osteomyelitis, when treated appropriately and promptly, has few long-term complications. If the diagnosis is delayed and inadequate treatment given, serious long-term sequelae may occur, making the need for prompt radiological diagnosis all too apparent. False-positive diagnoses need to be avoided as the required oral and intravenous antibiotic therapy carries a risk of adverse drug-related complications, considerable discomfort and expense.

The lower extremity is affected in about 65% of cases in children, with boys being afflicted twice as often as girls. Acute limp is a common presentation of lower extremity osteomyelitis but may also be a manifestation of vertebral body involvement. Haematogenous spread is generally more common in young children than in adults and is the main mode of spread in childhood. Infection from direct penetration is relatively rare, a notable exception being a *Pseudomonas* infection of the foot if the penetration is through the shoe, a condition often referred to as "sneaker osteomyelitis". The usual primary focus of osteomyelitis lies in the metaphysis of long bones because of the rich vascular supply to these regions. Certain other regions of the skeleton have an analogous vascular network and provide favourable conditions for infection. These are known as "metaphyseal equivalent" sites. The most important of these sites with regard to limping are the vertebral end-plate (discitis), iliac bone adjacent to the sacro-iliac joint, iliac crest, acetabular roof, anterior superior iliac spine, pubic bone, ischium, femur adjacent to the greater trochanter, patella, the tibia adjacent to the tibial tubercle, talus, posterior calcaneus and tarsal navicular. Retropharyngeal abscess may be associated with cervical osteomyelitis.

Cartilage impedes the spread of osteomyelitis much more effectively than the periosteum, making it most unusual for infection to spread through the cartilage to involve a joint. When a portion of the metaphysis is enclosed within the joint capsule, septic arthritis may ensue.

In infants up to 1 year of age, metaphyseal vessels pass freely into the cartilaginous epiphysis. After 1 year of age, however, metaphyseal vessels no longer pass through the growth plate but turn proximally to enter large sinuses beneath the growth plate. In neonates, therefore, blood-borne bacteria can directly infect the subarticular bone and then the joint. In children aged 1–16 years, the epiphyseal plate acts as a barrier and the infection is characteristically metaphyseal. Rarely, primary epiphyseal osteomyelitis may occur. Diaphyseal location tends to occur only in older children. This is usually a chronic low-grade osteomyelitis with organised lamellar new bone formation which is often difficult to distinguish from Ewing's sarcoma.

8.9.1
Presentation

Typically the child presents with fever, pain in the affected area and, if the location is in the spine, sacro-iliac joint or leg, with a limp or refusal to walk. (GAVALES and POTTS 1992). Occasionally mild symptoms only are present with relatively little in the way of systemic manifestations, especially if a short course of antibiotic therapy is given for some other suspected cause of fever. Children with chronic infection generally have local, diffuse pain without systemic symptoms. In both acute and chronic cases there is localised tenderness and there may be oedema and erythema. In contrast to septic arthritis, osteomyelitis produces only mild limitation of movement.

Laboratory investigations are often helpful, with an elevated white blood cell count and erythrocyte sedimentation rate (ESR). C-reactive protein may rise prior to ESR elevation and is useful acutely. In low-grade chronic osteomyelitis, these biochemical and haematological markers may be virtually normal. Culture of material directly from the infected site is the ideal way of establishing the causative organism but blood cultures and any appropriate joint fluid aspirate may yield an answer and avoid unnecessary intervention. *Staphylococcus aureus* accounts for just over half of cases and various strains of *Streptococcus* account for some 10%. In patients with sickle-cell disease *Salmonella* accounts for most cases. The main differential diagnoses are listed in Table 8.5.

8.9.2
Diagnostic Imaging

When the clinical presentation is suggestive, treatment is often initiated without radiological confir-

Table 8.5. Principal differential diagnoses of osteomyelitis

Septic arthritis
Cellulitis
Acute rheumatic fever
Malignancy

Table 8.6. Characteristic features of osteomyelitis on plain film radiography

Bone destruction
Sequestration
Cloaca
Involucrum
Soft tissue mass
Periosteal new bone

Table 8.7. Distinguishing features on scintigraphy of infection

	Angiographic phase	Blood pool	Late image focal lesion
Cellulitis	+	+/–	–
Osteomyelitis	+	+	+
Septic abscess	+	+	–

mation. Usually, plain radiographs will demonstrate no change for 7–14 days. Soft tissue gas collections or radiopaque foreign bodies are rare (SCHAUWECKER and BRAUNSTEIN 1990). The characteristic features of osteomyelitis on plain film radiography are listed in Table 8.6.

Skeletal scintigraphy provides positive evidence of infection within 24–72h (Fig. 8.43, Table 8.7). Phosphate radiotracers localise infection by the associated focal increase in blood flow and increased bone turnover (TUSON et al. 1994). False-negative results are more likely in the very young, especially in infants less than 6 weeks old. Other radiotracers may be used such as technetium-99m or indium-111 labelled white cells and may be helpful in difficult areas but are not needed with acute presentation, the clinical and laboratory findings together with the MDP scintigraphy being sufficient. Rarely, the area of infection presents as photopenia due either to tamponade of the blood supply secondary to the pressure of the pus, or to the abscess itself if big enough. This finding, especially in the femoral head, carries a poor prognosis.

Osteoporosis is an early radiological sign. Soft tissue swelling is present in the early stages but may

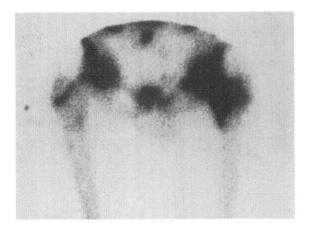

Fig. 8.43. Scintigram of proximal femoral osteomyelitis

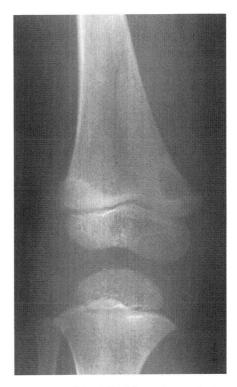

Fig. 8.45. Osteomyelitis of distal femoral metaphysis

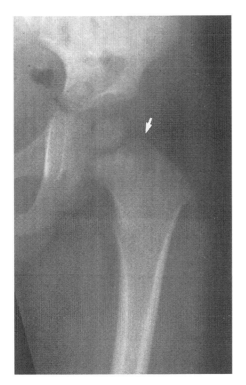

Fig. 8.44. Osteomyelitis (*arrow*) of proximal femoral metaphysis, lateral aspect

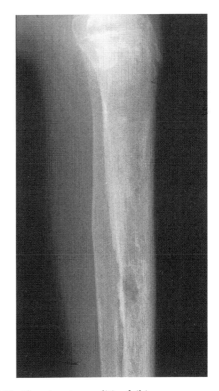

Fig. 8.46. Chronic osteomyelitis of tibia

be subtle. Fat planes may be displaced and their clarity lost. In most cases, the first bony abnormality is an area of bone destruction (Figs. 8.44, 8.45). More chronic osteomyelitis can produce a permeative pattern (Fig. 8.46) or in rarer situations a sclerotic reaction. Pus penetrates the cortex via a cloaca and extends beneath the periosteum, which it elevates. This firstly deprives the outer layer of cortex of its blood supply and then causes new bone to be laid down beneath the elevated periosteum, forming what is known as the involucrum. In children, this involucrum is prominent as the periosteal attachment to bone is less secure.

Early metaphyseal destruction occurs with progressive periosteal reaction. This may produce a Codman's triangle, making differentiation from malignancy difficult. Bone deprived of its blood supply may not be resorbed, resulting in devitalised fragments or sequestra which are dense on radiography. Vital bone around the site appears osteoporotic as disuse demineralisation of the perfused bone rapidly ensues.

High-resolution ultrasound has demonstrated periosteal reaction and subperiosteal abscess formation in long bones before any detectable change on plain film radiography (ABERNETHY et al. 1993; ABIRI et al. 1989; WRIGHT et al. 1995). MRI, as it becomes more freely available, will serve to demonstrate early soft tissue change and abscess formation (ABERNETHY and CARTY 1997). Diagnostic criteria for MRI in diagnosing osteomyelitis are findings of decreased intensity in the bone marrow cavity on short spin-echo sequences (T1 weighting) along with increased signal intensity in the bone marrow cavity on long TR/TE sequences (T2 weighting). Increased signal intensity of the soft tissues on long TR/TE sequences with poorly defined margins is considered indicative of oedema and/or nonspecific inflammatory change. Well-demarcated collections of decreased signal intensity on T1-weighted images and increased signal intensity surrounded by zones of decreased signal intensity on T2-weighted images are considered indicative of soft tissue abscesses. Decreased signal intensity on short TR/TE sequences in the area of the joint capsule or tendon sheath is consistent with synovial effusions and fluid in the tendon sheath. Biopsy of an affected area may be carried out under fluoroscopic, CT or even MRI guidance and can confirm a suspected diagnosis of infection as well as reveal the causative organism (UNGER and MOLDOFSKY 1988). An appropriate diagnostic imaging pathway in cases of suspected osteomyelitis is summarised in Fig. 8.47.

Septic arthritis has already been discussed in relation to the hip, but the general principles and imaging features apply to any joint (FINK and NELSON 1986).

Cellulitis is often an associated feature of osteomyelitis. This can be demonstrated with ultrasound, which will demonstrate soft tissue thickening and identify related lymphadenopathy.

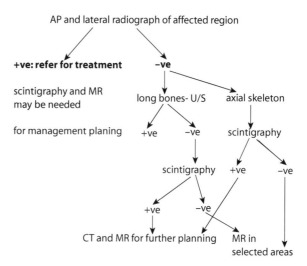

Fig. 8.47. Pathway for the investigation of osteomyelitis

Subacute osteomyelitis (Brodie's abscess) represents a subacute, localised form of osteomyelitis (LOPES et al. 1997). Its onset is often insidious with mild or absent systemic manifestations. The lesion is often localised in the metaphysis of tibia or femur and typically has a well-demarcated boundary surrounded by reactive sclerosis. Sequestra are unusual. A bone abscess may extend across the epiphyseal plate but will seldom develop in and remain localised to the epiphysis.

8.10
Bone Tumours

The child with a bone tumour may present to the emergency room because of limp due to chronic pain or because of a pathological fracture through the lesion. Recognition of the lesion so as to permit appropriate referral for further investigation and treatment is all that is required in an emergency department. Skeletal tumours in children have a predilection for the metaphyseal areas of long bones, especially the knee and the proximal femur. Tumours near growth plates may interfere with growth whereas other tumours such as haemangiomas may accelerate growth. Plain radiography will show most lesions and often the radiographic pattern is so typical that a diagnosis may be made (MAKLEY and CARTER 1986). Further imaging by CT, MRI and scintigraphy is then used appropriately for staging and treatment planning. The soft tissue component of malignant lesions is best appreciated on CT or MRI.

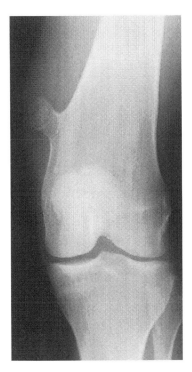

Fig. 8.48. Solitary bony exostosis

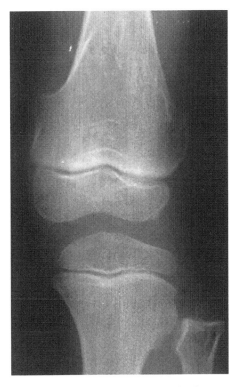

Fig. 8.49. Typical appearances of diaphyseal aclasia

8.10.1
Benign Lesions

8.10.1.1
Osteochondroma

Osteochondromas are also known as bony exostoses when they are pedunculated. The radiographic appearance is that of a bony lump with a sclerotic margin and sharp demarcation from normal bone (Fig. 8.48). They typically arise from the metaphyseal region, projecting away from the joint, and have a predilection for the bones around the knee, hip and proximal humerus. When multiple the disorder is confusingly referred to as diaphyseal aclasia (Fig. 8.49). This form follows an autosomal dominant pattern of inheritance. The lesions may present with localised pain due to trauma or localised mechanical attrition of tendons. If large they may need to be surgically removed. The child may, however, simply present with a palpable lump. Plain radiographs are so characteristic that further imaging is seldom required. Ultrasound or MRI will show the cartilaginous component and relationship to the neurovascular bundle if this is anatomically important.

8.10.1.2
Osteoid Osteoma

Typically presenting with dull pain that is worse at night and relieved effectively by aspirin, osteoid osteoma is most frequently found in the femur and tibia though the fibula, spinal appendages and phalanges may also be involved. The classical history of pain relief by aspirin is now seldom proffered as aspirin is no longer given to children because of the association with Reye's syndrome. Paracetamol, now used as an alternative, does not relieve the pain to the same degree. If the lesion is not demonstrated on the plain film, scintigraphy should be done with cross-sectional CT over the hot area (Fig. 8.50).

Osteoid osteoma is unusual below the age of 5 years and is 3 times more common in boys. There is a central core or nidus composed of osteoid and vascular fibrous tissue surrounded by sclerotic bone. On plain radiographs there is typically a central small lucency corresponding to the nidus, surrounded by dense fusiform sclerotic bone. Plain film tomography or CT will demonstrate the central nidus more clearly and scintigraphy will show increased local tracer uptake. CT-guided biopsy will confirm the diagnosis if required and can be used to

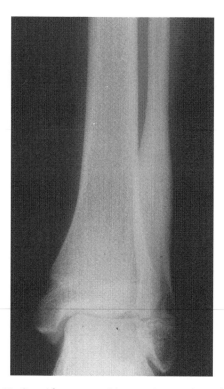

Fig. 8.50. Osteoid osteoma with extensive new bone formation in the fibula. The nidus is not visible

Table 8.8. Tumours of the lower body in children

Benign
Osteochondroma
Osteoid osteoma
Osteoblastoma
"Tumour-like" disorders
   Simple bone cyst
   Aneurysmal bone cyst
   Fibrous dysplasia
   Eosinophilic granuloma

Malignant
Primary
   Osteogenic sarcoma
   Ewing's sarcoma
   Adamantinoma

Secondary
   Neuroblastoma
   Embryonal rhabdomyosarcoma
   Retinoblastoma
   Medulloblastoma

Lymphoma/Leukaemia

resect the lesion by core biopsy, an effective and relatively minimally invasive form of therapy.

8.10.1.3
Osteoblastoma

Osteoblastoma is histologically very similar to osteoid osteoma but radiologically is larger (>1.5 cm) and more prone to arise in the medulla rather than the cortex. It is classically located in the spinal appendages.

8.10.1.4
Fibrous Dysplasia

Fibrous dysplasia is relatively common in childhood and has a predilection for the proximal femur and tibia, usually arising in the metaphysis. It may be found as an incidental finding. Coarsening of the bony architecture is noted with some remodelling. Advanced cases in the proximal femur can produce the classical "shepherd's crook" deformity of the femoral neck, which if severe enough may progress to pathological fracture through the lesion.

8.10.1.5
Simple Bone Cyst

Simple bone cysts are sharply defined with sclerotic margins. They are typically located in the proximal femur in the lower limb and the humerus in the upper limb. Although plain radiographic appearances are typical, CT will confirm a fat-fluid level if required. Secondary pathological fracture may present with localised pain. The lesion arises in the metaphysis and migrates to the diaphysis with growth. It is typically unilocular with sharp margins. If there is a fracture through the lesion a fragment of bone may be displaced into the lesion, a sign which is often alikened to a "falling leaf" (BAKER 1990).

8.10.1.6
Aneurysmal Bone Cyst

Arising in the long bones and posterior spinal elements, aneurysmal bone cysts are often eccentrically located initially; however, after epiphyseal closure they may appear more centrally located, traverse the epiphysis and mimic giant cell tumour. These lesions most commonly involve the distal femur, proximal tibia and proximal humerus. They have a multilocular appearance and can appear very aggressive. The lesion expands the bone.

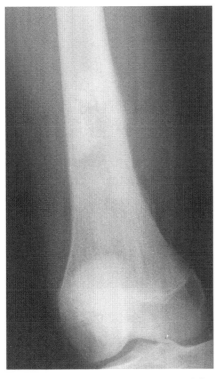

Fig. 8.51. Typical appearance of healing eosinophilic granuloma in the mid shaft of the femur

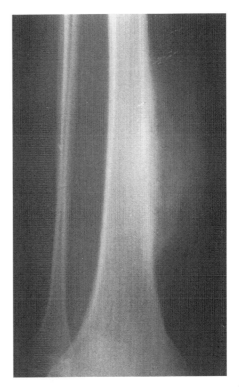

Fig 8.52. Typical appearance of osteogenic sarcoma with destruction of the cortex and a soft tissue mass

8.10.1.7
Eosinophilic Granuloma

Eosinophilic granuloma is one of the lesions of Langerhan's cell histiocytosis. In the long bones, eosinophilic granuloma presents as a destructive lesion that is often very aggressive looking. It may have a surrounding soft tissue mass. There is poor demarcation from normal bone and the geographical pattern seen in the skull is not seen. With repair, there is often prolific new bone (Fig. 8.51).

8.10.2
Malignant Lesions

Although malignant bone tumours usually present with well-established radiographic changes at presentation, occasionally the pain precedes the obvious radiographic changes and the diagnosis may be missed. The implications of missing such a lesion are so disastrous that an awareness of their possible presentation to an emergency department is essential. Early treatment is aggressive but at least offers the potential for long-term survival. The two most important primary lesions are osteogenic sarcoma and Ewing's sarcoma (BOYKO et al. 1987). Clinical presentation is with pain, usually of insidious onset, acute pain due to pathological fracture, or a palpable lump.

8.10.2.1
Osteogenic Sarcoma

Osteogenic sarcoma is more common in males, with its maximum incidence in the second and third decades. Cortical destruction and periosteal reaction are the early features (Fig. 8.52). Located eccentrically in the long bone metaphyses, these lesions classically present around the knee. The periosteum may be elevated in such a way as to produce a Codman's triangle (Fig. 8.53) due to tumour tissue, but the pattern of periosteal reaction may be layered or sunburst. A soft tissue mass is usually present. The differential diagnosis is from osteomyelitis or stress fracture if the periosteal reaction is very organised. MRI of the lesion, CT of the chest and scintigraphy of the rest of the skeleton are required for staging. Scintigraphy will identify skeletal metastases and skip

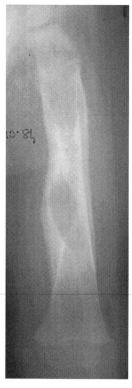

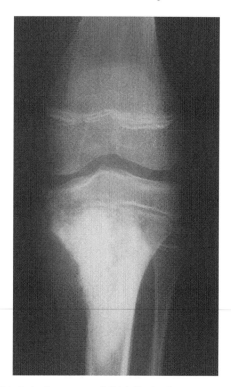

Fig. 8.54. Ewing's tumour of tibial diaphysis

Fig. 8.53. Codman's triangle of osteogenic sarcoma

lesions. Although CT of the chest is utilised for initial staging, thereafter plain film chest radiography is adequate for follow-up of chest lesions. Metastases from osteogenic sarcomas are often denser than metastases from other primary tumours, reflecting their bony origin. Rarely they may cavitate within the chest and cause a pneumothorax, the child presenting as an emergency with chest pain and breathlessness.

8.10.2.2
Ewing's Sarcoma

Ewing's sarcoma differs from osteogenic sarcoma in many ways. These patients, unlike those with osteogenic sarcoma, will often present systemically unwell with fever and leucocytosis as well as with localised pain and swelling. The diaphyses of long bones are more typically affected (Fig. 8.54) but other favoured sites include the vertebra, ribs, pelvis and scapula. On plain film radiography there may be periosteal new bone formation, but the underlying bone has a permeative or moth-eaten pattern with a broad transition zone between normal and abnormal bone. There is often a relatively large soft tissue compo-

nent which may not be fully appreciated on plain radiography. CT, MRI and scintigraphy will be required. These tumours also metastasize to the chest. When the primary lesion involves the iliac blade, the bone often appears sclerotic due to the attenuation of the x-ray beam by the large soft tissue mass.

8.10.2.3
Metastases

Metastases may be identified on plain film radiography from tumours such as neuroblastomas. In general in the emergency situation the child is known to have a tumour and the more difficult problem is to distinguish a benign cause of the pain from malignant disease. Radiographs of the painful area should be taken as for all children presenting with bone pain (Figs. 8.55, 8.56). If a metastasis is identified, the primary will usually be clinically detectable or identifiable by abdominal ultrasound. The lesions are destructive, may cause pathological fractures and are usually associated with localised osteopenia. Further investigation depends on local protocol. Scintigraphy is an ideal imaging modality in this situation to identify widespread bony disease prior to radio-

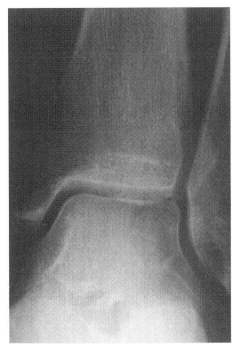

Fig. 8.55. Subtle talar metastasis from teratoma primary (courtesy of Dr. C.B. Loughrey)

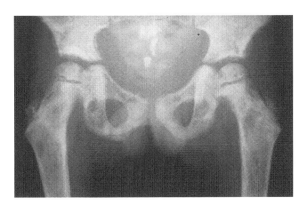

Fig. 8.56. Diffuse sclerotic metastasis from medulloblastoma

graphic changes. With secondary neuroblastoma scintigraphy will demonstrate increased uptake at the affected metaphyses (APPLEGATE et al. 1995). Iodine-123 metaiodobenzylguanidine scans have a special affinity for neural crest lesions and have a specific role in this situation.

8.11
Conclusion

Most clinicians will be able to identify the cause of a limp after careful history taking, clinical examina-

tion and appropriate plain film radiography. There are, however, many conditions where additional imaging will bring " added value" to the diagnostic pathway. A good understanding of the pathological processes and the available imaging modalities will enhance the clinician's ability to arrive at the correct diagnosis quickly and without unnecessary irradiation of the patient. By using the outlined regional approach, the possible diagnoses can be narrowed down to a likely few whilst remembering the rarer but serious pathologies of tumour, infection, etc. To paraphrase an old radiological aphorism, "You look for what you know and you see what you look for, as long as the correct imaging pathways are utilized."

References

Abbott GT, Carty H (1993) Pyogenic sacroiliitis, the missed diagnosis? BJR 66:120–122
Abernethy LJ, Carty H (1997) Modern approach to the diagnosis of osteomyelitis in children. BJHM 58(9):64–468
Abernethy LJ, Lee YCP, et al. (1993) Ultrasound localisation of subperiosteal abscesses in children with late acute osteomyelitis. J Pediatr Orthop 13:766–768
Abiri MM, Kirpekar M, et al. (1989) Osteomyelitis, detection with ultrasound. Radiology 172:509–511
Applegate K, Connolly LP, et al. (1995) Neuroblastoma presenting clinically as hip osteomyelitis: a "signature" diagnosis on skeletal scintigraphy. Pediatr Radiol 25[Suppl 1]:S93–96
Baker DM (1990) Benign unicameral bone cyst – a study of 45 cases with long term follow up. Clin Orthop Relat Res 71:140–151
Barton LL, Dunkle LM, et al. (1987) Septic arthritis in childhood. Am J Dis Child 141:898–900
Berman L, Fink AM, et al. (1995) Technical note: identifying and aspirating hip effusions. BJR 68:306–310
Blumhagen JD (1994) The child with a limp. In: Hilton SW (ed) Practical pediatric radiology. Saunders, Philadelphia, p 445
Boyko OB, Cory DA, et al. (1987) MR imaging of osteogenic sarcoma and Ewing's sarcoma. AJR 148:317–322
Busch MT, Morrisey RT (1987) Slipped capital femoral epiphysis. Orthop Clin North Am 18:637–647
Carty H, Maxted M, et al. (1984) Isotope scanning in the "Irritable Hip Syndrome" Skeletal Radiol. 11:32–37
Cotton A, Flipo RM, et al. (1995) Pigmented villonodular synovitis of the hip: a review of radiographic features in 58 patients. Skel Radiol 24(1):1–6
Dabney KW, Lipton G (1995) Evaluation of limp in children. Curr Opin Pediatr 7:88–94
De Smet AA, Fisher DR, et al. (1990) Value of MR imaging in staging osteochondral lesions of the talus (osteochondritis dissecans): results in 14 patients. AJR 155:555–558
Dorr U, Zeiger M, et al. (1988) Ultrasonography of the painful hip. Prospective study in 204 patients. Pediatr Radiol 19:36–40
du Lac P, Panuel M, Devred P, Bollini G, Padovani J (1990) MRI of disc space infection in infants and children. Report of 12 cases. Pediatr Radiol 20:175–178

Fink CW, Nelson JD (1986) Septic arthritis and osteomyelitis in children. Clin Rheum Dis 12:423–425

Fixen JA (1998) Problem feet in children. J R Soc Med 91:18–21

Gavales M, Potts H (1992) Bone infection in the limping child in the accident and emergency department. Arch Emerg Med 9:323–325

Gopakumar TS, Vaishya R, et al. (1992) The role of ultrasound and bone scanning in the management of irritable hips. Eur J Radiol 15:113–117

Harcke HT, Grisson LE (1990) Performing dynamic sonography of the infant hip. AJR 155:837–844

Henderson RC, Renner JB, et al. (1990) Evaluation of magnetic resonance imaging in Legg-Calve-Perthes disease. A prospective, blinded study. J Pediatr Orthop 10:289–297

Howard CB, Eihoran M, et al. (1993) The use of ultrasound in children with pain around the hip and thigh. Isr J Med Sci 29(2–3):77–81

Ippolito E, Tudisco C, et al. (1987) The Long term prognosis of unilateral Perthes' disease. J Bone Joint Surg 69B:243–250

Jones JR, Paterson DC, et al. (1990) Remodelling after pinning for slipped capital femoral epiphysis. J Bone Joint Surg 72:568–573

Kaniklides SE, Sahlstedt B, et al. (1996) Conventional radiography and bone scintigraphy in the prognostic evaluation of Legg-Calve-Perthes disease. Acta Radiol 37(4):561–566

Kearney SE, Carty H (1997) Pelvic musculoskeletal infection in infants-diagnostic difficulties and radiological features. Clin Radiol 52(10):782–786

King SJ, Carty HML, et al. (1996) Magnetic Resonance imaging of knee injuries in children. Pediatr Radiol 26:287–290

Laliotis N, Pennie BH, et al. (1993) Toddler's fracture of the calcaneum. Injury 24(3):169–170

Laur T, Chung T, et al. (1996) Musculoskeletal magnetic resonance imaging: how we do it. Pediatr Radiol 26(10):695–700

Lopes TD, Reinus WR, et al. (1997) Quantitative analysis of the plain radiographic appearance of Brodie's abscess. Inves Radiol 32(1):51–58

Major NM, Helms CA (1996) Absence or interruption of the supra-acetabular line: a subtle plain film indicator of hip pathology. Skel Radiol 25(6):525–529

Makley JT, Carter JR (1986) Eosinophilic granuloma of bone. Clin Orthop 204:27–44

Marchal GJ, Van Holsbeeck MT, et al. (1987) Transient synovitis of the hip in children. Role of US. Radiology 162:825–828

Mellick LB, Reesor K (1990) Spiral tibial fractures in children. A commonly accidental spiral long bone fracture. Am J Emerg Med 8:234–237

Micheli LJ, Fehlandt AF Jr (1994) Stress fractures. In Letts RM (ed) Management of pediatric fractures. New York, Churchill Livingstone

Mirrales M, Gonzales G, et al. (1989) Sonography of the painful hip in children. 500 consecutive cases. AJR 152:579–582

Nicholson DA, O'Keefe D (1995) Foot. In: Nicholson DA, Driscoll PA (ed) ABC of emergency radiology, BMJ, London, p 23

Oestreich AE, Maze WA, et al. (1987) The anteater's nose- a direct sign of calcaneo navicular coalition on the lateral radiograph. J Paediatr Orthop 7:709–711

Ranner G,, Ebner F, et al. (1989) Magnetic resonance imaging in children with acute hip pain. Pediatr Radiol 20:67–71

Renshaw TS (1995) The child who has a limp. Pediatr Rev 16(12):458–465

Rosenborg M, Mortensson W (1986) The validity of radiographic assessment of childhood transient synovitis of the hip. Acta Radiol (Diagn) 27:85–89

Schauwecker DS, Braunstein EM (1990) Diagnostic imaging of osteomyelitis. Infect Dis Clin North Am 4:441–463

Shravat BP, Harrop SN (1996) Toddler's fracture. J Accid Emerg Med 13:59–61

Spence LD, Kaar K, et al. (1994) The role of bone scintigraphy with pinhole collimation in the evaluation of symptomatic paediatric hips. Clin Rad 49:820–823

Thompson GH, Salter RB (1987) Legg-Calve-Perthes disease. Current concepts and controversies. Orthop Clin North Am 18:617–635

Tran-Minh VA, Pracos JP, et al. (1993) Sonography of the hip and soft tissues of the thigh in children. Radiol Men 85:247–251

Tolat V, Carty H, et al. (1993) Evidence for a viral aetiology of transient synovitis of the hip. J Bone Joint Surg 75(6):973–974

Tuson CE, Hoffman EB, et al. (1994) Isotope scanning for acute osteomyelitis and septic arthritis in children. J Bone Joint Sur (Br Vol) 76(2):306–310

Unger E, Moldofsky A (1988) Diagnosis of osteomyelitis by MR imaging. AJR 150:605–610

Weiner DS (1993) Pediatric orthopaedics, Churchill Livingstone, New York

Wright NB, Abbott GT, et al. (1995) Ultrasound in children with osteomyelitis. Clin Radiol 50(9):623–627

Further Reading

Marcelis SD, Daenen B, Ferrar MA, Dondelinger RF (eds) (1996) Peripheral musculoskeletal ultrasound atlas. Thieme Medical, New York, pp 118–189

Blumhagen MD (1994) The child with a limp. In: Practical pediatric radiology 2nd edn (Hilton SW, Edwards DK) (eds), WB Sounders, Philadelphia

Swischuk LE, John SD (1995) Differential diagnosis in pediatric radiology, 2nd edn. Williams and Wilkins, Baltimore

Rumack CM, Wilson SR, Charboneau JW (1998) Diagnostic ultrasound, 2nd edn, vol 2. Mosby, New York

Greenspan A (1997) Orthopaedic radiology, a practical approach, 2nd edn. Lippincott-Raven, Philadelphia

9 Fractures and Musculoskeletal Trauma

W. Ramsden

CONTENTS

9.1
Introduction

This chapter will discuss trauma to the paediatric appendicular skeleton, in which the initial aim of imaging is to define the nature and extent of injury and facilitate appropriate management. This primary aim is inseparable from the pursuit of related lesions and any potential or actual complications. A negative initial survey may allow reassurance, or possibly prompt further investigation of unexplained clinical findings.

The various imaging techniques available will be reviewed, and guidance given as to which situations may require more sophisticated investigations after initial plain radiographs. Fracture types and their

W. Ramsden, BM, FRCR, Consultant Paediatric Radiologist, St. James's University Hospital, Beckett Street, Leeds LS9 7TF, UK

causation are discussed, as are specific injuries and their associations in both the upper and lower limbs. Particular reference will be made to the normal and abnormal appearances of the developing skeleton, especially with regard to epiphyseal injuries.

9.2
Clinical Presentation of Fractures

Children with appendicular fractures are usually frightened and obviously in pain. They tend to guard the affected limb and will not move it. Local tenderness and deformity are good signs of bony injury, and if a child is not bearing weight, suspicion of a lower limb fracture is raised. Soft tissue swelling and bruising are less accurate clinical indicators.

A history of trauma is usually obtainable, although it may not have been witnessed by another person. If the history is incomplete, unlikely or changes, then it should be carefully checked to ensure the injury is truly accidental. Other factors which may raise suspicion of non-accidental injury include delayed presentation, numerous previous attendances, the child's general appearance and inclusion on the at-risk register.

9.3
Imaging Techniques

9.3.1
Plain Radiography

Plain radiographs remain the mainstay of imaging appendicular trauma, and in most cases will be all that is required. However, general guidelines are required for optimum utilisation, and despite these, delayed views or other techniques may still be required to demonstrate a bony injury.

Views in at least two planes are required in all suspected fractures of the appendicular skeleton (Fig. 9.1), with adequate coverage of the injured area.

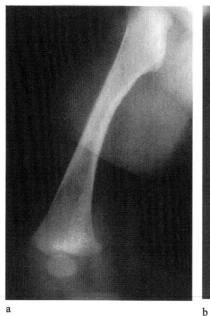 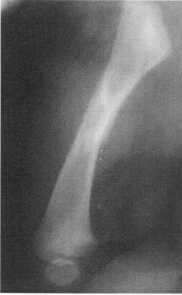

Fig. 9.1. a Fracture of the femoral diaphysis, "invisible" on initial view. **b** Effect of minor angulation of the beam

a   b

In long bone fractures, the joints above and below the site of injury should be included, especially where one of paired bones has been fractured and an associated injury or dislocation of the other bone must be excluded. Although biplanar views are a minimum requirement, certain areas with much bony overlap, such as the carpus, will require more projections.

Stress views are rarely used in paediatric practice, as forces which cause ligamentous injuries in adults more often lead to fractures in children. This is due to the relative strength of ligaments compared with immature bone.

Repeat radiographs are sometimes useful in children with continuing symptoms and negative initial investigations. Subtle stress injuries may be demonstrated by the appearance of a periosteal reaction at the fracture site, although it should be noted that this will take at least 5 days to appear and may not change management based upon the initial clinical impression.

Delayed radiographs may be used to assess the results of therapy or to pursue specific complications of certain injuries such as avascular necrosis. However, the caveat that additional examinations should only be ordered to guide management or give a prognosis must be borne in mind, as part of an overall strategy to minimise radiation dose in paediatric radiography. In addition, appropriate gonadal protection (not on initial pelvic radiograph), good collimation and the avoidance of repeat views should

be practised. Occasionally fluoroscopy is of value to obtain a non-standard but useful view of an injury, without the need for multiple exposures.

9.3.2
Further Studies

Although plain radiography is virtually always the first imaging method used in paediatric appendicular trauma, occasionally other modalities such as ultrasound are preferred, for example, in soft tissue trauma. Ultrasound may also usefully follow plain radiography in the detection of subtle periosteal elevation and joint effusions and the confirmation of transphyseal injuries when an entirely cartilaginous epiphysis is displaced from the adjacent metaphysis in an infant (Fig. 9.2).

Scintigraphy may be used to investigate continuing symptoms in the face of negative radiography in specific situations such as suspected stress injuries and scaphoid fractures. It may also confirm or refute multiple or distant bony lesions in a child with a pathological fracture through a pre-existent abnormality.

The role of computed tomography (CT) in limb fractures is centred upon complex areas where plain radiographs may be unable to define an injury clearly. Examples include the hindfoot, carpus and pelvis. Its use in the latter situation also allows visualisation of associated visceral injuries.

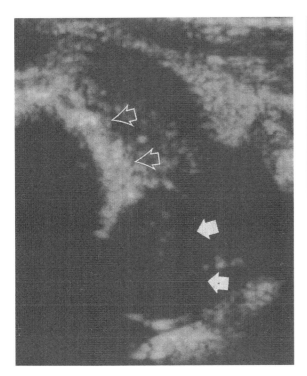

Fig. 9.2. Sonogram of the distal humerus in an infant, demonstrating posterior displacement of the unossified capitellar epiphysis (*closed arrows*) with respect to the distal humeral metaphysis (*open arrows*)

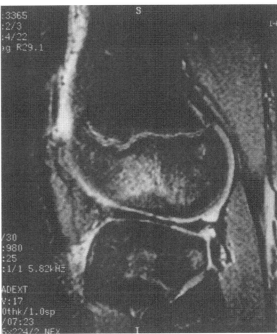

Fig. 9.3. Sagittal MRI (STIR sequence) demonstrating bone bruise in distal femoral epiphysis

Magnetic resonance imaging (MRI) has a limited initial role, but in common with ultrasound is extremely useful in defining the position of entirely cartilaginous epiphyses in the very young (OHASKI et al. 1997). Further uses are investigation of muscle, tendon and ligamentous injuries, as well as the visualisation of lesions such as stress fractures not demonstrated on plain radiography.

As well as standard T1- and T2-weighted sequences, short-tau inversion recovery (STIR) is also very useful in the detection of subtle non-specific oedema in both bone and adjacent soft tissue (Fig. 9.3). An inversion pulse is timed to cancel out the signal from fat, and although the images are noisy with poor detail, they act as an excellent guide to the general site of pathology, which may be followed up with other sequences.

9.4
Fracture Types

Fractures are classified as either simple or open, the difference being that the skin is breached in the latter with consequent danger of infection. Further terms applied are comminution, indicating a higher energy injury with more than two bony fragments and complex, where there is associated damage to neighbouring structures.

When fractures are described, any degree of displacement should be noted, with a rough estimate made of the degree of contact of opposing bone surfaces. The direction and degree of any angulation should also be described, despite children's known capacity for remodelling as healing occurs. However, it should be noted that rotation will not remodel. Intra-articular extension and disruption of joint surfaces are other important factors with regard to treatment and prognosis, and these too must be confirmed or excluded. In children such extension will frequently involve unfused epiphyses, which are discussed in detail later. With regard to joint injuries, dislocation implies complete loss of congruity between articular surfaces, whilst subluxation is incomplete loss of contact. Either may occur with or without an accompanying fracture.

Pathological fractures may occur in children, through bone already weakened by a pre-existent lesion. Such lesions are often occult until revealed by trauma; examples include simple cysts, eosinophilic granulomata and malignant bone tumours (Fig. 9.4). An unexplained lucency, area of sclerosis or periosteal reaction in the vicinity of an acute fracture should raise suspicion of a pre-existent lesion. A

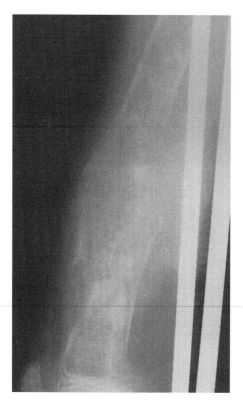

Fig. 9.4. Pathological fracture through an osteosarcoma of the femur

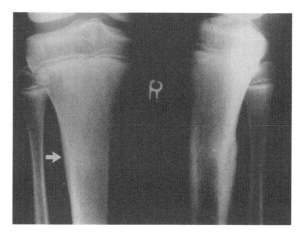

Fig. 9.5. Stress fracture of proximal tibial metaphysis. Subtle bone sclerosis (*arrowed*) and cortical thickening are the only signs visible on the AP view

fracture involving a simple cyst may display a pathognomic "fallen fragment" sign on plain radiography as a cortical fragment lies in the fluid-filled cavity.

Fractures also occur through areas of acute or chronic osteomyelitis, leading to a "floating" epiphysis in neonates as minor trauma separates it by disrupting a weakened, infected metaphysis. Confusion may occur in very young children when the epiphysis is non-ossified, and its displacement is due to pathological fracture not apparent on plain radiographs (CRAWFORD 1976). This situation poses the same problems as fractures involving the non-ossified epiphyses and in both situations ultrasound or MRI may be used to visualise cartilage directly. In pathological fractures through an area of suspected osteomyelitis both these modalities are more sensitive to bone infection than are plain radiographs owing to earlier visualisation of signs such as subperiosteal pus.

Pathological fractures also occur in children with generalised bony abnormalities in conditions such as osteogenesis imperfecta and meningomyelocele. Such injuries may occur with minimal trauma, and subsequent radiography may show subperiosteal

haemorrhage with calcification, marked callus formation at fracture sites and quick healing following immobilisation. Acquired changes in metabolic bone disease are another cause of pathological fractures. An example is renal osteodystrophy, affected children being prone to epiphyseal injuries, especially of the proximal humerus, proximal femur and distal radius.

Children are also prone to stress injuries due to repeated and prolonged action of muscle upon bone which has not yet accommodated itself to these forces (DAFFNER and PAVLOV 1992). The signs of these injuries may be extremely subtle on initial plain radiography, and the diagnosis should still be considered in the face of a suggestive clinical history. Positive findings which may be seen on initial radiographs include focal periosteal reaction, a break in the bone cortex or a sclerotic band (Fig. 9.5). Even follow-up radiographs may only be positive in approximately 50% of cases and some will be pursued with either isotopes or MRI. On MRI, the usual finding is a low-signal band perpendicular to the bone cortex on all sequences. MRI may also reveal a large amount of surrounding oedema, which should not cause disproportionate anxiety if the imaging findings are consistent with stress injury overall.

Avulsion injuries form another important subgroup, where a fragment of bone is pulled off by sudden contraction of an attached muscle, or by traction from a ligament or tendon. In children these are commonest around the pelvis and elbow (CARTY 1994). Unfused epiphyses are particularly vulnerable in this respect, a subject to be discussed in a later section.

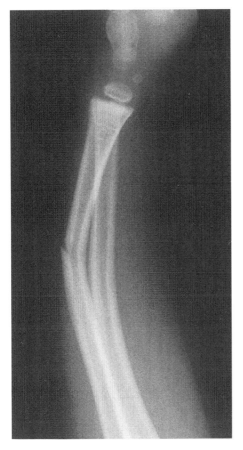

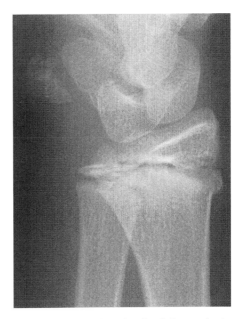

Fig. 9.7. Torus fracture of the distal radial metaphysis

Fig. 9.6. Plastic bowing of the ulna and greenstick fracture of the radius

9.4.1
Paediatric Fractures

Children's bones are weaker but more flexible and malleable than those of adults, which contributes to the occurrence of specific fracture types not found in the mature skeleton.

Occasionally, a long bone may bend, not break, and the injury may just show as a subtle overall increase in curvature, or even as a delayed periosteal reaction in young children when no initial fracture was diagnosed. Such plastic bowing fractures are most often seen in the forearm bones (Fig. 9.6) and are due to longitudinal force transmitted along the shaft of the bone. Although no fracture line is apparent radiographically, histologically multiple oblique microfractures are seen at the site of greatest bone compression (BORDEN 1975). A balance of forces producing bowing of both radius and ulna is relatively uncommon, and usually the non-bowed bone fractures. Dislocation of the non-bowed intact radius or ulna must also be excluded, as with standard

Monteggia and Galeazzi fractures. Young children slowly remodel these deformities, but this process is reduced in older children who many need orthopaedic reduction of bowing to allow treatment of an accompanying fracture or dislocation and restoration of full forearm movements.

A torus fracture ("lead pipe") (Fig. 9.7) occurs due to the buckling of a bone's cortex on the concave side of a bending force. Both this and the commoner greenstick injury are incomplete fractures. In the latter, the break of bone cortex and overlying periosteum occurs on the convex side of the bone. Buckling of the concavity of the injury may accompany this.

Paediatric fractures tend to heal quickly, with bony continuity being restored by approximately 3 weeks in a neonatal spiral upper limb fracture although the fracture is identifiable for longer. Children have a large capacity for remodelling fracture deformity, and the length of time an old injury remains detectable depends on the initial disruption.

Metaphyseal "corner" or "bucket handle" fractures are injuries seen in infants which have a high correlation with abuse. They are dealt with in another chapter.

9.4.2
Epiphyseal Separations

A knowledge of epiphyseal anatomy is important in the assessment of paediatric trauma, with regard to

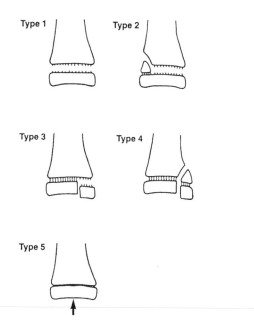

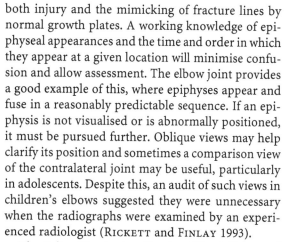

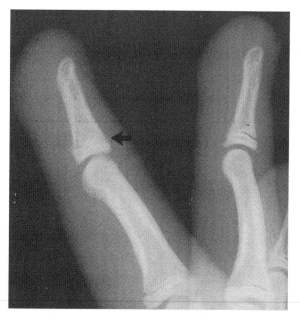

Fig. 9.8. Salter-Harris classification of fractures involving the epiphyseal plate

Fig. 9.9. Salter-Harris type 5 fracture of distal phalangeal epiphysis (*arrow*). Note normal epiphyseal plate of adjacent digit for comparison

both injury and the mimicking of fracture lines by normal growth plates. A working knowledge of epiphyseal appearances and the time and order in which they appear at a given location will minimise confusion and allow assessment. The elbow joint provides a good example of this, where epiphyses appear and fuse in a reasonably predictable sequence. If an epiphysis is not visualised or is abnormally positioned, it must be pursued further. Oblique views may help clarify its position and sometimes a comparison view of the contralateral joint may be useful, particularly in adolescents. Despite this, an audit of such views in children's elbows suggested they were unnecessary when the radiographs were examined by an experienced radiologist (RICKETT and FINLAY 1993).

The Salter-Harris classification (Fig. 9.8) is used for epiphyseal injuries because it has both therapeutic and prognostic significance. Injuries are graded 1–5, with the injuries' consequences becoming increasingly serious as the number rises.

Type 1 injuries involve the separation of the intact epiphysis from the underlying metaphysis, and although significant displacement may need reduction, if this is obtained prognosis is good. The commonest injury is the type 2 fracture, where the intact epiphysis carries a small metaphyseal fragment with it; if treated correctly, this, too, has a good prognosis. Both type 3 and type 4 injuries have separation of part of the epiphysis from the remainder, with a metaphyseal fragment accompanying it in the

case of type 4 injuries. The most serious grade, type 5 (Fig. 9.9), is rare, and occurs when part or all of the epiphysis and growth plate are crushed. These injuries can be very difficult to detect if undisplaced. Disturbance of subsequent growth is the major concern in epiphyseal injuries (Fig. 9.10), and thus accurate diagnosis and appropriate management are essential, especially in the higher grades or displaced fractures. Accurate reduction of intra-articular fractures is particularly important. However, prognosis has been shown to be worse in the lower limb, irrespective of Salter-Harris classification (ROGERS and POZNANSKI 1994).

A large series of epiphyseal injuries showed the distal radius and phalanges of the hand to be the sites most commonly affected. The same series showed the Salter-Harris type 2 to be the commonest injury, accounting for nearly three-quarters of the total (MIZUTA et al. 1987).

Epiphyseal injuries may also be stress induced, and although epiphyses may not be displaced, metaphyseal irregularity and sclerosis with physeal widening may occur. Adolescent gymnasts are prone to these injuries in their distal ulnar and radial epiphyses (Fig. 9.11). Slipped upper femoral epiphysis represents another example of such an injury, and is often missed in its early stages.

Plain radiographs are sufficient for imaging the vast majority of these injuries. The signs to look for

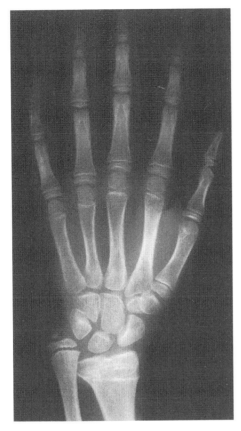

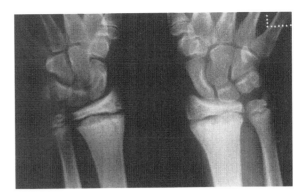

Fig. 9.11. Epiphyseal separations at the wrists of an adolescent gymnast

Fig. 9.10. Growth arrest affecting distal radius following previous epiphyseal injury

are displacement of the epiphysis, widening of the growth plate and loss of definition of the normally clear opposing surfaces of epiphysis and metaphysis (KAO and SMITH 1997). Sometimes small "lamellar" bone fragments may be seen in the physis, their source being the partially disrupted zone of provisional calcification.

Computed tomography may be used to back up plain radiographs in planning treatment of complex fractures, particularly those involving articular surfaces, and is especially helpful at the knee and ankle. CT or MRI may be needed in the long term to investigate any problems with growth arrest and to demonstrate bony or fibrous bridging across the physis in the latter situation. If possible, images should be acquired in a plane perpendicular to the fracture so detail is not lost, although thin sections and reconstruction may suffice instead.

A multiplanar capability is a major advantage of MRI, which is now the method of choice for demonstrating unossified epiphyses and physeal bridges in growth arrest. MRI also allows excellent demonstration of associated cartilage, soft tissue and ligaments,

which is important because many epiphyseal injuries at the knee are accompanied by ligamentous injury. Gradient-echo images are best in epiphyseal injury as the growth plate is hyperintense, in contrast to hypointense bone.

9.5
Injuries to the Upper Limb

9.5.1
Clavicular Fractures

A large series reported an incidence of 2.7 clavicular fractures per 1000 live births, making it the bone most commonly fractured at parturition (OPPENHEIM et al. 1990). Risk factors associated with clavicular fractures in the newborn are shoulder dystocia and high birth weight. These fractures may be associated with brachial plexus injuries, and although all such lesions healed uneventfully in the series quoted, their possible occurrence must be noted. The prognosis of the clavicular fracture itself is also very good.

The clavicle is also commonly fractured in childhood, and the middle third is usually affected, characteristically due to a fall on an outstretched hand. Radiographs often show a greenstick-type fracture with an abrupt kink in the clavicular contour. In a foreshortened frontal view, such as on a chest radiograph, the curvature of the normal bone may occasionally mimic injury.

The ligaments of the acromioclavicular joint are strong in children and separation relatively uncommon (LEE 1980). The injury is effectively confined to teenagers, and when suspected is best demonstrated by an erect radiograph taken with the child holding

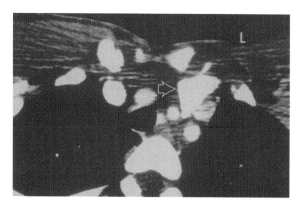

Fig. 9.12. Contrast-enhanced CT scan demonstrating posterior dislocation of left sternoclavicular joint. The dislocated medial clavicle is *arrowed*. Note its close proximity to underlying vessels

weights in their hands. Sternoclavicular joint dislocation may occur when a fall on the shoulder transmits force medially along the axis of the clavicle. Although anterior displacement of the medial clavicle is commoner, it is posterior dislocation which is more significant as vascular structures posterior to the involved sternoclavicular joint may be affected.

Plain radiographs of the sternoclavicular joints are rarely helpful, but CT is particularly useful in defining such injuries and the proximity of the medial clavicle to the vessels prior to surgical correction (Fig. 9.12).

9.5.2
Injuries to the Shoulder Girdle and Proximal Humerus

Scapular fractures and shoulder dislocation are both uncommon in childhood. With regard to the latter, anterior dislocation is the usual occurrence and an associated fracture dislocation extremely rare. Despite the rarity of dislocation, every attempt must be made to obtain views in two planes, although a transthoracic lateral radiograph may prove difficult to read compared with an axial film, if the latter is precluded by pain, swelling or movement. If there is serious concern regarding dislocation, then CT should be done (OBREMSKEY and ROUTT 1994).

Proximal humeral fractures are commoner than shoulder dislocation, often traversing the growth plate to give a Salter-Harris type 1 or 2 injury (MACNICOL 1994). The former usually occurs as a birth injury and the latter later in childhood, just prior to growth plate closure. Such injuries were

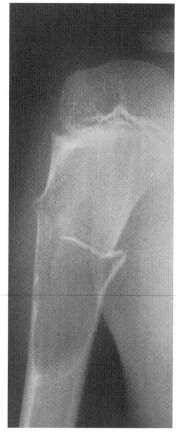

Fig. 9.13. Pathological fracture of proximal humeral metaphysis via simple bone cyst

classified by Neer according to the degree of displacement, as follows:

Type 1: displaced by 5 mm or less
Type 2: displaced by between 5 mm and one-third of shaft diameter
Type 3: one-third to two-thirds shaft displacement
Type 4: more than two-thirds shaft displacement

The type 1 injury is easy to miss owing to its minimal displacement. Although closed reduction has been suggested for type 3 and 4 fractures, satisfactory results and remodelling have occurred without (HOHL 1976).

The normal growth plate of the proximal humerus has an irregular contour demonstrated on the standard AP radiograph and is frequently mistaken for a fracture. Despite this, transverse and torus fractures of the proximal humerus may occur, with the surgical neck being the most frequent site of injury. As this region is one of the commonest to harbour simple bone cysts, pathological fractures will also occur (Fig. 9.13). As fractures are identified more

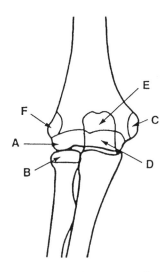

	Appears	Fuses
A. Capitellum	1-3 yrs	17-18 yrs
B. Radial Head	5-6 yrs	16-19 yrs
C. Medial Epicondyle	5-8 yrs	17-18 yrs
D. Trochlea	11 yrs	18 yrs
E. Olecranon	10-13 yrs	16-20 yrs
F. Lateral Epicondyle	10-12 yrs	17-18 yrs

Fig. 9.14. Appearance and fusion of elbow joint epiphyses

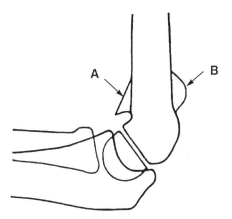

Fig. 9.15. The anterior (A) and posterior (B) fat pads of the distal humerus

distally, the possibility of an associated radial nerve injury must also be considered.

9.5.3
Injuries to the Distal Humerus and Elbow

9.5.3.1
Developmental Anatomy

At the elbow six epiphyses have to be accounted for initially they are cartilaginous, then ossified and finally fused as the growth plates are obliterated. The appearance and fusion of these epiphyses follow a set pattern, as illustrated in Fig. 9.14.

When imaging of the elbow is reviewed, any deviation from the expected sequence of ossification should prompt a search for an avulsed, malpositioned epiphysis.

9.5.3.2
Imaging the Elbow Joint

Radiographs remain the initial imaging study, and it is vital that good quality frontal and true lateral radiographs are obtained. Acquisition of the latter requires superimposition of the humeral epicondyles to display the joint space at a perpendicular to the humerus. Oblique projections are occasionally needed for injuries such as subtle radial head fractures, but these are not routine. However, if standard projections are not obtainable due to the child's pain, and obliques are all that are available, it may be helpful to radiograph the contralateral elbow in the same position. As much of the joint is cartilaginous in young children, allowance must be made for this when assessing the alignment of the humerus and forearm bones.

The lateral radiograph allows the presence or absence of a joint effusion to be investigated by its indirect effect upon fat pads lying anterior and posterior to the humeral metaphysis (Fig. 9.15). Although the anterior fat pad may be seen normally, if it is elevated, or if the fat in the olecranon fossa is at all visible, then an effusion is diagnosed and the suspicion of bony injury is increased. Although an elbow effusion may be due to an occult fracture, if a displaced epiphysis is excluded, other bony injuries are likely to be less serious and treated conservatively. A follow-up radiograph is rarely useful, and if it demonstrates a fracture, it is most often an undisplaced fracture of the radial head. In the elbow, as in all joints, if the capsule is ruptured then loss of fluid may negate the usual signs of effusion despite a serious injury.

The complexity of the elbow joint means that it is one of the most amenable to other forms of imaging when plain radiographs are insufficient. Ultrasound is especially useful in demonstrating unossified epiphyses which may be separated or dislocated from the underlying metaphysis.

Computed tomography may be used to clarify complex epiphyseal injuries, with 2D or even 3D reconstruction to aid treatment.

Magnetic resonance imaging combines the best features of both ultrasound and CT with excellent demonstration of non-ossified bone allied to its multiplanar capability, which is useful for evaluating complex fractures. A recent study (BELTRAN et al. 1994) showed MRI to be particularly useful in investigating fractures involving the non-ossified distal humeral epiphysis, with special reference to intra-articular extension; exclusion of this feature meant several patients were spared surgical intervention. In those patients who did have intra-articular extension, MRI allowed assessment of joint surface congruity, which is important as displacement of 2 mm or more often requires surgical treatment.

As the elbow may be fixed in flexion at the time of imaging, it is useful to use the humeral diaphysis as a fixed reference point for scanning in the axial, coronal and sagittal planes, from which malalignment of the distal fracture fragments may be judged.

9.5.3.3
Fractures of the Distal Humerus and Elbow

In infants whose elbow epiphyses have not yet ossified, the diagnosis of a transphyseal injury can be difficult and the posterior displacement of the non-ossified distal humeral fragment may lead to an erroneous diagnosis of elbow dislocation. However, signs of the correct diagnosis are available on the plain film, such as posteromedial displacement of the normally related proximal forearm bones with respect to the distal humerus or an associated distal humeral metaphyseal fragment. If doubt remains, ultrasound can accurately assess displacement of the non-ossified distal humeral epiphysis (WELK and ADLER 1992), as can MRI (Fig. 9.16). MRI has the further advantage of distinguishing Salter-Harris 2 from Salter Harris 4 epiphyseal fractures; this is important, as the latter may require operative reduction and fixation if displaced by more than 2 mm. Optimal MRI techniques are T1-weighted and gradient-echo sequences obtained in the coronal and sagittal planes.

It should be noted that transphyseal injury has an association with abuse in infants and toddlers (NIMKIN et al. 1995).

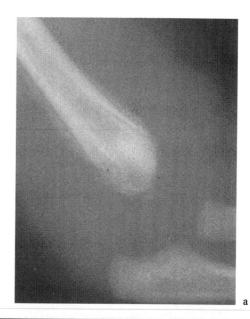

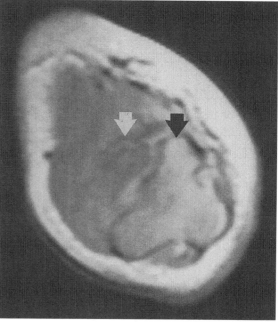

Fig. 9.16. a Lateral radiograph and **b** axial MR (TR 1800 TE 25) scan of fracture through distal humeral physis in a neonate. The MR scan demonstrates posterior displacement of the wholly cartilaginous epiphysis (*black arrow*) with respect to the metaphysis (*white arrow*)

Supracondylar fractures in children result from a fall onto an outstretched hand and the peak incidence is at around 8 years. The fracture line is commonly transverse and passes just proximal to the bony masses of the capitellum and trochlea with the distal fragment usually displaced posteriorly. Brachial artery damage occurs with displaced fractures.

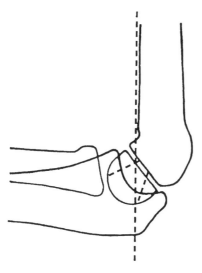

Fig. 9.17. The anterior cortical line of the distal humerus

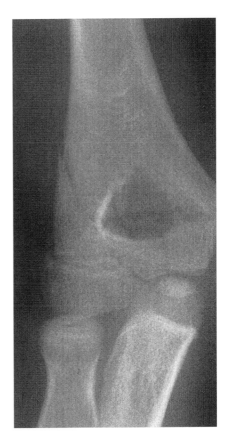

Fig. 9.19. Complex fracture of the distal humerus with inferior extension toward the elbow joint

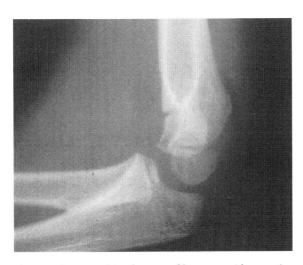

Fig. 9.18. Supracondylar fracture of humerus with posterior displacement of the capitellum and joint effusion

Undisplaced or minimally displaced fractures may be subtle on plain radiographs, with only minor cortical irregularity visible. The fracture becomes more obvious as displacement increases, and on the lateral view a line drawn along the anterior cortex of the distal humerus should bisect the middle third of the capitellum (Fig. 9.17). If it does not, there is a supracondylar fracture (Fig. 9.18). Check radiographs are important to ensure a good result if an angulated or displaced fracture is manipulated.

The initial radiograph may reveal a less common variant of the standard injury (Fig. 9.19). This frac-

ture has an additional transcondylar component running distally and encroaching upon the humeral articular surface. These fractures are difficult to diagnose and treat in young children and will need reduction and pinning, involving an open operation if there is significant displacement. If the transcondylar fracture is missed, mal- or non-union of the humeral condyle may occur (BEATY and KASSER 1995).

Fractures of the condyles and epicondyles of the distal humerus are also seen in children. Fracture of the lateral condyle (Fig. 9.20) frequently involves the capitellum, part of the adjacent trochlea and an associated bony fragment from the lateral aspect of the distal humeral metaphysis. In young children, where the capitellar epiphysis may be the only one ossified, the full extent of such an injury may not be appreciated; scrutiny of its relationship to the distal humeral metaphysis may alert the radiologist to the true situation.

Fractures of the medial condyle are uncommon in children and when they do occur they may be missed due to non-ossification of the trochlea or misdiag-

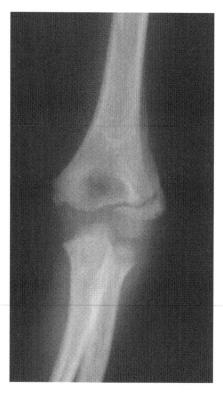

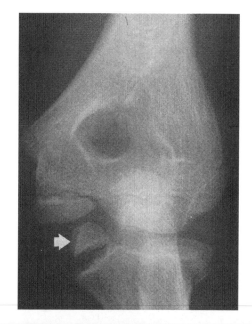

a

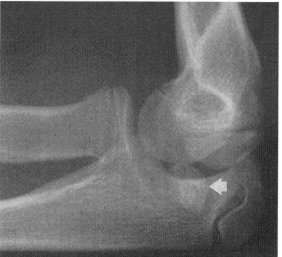

b

Fig. 9.20. Healing fracture of the lateral condyle of the distal humerus

nosed as epicondylar fractures. If plain radiographs are unhelpful, MRI can be used to pursue the diagnosis. The fracture is important; if the vascular supply to the trochlea is damaged, it may subsequently undergo avascular necrosis.

Avulsion of the medial epicondyle occurs more frequently and ranges from minor separation to major displacement. A serious complication of the latter is entrapment of the avulsed epicondyle within the elbow joint (Fig. 9.21) during dislocation, although the latter may have reduced spontaneously prior to radiography.

If the child has an ossified epiphysis, a careful check of its position must be made on the plain radiographs, both AP and lateral, to ensure it is not intra-articular. Symptoms referable to the area may also be caused by a chronic traction injury of the medial epicondyle "little leaguer's elbow". Lateral epicondylar avulsions can also occur but a trapped intra-articular fragment is uncommon with this injury.

The elbow joint is the most commonly dislocated in childhood (ASHER 1976), the usual pattern being displacement of the radius and ulna posterolaterally with respect to the distal humerus due to a fall on the outstretched arm. The humeroradial joint may dislo-

Fig. 9.21. a Frontal and **b** lateral radiographs demonstrating intra-articular entrapment of an avulsed medial epicondyle (*arrow*) following reduction of elbow dislocation

cate alone, with tearing of the lateral collateral ligament, or both forearm bones may dislocate with regard to the humerus and the medial collateral ligament is also torn. Post-reduction views are especially important in this situation due to associated fractures of the medial epicondyle, which may be the source of an intra-articular bone fragment. Neurovascular injuries can occur in association with elbow dislocation, as can heterotopic bone formation, contractures and ankylosis (KARASICK et al. 1991).

Pulled elbow occurs after a sudden pull on the extended, pronated arm of a young child and is most likely due to momentary separation of the radiocapitellar joint followed by interposition of part of the anterior joint capsule. The usual finding on plain radiographs is a pronated oblique view instead of a standard lateral elbow as the child will not allow supination, although the latter subsequently forms part of the reduction manoeuvre. In pulled elbow the oblique radiograph should be otherwise normal and the capitellum and radius normally aligned (BRETLAND 1994).

9.5.4
Injuries of the Forearm Bones

Fractures of the olecranon may be transphyseal, metaphyseal or combined. These injuries are all uncommon and may occur either in isolation or in association with a radial neck fracture when a valgus force is applied to an extended elbow (DORMANS and RANG 1990). Sometimes the growth plate of the olecranon can be confused with a fracture line and the epiphysis may be bipartite. Fusion occurs at 16–20 years of age.

A fragmented and ragged appearance of the olecranon epiphysis may indicate a stress injury in young gymnasts and is often accompanied by growth plate widening.

Fractures of the proximal radius usually occur in the metaphysis or radial neck in children, at the insertion of the annular ligament. These are most often Salter-Harris type 1 or 2 lesions, and in young children there may be confusion with radiohumeral dislocation as a cartilaginous radial head remains congruous with the capitellum whilst the bony metaphysis is displaced. Such radiographic confusion may be reduced by the use of ultrasound or MRI. These injuries are accompanied by other elbow fractures, most commonly of the olecranon, in approximately 50% of cases.

The shafts of the radius and ulna may break either together or alone. In the latter instance it is most important that the radiologist searches for an associated dislocation affecting the non-fractured forearm bone, as the shortening of its partner puts it under much stress. To this end, adequate views of the wrist and elbow joints must be obtained and congruity of the radiocapitellar and distal radioulnar joints confirmed. In the case of the former, a line drawn along the axis of the proximal radius should bisect the capitellum, whatever the plane of the radiograph.

A Monteggia injury occurs when there is an ulnar fracture associated with dislocation of the radial head (Fig. 9.22). The radial head usually dislocates anteriorly, although posterior and lateral displacements also occur. The injury is less common in children than adults (GLEESON and BEATTIE 1994) but its recognition is crucial as an unreduced radial head dislocation can lead to impaired elbow movements, nerve palsies and degenerative arthritis. Rarely, radial head dislocation can accompany fractures of both forearm bones.

In the Galeazzi injury the radial shaft is fractured and this is associated with dislocation of the distal radio-ulnar joint (Fig. 9.23). It should be noted that

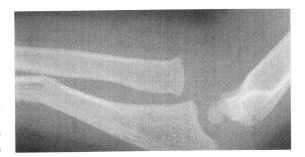

Fig. 9.22. Monteggia fracture dislocation

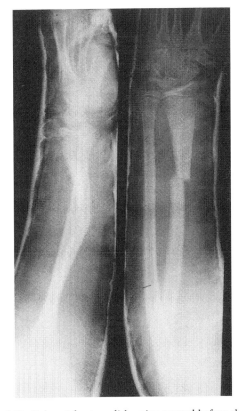

Fig. 9.23. Galeazzi fracture dislocation treated before abnormality of distal radioulnar joint was recognised

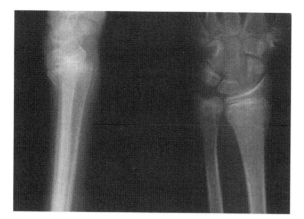

Fig. 9.24. Salter-Harris type 2 epiphyseal injury of the distal radius

greenstick or bowing fractures can also produce these patterns of injury.

Fractures of both forearm bones, without dislocation, occur more commonly. In young children these are most commonly greenstick injuries, with the intact periosteum on the unbroken side acting like a hinge. The median nerve can occasionally become entrapped in forearm fractures, and radiological markers have been noted in the few cases reported. In a patient with appropriate symptoms and signs a bony canal on the anterior surface of a bone is suggestive, as is incongruent reduction of a previous fracture (AL-QUATTAN et al. 1994).

Greenstick injuries of the distal forearm bones are usually detectable on plain radiographs, although elevation of the pronator quadratus fat pad may not occur as a supportive sign (ZAMMIT-MAEMPEL et al. 1988). Another common fracture of children's wrists is the Salter-Harris type 2 separation of the distal radial epiphysis (Fig. 9.24). Although fractures of the distal radius may often be accompanied by fractures of the distal ulna or its styloid, isolated distal ulnar fractures are uncommon. For this reason, if a radiograph shows an apparently isolated ulnar fracture, a very careful search for an associated radial injury must be made, especially in the case of ulnar styloid fractures, which virtually never occur alone (STANSBERRY et al. 1990).

Dislocation of the distal radio-ulnar joint may occur as part of the Galeazzi fracture, but can occur in isolation, with the ulna displaced to either the volar or dorsal aspect of the radius. Good lateral radiographs of the wrist are essential to evaluate such injuries, and a careful search must be made for an associated radial shaft fracture. CT may be required to confirm the dislocation.

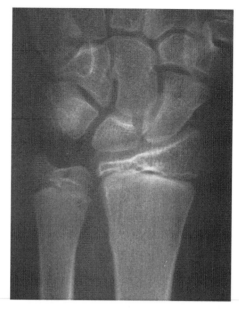

Fig. 9.25. Fracture of the distal pole of the scaphoid (and buckle fracture of radial diaphysis)

9.5.5
Fractures of the Carpus and Hand

Carpal fractures are far less common in children than in adults, but they do occur. As in adults the scaphoid is the most commonly fractured bone (SIMMONS and LAVALLO 1988) and initial evaluation should be with a standard radiographic series. Scaphoid fractures occur in adolescents, but are extremely rare under 10 years of age. The distal third of the bone is most commonly involved in children (Fig. 9.25), and although non-union of fractures and avascular necrosis have been reported (CAPUTO et al. 1995), they are very uncommon. The traditional approach to follow-up imaging in patients with continuing symptoms and normal initial radiographs has been to re-x-ray the treated patient at 10 days, when the fracture line may have become visible. Scintigraphy may be used to pursue a suspected fracture even further (Fig. 9.26), but a significant number of positive scans will never be radiographically confirmed, leading to the possibility of overdiagnosis and overtreatment (TIEL-VAN BUUL et al. 1993). Having said this, scintigraphy may demonstrate an unsuspected injury to another of the carpal bones, and thus explain a child's continuing pain.

Magnetic resonance imaging has been performed shortly after trauma presumed to involve the scaphoid. In a small series of skeletally immature patients, MRI detected three times the number of

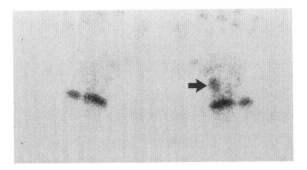

Fig. 9.26. Scintigraphic confirmation of left scaphoid fracture (*arrow*)

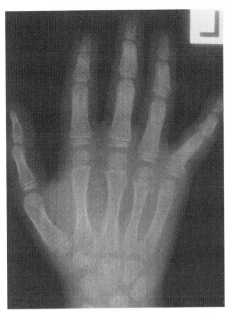

Fig. 9.27. Salter-Harris type 2 epiphyseal injury of the proximal phalanx of the little finger

fractures seen on initial radiographs, although all fractures later became apparent on delayed views (COOK et al. 1997). Perhaps more usefully, a normal MRI can exclude fracture soon after injury.

Marrow oedema in the scaphoid which has not progressed to fracture and extensor tenosynovitis may also be detected on MRI, both of which might explain symptoms in patients without fractures.

The triquetrum is the second most commonly fractured bone in the carpus, usually due to a fall on the outstretched hand causing a ligamentous avulsion or impingement of the ulna. A posterior flake may be visible on the lateral radiograph of the wrist but fractures of this partly cartilaginous bone during development may be subtle. Oblique views are advocated to pursue suspected fractures further, as a missed injury can lead to continued pain and fracture non-union (LETTS and ESSER 1993).

Fractures of other carpal bones and carpal and carpometacarpal dislocations are all very uncommon in children. Where unusual carpal fractures are suspected, but poorly visualised on plain radiographs, CT may help define injuries better. The most commonly affected carpometacarpal joint is that of the thumb. The Bennett fracture-dislocation occurs at this site and radiographs show a small fragment of bone remaining in contact with the adjacent trapezium whilst an oblique fracture, which reaches the joint surface, carries the rest of the thumb metacarpal proximally and laterally. This is equivalent to a Salter-Harris type 3 injury prior to growth plate fusion, where a fragment of the epiphysis is retained in place by the deep ulnar ligament.

However, fractures of the metacarpals do occur, particularly greenstick injuries, which often involve the neck of the little finger metacarpal. A Salter-Harris type 2 fracture may occur through the base of the thumb metacarpal. It must be remembered that other metacarpals, in particular that of the

index finger, can have accessory ossification centres at their bases whose growth plates may mimic fractures.

Dorsal dislocation of the metacarpophalangeal joint of the thumb is the commonest dislocation in children's hands, and as in all dislocations, a careful search must be made for any associated fracture on pre- and post-reduction films. A more significant injury of this joint is rupture of the ulnar collateral ligament due to excessive radial force. In children this often causes avulsion of a bony fragment from the base of the proximal phalanx, usually giving a Salter-Harris type 2 fracture in those aged 5–11 years and a type 3 or 4 fracture in adolescents. The tendency towards fracture rather than ligamentous injury in children means stress views are rarely needed.

Dislocations of the other metacarpophalangeal joints are almost always posterior, and the index finger is most commonly affected. There may be associated interposition of the volar plate, which will prevent closed reduction.

The Salter-Harris type 2 fracture at the base of the proximal phalanx of the little finger is the commonest fracture of all in children's hands (Fig. 9.27). Subtle greenstick or buckle fractures in this region are frequently missed on plain radiographs, and special attention should be paid to this area when the little finger is injured.

Fractures of the shafts of the proximal and middle phalanges of the digits are less common than in

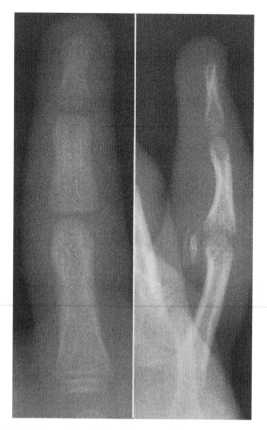

Fig. 9.28. Frontal and lateral views of epiphyseal avulsion affecting middle phalanx of ring finger. Note the avulsed fragment is invisible on the AP view, but the epiphysis is missing

adults, but fractures of the necks of these bones are commoner, and are often accompanied by rotation of the distal fragment, which will need correction. Significant injuries may traverse the condyles of these bones with intra-articular extension and good quality radiographs must be obtained to ensure that such injuries are not missed as they will need at the least immobilisation and possibly internal fixation.

Epiphyseal displacement occurs from the bases of both middle and distal phalanges and may be missed on inadequate radiographs as the avulsed fragment is obscured (Fig. 9.28). To avoid missing such injuries, good AP and lateral views of the involved digit must be obtained and the radiologist must account for all the ossified phalangeal epiphyses. If one is "missing", this fact should not be passed over, and instead a careful search should be made for an avulsed epiphysis. It is good practice to radiograph just the affected digit, as this minimises radiation exposure and concentrates the mind upon the affected area.

In both request and report, the digits of the hand should be referred to by name to avoid any confusion as to which is involved.

Dorsal dislocations of the proximal and distal interphalangeal joints occur and may be reduced prior to the patient attending the Accident and Emergency Department. Radiographs should be obtained in such cases to exclude underlying fracture, even if the patient has good joint movement.

Fractures of the distal phalanges are often painful, but relatively unimportant injuries, and the treatment of associated soft tissue damage frequently takes precedence (McRae 1981). Forced flexion at the distal interphalangeal joint in an extended finger can result in a "mallet finger" due to avulsion of the long extensor tendon. Although the injury is readily diagnosed clinically, radiographs should be obtained as a bone fragment is avulsed in some cases, leading to a Salter-Harris type 3 injury, although its initial management does not differ from that of injury to the tendon alone.

9.6
Injuries to the Pelvis and Lower Limb

9.6.1
Pelvic Fractures

Children's pelvic fractures encompass a wide range of severity, from avulsion injuries to major disruptions of the pelvic ring and, excepting the avulsions, they are uncommon. As the result of a large series reported from Toronto, a four type classification was suggested (Torode and Zieg 1985). Type 1 pelvic fractures comprised avulsion injuries, whilst type 2 were isolated fractures of the iliac wing. Fractures of the pelvic ring were subdivided into types 3 and 4, the former being simple ring fractures and the latter ring disruptions. Not surprisingly, the outcome was worse in higher stage injuries, and patients with ring disruption have the highest incidence of long-term morbidity (Garvin et al. 1990).

Avulsion injuries may be acute or chronic and usually occur in adolescents as a result of sporting activity. The chronic lesions are due to repetitive traction on a developing apophysis whilst acute injuries follow sudden contraction of an attached muscle. The hamstrings and adductors are attached to the ischial tuberosity and this is the most commonly affected area (Fig. 9.29). Sartorius and the straight head of Rectus femoris are attached to the anterior superior and anterior inferior iliac

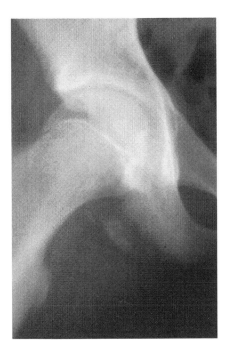

Fig. 9.29. Avulsion injury of the ischial tuberosity

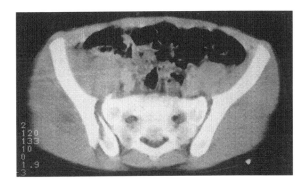

Fig. 9.30. CT scan demonstrating fracture of the right ilium with extension into the sacro-iliac joint

spines. These, too, are areas where avulsions may occur.

Most acute avulsion injuries will be shown on a standard AP pelvic radiograph although anterior inferior iliac spine injuries may need an additional oblique view. Chronic injuries may be subtle, especially when in the region of the ischial tuberosity, and areas of radiolucency with periosteal reaction may be mistaken for lesions such as Ewing's sarcoma (SUNDAR and CARTY 1994). On the other hand, these injuries may be impressively florid, mimicking bone-forming tumours such as osteogenic sarcoma. Familiarity with the appearances of these lesions and an appropriate history are important factors in making the correct diagnosis.

Fractures grouped within types 2–4 most commonly occur when children are pedestrians struck by a car. Interestingly, pelvic fractures in children are far less common than in adults following falls from a height (ROSHKOW et al. 1990). Major trauma protocols include a pelvic radiograph as part of an initial series, but in this specific situation in children it is recommended that the need for pelvic radiographs is assessed on a case-by-case basis. In isolated fractures of the iliac wing, associated soft tissue injuries are less common than in types 3 and 4 and the prognosis is good. As with type 1 injuries, plain radiographs are usually sufficient to define the bony lesion, although further imaging such as ultrasound or CT (Fig. 9.30) may be required to investigate suspected soft

tissue or visceral damage. CT has the further advantage of demonstrating the haematoma and extent of bleeding.

The type 3 group includes patients with pubic symphysis disruption and fractures of the pubic rami. Wide diastasis of the pubic symphysis can occur to approximately 2.5 cm without sacro-iliac joint instability, possibly due to the elasticity of the child's pelvis. Nevertheless, prior to diagnosing an isolated fracture of the pelvic ring, a careful search must be made for a second injury.

When the pelvic ring is fractured in two places and an unstable segment results, the patient falls into the most severely injured group, type 4. These injuries include bilateral fractures of the pubic rami, fractures involving both anterior and posterior elements, and fractures of the anterior structures and acetabular part of the ring.

Abdominal and genito-urinary injuries are far more common in association with type 3 and 4 fractures. Intrapelvic and retroperitoneal haematomas were the commonest local association in a recent series, and haemorrhage the commonest cause of death (RIEGER and BRUG 1997). There was also a significant incidence of urethral injury and rectal and vaginal tears, and to a lesser extent, bladder rupture. Although haematuria may often occur without significant urinary tract injury, further signs suggestive of urethral trauma in males should be investigated with a urethrogram prior to any attempt at catheterisation. Damage to the posterior urethra is usually associated with fractures of the pubic bones or major diastasis of the symphysis. Lacerations of the liver and spleen are the commonest associated abdominal injuries.

Plain radiography is the initial investigation in these patients. Work in adults has shown that the causative force and extent of ring fractures can usually be accurately assessed on an AP pelvic radiograph (YOUNG et al. 1986). In YOUNG et al.'s series, pelvic ring fractures were subdivided by causation into AP compression, lateral compression, vertical shear and complex fractures. AP compression caused vertically orientated fractures of the pubic rami or diastasis of the symphysis pubis associated with varying degrees of sacro-iliac joint damage. Lateral compression was associated with horizontal fractures of the pubic rami, sacral fractures and lesser numbers of iliac wing fractures and central dislocations of the hip.

Vertical shearing forces cause the sacrum to be forced down between the iliac wings, with varying numbers of associated vertically orientated fractures. Complex injuries were those in which at least two different forces had been applied.

In many cases, therefore, the fracture patterns demonstrated on plain radiography with their implied causative forces will guide appropriate realignment; nevertheless, many patients will proceed to CT, either to better define bony injury or to investigate suspected visceral trauma or both. CT allows fracture patterns to be more clearly defined than on plain radiographs, gives better definition of the state of the pelvic ring and helps surgical planning. It is particularly useful in assessment of the sacrum and sacro-iliac joints, areas in which plain radiography is at is weakest (KESHISHYAN et al. 1995). It is essential that the scan is viewed using both bone and soft tissue windows, and intravenous contrast injection is an important adjunct for examination of the viscera.

Two-dimensional CT may be performed using 5-mm contiguous axial slices through the affected part of the pelvic ring, but 3D reconstructions require thinner (3-mm) overlapping slices. Although the latter are associated with a higher radiation dose to the pelvis, in both 2D and 3D work the mAs can be significantly reduced without compromising the effectiveness of the study. In a series of children undergoing CT for pelvic or acetabular trauma, 2D and 3D reformatting was useful in significant numbers in improving fracture definition, guiding management and selecting an operative approach and hardware (MAGID et al. 1992). However, it would not be necessary to go to such lengths in stable patients or those with simple injuries to the symphysis or anterior ring.

Stable patients with type 3 or 4 fractures who do not undergo CT should have the abdominal and pelvic viscera examined sonographically. Portable ultrasound also provides a quick means of detecting intraperitoneal free fluid or major visceral injury whilst a child is being resuscitated in the Accident and Emergency Department.

It has been shown that children with additional bony injuries besides their pelvic fracture have an increased likelihood of head and abdominal trauma (VAZQUEZ and GARCIA 1993). This should be borne in mind when imaging studies are planned, and if CT of the pelvis is undertaken, consideration should be given to scanning the head or abdomen at the same visit, if there is clinical suspicion of further injury elsewhere. Thoracic trauma also occurs in a significant number of children with pelvic fractures (18.5% in the series reported by RIEGER and BRUG in 1997).

9.6.2
Injuries to the Hip and Proximal Femur

Acetabular fractures are rare in children, but an important difference from adults is the potential for damage to the triradiate cartilage and subsequent growth disturbance. A plain AP pelvic radiograph is the usual imaging starting point, but further imaging should be by CT, rendering multiple radiographic projections redundant. Protocols are similar to those applied in the pelvis. The major advantages are direct visualisation of cartilage, delineation of complex fracture lines and localisation of intra-articular fragments (Fig. 9.31).

Many children with acetabular fractures will have an associated hip dislocation; most such cases comprise posterior dislocations, but central dislocations also occur, as do anterior and rarely obturator dislocations. Prompt recognition of hip dislocation is important as reduction delayed beyond 24h increases the risk of subsequent avascular necrosis of the

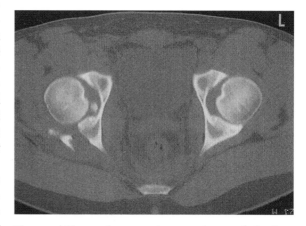

Fig. 9.31. CT scan demonstrating posterior acetabular fracture of right hip with intra-articular bone fragment

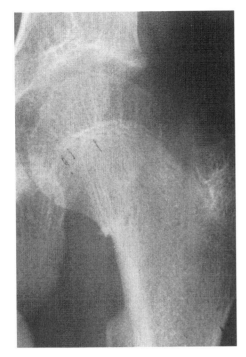

Fig. 9.32. Transcervical fracture of the femoral neck

femoral capital epiphysis. Other complications include an associated chondral or osteochondral fracture fragment preventing satisfactory reduction of the femoral head into the acetabulum, recurrent dislocation, progressive subluxation and heterotopic ossification (HEEG et al. 1989; MOSELEY 1992). A careful search for associated fractures must be made on the initial radiographs, particularly of the femur and pelvis, and also the patella if an anterior impact has forced the femur backwards.

Fractures of the femoral head and neck account for under 1% of all paediatric fractures and their incidence in children is less than 1% of that in adults. Proximal femoral fractures have been subdivided into five groups based upon their location: through the growth plate (type 1), transcervical fractures (type 2) (Fig. 9.32), basal (type 3), intertrochanteric (type 4) and, finally, subtrochanteric (type 5) injuries (AZOUZ et al. 1993).

The child's special osseous and vascular anatomy in this region mean that these uncommon fractures are associated with significant complications such as avascular necrosis, premature growth plate fusion, varus deformity and non-union. Generally, these complications are more frequent and more serious than in adults. Scintigraphy provides a means of diagnosing avascular necrosis at an early stage, thus enabling an accurate prognosis to be given.

Type 1 injuries are defined as an acute traumatic separation of a previously normal epiphysis and although the least common of the group, have the highest rate of complications (HUGHES and BEATY 1994). This fracture may or may not be accompanied by dislocation of the femoral head from the acetabulum. In young children significant trauma is needed to produce this injury, and it may also be seen in neonates with birth trauma secondary to a breech or foot presentation. Children with systemic conditions such as chronic renal failure and myelodysplasia are also prone to this injury, which is distinct from the gradual slip of the femoral capital epiphysis occurring in adolescence.

As in all femoral neck fractures, initial imaging of the type 1 injury should include both AP and lateral views of the affected hip. This allows assessment of the position of the femoral capital epiphysis from front to back as well as side to side and judgement of any growth plate disruption, although fracture displacement is often gross and easy to see. In neonates, ultrasound may be used as an adjunct in suspected birth injury where differentiation from a congenital hip dislocation may be difficult on a plain radiograph alone.

The transcervical and basal femoral neck fractures comprise the commonest and next commonest respectively. They generally have a good prognosis if non-displaced, although displacement leads to a significant increase in subsequent avascular necrosis. The fewest complications are seen with fracture types 4 and 5.

If there is no history of injury, or a history of insignificant trauma, insufficiency fractures due to generalised bone weakening and pathological fractures due to localised bone abnormalities must be considered. In the latter situation, unicameral bone cysts, fibrous dysplasia and underlying malignancies cause significant numbers of pathological fractures.

9.6.3
Fractures of the Mid and Distal Femur

Femoral fractures are seen as birth injuries in breech babies delivered vaginally, and in rare cases, in breech babies delivered by Caesarian section. These may occur in the midshaft, but distal metaphyseal fractures have also been reported in breech babies delivered by section (VASA and KIM 1990).

Fractures of the femoral diaphysis in children are common, and usually easily diagnosed on plain

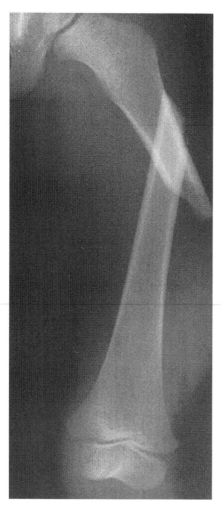

Fig. 9.33. Femoral fracture demonstrating angulation and overlap due to pull of surrounding muscles

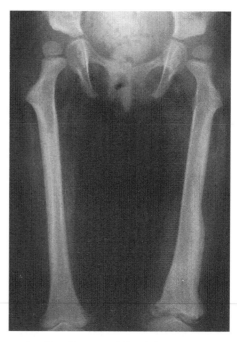

Fig. 9.34. Healing fracture of distal femur in a child with myelomeningocele

radiographs provided two views are obtained at right angles. The pull of surrounding muscle frequently causes overlap of fracture ends and associated angulation (Fig. 9.33). In older children, major trauma such as occurs in road traffic accidents is often the cause of femoral fracture, whilst in younger children lesser forces may be sufficient to produce the injury. Oblique or spiral femoral fractures are the result of twisting forces whilst a transverse fracture may be caused by a direct blow. Stress fractures may also occur in the shaft and neck of the femur in children, although they are uncommon. Those in the femoral diaphysis may occur at any site, and run a greater risk of displacement than those occurring in children's femoral necks. They can present as hip, thigh or knee pain, and may be misdiagnosed as bone tumours on initial plain radiographs (MEANEY and CARTY 1992).

The fracture line may or may not be visible; if it is not, plain radiographic features pointing to the cor-rect diagnosis are an absence of cortical bone destruction and an uninterrupted periosteal reaction which is localised to the bone cortex traversed by the stress fracture. The diagnosis is supported by a sharply defined area of increased activity on bone scintigraphy and no soft tissue mass on either CT or MRI, although the latter investigations may be reserved for cases where plain radiographs and isotopes have not proved diagnostic. Delayed radiographs should be obtained at an interval of 2–3 weeks to look for evidence of repair and ensure there is no evidence of cortical destruction, which would require biopsy.

A common variant which may cause confusion on imaging studies is minor avulsion produced by the pull of the adductor insertions upon the medial aspect of the distal femoral metaphysis. The affected area may show cortical irregularity and be confused with malignancy. It is important that this phenomenon is recognised and in common with suspected stress fractures not biopsied, as active callus formation may be very difficult to distinguish from bone tumour pathologically.

Distal femoral metaphyseal injuries (supracondylar fractures) are uncommon in young children but may occur in metabolic bone disease or neurological conditions such as myelomeningocele (Fig. 9.34). Children with these underlying abnormalities may also present with impaction fractures, e.g. of the proximal tibia.

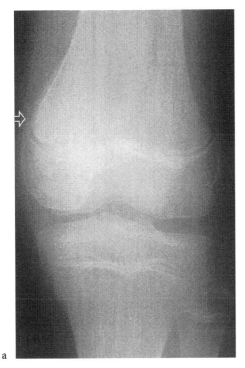
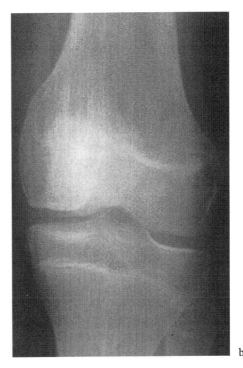

Fig. 9.35. a Healing fracture of medial aspect of distal femur involving the growth plate (*arrow*). **b** A delayed radiograph demonstrates premature fusion of the epiphysis consequent upon the injury

Displaced supracondylar fractures occur as a result of significant trauma such as motor accidents, and angulation of the distal fragment may occur secondary to the pull of posterior musculature.

Ossification is visible in the distal femoral epiphysis at term, and the associated physis is the largest and fastest growing in the body, making the greatest contribution to the eventual length of the femur. Although injuries to this area are relatively uncommon, they are important with regard to complications such as angulation and leg length discrepancy which may follow damage to the growth plate (Fig. 9.35).

Although the commonest injury is the Salter-Harris type 2, the classification does not always provide an accurate guide to the likelihood of subsequent problems and other factors such as young age, greater trauma or displacement and inadequate reduction may increase the risk (BEATY and KUMAR 1994). Plain radiographs may demonstrate a triangular fragment of metaphyseal bone (Thurston-Holland sign) associated with Salter-Harris type 2 fractures, and may also show fracture lines traversing the partly ossified epiphysis.

Compression injuries are suggested by a decrease in the normal width of the growth plate, usually 3–5 mm until the age of 8–10 years. This provides a good example of when a comparison view may prove useful.

Further imaging may grade fractures of these partly ossified regions more accurately. A case report regarding a Salter-Harris type 4 fracture of the distal femoral epiphysis in a 9-year-old showed that both CT and MRI could be used in a complementary fashion to pursue initial plain radiographic findings. Five-millimetre axial CT slices were used to identify separated bony fragments whilst MRI demonstrated significant chondral (Fig. 9.36) and meniscal injury. Gradient-echo imaging was particularly good at demonstrating fracture lines (WHITE et al. 1994). These modalities may also be used to pursue physeal bars in children who develop growth arrest or angulation as a consequence of their fractures.

9.6.4
Injuries Around the Knee

9.6.4.1
Fractures Around the Knee

The knee will be discussed in three sections, namely fractures, ligamentous and cartilaginous injuries, and patellar lesions. There is much overlap in the imaging appearances, which may reflect injury to both bone and associated soft tissues.

The distal femoral and proximal tibial epiphyses may remain unfused until the late teens, as may the

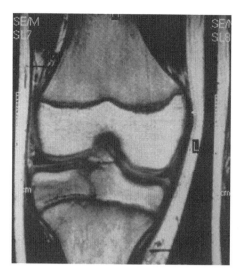

Fig. 9.36. Coronal T1-weighted MR scan showing an osteochondral fracture of the proximal tibial epiphysis

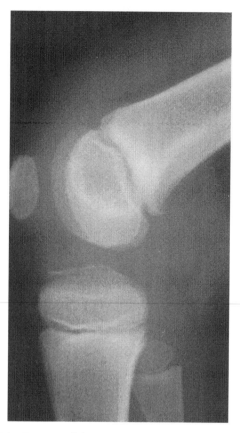

Fig. 9.37. Fracture of the anterior tibial spine (not visible on AP view)

tibial tuberosity prior to its fusion with the proximal tibial epiphysis. The standard radiographic series consists of AP and lateral projections of the joint, and it is uncommon to require further plain radiographs in children. A joint effusion may be demonstrated as an oval soft tissue density immediately posterosuperior to the upper pole of the patella on the lateral radiograph, reflecting increased fluid within the suprapatellar pouch. Occasionally a horizontal beam lateral view will demonstrate the fat-fluid level of a lipohaemarthrosis at the same location, due to an underlying fracture.

If the history of knee trauma is uncertain, and imaging negative, referred pain from the hip should be considered.

Fractures of the anterior intercondylar eminence of the tibia are functionally similar to disruption of the partly attached anterior cruciate ligament, but the former is the commoner of the two in children, usually following a hyperextension injury (EL-KHOURY et al. 1997). The fracture has been graded into three types by Meyers and McKeever, from non-displaced (type 1), to elevation with a posterior hinge (type 2) and, finally, displaced and even rotated (type 3). The distinction matters, as irreducible type 2 fractures and all type 3 injuries require operative fixation (BEATY and KUMAR 1994).

The radiographic abnormalities may be subtle, with just a small displaced calcific fragment on the lateral view (Fig. 9.37) reflecting disruption of underlying epiphyseal cartilage. The lesion may be missed on the AP radiograph as the knee is flexed. A tunnel view may help if the injury is suspected clinically, yet

not shown on AP or lateral projections. A more definite diagnosis may be made using MRI.

Fractures of the main proximal tibial epiphysis account for only 3% of lower extremity epiphyseal injuries, owing to a paucity of ligamentous attachments. The usual pattern of injury is a hyperextension force which displaces the tibial metaphysis posteriorly. A Salter-Harris type 2 fracture is the most common type of injury and if there is little displacement, it may be difficult to appreciate on plain radiographs. A small fleck of bone adjacent to the metaphysis may aid diagnosis. MRI may prove useful in difficult cases, rather than the previously advocated stress radiographs, and is certainly kinder in a child who is in pain.

As in injuries to the distal femoral growth plate, the commonest complications are angular deformity and limb length discrepancy, although displaced fractures have the additional risk of damaging the relatively fixed popliteal artery, which lies close to the tibial epiphysis.

Avulsion of the tibial tuberosity is an uncommon injury most often seen in male adolescents, and usually occurs whilst jumping or playing sport. This injury is differentiated radiographically from Osgood-Schlatter's disease by some authors who state that the latter does not involve the physis (OGDEN et al. 1980), whilst others suggest a closer association between the two conditions. It is widely agreed that the chronic condition results from micro-avulsions caused by repeated traction injuries to the tibial tuberosity.

The lateral radiograph provides a guide to the size and displacement of the avulsed fragment, although it should be noted that the normal epiphysis can appear irregular. Proximal displacement of the patella may also be seen, depending on the position of the tibial tuberosity.

Severe trauma may result in the uncommon "floating knee injury", where the joint is flail due to fractures of the femoral and tibial shafts above and below it. These are commonly accompanied by other injuries.

Major trauma may also cause knee joint dislocation, although this is rare in children as such force will usually cause a displaced fracture of the unfused distal femoral epiphysis (GORTLAND and BENNER 1976). Dislocation may lead to the tibia being displaced laterally, medially, posteriorly or, most commonly, anteriorly. These injuries usually result in disruption of the cruciate ligaments, and damage to the popliteal artery and peroneal nerve can also occur. Dislocation will be obvious on plain radiographs, although some will be reduced at the site of the accident. Angiography is required if there is any suggestion of vascular injury, as its repair will take precedence over all else.

9.6.4.2
Injuries to the Knee Ligaments and Menisci

In contrast to the majority of the injuries discussed in the previous section, trauma to the ligaments and menisci is best imaged using MRI, although indirect signs of such injuries visible on plain radiographs may still prove useful.

In two major studies of MRI of the traumatised paediatric knee, injuries of the medial meniscus were shown to be the commonest lesions, followed by those of the lateral meniscus, which in turn were commoner than tears of the anterior cruciate ligament (ZOBEL et al. 1994; KING et al. 1996). Tears of the menisci are significantly less common than in adults. Both studies noted a variety of injuries associated with medial meniscal lesions and anterior

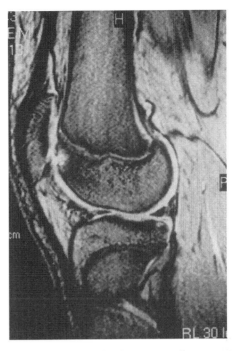

Fig. 9.38. Sagittal T2-weighted MR scan of post-traumatic osteochondritis dissecans in an unusual post-patella location with surrounding resolving bone bruise

cruciate ligament tears, but only the earlier study found associated lesions with lateral meniscal injuries. However, both noted significant numbers of discoid lateral menisci when this area was traumatised. Posterior cruciate ligament injuries were restricted to a single case in each series. Associated injuries affecting the medial and lateral collateral ligaments and osteochondral fractures [including osteochondritis dissecans (Fig. 9.38)] were also detected, as was bone marrow oedema.

A recommended protocol in these circumstances would include sagittal and coronal T1-weighted images, coronal T2-weighted images and sagittal T2-weighted gradient-echo images with thin 3-mm slice thickness at a spacing of 1 mm. Intact ligaments usually have uniform low signal intensity, and definite tears show disruption or deformity and increased signal intensity (Fig. 9.39). Possible tears show as increased signal alone.

In the case of the menisci, a definite tear shows as high signal traversing the normal low signal to reach an articular surface, or meniscal deformity. Equivocal meniscal injuries are those in which there is high signal that does not definitely reach an articular surface, although such menisci are often found to be normal at arthroscopy. When KING et al. (1996) compared the meniscal findings at MRI with subse-

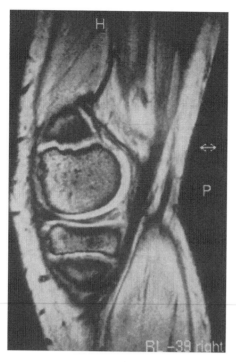

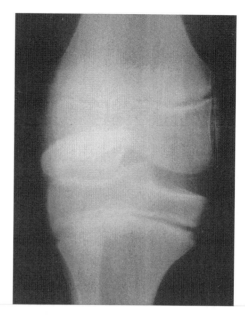

Fig. 9.40. Sleeve fracture with proximal displacement and rotation of the patella

Fig. 9.39. Sagittal T2-weighted MR scan demonstrating menisceal tear (lying posteriorly)

quent arthroscopy in 26 patients, a sensitivity of 100% and a specificity of 89% were quoted for tears if the equivocal menisci were regarded as positive. Using the same criteria, ZOBEL et al. (1994) also quoted sensitivities and specificities above 80% for meniscal tears.

Both of the aforementioned studies make the point that false-positive MRI findings tend to derive from the posterior horns of the menisci, and that intrasubstance tears not visible arthroscopically may also contribute to the false-positive rate.

An example of an injury with an associated useful plain radiographic sign is the Segond fracture, which, although primarily an adult occurrence, may also be seen in older children and adolescents. The plain radiograph reveals an avulsion fracture of a fragment of bone from the lateral aspect of the proximal tibia owing to the transmission of abnormal force through the lateral capsular ligament of the knee. Although the fracture itself is not significant, the plain radiographic finding must not be dismissed as the forces which cause it are associated in all cases with disruption of the anterior cruciate ligament and/or meniscal tears.

The true extent of the ligamentous injury is best revealed by MRI, although the Segond fracture may be seen in only a third of cases (WEBER et al. 1991). In all cases in the study by Weber et al., bone marrow oedema adjacent to the insertion of the lateral capsular ligament helped reveal the nature of the injury.

9.6.4.3
Injuries to the Patella

The patella is not visible on plain radiographs until it ossifies at approximately 5 years of age. Ossification can occur from more than one centre, leading to bipartite or an even more fragmented composition of the normal bone which may be confused with fracture. The additional ossification centres are located at the superolateral aspect of the patella and have smooth cortical margins. Multipartite patellae are often, but not always, bilateral.

Fractures of the patella in children are uncommon, and the majority are due to road traffic accidents. In a recently reported series (MAGUIRE and CANALE 1993) the main fracture types were comminuted (including stellate fractures) and transverse. Small chip fractures were a little less common, but occurred more often than vertical fractures. A rarer subgroup comprises "sleeve" fractures (Fig. 9.40), where hyperextension injury leads to avulsion of cartilage from the lower pole of the bone. These fractures may occur during sporting activity, owing to forceful contraction of the quadriceps muscle against a partly flexed knee joint. Such fractures are important, as a small bony avulsion and high patella seen on plain radiography may represent a far larger cartilaginous injury. Standard patellar fractures are generally visible on plain radiographs, with the addition of specialised patellar views if necessary.

The degree of displacement should be noted and may be underestimated if the radiograph is taken in extension. Many patellar injuries are due to road accidents, and a check for fractures of the ipsilateral femur and/or tibia should be made as nearly 20% of such patients will suffer these associated injuries.

A small series of sleeve fractures were evaluated using MRI (BATES et al. 1994), which allows direct visualisation of the avulsed cartilaginous fragment and assessment of displacement or intra-articular extension. Rupture of the inferior patellar tendon without bony injury, which also prevents extension of the knee joint, will also be revealed using this modality.

Dislocation of the patella is not unusual, may be recurrent and usually first occurs in adolescence. Risk factors predisposing to this injury include patella alta and a flatter than normal sulcus between the femoral condyles, which reduces their stabilising influence. It has been suggested that dysplasia of the femur's patellar surface may be related to patella alta, as the stimulus to develop a deep sulcus is not present. Direct ultrasonic measurements of the femoral articular cartilage have confirmed a flatter intercondylar sulcus in patients suffering from patellar dislocation compared with normal knees (NIETOSVARRA and AALTO 1997). The patellofemoral relationship and osseous intercondylar sulcus may also be assessed on a "skyline" radiograph.

The patella dislocates laterally, often whilst playing sport, and is frequently relocated prior to the patient attending hospital. The risk of associated osteochondral fractures is well known, but their incidence has been revised upwards to 39% in a recent series (NIETOSVARRA et al. 1994). These fractures were equally split between capsular avulsions of the medial patellar margin and intra-articular fracture fragments from the lateral femoral condyle and/or patella itself. They most likely occur when the patella relocates with the knee in flexion, and the medial patellar facet slides back over the lateral femoral condyle.

If the patella is still fully dislocated when the patient attends for plain radiographs, it will be vis-

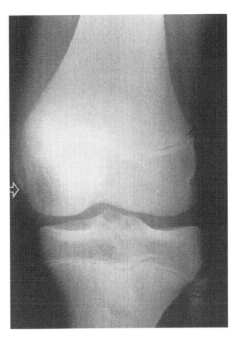

Fig. 9.41. Osteochondral fracture (*arrow*) due to previous patellar dislocation

ible on standard views of the knee. If the patella has relocated, a "skyline" view should be performed as this may reveal a fracture of the bone's medial aspect, in itself suggestive of a relocated dislocation. Although the radiographs may reveal an associated osteochondral fracture (Fig. 9.41), they may be subtle or purely chondral in nature. In such cases, either CT or MRI may be used to pursue them further.

9.6.5
Fractures of the Tibia and Fibula

Acute fracture of the proximal tibial metaphysis usually occurs secondary to rotatory and valgus stress and is most often seen in younger children. The commonest pattern of injury is a medial greenstick fracture with an intact fibula. The main complication of this injury occurs in the healing phase, when overgrowth of the medial part of the proximal tibia can cause persistent valgus deformity. Plain radiographs are used both to detect the initial injury and to monitor healing. In cases of more forceful trauma a further potential complication in this area is damage to the anterior tibial artery, which is fixed as it crosses the interosseous membrane.

In older children stress injuries of the tibia occur in relation to sporting activity, at the junction of either the middle and proximal or the middle and distal thirds of the bone. These lesions generally affect the posterior cortex, and as with stress injuries elsewhere, may be subtle on initial presentation. Their presence may be suspected clinically, and follow-up plain radiographs, scintigraphy or MRI may all be used to pursue the diagnosis.

The "toddler fracture" (Fig. 9.42) is an undisplaced oblique fracture of the distal tibia which presents in pre-school children as limping or refusal to bear weight. Initial radiographs may be negative, and if a history of trauma is difficult to obtain there may be confusion with other causes of limp, such as early osteomyelitis, should the child have a co-incident infection elsewhere. The diagnosis may become clear on a delayed radiograph as a periosteal reaction, callus or the fracture itself becomes visible. However, clinical anxiety may require earlier confirmation of the diagnosis, and scintigraphy is a useful method to pursue this. In toddler's fracture the bone scan shows increased activity over most or all of the affected tibia. This contrasts with the common differential diagnosis of osteomyelitis, which demonstrates a localised increase in activity, typically in the metaphysis (DE BOECK et al. 1991).

Fractures of the tibial diaphysis range from greenstick to displaced depending on the degree of trauma and may or may not be accompanied by a fibular fracture. They are assessed on plain radiographs, and apart from the valgus deformity, which can occur proximally due to overgrowth, are also prone to malalignment if angulation and rotation are not corrected. Although some malalignment may correct in younger children, this is less likely in adolescents, and since rotation will not realign it should be noted if seen on initial radiographs.

Pathological fractures also occur in the tibia, most commonly in the metaphyses secondary to solitary bone cysts. Other causes of pathological fracture which may be seen elsewhere include osteogenesis imperfecta and renal bone disease with associated brown tumour, although the latter is more commonly seen in primary hyperparathyroidism. A lesion which may be confused with a pathological fracture is a congenital pseudo-arthrosis of the tibia, especially in the absence of cutaneous evidence of neurofibromatosis. A clue may be obtained from the site of the lesion as pseudo-arthroses are most often seen at the junction of the mid and lower thirds of the bone. The fibula may also be involved (Fig. 9.43).

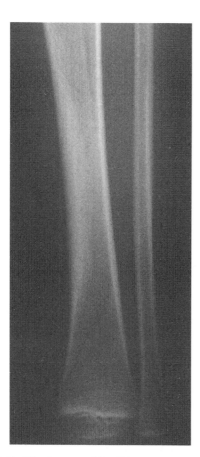

Fig. 9.42. Toddler fracture of the tibia

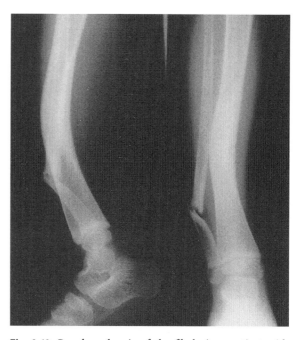

Fig. 9.43. Pseudo-arthrosis of the fibula in a patient with neurofibromatosis

Fractures of the fibula may occur in isolation due to direct trauma, but it may also break with the tibia, and a careful examination should be made of the latter before diagnosing an isolated fibular fracture on plain radiographs. The lateral collateral ligament of the knee joint is partly inserted into the head of the fibula, and isolated avulsion fractures can occur. However, this lesion can be confused with the more serious Segond fracture and the source of a laterally placed avulsion fragment should be confirmed on the plain radiograph if possible.

Fractures of the fibular neck have an association with those of the medial malleolus of the ankle as part of the Maisonneuve fracture. This injury is due to external rotation of the talus whilst the foot is everted or neutral, and is another reason for caution in diagnosing an isolated fibular fracture.

Stress injuries of the fibula also occur, usually in the lower third of the bone. In common with those of the tibia, they are typically secondary to sporting activity.

9.6.6
Ankle Injuries

Accessory ossicles are common at the ankle joint (Fig. 9.44) and can be confused with fractures in cases of trauma. In a recent series (CARTY 1992) more than 200 children's ankle radiographs were analysed and the incidence of accessory ossicles at each of the malleoli calculated at 5.2%. This represents an increase for the lateral malleolus compared with previous reports, and ossicles at both malleoli were noted to be commoner in boys. In plain radiographic assessment, errors are reduced by familiarity with these variants, checking of an ossicle's cortical edge for smoothness or irregularity, and in the case of the lateral malleolus, checking for a fibular groove into which an ossicle would fit. The latter is best seen on the lateral view of the ankle; this view also provides the best radiographic means of seeing a joint effusion, which presents as a soft tissue opacity immediately anterior to the joint. Further signs suggestive of an ossicle rather than a fracture are absence of soft tissue swelling over the malleolus and no periosteal reaction on delayed radiographs. It should also be noted that in adolescents the distal tibial and fibular physes close at approximately the same age, and if one is fused but the other not, the suspicion of an epiphyseal injury is raised (DAFFNER 1994).

The standard radiographic examination of the ankle consists of an anteroposterior view in ap-

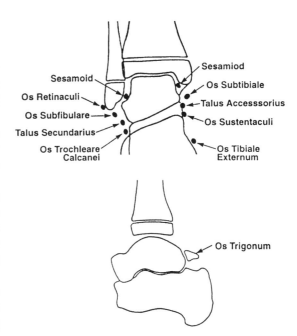

Fig. 9.44. Accessory ossicles of the ankle joint (frontal and lateral views)

proximately 20° of internal rotation to profile the ankle mortice and a "lateral" at right angles to this. Apart from checking for fracture lines and effusions, the symmetry of the talus between the malleoli should be noted, as should any talar tilt. The distance between the lateral border of the tibia and medial border of the fibula in a child should not greatly exceed 5 mm at the ankle. If it does, disruption of the inferior tibiofibular joint should be suspected.

Efforts have been made to reduce extremity radiographs in children felt unlikely to have fractures clinically, and in a recent series (CHANDE 1995) a set of decision rules were applied to radiography of children's ankle joints following trauma. The rules were derived from those applied in adults (Ottawa Ankle Rules), and led to radiographs only being obtained in those who had pain near the malleoli and either inability to bear weight immediately after the injury or bony tenderness at the posterior edge or tip of either malleolus. Application of these rules to 71 children led to fracture detection in 21% and no known missed fractures, whilst decreasing the radiographs ordered by 25%. Such rules may help decrease inappropriate examinations and radiation dose, but the sample was relatively small, and there was no follow-up information on those who were not radiographed.

Rules may provide useful guidance but cannot completely replace clinical acumen, and particularly in the case of injuries which may involve the growth plate, clinical suspicion should be pursued radiographically.

The predominant fractures found at the ankle in children are Salter-Harris type epiphyseal injuries and avulsions from the tip of the lateral malleolus, although the earlier comment with regard to accessory ossicles should be noted with respect to the latter. It should also be borne in mind that in the developing skeleton the physis is more likely to fail than ligaments. Two more extensive fractures tend to occur around the transitional period in which the distal tibial epiphysis fuses with the metaphysis, the first being the triplane fracture, which tends to occur earlier in this period than the second, the Tillaux fracture (ARMSTRONG 1992).

In the triplane fracture there is vertical fracture of the tibial epiphysis in the sagittal plane, horizontal fracture through the lateral part of the physis in the axial plane and an oblique coronal fracture through the metaphysis. On a frontal radiograph, appearances suggest a Salter-Harris type 3 fracture of the epiphysis (Fig. 9.45a), whilst the lateral radiograph resembles a type 2 injury because of the metaphyseal fracture (Fig. 9.45b).

Such confusion is highly suggestive of a triplane fracture, which overall accounts for 6% of all distal tibial epiphyseal injuries and is difficult to fit into a standard Salter-Harris classification. It tends to occur laterally, as this is often the last part of the distal tibial physis to fuse. Such an injury requires accurate anatomical reduction and CT (Fig. 9.46) with multiplanar reformatting is very useful to define the fracture anatomy completely prior to treatment

The Tillaux fracture (Fig. 9.47) is a less complex injury at a similar location, where a Salter-Harris type 3 injury occurs to the anterolateral aspect of the distal tibial physis owing to external rotation. The bony attachment of the anterior tibiofibular ligament to the epiphysis is stronger than that of the epiphysis to the rest of the tibia and the fracture line crosses the physis until it meets its fused part, whereafter it passes through the epiphysis into the joint. The injury is usually visible on plain radiographs, but its demonstration is subject to the x-ray beam being parallel to the fracture and oblique views may be necessary. Growth arrest is not a factor in this injury as most of the epiphysis is already fused, the main aims of treatment being restoration of joint congruity and ensuring there is no persistent diastasis at the inferior tibiofibular joint.

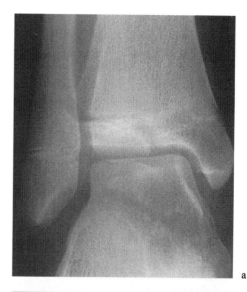

a

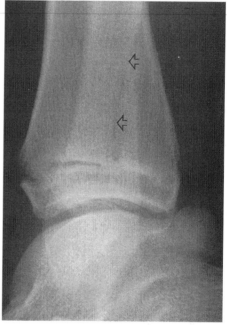

b

Fig. 9.45. a AP and b lateral radiographs of a triplane fracture of the ankle. The subtle superior limb is only visible on the lateral view (*arrows*)

Aside from the serious injuries described, the commonest fractures at the ankle in children are Salter-Harris type 1 and 2 fractures of the distal fibula due to supination inversion injuries. These fractures may be subtle on plain radiographs, and just show as minimal growth plate widening.

A supination-plantar flexion mechanism may result in Salter-Harris type 1 and 2 fractures of the distal tibial epiphysis. More serious Salter-Harris type 3 or 4 injuries can occur at the medial malleolus due to forced inversion of the ankle. Initially they

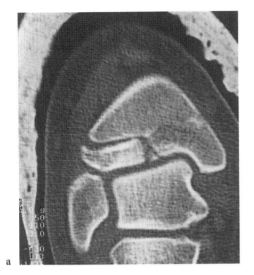

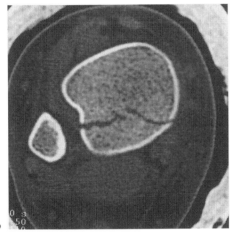

Fig. 9.46. a Coronal CT scan via the ankle and b axial scan through the distal tibia and fibula, confirming triplane fracture

may appear as type 3 fractures, but radiographic review may reveal a small attached metaphyseal flake indicative of a type 4 injury. These are significant injuries due to their potential for subsequent growth arrest, which may be delayed, and thus serial follow-up radiographs will be required (GRIFFIN 1994). The association between fractures of the medial malleolus and fibular neck in the Maisonneuve fracture should also be remembered, in which there is also disruption of the intra-osseous membrane to the level of the fibular fracture.

9.6.7
Fractures of the Foot

A plain radiographic survey in children with trauma to the foot should initially consist of dorsoplantar,

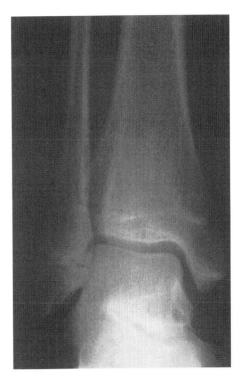

Fig. 9.47. Tillaux fracture of the ankle

oblique and lateral views. In complex injuries to the hindfoot, CT has, to a large extent, supplanted additional radiographic projections. Scans should be obtained as 3-mm slices reconstructed every 2 mm, which will allow multiplanar reformatting.

There are several important normal variants in the bony anatomy of the developing foot of which the reporting radiologist should be aware if they are not to be misinterpreted as fractures. An example is the os trigonum, which is an accessory bone derived from a secondary ossification centre lying immediately posterior to the body of the talus, and present on review in 10% of children's ankle radiographs in a large series (CARTY 1992). It usually fuses with the talus, but when it does not, the intervening cartilage may be misinterpreted as a fracture. There are further accessory ossicles which may cause confusion, but it should be noted that both they and their opposing bone surface are generally smooth rather than jagged, sometimes with reciprocal contours.

Apophyses are another source of potentially confusing appearances. That of the calcaneus may frequently have a sclerotic and segmented appearance during normal development which is misinterpreted as either osteochondritis or fracture. That at the base of the little toe metatarsal may be wrongly identified as a fracture fragment, although if it is remembered

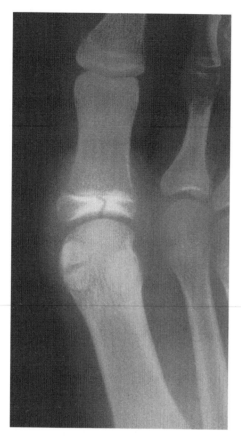

Fig. 9.48. Salter-Harris type 3 epiphyseal injury of the proximal phalanx of the great toe

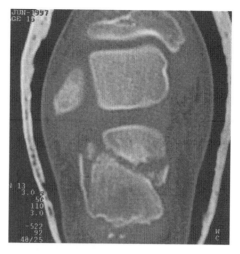

Fig. 9.49. Coronal CT scan demonstrating comminuted fracture of the calcaneus. The extent of the injury was poorly shown on plain radiographs

that the growth plate orientation is oblique, and that of fractures usually transverse, such confusion should not arise. There may be a bifid epiphysis at the base of the proximal phalanx of the great toe which can mimic a Salter-Harris type 3 epiphyseal injury, but does not have separation of the epiphyseal components and physeal widening seen in true fractures (Fig. 9.48) (KARASICK 1994).

Talar fractures are uncommon in children, possibly as much of the bone is composed of cartilage. The commonest form of injury is due to forced dorsiflexion of the ankle leading to impingement of the bone upon the distal tibia. Such injuries are frequently minimally displaced and often missed, yet may still lead to subsequent osteonecrosis. However, this complication is commoner in severer lesions such as displaced neck fractures, crush injury or dislocation. It can also occur as a consequence of open reduction of a fracture. Evidence of delayed osteonecrosis may not be visible for 6 months, so careful follow-up is needed, and supplementing plain radiographs with bone scintigraphy in suspicious cases may help make the diagnosis. Osteochondritis dis-

secans of the talar dome represents an osteochondral fracture which may not be detected acutely.

The calcaneus is the most frequently fractured tarsal bone in children, and although traditionally associated with falls from a height, a review of 45 children who had had such falls (ROSHKOW et al. 1990) found only one such occurrence, albeit bilateral. Calcaneal fractures tend to involve the tuberosity and avoid the posterior facet, so most are classified as extra-articular injuries. They may be very difficult to delineate radiographically, and as mentioned previously, both CT (Fig. 9.49) and scintigraphy may be used to investigate suspected fractures further. It should be noted that the use of Bohler's angle to aid detection of calcaneal fractures, as is done in adults, is not reliable in children.

Scintigraphy was shown to be particularly useful in calcaneal fractures in children aged under 3 years in a series of seven cases (LALIOTIS et al. 1993). In young children who present with acute limp or failure to bear weight an injury of the calcaneus should be considered in the differential diagnosis even in the absence of a history of trauma. Such injuries may be stress fractures, and in the study of Laliotis et al. only a minority were visible on initial plain radiographs (Fig. 9.50a). The majority of calcaneal fractures were diagnosed scintigraphically (Fig. 9.50b) once infection had been excluded by normal temperature, full blood count and ESR.

A pseudocyst of the calcaneus is a normal variant which is not infrequently seen in children radiographed following trauma. It appears as a lucent area within the calcaneus and is devoid of normal trabe-

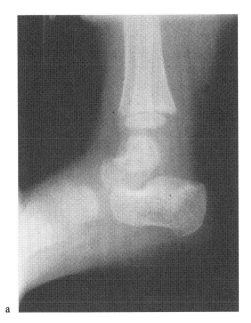

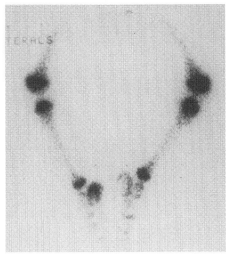

a

b

Fig. 9.50. **a** Plain radiograph and **b** bone scintigram of right calcaneal fracture in a young child. The injury is clearly demonstrated only by the isotope examination. The radiograph is a late film and the fracture line is sclerotic

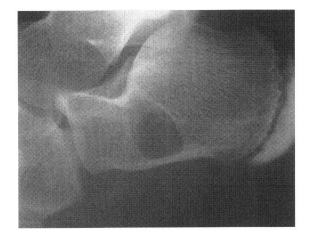

Fig. 9.51. Cyst or pseudocyst of the calcaneus

ossicles mentioned earlier and, if present, is bilateral in the majority of patients. Fractures of the body of the navicular make up the third group, and in young athletes these are often stress injuries which may be difficult to detect. Usually they are either partial or complete fractures in the sagittal plane in the centre of the bone. If scintigraphy utilised in patients with mid foot pain shows increased activity in the navicular region, a CT scan should be performed to confirm the diagnosis (PROKUSKI and SALTZMAN 1997).

Stress injuries also occur in the shafts of the metatarsals, often in runners and dancers (CARTY 1994). The latter group also suffer from spiral fractures of the little toe metatarsal as they "roll off" demipointe (GRIFFIN 1994). The stress injuries are frequently subtle on initial radiographs and are only clearly revealed on delayed films as periosteal reaction and sclerosis develop around the fracture.

Fractures of the metatarsals and phalanges are commoner than those of the hind and mid foot, and are frequently of greenstick or torus pattern. Epiphyseal fractures are not rare, an example being the Salter-Harris type 2 injury which can occur at the base of the great toe metatarsal after jumping from a height.

Acknowledgements. The manuscript was typed by Mrs. V. Donaldson and Miss N. Paggiosi. Radiographs were loaned by Dr. A.P. Coral, Dr. W.P. Butt, Mr. B.W. Scott and Prof. H. Carty.

culae. It weakens the bone and may be the site of overt pathological fracture or microfractures. Radiographically, it is not possible to distinguish this lesion from a simple cyst (Fig. 9.51).

The navicular can fracture in three ways. Fractures of the dorsal cortex are due to avulsion of the capsule of the talonavicular joint and are shown on a lateral radiograph. Avulsion of the navicular tuberosity is due to forceful tibialis posterior contraction, revealed as a medial bony fragment which is rarely displaced. This may be confused with an accessory navicular but the latter shows the characteristics of

References

Al-Quattan MM, Clarke HM, Zimmer P (1994) Radiological signs of entrapment of the median nerve in forearm shaft fractures. J Hand Surg [Br] 19:713–719

Armstrong PF (1992) Serious fractures and joint injuries involving the foot and ankle. Instruct Course Lect 41:413–420

Asher MA (1976) Dislocations of the upper extremity in children. Orthop Clin North Am 7:583–591

Azouz EM, Karamitsos C, Reed MH, Baker L, Kozlowski K, Hoeffel J-C (1993) Types and complications of femoral neck fractures in children. Pediatr Radiol 23:415–420

Bates DG, Hresko MT, Jaramillo D (1994) Patellar sleeve fracture: demonstration with MR imaging. Radiology 193:825–827

Beaty JH, Kumar A (1994) Fractures about the knee in children. J Bone Joint Surg Am 76:1870–1880

Beaty JH, Kasser JR (1995) Fractures about the elbow. Instruct Course Lect 44:199–215

Beltran J, Rosenberg ZS, Kawelblum M, Montes L, Bergman AG, Strongwater A (1994) Pediatric elbow fractures: MRI evaluation. Skeletal Radiol 23:277–281

Borden S IV (1975) Roentgen recognition of acute plastic bowing of the forearm in children. Am J Roentgenol 125:524–530

Bretland PM (1994) Pulled elbow in childhood. Br J Radiol 67:1176–1185

Caputo AE, Watson HK, Nissen C (1995) Scaphoid nonunion in a child: a case report. J Hand Surg [Am] 20:243–245

Carty H (1992) Accessory ossicles at the lateral malleolus: a review of the incidence. Eur J Radiol 14:181–184

Carty H (1994) Sports injuries in children – a radiological viewpoint. Arch Dis Child 70:457–460

Chande VT (1995) Decision rules for roentgenography of children with acute ankle injuries. Arch Pediatr Adolesc Med 149:255–258

Cook PA, Yu JS, Wiand W, Cook AJ II, Coleman C, Cook AJ (1997) Suspected scaphoid fractures in skeletally immature patients: application of MRI. J Comput Assist Tomogr 21:511–515

Crawford AH (1976) Fractures about the knee in children. Orthop Clin North Am 7:639–656

Daffner RH (1994) Ankle trauma. Semin Roentgenol 29:134–151

Daffner RH, Pavlov H (1992) Stress fractures: current concepts. AJR 159:245–252

De Boeck K, Van Eldere S, De Vos P, Mortelmans L, Casteels-Van Daete M (1991) Radionuclide bone imaging in toddler's fracture. Eur J Pediatr 150:166–169

Dormans JP, Rang M (1990) Fractures of the olecranon and radial neck in children. Orthop Clin North Am 21:257–267

El-Khoury GY, Daniel WW, Kathol MH (1997) Acute and chronic avulsive injuries. Radiol Clin North Am 35:747–766

Garvin KL, McCarthy RE, Barnes CL, Dodge BM (1990) Pediatric pelvic ring fractures. J Pediatr Orthop 10:577–582

Gleeson AP, Beattie TF (1994) Monteggia fracture-dislocation in children. J Accid Emerg Med 11:192–194

Gortland JJ, Benner JH (1976) Traumatic dislocations in the lower extremity in children. Orthop Clin North Am 7:687–700

Griffin LY (1994) Common sports injuries of the foot and ankle seen in children and adolescents. Orthop Clin North Am 25:83–93

Heeg M, Klasen HJ, Visser JD (1989) Acetabular fractures in children and adolescents. J Bone Joint Surg Br 71:418–421

Hohl JC (1976) Fractures of the humerus in children. Orthop Clin North Am 7:557–571

Hughes LO, Beaty JH (1994) Fractures of the head and neck of the femur in children. J Bone Joint Surg Am 76:283–292

Kao SCS, Smith WL (1997) Skeletal injuries in the pediatric patient. Radiol Clin North Am 35:727–746

Karasick D (1994) Fractures and dislocations of the foot. Semin Roentgenol 29:152–175

Karasick D, Burk DL Jr, Gross GW (1991) Trauma to the elbow and forearm. Semin Roentgenol 26:318–330

Keshishyan RA, Rozinov VM, Malakhov OA, Kuznetsov LE, Strunin EG, Chogovadze GA, Tsukanov VE (1995) Pelvic polyfractures in children radiographic diagnosis and treatment. Clin Orthop Relat Res 320:28–33

King SJ, Carty HML, Brady O (1996) Magnetic resonance imaging of knee injuries in children. Pediatr Radiol 26:287–290

Laliotis N, Pennie BH, Carty H, Klenerman L (1993) Toddler's fracture of the calcaneum. Injury 24:169–170

Lee FA (1980) Skeletal trauma. In: Gwinn JL, Stanley P (eds) Diagnostic imaging in pediatric trauma. Springer, Berlin Heidelberg New York, p 187

Letts M, Esser D (1993) Fractures of the triquetrum in children. J Pediatr Orthop 13:228–231

Macnicol MF (1994) Indications for internal fixation. In: Benson MKD, Fixsen JA, Macnicol MF (eds) Children's orthopaedics and fractures. Churchill Livingstone, Edinburgh, p 709

Magid D, Fishman EK, Ney DR, Kuhlman JE, Frantz KM, Sponseller PD (1992) Acetabular and pelvic fractures in the pediatric patient: value of two- and three-dimensional imaging. J Pediatr Orthop 12:621–625

Maguire JK, Canale ST (1993) Fractures of the patella in children and adolescents. J Pediatr Orthop 13:567–571

McRae R (1981) Practical fracture treatment, 1st edn. Churchill Livingstone, Edinburgh

Meaney JEM, Carty H (1992) Femoral stress fractures in children. Skeletal Radiol 21:173–176

Mizuta T, Benson WM, Foster BK, Paterson DC, Morris LL (1987) Statistical analysis of the incidence of physeal injuries. J Pediatr Orthop 7:518–523

Moseley CF (1992) Fractures and dislocations of the hip. Instruct Course Lect 41:397–401

Nietosvarra Y, Aalto K (1997) The cartilaginous femoral sulcus in children with patellar dislocation: an ultrasonographic study. J Pediatr Orthop 17:50–53

Nietosvaara Y, Aalto K, Kallio PE (1994) Acute patellar dislocation in children: incidence and associated osteochondral fractures. J Pediatr Orthop 14:513–515

Nimkin K, Kleinman PK, Teeger S, Spevak MR (1995) Distal humeral physeal injuries in child abuse: MR imaging and ultrasonography findings. Pediatr Radiol 25:562–565

Obremskey W, Routt MLC Jr (1994) fracture-dislocation of the shoulder in a child: case report. J Trauma 36:137–140

Ogden JA, Tross RB, Murphy MJ (1980) Fractures of the tibial tuberosity in adolescents. J Bone Joint Surg Am 62:205–215

Ohaski K, Brandser EA, El-Khoury GY (1997) Role of MR imaging in acute injuries to the appendicular skeleton. Radiol Clin North Am 35:591–614

Oppenheim WL, Davis A, Growdon WA, Dorey FJ, Davlin LB (1990) Clavicle fractures in the newborn. Clin Orthop Relat Res 250:176–180

Prokuski LJ, Saltzman CL (1997) Challenging fractures of the foot and ankle. Radiol Clin North Am 35:655–670

Rickett AB, Finlay DBL (1993) Audit of comparative views in elbow trauma in children. Br J Radiol 66:123–125

Rieger H, Brug E (1997) Fractures of the pelvis in children. Clin Orthop Relat Res 336:226–239

Rogers LF, Poznanski AK (1994) Imaging of epiphyseal injuries. Radiology 191:297–308

Roshkow JE, Haller JO, Hotson GC, Sclafani SJA, Mezzacappa PM, Rachlin S (1990) Imaging Evaluation of children after falls from a height: review of 45 cases. Radiology 175:359–363

Simmons BP, Lavallo JL (1988) Hand and wrist injuries in children. Clin Sports Med 7:495–512

Stansberry SD, Swischuk LE, Swischuk JL, Midgett TA (1990) Significance of ulnar styloid fractures in childhood. Pediatr Emerg Care 6:99–103

Sundar M, Carty H (1994) Avulsion fractures of the pelvis in children: a report of 32 fractures and their outcome. Skeletal Radiol 23:85–90

Tiel-van Buul MMC, van Beek EJR, Broekhuizen AH, Bakker AJ, Bos KE, van Royen EA (1993) Radiography and scintigraphy of suspected scaphoid fracture. J Bone Joint Surg Br 75:61–65

Torode I, Zieg D (1985) Pelvic fractures in children. J Pediatr Orthop 5:76–84

Vasa R, Kim MR (1990) Fracture of the femur at cesarean section: case report and review of literature. Am J Perinatol 7:46–48

Vazquez WD, Garcia VF (1993) Pediatric pelvic fractures combined with an additional skeletal injury is an indicator of significant injury. Surg Gynaecol Obstetr 177:468–472

Weber WN, Neumann CH, Barakos JA, Petersen SA, Steinbach LS, Genant HK (1991) Lateral tibial rim (Segond) fractures: MR imaging characteristics. Radiology 180:731–734

Welk LA, Adler RS (1992) Case report 725. Skeletal Radiol 21:198–200

White PG, Mah JY, Friedman L (1994) Magnetic resonance imaging in acute physeal injuries. Skeletal Radiol 23:627–631

Young JWR, Burgess AR, Brumback RJ, Poka A (1986) Pelvic fractures: value of plain radiography in early assessment and management. Radiology 160:445–451

Zammit-Maempel I, Bisset RAL, Morris J, St C. Forbes W (1988) The value of soft tissue signs in wrist trauma. Clin Radiol 39:664–668

Zobel MS, Barrello JA, Siegel MJ, Stewart NR (1994) Pediatric knee MR imaging: pattern of injuries in the immature skeleton. Radiology 190:397–401

10 Emergency Imaging in Non-accidental Injury

P. RAO

CONTENTS

10.1 Introduction

The terms non-accidental injury (NAI) and child abuse describe a spectrum of injuries ranging from the well-publicised physical and sexual abuse to the less frequently documented emotional abuse, neglect, deprivation and abandonment. Literature on the presentation and radiology of the abused child is extensive, dating back to 1860, when Tardieu published what is thought to be the first article on the concept of the battered child (SILVERMAN 1972). Major contributions were made earlier this century by John CAFFEY (1946, 1972, 1974). The past two decades have seen a marked increase in the use of diagnostic imaging in the assessment of traumatised and critically ill patients. Whilst the plain radiograph and skeletal survey are essential in the initial radiological work-up of patients suspected of NAI, cross-sectional imaging with ultrasound, computed tomography (CT) and magnetic resonance imaging (MRI) has increased both the rapidity and the accuracy of assessment of the full extent of the injuries sustained. Imaging plays a key role in both the initial and the long-term management of the abused child. It is important that the imaging findings are not taken in isolation but are considered together with the clinical history and presentation. This will help to distinguish between abuse and accidental trauma. It must be remembered that the physical signs of abuse may be absent and that the radiological abnormalities alone may provide the initial or only evidence that abuse has taken place.

Knowledge and understanding of the types of forces and mechanisms used to inflict the various injuries on the child is important. Correlation with the child's age and stage of development is of utmost importance as the significance of injuries varies with both. Familiarity with typical accidental injuries of childhood is also of prime importance in distinguishing between accidental and non-accidental trauma and to prevent inappropriate diagnosis of NAI.

This chapter will discuss the emergency radiology of the abused child, concentrating on initial presentation and management of the child. This will be followed by a more detailed discussion of the types and mechanisms of injury, their radiological evaluation, and the imaging findings likely to be encountered by the radiologist dealing with NAI.

P. RAO, BSc Hons, MB BS, MRCP, FRCR, Lecturer in Paediatric Radiology, Royal Liverpool Children's NHS Trust, Alder Hey, Eaton Road, Liverpool, L12 2AP, UK

10.2
Clinical Presentation

The spectrum of injuries potentially sustained by the abused child who presents as a medical emergency is wide, ranging from what are initially considered to be minor vague symptoms to severe damage resulting in shock. The child may present with the same symptoms and signs as those with accidental trauma or true medical illness. Often multiple injuries are present which are not always immediately apparent. Presentation of the obtunded child is a medical emergency and the immediate concern is to resuscitate the child and ensure cardiovascular stability. The initial diagnosis is often that of a medical emergency such as meningitis or status epilepticus, especially if overt superficial injury is absent. During resuscitation injuries may become apparent, such as subtle bruising or a torn frenulum, pointing to the diagnosis. Some obtunded children who are abused have no overt injury and the diagnosis is only made by imaging findings.

A small number of abused children present with abdominal trauma. There is no place for radiological investigations in haemodynamically unstable children suspected of major organ injury; immediate surgery is required. Hypotension is an unreliable predictor of major organ injury in the paediatric population as children are able to maintain a normal blood pressure despite significant blood loss (STEIN et al. 1994).

Once an obtunded child is resuscitated and stabilised, a more detailed head and body examination is carried out. Plain radiography is performed at this stage. A set protocol of trauma films should be taken. These may vary slightly between departments but the lateral cervical spine, chest and abdomen are regarded in most centres as standard films in a trauma victim, particularly if no history is available or the patient is unconscious. In the unconscious child without a history of trauma, the first imaging should be head CT. Further radiographs should be guided by the clinical history and examination. The sequence of further diagnostic imaging is usually determined by the initial neurological examination of the child. Injury to the brain assessed by the Glasgow Coma Scale takes priority over other injuries. Once the patient is neurologically and haemodynamically stable, a search for other non-life-threatening injuries can be instituted.

Diagnosing NAI is relatively straightforward if the typical soft tissue or skeletal injuries of NAI exist. Diagnostic difficulties occur in the absence of these external markers of abuse. Suspicions should be aroused in the following circumstances:

1. The presence of an inappropriate or clearly implausible history.
2. The presence of an inconsistent or conflicting history.
3. Delay in seeking medical help if a healing fracture is found on skeletal survey.
4. Delay in seeking medical help such that a child presents in a dehydrated or cachectic state.
5. Radiographic evidence of trauma exceeds that expected from the clinical history.

Other suspicious situations, which in the absence of appropriate clinical circumstances may require further investigation, are:

1. Abdominal trauma of unknown cause
2. Gastric outlet obstruction after the peak age for pyloric stenosis
3. Pancreatitis and pancreatic pseudocysts
4. Suspicious burns
5. Failure to thrive
6. History of previous trauma to this child or a sibling or any other suspicion of neglect and abuse

The diagnosis of NAI may thus become apparent as the history unfolds or during the examination but occasionally only becomes evident after investigations have been performed.

If NAI is suspected, a full skeletal survey is performed after the patient has been stabilised. This should be done during normal daylight hours and not as an emergency in the middle of the night. The child will be in a place of safety in hospital. If the child has an obvious femoral fracture requiring Gallows traction, the lower limbs should be radiographed before the traction is applied so that the child is not disturbed by its removal. The rest of the survey should be completed the next day. The skeletal survey has three main purposes: to demonstrate a fracture presenting clinically, to demonstrate occult fractures and to date fractures. A recommended schedule of images is given in Table 10.1 and discussed in Sect. 10.4.10.

10.3
Skull and Brain Injuries in NAI

Non-accidental injury is the leading cause of serious head injury in infants (American Academy of Pediatrics 1993; CARTY and RATCLIFFE 1995). Clinical presentation may be non-specific, with vague symp-

Table 10.1. Skeletal survey

AP chest
AP both upper limbs
AP both lower limbs
Abdomen and pelvis
Coned AP and lateral of knees and ankles
Lateral thoracolumbar spine
AP and lateral skull – add a Townes view if there is occipital
    injury
AP hands and feet if clinically suspicious

Table 10.2. Features of skull fractures found more commonly
in NAI than in accidental trauma

Complex fractures
Diastatic fractures measuring more than 3 mm wide
Multiple fractures
Fractures involving both sides of the skull
Fractures of differing ages
Depressed fractures, especially of the occiput

toms such as lethargy and poor feeding, and in the absence of external signs such as bruising, the diagnosis may be missed. A child presenting with fits or collapse in the absence of other manifestations of NAI often has a presumed diagnosis of meningitis or near-miss sudden infant death syndrome (SIDS). Approximately 10% of all neurological disease in children is caused by abuse. This figure increases to 64% in infants less than 11 months of age in whom acute head trauma is identified on CT (BILLIMIRE and MEYERS 1985).

The most common eye injuries in abuse are retinal haemorrhages, peri-orbital oedema, retinal detachment and lens subluxation often resulting in permanent visual defects. Between 50% and 80% of cases of shaking in child abuse entail retinal haemorrhages (STANTON 1979; CARTER and McCORMICK 1983; HADLEY et al. 1989). This emphasises the need for fundoscopy in all children who present obtunded and not just those in whom abuse is already suspected. Retinal haemorrhages are extremely uncommon in accidental head trauma (EISENBREY 1979). Those associated with birth delivery resolve completely within 4 weeks.

10.3.1
Skull Fractures

Skull fractures require impact trauma to the head. There may be clinical evidence of a scalp haematoma but rarely the development of a haematoma is delayed. In children haemorrhage into the subgaleal space may become haemodynamically significant. Subgaleal haematomas and scalp contusions are useful indicators of the impact point against the calvarium and may assist in identifying subtle fractures. Subgaleal blood may be a sign of both skull fracture and epidural haematoma. Haemorrhage can also occur between the periosteum and the outer table of the calvarium. This subperiosteal haemorrhage or cephalhaematoma is delimited by the sutures and can lead to alteration of the shape and thickness of the calvarium focally.

The types and pattern of skull fracture occurring in abuse and accidental trauma do not necessarily differ. There is no one type of fracture that is pathognomic of abuse (CARTY 1991). Skull fractures which are not usually seen in uncomplicated accidental trauma and which are more suspicious of abuse are shown in Table 10.2. Skull fractures in abused children are often complex or multiple, depressed or wide and sometimes increase in width (Fig. 10.1). Non-parietal fractures, especially occipital fractures, occur more commonly in abuse than in accidental injury. Any type of fracture can occur (Fig. 10.2). The presence of a skull fracture of any type must be correlated with the clinical history. Dating skull fractures is difficult as they do not heal by callus formation. If the edges are rounded and smooth, the fracture is usually more than 2 weeks old.

Minor accidental falls or short falls are very rarely associated with serious or fatal injury (MUSEMECHE et al. 1991; KRAVITZ et al. 1969; REIBER 1993). Simple skull fractures in accidental trauma have a very low risk of intracranial sequelae (THORNBURY et al. 1983; HARWOOD-NASH et al. 1971; LLOYD et al. 1997). If major injury is present with an incompatible history of only minor trauma, the history is likely to be unreliable and inaccurate and NAI must be suspected (REIBER 1993; CHADWICK et al. 1991).

10.3.2
Cerebral Manifestations of NAI

In NAI the two main mechanisms of injury causing brain damage are impact injuries (including acceleration-deceleration forces) and whiplash shaking injuries. The primary injury may be complicated by pathophysiological responses leading to the secondary injury – hypoxic ischaemic damage (BROWN and MINNS 1993). Shaking is most common in infants

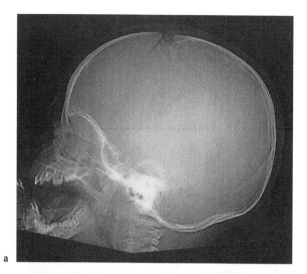

a

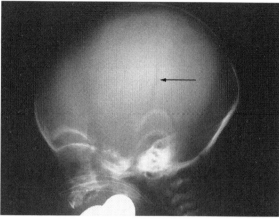

Fig. 10.2. Lateral skull view of a 3-month-old abused infant demonstrates a diastatic fracture extending through the temporal and parietal regions (*arrow*)

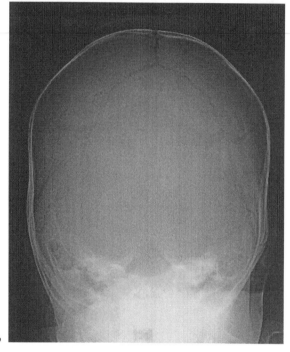

b

Fig. 10.1 a,b. Lateral and Townes skull radiographs in an 8-month-old abused infant demonstrating diastatic biparietal fractures

small brain relative to the size of the cranium means that as whiplashing occurs, the brain can swirl in different directions, generating shearing forces within the skull and brain. These, with added rotation, are important in producing the brain injury and associated subdural haematoma (CARTY and RATCLIFFE 1995; CARTY 1991; CAFFEY 1972; OMMAYA et al. 1968; DYKES 1986; NEWTON 1989). The general consensus is that shaking alone can cause the brain injury but that an associated impact injury often occurs. The head may strike a solid object during the shake or the child may be thrown away or slammed down onto a surface at the end of the shake. The surface may be hard or soft, such as a bed. The end result is a skull fracture (ELLISON et al. 1978; HADLEY et al. 1989) and this is often the last event in a shake. In abuse the major complications of intracranial injury are subdural haematoma, cerebral oedema and hypoxic ischaemic encephalopathy. Less commonly intracerebral haemorrhage, intraventricular haemorrhage, extradural haemorrhage and shear injuries with petechial bleeds occur.

10.3.3
Subdural Haematoma

Subdural haematoma is caused by trauma associated with rotation between the brain and dura causing shearing of the bridging veins in the subdural space (GUTHKELCH 1971). Though it has been suggested that subdural haematomata may occur in trivial trauma (AOKI and MASUZAMA 1984), this is not widely accepted, and the more generally held view is

under 1 year of age but can occur in older children (KLEINMAN 1990). The child is often held by the rib cage and squeezed, resulting in fractured ribs and high central venous pressure, one cause of the retinopathy. Several authors have investigated the mechanism of production of subdural haematoma during whiplash shaking (GUTHKELCH 1971; CAFFEY 1972, 1974; OMMAYA et al. 1968). The infant's large head relative to its body and weak neck muscles results in poor head control with little support. The

Table 10.3. CT and MRI of intracranial haemorrhage (density/signal compared to cortex)

Time	NECT density	CECT density	T1 W signal	T2 W signal	GRE signal
4–6 h	Increased	–	Isointense	Increased	Decreased
7–72 h	Increased	–	Isointense	Decreased	Much decreased
4–7 days	Increased/isointense	–	Isointense (centre) Increased (rim)	Decreased	Much decreased
1–4 weeks	Decreased/isointense	Rim enhancing	Increased	Increased	Decreased
Chronic	Decreased	–	Decreased	Decreased	Decreased

Based on information from Osborn AG, Tong KA (eds) (1996) Handbook of neuroradiology: brain and skull, 2nd edn. Mosby, St. Louis, Chap. 19, and from Mattle HP, O'Reilly GV, Edelman RR, Johnson KA (1990) Brain: spontaneous haemorrhage. In: Edelman RR, Hesselink JR (eds) Clinical magnetic resonance imaging. Saunders, Philadelphia, Chap. 16.
NECT, Non-enhanced CT; CECT, contrast-enhanced CT; T1 W, T1-weighted; T2 W, T2-weighted; GRE, gradient echo.

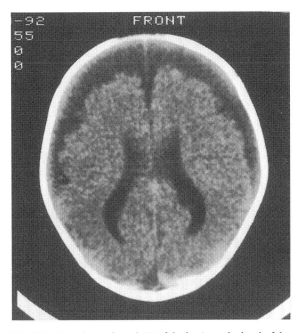

Fig. 10.3. Unenhanced axial CT of the brain at the level of the bodies of the lateral ventricles in a 7-month-old child demonstrating bilateral chronic low-density subdural haematomata extending over both frontoparietal regions. Fresh high-density subdural blood is also noted posteriorly

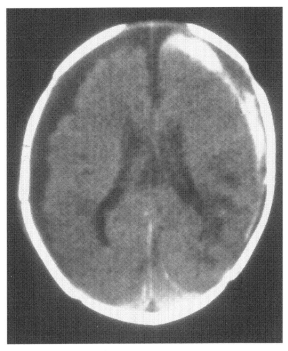

Fig. 10.4. Unenhanced axial CT of the brain at the level of the lateral ventricles in a 10-month-old abused child demonstrating bilateral subdural haematomata of differing ages. A chronic low-density subdural collection is present on the right. On the left, there is both high and low density, indicating subdural bleeds of differing ages. Fresh interhemispheric fissure subdural blood is also noted posteriorly

that the causative force is significant. In the appropriate clinical setting accidental subdural haematomata can occur but the history is compatible. Features of subdural haematomata that are suspicious and suggest NAI are:

1. Presence of a subdural haematoma in the absence of skull fracture or an apparent history of trauma implying a shaking injury.
2. Bilateral subdural haematomata (Fig. 10.3). Accidental subdural haematomata are usually unilateral and under the injury site.
3. Subdural haematomata of differing ages (Fig. 10.4). The density of blood on CT and MRI varies with the age of the haematoma (Table 10.3).
4. Subdural haematoma in the presence of retinal haemorrhages implying acceleration-deceleration forces.
5. Acute interhemispheric fissure subdural haematoma (falx haemorrhage), seen as a bright, irregularly thickened falx (Fig. 10.5).

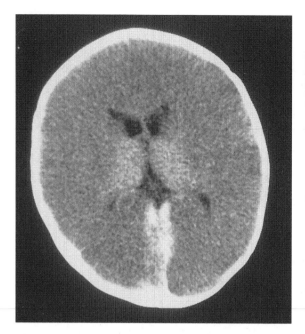

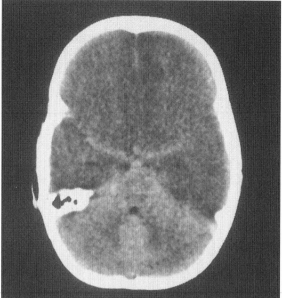

Fig. 10.5. Unenhanced axial CT of the brain in an 8-month-old abused infant demonstrating acute posterior inter-hemispheric fissure subdural blood (falx haemorrhage). The falx posteriorly is thickened, irregular and bright. The brain parenchyma demonstrates the CT appearances of "acute reversal"

Fig. 10.6. Unenhanced axial CT of the brain in an abused child at the level of the fourth ventricle demonstrating the features of "acute reversal". There is decreased density of the cerebral grey and white matter and loss of grey white matter differentiation with sparing of the cerebellum and brainstem

In accidental trauma subdural blood does not usually extend into the falx. The normal falx is thin in the centre, except near the vertex, and expands into a triangle anteriorly and posteriorly where it merges into the superior sagittal sinus. In acute interhemispheric fissure subdural, there is thickening and irregularity of the falx on lower sections at or just above the ventricles, or unilateral thickening posterior to the corpus collosum. An acute interhemispheric fissure subdural is highly associated with NAI (OSBORN et al. 1980; ZIMMERMAN et al. 1982). Care must be taken to differentiate falx haemorrhage from a normal falx that looks bright against an abnormally low-density brain. A normal falx is smooth and sharp. On follow-up scans a true falx haemorrhage will show a sequential change in density. Subarachnoid blood is located anteriorly in the interhemispheric fissure and forms an irregular zig-zag pattern as hyperdense blood fills the sulci. Diffuse falx calcification does not occur in infants and does not cause confusion. A subdural haematoma producing more mass effect than can be accounted for by its size alone indicates the presence of brain swelling and there may also be contusions and diffuse axonal injury. A subdural haematoma may be later complicated by the formation of neomem-branes, which develop within 2–3 weeks after initial haemorrhage.

10.3.4
Hypoxic Ischaemic Encephalopathy

Hypoxic ischaemic injury to the brain is a consequence of the primary insult. The reversal sign (HAN et al. 1989) describes a distinctive CT appearance in which there is diffusely decreased density of the cerebral grey and white matter with decreased or lost grey-white matter differentiation and a relative increase in density of the thalami, brainstem and cerebellum (Fig. 10.6). Although it is highly associated with child abuse it can result from a variety of other causes such as drowning, fits, status asthmaticus, cardiac arrest, electrocution and accidental injury. In these circumstances it is not associated with cerebral bleeding unless there is a haemorrhagic diathesis. It carries a poor prognosis with irreversible brain damage irrespective of the cause. Pathologically, possible explanations for the reversal sign include preserved brain tissue, petechial haemorrhage and mineralized neurons for high-density areas on CT, and severe oedema and/or tissue destruction for low-density areas on CT (HAN et al. 1989). The presence of the reversal sign with interhemispheric fissure subdural blood is highly suggestive of a shaking injury of NAI. Complications of the brain injury of NAI include obstructive hydrocephalus from arachnoiditis, communicating hydrocephalus from alteration in cerebrospinal fluid (CSF) dynamics, cerebral atrophy, cerebral infarction and multicystic encephalomalacia. Clinically the spectrum of disabilities is wide, ranging from mild developmental delay, clumsiness and attention disorders to motor and intellectual impairment, hemiplegia, quadriplegia and cerebral palsy and blindness with gross mental and physical handicap.

10.3.5
Diffuse Brain Swelling

Diffuse brain swelling is a common CT finding in head-injured children (BRUCE et al. 1981) and is the cause of death in most fatal cases of NAI. Brain swelling may be focal or diffuse throughout both hemispheres and is caused by the acute traumatic event as well as by secondary injury from hypoxia, hypotension, hypercarbia, intracranial hypertension and seizures (ROUSE and EICHELBERGER 1992). It is associated with diffuse axonal injury, hyperaemic swelling and true cerebral oedema. At CT there is obliteration of the CSF spaces and sulci, loss of the basal cisterns and compression and effacement of the lateral ventricles (Fig. 10.7). The increased water content due to brain oedema causes the decrease in CT attenuation. Focal areas of white matter oedema may exist. Oedema may conform to a vascular territory. A vascular distribution has also been described in cases attributed to a combination of strangulation and shaking (KLEINMAN 1990; BIRD et al. 1987). In hyperaemic oedema, brain attenuation increases (BRUCE et al. 1981).

10.3.6
Imaging of Skull and Brain Injuries

Patients who are undergoing neurological imaging may have multisystem injury in association with head injury and thus may be both neurologically and haemodynamically unstable. Prior to undergoing any further imaging, the patient must be resuscitated and rendered haemodynamically stable and monitoring must continue for the duration.

The presence or absence of a skull fracture is not a reliable indicator of intracranial injury. A skull

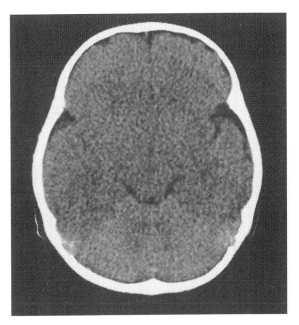

Fig. 10.7. Unenhanced axial CT of the brain demonstrating diffuse brain swelling. There is effacement of the ventricles and compression of the basal cisterns. The parenchyma is of diffusely decreased density with loss of normal grey — white matter differentiation

fracture may be absent even in the presence of severe intracranial injury. It is recommended that skull radiography in children over 2 years of age should only be performed to confirm a suspected depressed fracture or penetrating injury or where NAI is suspected. However, skull radiography should be performed in all children under 2 years of age with suspected head injury because of the greater probability of abuse in this younger age group (LLOYD et al. 1997) and the fact that a fracture may be missed on CT and intracranial trauma attributed to accident. Skull fractures, except those of the skull base, are usually obvious. Pneumocephalus secondary to basilar skull fractures is occasionally seen. Fluid levels in the paranasal sinuses, although a non-specific sign, or opacification or fluid levels in the mastoid air cells or middle ear may be due to basilar fractures with either haemorrhage or CSF leaks.

Cross-sectional neuroimaging is required in any obtunded or neurologically unstable child and in any child suspected to be the victim of abuse when a skull fracture is detected even in the absence of neurological signs. At present CT remains the most practical and cost-effective CNS imaging technique. It is the initial investigation of choice because it is non-invasive, is widely available and will exclude surgically correctable lesions. It is superior to MRI in demonstrating fractures and acute haemorrhage (COHEN et al. 1986; BALL 1989; SATO et al. 1989). Unenhanced scans should be performed, initially with 10-mm sections through the brain and a 512 × 512 matrix reconstruction, with thinner sections through the base of the brain if required. Ideally fast scanning with a CT acquisition time of less than 2s is required to decrease motion artefacts in children who are not intubated. In order that subtle abnormalities of brain parenchyma are not missed, all cranial CT scans must be of high quality and performed with adequate mAs. Too great a reduction in mAs, although minimising radiation dose to the infant, results in grainy, poor quality scans of limited diagnostic capability and makes it difficult to assess subtle signs of oedema. In general, intravascular contrast is not required. It may occasionally help to clarify the presence of a suspected isodense subdural. Skull radiographs must be performed in addition to CT to look for skull fractures. CT may miss fractures which lie in the plane of the beam even if images are reviewed on bone window settings. TSAI et al. (1980) found radiographic evidence of skull fractures in 5 of 12 abused children in whom the fracture could not be seen on CT.

Typically, acute subdural haematomata are of high attenuation on CT (Fig. 10.3, 10.4). If the patient is severely anaemic (haemoglobin 8–10g/dl) or if there is concurrent leakage of CSF into the subdural space, an acute subdural bleed can be isointense. The collection is concave as it conforms to the surface of the brain. Manipulation of window settings to increase contrast will permit easier detection of small thin collections of blood. A subdural haematoma is not related to skull sutures and is not limited by dural sutures in its extent. It is limited in spread by the falx and tentorium. There may be an associated mass effect on the brain parenchyma. Follow-up scans show characteristic changes in the density of the subdural collection with time and will detect rebleeds (Table 10.3).

Follow-up scans are indicated to assess complications such as hydrocephalus and venous infarction and in unstable cases with changing neurology.

High-resolution transfontanellar ultrasound (US) can and should be performed in addition to CT in neonates and small babies with a patent fontanelle. Subdural haematoma can be detected by US (LAM and CRUZ 1991; JASPAN et al. 1992) and can be differentiated from subarachnoid haemorrhage. Occasionally difficulties arise in distinguishing a small posterior interhemispheric subdural bleed from sagittal sinus thrombosis, which can occur as a complication of head trauma. US can be used to as-

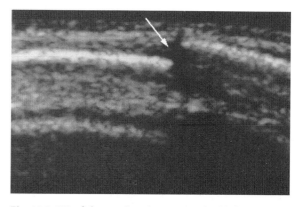

Fig. 10.8. US of the cranium in a 4-month-old abused child demonstrating a fracture of the right parietal bone (*arrow*). (Courtesy of Doz. Dr. M. Riccabona and Professor Dr. R. Fotter, Department of Paediatric Radiology, LKH University Hospital Graz)

sess the patency of the major venous sinuses. US may also detect vault fractures and may determine the degree of separation of the fracture ends (Fig. 10.8). Advantages of US are its portability and sensitivity in detecting cystic change due to shear injury at the grey-white matter junction. Disadvantages of US are that it is operator dependent, it cannot be used in older children and certain areas of the brain remain inaccessible to US, particularly the posterior fossa. US alone is not adequate to exclude intracranial injury in NAI.

The advent of MRI has made a huge impact in craniocerebral imaging (BALL 1989; SATO et al. 1989). In addition to having superior anatomical resolution, MRI can distinguish chronic subdural collections associated with ventricular dilatation from increased fluid in the CSF spaces due to cerebral atrophy. It is more sensitive in detecting small horizontally orientated subdural haematomata because of the multiplanar facility, and in detecting subdural haematomata of differing ages. It is highly sensitive in the detection of parenchymal shearing injuries, cortical contusions and subtle focal or diffuse cerebral oedema (BALL 1989; SATO et al. 1989). Several studies have shown that not only is MRI more sensitive than CT in detecting them but it demonstrates them earlier (GENTRY et al. 1988; KELLY et al. 1988; LEVIN et al. 1987; HESSELINK et al. 1988).

Disadvantages of MRI are its lack of widespread availability, length of scan time and requirements for anaesthesia in young children. It is limited in its ability to demonstrate calvarial fractures and pneumocephalus and is not as good as CT in demonstrating subarachnoid blood. Realistically the increase in sensitivity in the detection of certain lesions is not necessarily of benefit to the patient in the acute trauma setting. Studies assessing the potential value of MRI in the acute setting are still ongoing and the degree to which MRI alters patient management compared with the information derived from CT is not yet defined. At present MRI is reserved for the following cases:

1. If CT is equivocal or normal in the presence of abnormal neurology
2. In patients suspected of having brainstem lesions
3. In evaluating patients with suspected vertex or infratemporal extra-axial haematoma
4. In assessing the patency of major venous sinuses
5. To clarify questionable areas of haemorrhage identified on the initial CT scan. The appearance of haemorrhage on MRI depends on the time after trauma at which the scan is performed (Table 10.3).

It is recommended that MRI should be performed in all suspected NAI cases but the timing of MRI should be tailored to the clinical condition of the patient. Non-urgent scans can be performed when the patient is stable and are particularly useful for detecting the number and age of subdural bleeds. Follow-up MRI scans are performed to assess for sequelae of brain injury such as gliosis.

10.4
Skeletal and Soft Tissue Injuries in NAI

Skeletal injuries in NAI occur most commonly under the age of 3 years (LODER and BOOKOUT 1991; KEMPE et al. 1962; CARTY 1993a) although some authors quote 1 year (AKBARNIA et al. 1974; KOGUTT et al. 1974). The incidence of bony injuries has been variously reported as between 11% and 55% (BROWN and MINNS 1993; CARTY 1989). Under one year of age, when infants are not yet fully mobile, accidental fractures may occur but are rare (WORLOCK et al. 1986). In the presence of an absent or inappropriate history, NAI must be suspected.

Skeletal injuries can be divided into those occurring frequently but with a low specificity for abuse and those occurring less frequently but with a high specificity for abuse (Tables 10.4, 10.5).

10.4.1
Metaphyseal Fractures

The classical metaphyseal fracture, also known as the corner or bucket handle fracture, is highly character-

Table 10.4. Fractures considered to have a high specificity for abuse

Metaphyseal fractures
Rib fractures
Scapular fractures
Fractures of the outer end of the clavicle
Fractures of differing ages
Vertebral fractures or subluxation
Digital injuries in non-mobile children
Bilateral skull fractures
Complex skull fractures

Table 10.5. Fractures frequent in NAI but of low specificity

Mid-clavicular fractures
Simple linear skull fractures
Single long bone fractures

istic of and specific for abuse although the less specific diaphyseal fracture is reported to occur 4 times as frequently (LODER and BOOKOUT 1991; MERTEN et al. 1983).

Metaphyseal fractures are most commonly seen in non-mobile abused infants but may occur up to about 2 years of age. The twisting and shearing forces required to produce such fractures are not those generated in simple accidental falls. Metaphyseal fractures are most frequent around the knees and ankles but are also seen at the shoulders, elbows, wrists and hips and these areas must be carefully scrutinised on the plain radiograph (Fig. 10.9). Metaphyseal fractures may only be visible on one projection and must not be dismissed because of their non-visibility if only one projection is viewed. Subtle metaphyseal fractures, when healed, may appear as a subtle loss of the normal contour with a "squaring off" of the contour. Alternatively, there may be cloaking of the bone by periosteal new bone that is totally out of proportion to the initial injury. The appearances during fracture repair depend on the initial disruption.

The importance of good quality radiographs cannot be overstated. The most subtle metaphyseal fracture is the metaphyseal lucent line (CARTY 1989; KLEINMAN and MARKS 1996) (Fig. 10.10). It repairs without periosteal new bone and can easily be overlooked on suboptimal radiographs which are not of the correct exposure or if the limbs are poorly positioned. Metaphyseal fractures must be distinguished from accidental torus fractures that commonly occur at the metadiaphyseal junction (KLEINMAN et al. 1991b). Metaphyseal fractures may occur during shaking, but direct wrenching or twisting force to the

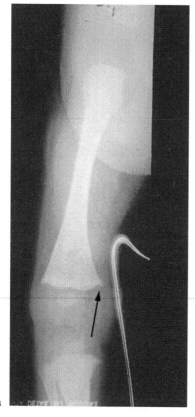
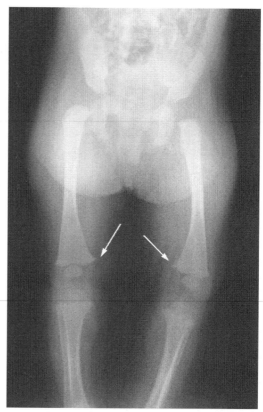

a   b

Fig. 10.9. a Radiograph of right knee of an abused infant demonstrating the classical metaphyseal or corner/bucket handle fracture of the distal femoral metaphysis (*arrow*). **b** Radio-graph of both lower limbs of an abused infant demonstrating bilateral bucket handle fractures of both distal femoral metaphyses (*arrows*)

limb using the extremities as "handles" is also a well-recognised mechanism. Periosteal new bone may not be seen with small corner fractures because subperiosteal bleeding does not occur and the fracture is entirely intracapsular (bleeding and periosteal elevation are essential for the formation of periosteal new bone).

10.4.2
Diaphyseal Fractures

Diaphyseal fractures occurring in the long bones are most frequently seen in the femur, humerus and tibia (Fig. 10.11). Variable frequencies and fracture patterns have been quoted (Loder and Bookout 1991; Akbarnia et al. 1974; Kogutt et al. 1974; King et al. 1988). There is no pattern or type of diaphyseal fracture specific to NAI although transverse fractures are stated to be the most frequent. The significance of diaphyseal fractures increases when:

1. They are multiple.
2. They are of differing ages.
3. They are bilateral.
4. There is a fracture through callus.
5. They are found in a state of healing, implying a failure to seek medical attention.
6. They are in association with fractures which have a high specificity for abuse.

Spiral fractures are more common than transverse fractures in both accidental and non-accidental injury. Spiral fractures of the long bones are produced by a twisting force and are always suspicious of abuse but must be viewed in the light of the clinical history. Some studies quote an increased frequency of left-sided diaphyseal fractures, reflecting the greater frequency (87%) of right-handedness in the population (Edwards 1987; Hilton 1994). Transverse fractures may result from direct blows or from bending of the limb. Excluding supracondylar fractures of the humerus in toddlers, in the absence of an appropriate clinical history all humeral fractures should be re-

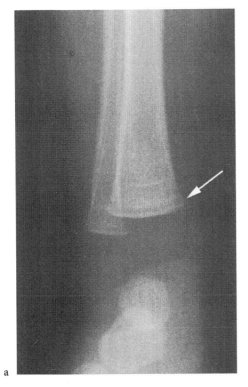

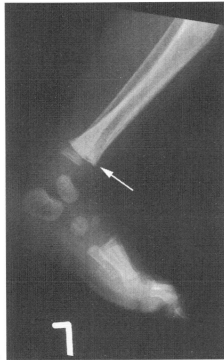

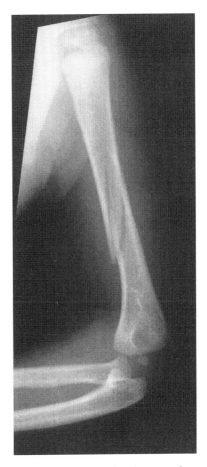

Fig. 10.11. Lateral radiograph of the humerus demonstrating an acute undisplaced oblique fracture through the midshaft of the humerus in this battered child

Fig. 10.10. a Radiograph of the distal tibia and fibula. The metaphyseal lucent line, the most subtle of metaphyseal fractures, is seen on this coned radiograph of the ankle (*arrow*). b Lateral radiograph of the ankle and foot demonstrating metaphyseal fractures of the distal fibula and tibia evident as a metaphyseal lucent line. There is also a corner fracture of the distal tibia (*arrow*)

garded as suspicious of abuse irrespective of fracture type (WORLOCK et al. 1986; MERTEN et al. 1983; THOMAS et al. 1991). However, it must be remembered that in the appropriate clinical setting supracondylar fractures may also occur in abuse.

In the non-mobile child any type of femoral fracture has a high incidence of abuse. Femoral fractures can still occur in abuse in the mobile child (THOMAS et al. 1991; BEALS and TUFTS 1983; ANDERSON 1982). Thus, in the absence of an appropriate history of trauma, any fracture of the femur or humerus is highly suggestive of abuse, particularly in the non-mobile child. The "toddler's fracture", which is a spiral fracture of the tibia, is a well-documented accidental fracture and should not be confused with abuse. Presentation of diaphyseal fractures is varied. The child may present with a swollen limb. The immobile child may cry incessantly and fail to use the limb in a normal way. The mobile child will refuse to weight bear or walk.

Impaction buckle fractures at the metadiaphyseal junction occur from impaction forces transmitted as the child is forcibly thumped down on its legs on a hard surface and are most common in the distal femora or proximal tibia (CARTY 1989; KOGUTT et al. 1974). They must be differentiated from accidental torus fractures which may occur at the same site but typically occur in the distal tibia (KLEINMAN et al. 1991b). In the non-mobile child abuse is the more likely cause.

10.4.3
Epiphyseal Fractures

Epiphyseal fractures and true Salter-Harris fractures are rare in NAI compared with accidental trauma, partly owing to the younger age group of abused children. In young children movement is largely prevented by the epiphysis being held tightly in position by the periosteum. The most common sites are the proximal femur and humerus (CARTY 1989). The mechanism of injury in humeral fractures is external rotation, usually of the forearm. In abuse the forearm is displaced medially; in accidental injury displacement is lateral (HILTON and EDWARDS 1994; EDWARDS 1987). Clinically the child presents with a markedly swollen and painful elbow and in the absence of an appropriate history NAI should be suspected. Fracture-separation of the epiphysis and dislocation is sometimes seen. This may be detected by US before becoming radiologically visible, particularly if the adjacent epiphysis is not ossified (CARTY 1993). Epiphyseal injuries, unlike diaphyseal and metaphyseal injuries, are commonly complicated by growth disturbances and orthopaedic deformity.

10.4.4
Periosteal New Bone

Periosteal new bone is seen as a normal physiological phenomenon between 6 weeks and 6 months of age. It is more prominent in the lower limbs than the upper limbs, is confined to the diaphysis and does not extend to the epiphysis. When present on the tibia it will usually also be present on the femur. Its detection is influenced by the degree of rotation of a limb. Physiological new bone always has a fine organised lamellar appearance. Outside this age pathological periosteal new bone in child abuse usually occurs during fracture repair, but it can occur in

the absence of a fracture and implies a gripping or twisting force (CARTY 1993; WORLOCK et al. 1986; CHAPMAN 1990; CAFFEY 1946) or acceleration-deceleration forces alone (CHAPMAN 1990; KLEINMAN 1987a). The periosteum is attached only loosely to the underlying bone in young children and separation subsequent to formation of a subperiosteal haematoma frequently follows trauma. The periosteum may be stripped off the cortex for the entire length of the shaft. In infants under 6 months of age it is sometimes difficult to distinguish between physiological and pathological causes of periosteal new bone especially in the absence of a visible fracture. Features of physiological periosteal new bone have already been described. In addition to these, such bone shows normal uptake on isotope bone scintigraphy whereas pathological periosteal new bone shows increased radioisotope uptake (STY and STARSHAK 1983). Florid periosteal reaction cloaking the bone and implying repetitive injury, very severe twisting or failure to immobilise the limb is a feature of abuse (Fig. 10.12). Clinically this may present as a hot swollen limb and mimic osteomyelitis, a particular problem in the emergency room. In abuse, the C-reactive protein or white cell count and the child's

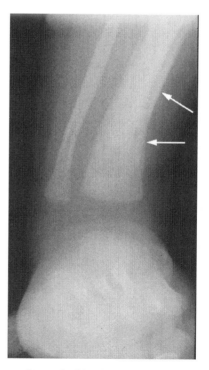

Fig. 10.12. Radiograph of the distal leg and ankle demonstrating healing fractures of the distal tibia and fibula associated with florid periosteal reaction of the medial and lateral sides of the tibia and extending to the metaphysis (*arrows*)

temperature are normal. If a mistaken diagnosis leads to surgery, no pus is found.

10.4.5
Digital Injury

The hand is frequently injured in child abuse. Common injuries are bruises, burns and lacerations but fractures themselves are relatively rare. Direct digital injury from trampling or squeezing or forced hyperflexion of the digits has been reported (NIMKIN et al. 1997). Accidental injuries in toddlers usually involve the phalanges alone and stem from trapping the finger in a door. Abusive fractures may affect the metacarpals and metatarsals as well as the digits. Although not specific for abuse, in young children these fractures provide additional documented evidence of possible child abuse trauma. There may be no soft tissue evidence of injury, suggesting that the fractures have resulted from torsion or twisting forces rather than from direct blows.

10.4.6
Spinal Injury

Spinal injury is comparatively rare in abuse and is usually due to hyperextension and hyperflexion injuries as a result of direct trauma or impaction forces sustained when the child is thumped down on its bottom or impacts against a surface when thrown away (CARTY 1989). Neck fractures may occur by hyperflexion/extension on falling. The most common injuries to the spine involve the vertebral bodies. The commonest sites for vertebral body compression fractures are the lumbar and thoracolumbar regions, and the findings range from minimal loss of height of the anterior aspect of the vertebral body to severe compression deformity and loss of disc space. The radiographic changes may be mistaken for infection, leukaemic infiltration or Langerhans cell histiocytosis. Complications include rupture of the spinal ligament and vertebral dislocations, disc herniation and avulsion of the posterior elements resulting in kyphosis, cord damage and paraplegia if the injury is high enough. The lateral spine radiograph demonstrates most of the fractures (Fig. 10.13). Young children and babies are prone to upper cervical spine injury due to increased flexibility of the supporting ligaments and joint capsules and more horizontal facet joints which are prone to displacement (PANG and WILBERGER 1982), how-

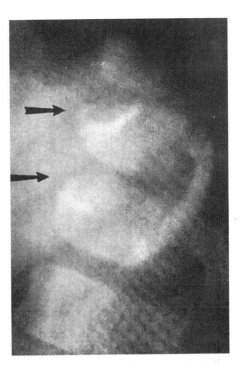

Fig. 10.13. Lateral radiograph of the thoracolumbar junction in an abused infant reveals varying degrees of notching of the anterosuperior endplates of T12 and L1 vertebral bodies (*arrows*) associated with surrounding sclerosis at T12. There is disc space narrowing at T11/T12 and T12/L1 levels

ever, such injuries are rarely seen in life, being found on occasion at post mortem. Obvious fractures and dislocations are usually detected on the standard lateral and frontal cervical spine views. If in doubt, flexion-extension views, CT or MRI will give further information. MRI is essential in the presence of abnormal neurology. CT and plain films will identify bony detail and detect avulsed fragments. CT planes must be chosen to ensure that they cover the plane of the fracture or lamina injuries may be missed.

10.4.7
Rib Fractures

In any case of suspected abuse a chest radiograph is mandatory. In any child admitted collapsed or obtunded a chest radiograph is performed to exclude pulmonary or cardiac causes. Demonstration of rib fractures in children, be they solitary or multiple, is highly suspicious of abuse (Fig. 10.14). The fractures are most frequent in the necks, posterior shafts and axillae, especially medial to the costotransverse articulation (CARTY 1989, 1993). Fractures at the neck

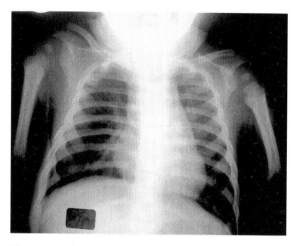

Fig. 10.14. Bilateral rib fractures in an abused infant seen clearly in the axillary (lateral) aspect of the right fifth to seventh and left fourth to sixth ribs. More subtle rib fractures are seen as minor alterations in the contour of the rib in the right eighth and left third ribs. A fracture of the right acromion process is also noted

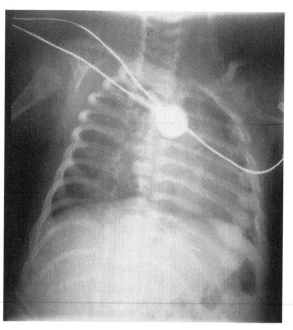

Fig. 10.15. Oblique chest radiograph taken 2 weeks after presentation demonstrating fractures with callus formation during healing. The oblique projection may help to demonstrate fractures not easily seen on the frontal radiograph

are typical of a squeezing chest injury. Anterior rib fractures, though less frequent than in other locations, also occur. In babies and infants the fracture mechanism usually involves squeezing and compression of the thorax during violent shaking (KLEINMAN 1990; CARTY 1993; CARTY and RATCLIFFE 1995). In children the forces sustained in cardiopulmonary resuscitation do not normally result in rib fractures (FELDMAN and BREWER 1984; SPEVAK et al. 1990). Further recognised mechanisms are throwing the child so that it impacts on a hard surface and causes compression of the ribs, kneeling or trampling on the chest and, in older children, direct assault by kicking or beating. If the fractures are in the lower ribs there may be damage to the liver or spleen. Direct forces applied to the chest wall with the child on a hard surface may be accompanied by lung contusion or laceration but relative to the incidence of fractures, the detection of lung damage is rare.

Almost 90% of abuse-related rib fractures occur in infants less than 2 years of age, and most are in those under 1 year of age – a reversal of the age distribution of accidental thoracic injuries (MERTEN et al. 1983). External signs of injury to the chest are rare. Other evidence of external injury to the body, fractures and/or bruising may be present if the child is also flung away either as the mechanism of injury or at the end of the shake. If a row of fractures involves the necks and lateral aspects of the ribs a flail chest may result.

Soon after the injury rib fractures may be undetectable because of superimposed lung contusion shadows, position of the fracture relative to the incident x-ray beam, poor quality radiographs or non-displacement (KLEINMAN and MARKS 1988). Rib fractures become easier to see during healing (CARTY 1993). A repeat chest radiograph should be obtained 7–10 days after presentation in cases of suspected abuse, the film being taken on the same exposure factors to enable direct comparisons to be made. Coned and oblique views of certain rib areas can be used in infants in whom there is a high suspicion of abuse but no abnormality is seen on the frontal chest radiograph (Fig. 10.15). Focal pleural thickening is a suspicious sign. Careful review of the ribs seen on radiographs of the upper arms will often reveal a fracture not visible on the frontal chest radiograph.

More subtle signs of rib fractures such as expansion and widening of the ribs frequently occur at the neck and are often overlooked. Fractures in this position are pathognomonic of abuse. As in adults, the first rib is protected by the overlying shoulder girdle and a fracture of this is rare in NAI. First rib fractures require a much greater force than that required to produce rib fractures elsewhere in the chest. First ribs tend to fracture laterally as opposed to posteriorly (STROUSE and OWINGS 1995). Fractures of the ribs close to the thoracic inlet may be accompanied by brachial plexus or vascular injury. Signs to look for on the chest radiograph which usually accompany subclavian vascular injury are fracture displacement and evidence of mediastinal haematoma, as already stated. Fractures of the lower rib cage may be associated with injury to intra-abdominal organs.

10.4.8
Clavicular and Scapular Injury

The quoted frequency of clavicular fractures in NAI is between 2% and 6% (KLEINMAN 1990). The clavicle is the most frequently injured bone in birth trauma. It is also frequently injured in accidental injury once the child reaches 3 years of age. The midshaft is the usual site of injury in accidental trauma. In abuse both the midportion and the medial and lateral aspects of the clavicle may be injured, fracture of the outer end of the clavicle in infants being highly associated with abuse. Differentiating abuse from birth trauma is normally not difficult. Clavicular injuries sustained at birth are isolated injuries and periosteal new bone is seen at about 11 days and mature callus at 1 month of age. Mid-shaft clavicular fractures in accidental trauma result from a fall on an outstretched hand, a mechanism that does not occur in infants until they become toddlers. Mid-clavicular fractures due to abuse probably also occur from a fall on the shoulder, the same mechanism that causes lateral tip injury. Accidental clavicular fractures are unusual under the age of about 3 years, so the finding of a mid-clavicular fracture in a child which is not a birth fracture attains a higher significance than in older children.

Clavicular fractures do not always present with immediate symptoms. The force of the accidental injury may not be appreciated and it is not perceived as being great enough to cause a fracture. The child then presents with continued pain focally at the fracture site or on limb movement. Delayed presentations due to continuing pain or swelling may be associated with radiographic evidence of a healing fracture. An isolated clavicular fracture not associated with any other injuries is of low significance once the child becomes a toddler.

Acromial injuries are the commonest scapular injury in abuse. Partial avulsion or complete fracture may occur (Fig. 10.16). Such fractures are rare and, though easily overlooked, are highly associated with

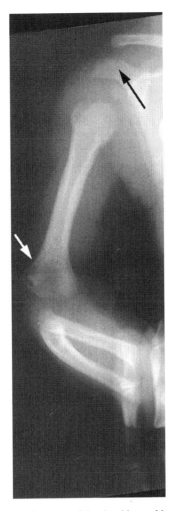

Fig. 10.16. AP radiograph of the shoulder and humerus in an abused child demonstrates an undisplaced fracture through the right acromion process (*black arrow*). There is also a metaphyseal fracture of the distal humerus (*white arrow*) and fine periosteal new bone along the medial shaft of the humerus

abuse. Sternal fractures or sternocleidomastoid dislocations are rare but highly specific for abuse. They are not evident on frontal chest radiographs but are detected on scintigraphy.

10.4.9
Soft Tissue Injuries

Bruising is a common clinical sign of abuse but abuse can occur in the absence of any soft tissue markers of injury, especially those involving acceleration-deceleration forces alone (KLEINMAN et al. 1991b). Multiple bruises of differing ages and bruises found in sites unlikely to be affected by accidental

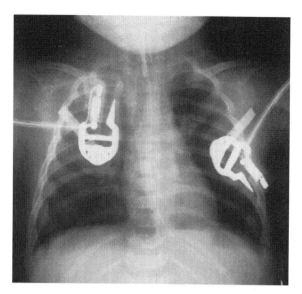

Fig. 10.17. Frontal chest radiograph of an abused child demonstrating lateral rib fractures and calcification in the soft tissues around the neck: "necklace calcification". [From Carty H (1993) case report. Child abuse: necklace calcification: a sign of strangulation. Br J Radiol 66: 1186—1188]

injury are considered typical of NAI. Careful scrutiny of the soft tissues on the radiograph may reveal disruption of the normal soft tissue planes at the site of the bruise. Calcified soft tissue haematomas may result and are usually seen in older children (CARTY 1991). "Necklace calcification" due to calcification in the soft tissues around the neck most probably represents fat necrosis following strangulation (CARTY 1993) (Fig. 10.17). Occult deep soft tissue injuries may have unusual clinical presentations and require CT or MRI to assess the full extent of the injury. Children who present with inflicted soft tissue injury, particularly if extensive or deep trauma is present, should be investigated for occult skeletal injury.

10.4.10
Imaging of Skeletal and Soft Tissue Injuries

The sequence of diagnostic imaging in the abused traumatised child is determined by the cardiovascular and neurological status of the child. Both these have to be stabilised before proceeding with further investigations. In appropriate situations, trauma films are often instituted as resuscitation is taking place. The main uses of radiology in the context of skeletal injury in NAI are to date fractures, to demonstrate occult fractures and to demonstrate and confirm a fracture presenting clinically.

The skeletal survey is a well-established and recognised investigation in child abuse. A recommended protocol of images is given in Table 10.1. Skeletal radiographs provide documented evidence and sometimes the only evidence that abuse has taken place. Each radiology department should have a departmental protocol defining the radiographic projections and exposure factors. These should be adhered to and strict quality control should be in place. Additional views should be obtained of any areas with questionable findings. In particular, coned AP and lateral views of the knees and ankles are required to adequately demonstrate these areas. A "babygram" film is not an adequate skeletal survey. In such a radiograph, the ankles are almost invariably bent and metaphyseal fractures are easily missed. For digital injuries high-detail well-collimated radiographs are essential to increase diagnostic probability. Oblique views of the hands are very useful for demonstrating buckle fractures, which may not be evident on the frontal view. Repeat radiographs after 2 weeks enhance detection of occult fractures in the healing phase and provide further important information on the number, character and age of injuries; such radiographs should include the chest, ankles and knees (KLEINMAN 1996). Skeletal surveys are of most value in the detection of fractures in infants under 2 years of age. The yield decreases with increasing age (NIMKIN et al. 1997). A child presenting as a sudden infant death syndrome (SIDS) should have a skeletal survey performed and reported, ideally by a paediatric radiologist, before the post-mortem is undertaken.

Sometimes the fractures demonstrated in life or death are pathognomic of abuse. The fractures are not usually the cause of death but are an indication of the presence of previous injury if they are old or the extent of a fatal assault. More usually it is the combination of the patient's age and clinical history together with the fracture type that indicate abuse as the probable cause. The presence of multiple fractures of different ages indicates that multiple episodes of trauma have occurred and is typical of abuse. Some fractures, particularly metaphyseal fractures, may not be palpable and will be missed if radiographs are not performed. If there is doubt about a lesion the pathologist should review the limb and obtain high-quality radiographs with the soft tissues removed prior to careful histopathological study of the lesion.

Scintigraphy. Skeletal scintigraphy has been used in suspected or proven NAI cases although this is not routinely practised. Some authorities advocate it as the screening method of choice (STY and STARSHAK 1983). It is of more value in older children, in whom skeletal injury is rarer. Scintigraphy may be used as the primary investigation in these children who show clinical evidence of musculoskeletal injury, with radiographs directed towards the abnormal areas. This avoids the need for unnecessary radiation exposure. Some series show an increase in sensitivity of between 25% and 50% in detecting soft tissue as well as bony injury (CONWAY et al. 1993). Scintigraphy has the advantage that the whole skeleton may be examined without the need for further radiation exposure, and fractures not seen on x-ray may be appreciated. The two techniques are complimentary. It is generally accepted that once an area of increased uptake is identified on scintigraphy, this area should be radiographed. When correctly performed and interpreted, scintigraphy is very sensitive in detecting bone trauma. However, this cannot always be achieved in young children. In children adequate high-quality images are usually only obtained under the following conditions:

1. Adequate patient immobilisation and/or sedation. Spurious asymmetry of isotope activity can be caused by restlessness of the infant during scanning.
2. Positioning without patient rotation.
3. Separate imaging of the lower limbs from the trunk.
4. The limbs on both sides of the body should be in the same position. This is of most importance for joints that cannot be positioned neutrally.
5. Use of a high-resolution technique (3-mm pinhole collimator views).
6. Adequate count density.
7. Separate images of the diaphysis and metaphysis are obtained to exclude the presence of metaphyseal corner fractures.

The reporting doctor must be familiar with the normal bone scan appearances in children. Metaphyseal fractures lie at the ends of actively growing bone and in regions of maximum normal radionuclide uptake, making it difficult to detect increased activity with minimally disrupted metaphyseal fractures. A further advantage of the isotope bone scan is that it assesses the entire skeleton and can detect fractures not apparent on the plain film. However, limitations of scintigraphy are that symmetrical fractures may be missed and it is relatively insensitive in the detection of skull and vertebral body fractures. It is also unable to determine the age and type of fracture. Scintigraphy should thus be considered a supplementary imaging technique in the following situations:

1. To resolve ambiguous lesions on radiography.
2. In the presence of a high clinical suspicion of abuse but a negative skeletal survey.
3. To demonstrate occult fractures before they become visible on plain radiographs.
4. In children with single fractures who otherwise have a negative skeletal survey but in whom clinical suspicion of abuse is high. Demonstration of further fractures would aid confirmation of NAI.

Reference must be made to the plain skeletal radiographs to ensure correct interpretation of lesions. The degree of isotope localisation is determined by the time scintigraphy is performed after the incident. Bone scans become positive within hours of an injury and the time evolution of scintigraphic features has a characteristic course (STY and STARSHAK 1983). In uncertain cases, if a repeat scan 3–4 days later fails to show any focal abnormality a fracture is effectively excluded. Repeat bone scans are not routine practice. Scintigraphy is most sensitive in detection of rib, scapular, spinal, diaphyseal and pelvic fractures. A lower sensitivity is seen with hairline skull fractures, and flat bones, old healed fractures and metaphyseal fractures and may be missed.

Ultrasound has been used to demonstrate subperiosteal haemorrhage, fracture separation of the epiphysis, occult long bone fractures and costochondral injuries before they are radiographically evident. It is a useful supplementary investigation, particularly when dating injuries (KLEINMAN 1987a; GRAIF et al. 1988; STREETS et al. 1990).

10.4.11
Dating of Fractures

Precise dating of fractures is not possible but an estimate can usually be performed (Table 10.6). The estimates are based on knowing the repair patterns following accidental injury when the time of injury

Table 10.6. Dating fractures (adapted from O'CONNOR and COHEN 1987)

	Bank	Peak
Soft tissue resolution	2–10 days	4–10 days
Early periosteal new bone	4–21 days	10–14 days
Loss of fracture line definition	10–21 days	14–21 days
Soft callus	10–21 days	14–21 days
Hard callus	14–90 days	21–42 days
Remodelling	3 months–2 years	

and its immediate and subsequent management are known. The shorter the time interval between the injury and the initial radiograph, the easier fracture dating becomes. Repair processes are lengthened when the initial injury is more severe. Florid periosteal reaction occurs with repeated trauma, severe trauma or failure to immobilise the limb.

10.5
Thoracic and Abdominal Injuries

Although of much lower frequency than skeletal and brain injuries in NAI, abdominal and thoracic injuries are associated with significant mortality and morbidity. Stated mortality rates are around 50% (CARTY 1991; COOPER et al. 1988; TOULOUKIAN 1968). The average age for blunt abdominal trauma and fatal visceral injury in NAI is 2 years. Children who present with intra-abdominal bleeding, particularly in the presence of shock, have a higher mortality. Important predictors of the type and severity of injury are vital signs and haematocrit on admission (COOPER et al. 1988).

In NAI the duodenum, pancreas and mesentery are more frequently injured than the liver, kidneys and spleen. In accidental trauma the solid organs are more commonly injured (SIVIT et al. 1989a; TOULOUKIAN 1968; COOPER et al. 1988). Most visceral injuries are not specific for abuse. The type and extent of injury must be assessed in the light of the history. In young children under 5 years of age, excluding motor vehicle accidents, significant accidental abdominal trauma is extremely rare and thus, if found, is highly suggestive of abuse. The mechanism of injury is a blunt, direct compressive force. Acute presentations are with signs of shock and hypovolaemia, peritonitis and an acute abdomen. The children are often more severely ill than with accidental trauma as there is frequently a delay in bringing the child to medical attention. The child may present more insidiously, often with longstanding symptoms of functional organ impairment, weight loss, vomiting, anorexia and no history of trauma. The magnitude of injury is underestimated. It is in this group that repeated presentations to the casualty department or GP are made, and if external signs of abuse are missing, the child may later return moribund or dead.

Vomiting is a non-specific sign occurring in both acute and chronic presentations. It is a feature of both abdominal and head injuries. An intracranial cause for vomiting must be sought if investigations for an abdominal cause prove negative. A significant number of children who have sustained blunt abdominal or thoracic trauma also suffer from cerebral injury which renders the physical examination less reliable and increases the need for diagnostic imaging.

10.5.1
Imaging of Thoracic and Abdominal Injuries

The initial clinical abdominal examination usually detects the presence of trauma. There may be visible external indicators of abuse such as bruising or abrasions. If the patient cannot be stabilised, imaging does not have a role. Hypotension is an unreliable predictor of major organ injury in the paediatric population as children are able to maintain a normal blood pressure despite significant blood loss (STEIN et al. 1994).

The sequence of investigations usually involves initial plain radiographs as per departmental trauma protocol with further cross-sectional imaging and contrast studies as required. The plain abdominal radiograph is not a sensitive or specific investigation in abdominal trauma. Its main purpose is in the demonstration of free air, which, if present is an indication for immediate surgery and no further imaging. Less than 30% of patients with ruptured viscera demonstrate free air on radiographs. Therefore, a normal radiograph does not exclude significant intra/extraperitoneal injury. Loss of the lateral psoas margins or displacement of the kidneys indicates retroperitoneal injuries.

CT is the investigation of choice in a child with abdominal or thoracic trauma and is indicated in the following situations:

1. Haemodynamic stability but potentially significant intra-abdominal injury by history
2. Significant initial fluid resuscitation requirements without an obvious source of blood loss
3. Multiple system injury, especially with head injury
4. Inability to perform an adequate abdominal examination
5. Haemoglobin below 10 g/dl that is not explained by an obvious source of blood loss
6. Haematuria associated with signs of abdominal injury

Several studies have evaluated the use of diagnostic peritoneal lavage, comparing it with CT in blunt abdominal trauma (ENGRAV et al. 1975; PARVIN et al.

1975; GILL et al. 1975; ALYONO and PERRY 1981; ALYONO et al. 1982; MCLELLAN et al. 1985; DAVIS and HOYT 1990; SHERCK and OAKES 1990). If diagnostic peritoneal lavage is being contemplated, CT should be performed first as the lavage fluid makes the interpretation of the significance of free fluid impossible.

Much has been written about the relative merits of CT and US in the imaging of abdominal trauma (SIVIT et al. 1989a; FILIATRAULT and GAREL 1995; KIRKS 1983; RAPTOPOULOUS 1994; TURNOCK et al. 1993; RANCE and BEAR 1980; SIVIT and EICHELBERGER 1995; KANE et al. 1991; JAMIESON et al. 1996). Advantages of US include its portability, speed of use, cost-effectiveness and bedside use. It can detect free fluid and parenchymal injuries. It is limited in the overall assessment of the abdomen by bowel gas and open wounds and bandages render some areas inaccessible. US is useful in the follow-up of patients to assess resolution of known lesions and the quantity of haemoperitoneum. The general consensus is that whilst US can give good information on solid organ injury, CT remains the gold standard for complete assessment of the whole abdomen and gives better anatomical and often functional definition and may reveal bony trauma. It has the further advantage of assessing bowel and mesenteric injuries.

Injured children do not usually require sedation in scanning the abdomen and pelvis. Sedation is contraindicated in the presence of neurological injury. Some children are too irritable to be scanned and if sedation is required, a general anaesthetic may be needed.

If bowel distension is required, water is the medium of choice. All scans should be performed with intravenous contrast, with a dose of 2 ml per kilogram, which also demonstrates renal function and vascular integrity. Optimal intravenous enhancement of solid abdominal organs is necessary to maximise contrast between normal and abnormal parenchyma and adjacent collections of blood (FEDERLE et al. 1981). Depending on patient size and particular organs of interest, slice thickness varies between 5 and 10 mm. Scanning should include the whole of the abdomen as the only sign of trauma may be small pockets of free fluid deep in the pelvis. In older children a small amount of fluid in the pouch of Douglas may be normal. The images should be reviewed on both soft tissue and wide window settings, which increases the sensitivity in detection of small amounts of extraluminal air.

Magnetic resonance imaging is not indicated in the acute setting except in suspected spinal cord injury or occasionally in assessing vascular integrity if mediastinal widening is present. Radioisotope studies of the kidneys are useful in follow-up studies as they provide information on function.

10.5.2
Liver Injuries

In abuse as opposed to accidental trauma the liver is injured more frequently than the spleen or kidneys. The left lobe is the most vulnerable part as it is compressed against the spine during direct blows. In accidental trauma the larger right lobe, especially the posterior segment, is more often injured (STALKER et al. 1986).

The most common liver injuries in abuse are subcapsular haematomas, parenchymal contusions and lacerations (CARTY 1991; RUESS et al. 1995), usually as a result of direct impact following deceleration from direct blows to the abdomen. Small contusions and lacerations can remain clinically silent, which makes estimation of the true incidence of liver injuries difficult. The presence of ascites due to liver injury is an indicator of major hepatic trauma. Further less frequent complications of hepatic injury are given in Table 10.7. A rise in blood transaminase levels is a reliable indicator of hepatic damage. Fresh subcapsular haematomas have a central high-density area of clotted blood surrounded by lower density non-clotted blood. Subcapsular haematomas are usually seen as low-density collections on both US and CT when the haematoma has organised. Hepatic lacerations are evident as irregular branching or linear regions of low attenuation against a background of normally enhancing liver parenchyma. Hepatic contusion appears as focal poorly marginated areas of low density (Fig. 10.18).

Table 10.7. Complications of hepatic injury

Subcapsular haematoma
Parenchymal contusions, lacerations, haematoma
Subphrenic abscess
Hepatic abscess from infection of haematoma
Disruption of hepatic duct
Biloma
Hepaticobiliary fistula
Hepatic portal vein thrombosis
Complete avulsion of common duct from its attachment to the duodenum
Ascites
Intraperitoneal bleed
Associated thoracic injuries – lung contusion, rib fractures

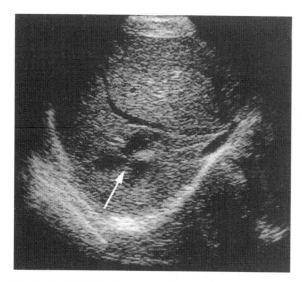

Fig. 10.18. US of the liver in an abused child who sustained severe non-accidental trauma to the right upper quadrant resulting in hepatic lacerations seen as irregular branching regions of low density in the hepatic parenchyma (*arrow*). (Courtesy of Doz. Dr. M. Riccabona and Professor Dr. R. Fotter, Department of Paediatric Radiology, LKH University Hospital Graz)

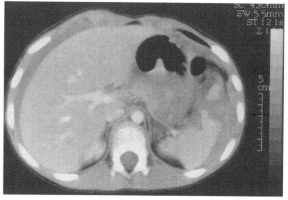

Fig. 10.19. Axial contrast-enhanced CT of the upper abdomen in a young abused child who sustained blunt injury to the left upper quadrant, demonstrating fragmentation of the spleen. There is also free fluid around the spleen and liver. At surgery, the splenic vessels were intact

Periportal lucency may represent haemorrhage, lymphatic oedema secondary to overhydration or extravascular fluid in the setting of reperfusion injury (PATRICK et al. 1992). It is seen in up to 80% of children with hepatic injury. Extensive periportal lucency is associated with physiological instability and a higher mortality (SIVIT et al. 1993). As with accidental trauma, the size and extent of injury on CT scans do not correlate with the need for surgery as many lesions resolve spontaneously.

10.5.3
Splenic Injuries

Splenic injury in NAI has a lower incidence compared with accidental trauma. The mechanism of abusive abdominal injury in infants and toddlers is direct compressive force over the midline. Injuries to the spleen are not usually caused by this mechanism of injury (CARTY 1991; KLEINMAN 1990). Injuries include parenchymal contusions and lacerations and subcapsular and intraparenchymal haematomas.

The initial plain radiograph, though usually normal, may reveal signs of intraperitoneal bleed, elevation of the left hemidiaphragm, pneumothorax, rib fractures and splenomegaly (KIRKS 1983). Enlargement of the splenic mass due to intra/perisplenic or

subcapsular haematoma displaces the gastric air bubble medially and the splenic flexure inferiorly. Patients with longstanding splenomegaly of any cause are at greater risk of rupture following even minor trauma. Both US and CT can identify splenic injuries but CT is the gold standard (JEFFREY et al. 1981) (Fig. 10.19). A diagnostic accuracy rate as high as 98% for CT evaluation of the spleen has been reported (WING et al. 1985). The well-enhanced spleen appears denser and of higher attenuation than intrasplenic contusion or haematoma or adjacent extraparenchymal bleed. Perisplenic blood must be distinguished from pleural fluid or blood in the left posterior costophrenic sulcus (SILVERMAN et al. 1985). Perisplenic blood does not indent the parenchyma whereas subcapsular splenic haematoma does. Injuries to the anterior and medial aspects of the spleen may be obscured by gastric atony and overdistension (GINALDI et al. 1976).

False-negative CT has been reported in cases of delayed splenic rupture (FAGELMAN et al. 1985; PAPPAS et al. 1987). This is rupture occurring more than 48h after blunt trauma in a previously haemodynamically stable patient following an initially normal CT scan (KLUGER et al. 1994).

Current management of splenic trauma is to conserve the spleen whenever possible and avoid splenectomy because of the risk of overwhelming sepsis in asplenic individuals (BALFANZ et al. 1976). The physiological condition of the patient and not the CT appearance determines the need for operative intervention in all solid organ trauma in both accidental and non-accidental injury (BRICK et al. 1987). Non-operative management in children is more successful than in adults. Children have a thicker splenic capsule and their splenic vessels are more responsive to haemodynamic changes, leading to spontaneous cessation of bleeding (MORSE and GARCIA 1994).

10.5.4
Renal Tract Injuries

The kidney is an infrequent site of injury in NAI. Injuries range from minor parenchymal contusions and lacerations to disruption of the renal parenchyma and collecting system or more major damage with capsular tear and renal fracture. More severe critical injuries include avulsion or thrombosis of the renal vessels or complete renal fragmentation (KIRKS 1983). Acute renal failure in the absence of direct trauma can occur as a consequence of massive bleeding which leads to rhabdomyolysis and subsequent myoglobinuria. There is a higher risk of injury in abused children who also have underlying unrelated structural renal abnormalities (KLEINMAN 1990).

Haematuria in general is a poor predictor of the presence or extent of renal damage, being a non-specific marker for injury to the liver, spleen and retroperitoneum. Both the presence and an increasing amount of haematuria are associated with significantly higher risks of abdominal trauma, multiple organ trauma and renal injury in the presence of clinical symptoms. There is a better correlation between the extent of urological injury and the degree of haematuria in blunt renal trauma than in penetrating injury. NICOLAISEN et al. (1985) concluded that blunt trauma patients who are in shock need evaluation whereas those with stable vital signs do not need further renal tract investigations.

Several studies have concluded that patients with microscopic haematuria do not all need investigating (KLEIN et al. 1988; GUICE et al. 1983; NICOLAISEN et al. 1985), but in spite of this most children will at least have a US examination. US of the kidneys in acute trauma is generally sensitive in detecting contusion and perirenal extravasation provided the kidneys are well visualised. No functional information is obtained. Intravenous urography (IVU) has been used in the past in acute renal trauma and generally identifies renal morphology and function and demonstrates extravasation (Fig. 10.20). CT is now considered to be the diagnostic imaging modality of choice. CT is judged to be more accurate in demon-

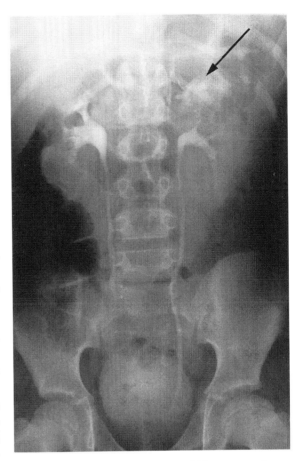

Fig. 10.20. IVU in a child who sustained blunt trauma from a kick to the left renal angle. This image taken at 10 min after injection of contrast demonstrates extravasation of contrast from the left upper pole in the contused kidney (*arrow*)

strating renal parenchymal injuries and perirenal collections (KIRKS 1983), can assess function and can diagnose renal vascular pedicle injuries. The kidneys are automatically imaged during contrast-enhanced CT. CT findings include segmental areas of reduced renal perfusion, cortical lacerations and perirenal and intrarenal haematoma (Figs. 10.21, 10.22). US is useful after the acute setting to follow resolution of collections.

The lower urinary tract is usually spared in NAI (KLEINMAN 1990). Direct blows against a full bladder may result in rupture of the bladder without an associated pelvic fracture. Gross haematuria almost always signifies bladder injury. The diagnosis of bladder leak or rupture may be made on contrast-enhanced CT provided the bladder is distended with contrast. Alternatively, contrast instilled into the bladder via a urinary catheter may demonstrate extravasation (Fig. 10.23).

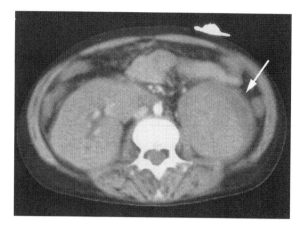

Fig. 10.21. Axial contrast-enhanced CT of the upper abdomen at the level of the kidneys demonstrates a low-density non-enhancing subcapsular haematoma of the left kidney (*arrow*)

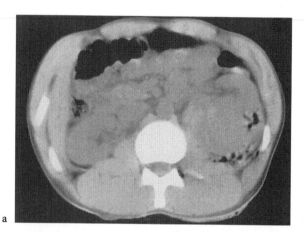

a

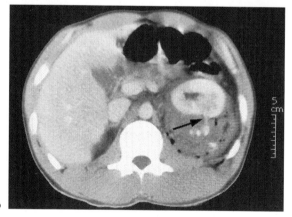

b

Fig. 10.22 a,b. Axial CT slices through the upper abdomen. **a** Without intravenous contrast. A large soft tissue mass is demonstrated in the left upper quadrant containing gas density. The left kidney is poorly delineated from the mass. **b** Following intravenous contrast enhancement, there is now clear delineation of the left kidney, which enhances, from the adjacent low-density non-enhancing haematoma. The site of renal injury as demonstrated by the site of leakage of contrast is clearly evident (*arrow*)

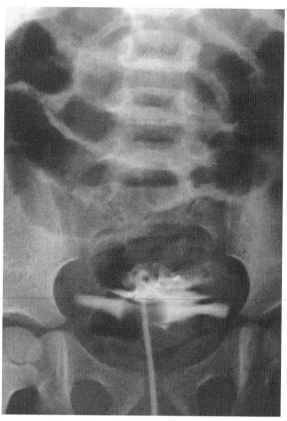

Fig. 10.23. Radiograph taken early during the course of instilling contrast into the bladder demonstrates contrast extravasation secondary to bladder rupture in an abused child who sustained a direct blow against a full bladder. There was no associated bony injury. (Courtesy of Doz. Dr. M. Riccabona and Professor Dr. R. Fotter, Department of Paediatric Radiology, LKH University Hospital Graz)

Posterior urethral injuries secondary to blunt trauma to the pelvis occur almost solely in boys because the bladder base and posterior urethra are fixed tightly to the pelvic floor and pubis. In girls the urethra is more mobile. Approximately 5% of boys with fractures of the anterior pubic ramus have a posterior urethral injury and 10%–20% of these also have associated bladder injury. Anterior urethral injuries are also more common in boys but are not usually associated with fractures of the bony pelvis. Urethral and genital injuries occur in sexually abused children in both sexes. Presentation is with blood at the urethral meatus, inability to void and progressive distension of the urinary bladder (GOLDMAN et al. 1997; NOE and JERKINS 1992; SANDLER et al. 1981). Visual evidence of trauma with bruising of the external genitalia and perineal haematoma may be present. Pelvic examination may reveal a mass due to pelvic haematoma. In boys suspected of urethral rupture, prior to passage of a urinary catheter, retrograde urethrography should be performed to demonstrate the urethra and prevent inadvertently converting a partial tear to a complete tear. Retrograde urethrography is not usually performed in girls as urethral injuries are much rarer. If such injuries are present they are frequently associated with significant coexistent injuries to the bladder neck and anterior vaginal wall (MERCHANT et al. 1984; NOE and JERLINS 1992; WILLIAMS 1975).

10.5.5
Pancreatic Injuries

Trauma is the most common cause of pancreatitis in children. Once accidental injury and hereditary pancreatitis have been excluded, acute haemorrhagic pancreatitis is highly suggestive of NAI. In the absence of a history of trauma in children a skeletal survey is advised as this may show other manifestations of abuse. Pancreatic injuries may present acutely with shock, abdominal pain and vomiting or more insidiously with weight loss, chronic abdominal pain and a palpable mass due to a pancreatic pseudocyst.

Early clinical diagnosis of pancreatic injury may be difficult (NORTRUP and SIMMONS 1972). As the gland is retroperitoneal, signs of peritonitis are classically absent. Often the clinical signs of injury evolve slowly and may be masked by associated injuries. The serum amylase is a non-specific indicator of pancreatic injury and raised levels are present in other conditions. The typical rise in amylase may be delayed for more than 24h post injury. Acute pancreatitis and pancreatic pseudocyst occur relatively commonly in blunt abdominal trauma in NAI compared with accidental trauma (CARTY 1991; SLOVIS et al. 1975); this is due to the effect of direct punches and kicks over the midline as the gland crosses the vertebral column (JEFFREY 1989; SIVIT et al. 1992a). The plain abdominal radiograph may show an abdominal mass in a patient with a pseudocyst. Transection, laceration or contusion usually occur at the junction of the body and tail. Seepage of active pancreatic enzymes into the tissue spaces ultimately leads to haemorrhagic pancreatitis.

Thin-section CT is considered the best imaging modality although it has been quoted as missing one-third of the injuries (CARTY 1991; KLEINMAN 1990; SIVIT et al. 1992a). In children, the pancreas is a small organ and there is a general paucity of surrounding retroperitoneal fat and little separation of the pancreatic fragments in injury (JEFFREY et al. 1983). Other sources of diagnostic error include unopacified bowel adjacent to the pancreas, streak artefacts simulating lacerations and haematoma arising from the spleen or left kidney around the pancreatic tail. Fluid in the lesser sac is common, being found in more than 70% of children with pancreatic injury compared with less than 1% of children without it (SIVIT et al. 1991). Its presence is a helpful sign in uncertain cases. These fluid collections may become secondarily infected.

Ultrasound is limited in the initial detection of pancreatic trauma but is useful in follow-up of injury, especially for serial evaluation of peripancreatic fluid collections that may evolve into pseudocysts (JEFFREY et al. 1986). US can detect extrapancreatic fluid collections. Diffuse or focal gland enlargement and pancreatic duct dilatation are common sonographic findings, being demonstrated in approximately half of patients. Decrease in gland echogenicity occurs in the presence of interstitial oedema. Peripancreatic extension of inflammation into the soft tissues can appear hypo- or hyperechoic (COLEMAN et al. 1983; SIEGEL et al. 1987).

On CT the appearance of acute pancreatitis ranges from a normal appearing gland to diffuse gland enlargement (BALTHAZAR 1989; BALTHAZAR et al. 1990; DONOVAN et al. 1982; KING et al. 1995). Pancreatic contours may remain smooth and regular. Intrapancreatic fluid collections may occur. Extrapancreatic changes are often the most evident. Gland enhancement in mild pancreatitis is usually normal whereas in severe disease heterogeneous enhancement is seen. Progression to pancreatic abscess and necrosis may occur and pancreatitis may be complicated by formation of pseudocysts. These are evident on CT as homogeneous round or oval well-encapsulated collections with an attenuation similar to water. Areas of high attenuation within the pseudocysts are due to haemorrhage or infection. When adequately performed, in the acute stages CT may demonstrate the low-attenuation laceration or fracture traversing the gland, fluid in the lesser sac and anterior pararenal space, thickening of the anterior renal fascia and free peritoneal fluid (DODDS et al. 1990; HERMAN and SIEGEL 1991; SIVIT et al. 1992a). The best indicator of pancreatic injury at CT is unexplained peripancreatic fluid in the absence of other visceral injury (SIVIT et al. 1992a). Peripancreatic fluid in the anterior pararenal space may dissect between the pancreas and splenic vein (LANE et al. 1994; SIVIT and KAUFMAN 1995).

Accompanying skeletal and soft tissue injuries may occur but the association with fat necrosis at distant sites is actually rare and plays no part in the acute setting.

10.5.6
Adrenal Injuries

Unsuspected adrenal injuries are occasional incidental findings when imaging for other abdominal or thoracic injuries. Unilateral adrenal haemorrhages usually occur on the right side (NIMKIN et al. 1994; SIVIT et al. 1992b). Adrenal haemorrhages become clinically apparent if bilateral and acute adrenocortical insufficiency results (RAPTOPOULOUS 1994). Signs to look for on CT are round or oval homogeneous low-attenuation masses within the gland, thickening of the ipsilateral diaphragmatic crus, infiltration of the surrounding fat with haemorrhage and the presence of free intraperitoneal fluid or blood (BURKS et al. 1992). Although adrenal haemorrhage may occur as an isolated injury, associated injuries to adjacent organs such as the kidneys, spleen and pancreatic tail should be sought (Fig. 10.24).

10.6
Hollow Viscus Injuries

Hollow viscus injuries are often fatal in child abuse because of the severity of the injuries and the delay in diagnosis. Bowel injuries occur with greater frequency in NAI compared with accidental trauma. Knowledge of the mechanism of injury increases the index of suspicion of bowel trauma. The three main categories of injury are mesenteric injuries, bowel disruption from partial or complete transection or perforation, and haematoma formation. The mortality is high. The mesenteric side of the bowel is more prone to vascular tears and the antimesenteric side to perforation. These injuries are more common in the small bowel, especially the jejunum, than in the colon or duodenum.

10.6.1
Duodenal and Jejunal Injuries

The duodenum, in particular the second and third parts, is the most frequent site of bowel injury in blunt abdominal trauma. Injury occurs from direct

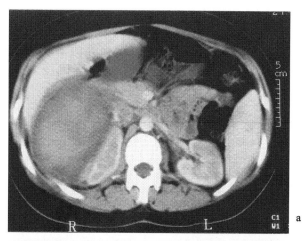

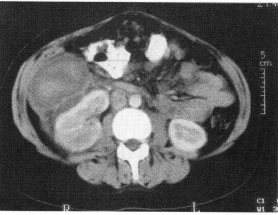

Fig. 10.24. a Contrast-enhanced axial CT through the upper abdomen demonstrating a large non-enhancing homogeneous low-attenuation mass in the right suprarenal region causing compression of the adjacent right kidney, which was a large right adrenal haematoma. **b** Contrast-enhanced axial CT through the upper abdomen again demonstrates a large right adrenal haematoma. There is compression of the injured adjacent right kidney, which demonstrates a subcapsular haematoma

compression as the duodenum passes over the vertebral column, from shear injury or from formation of a closed loop between the pylorus and the ligament of Treitz which results in a marked increase in intraluminal pressure (COX and KUHN 1996).

Intramural haematomas of the duodenum and jejunum are the most frequent gastrointestinal injuries sustained in abuse and are typically located in the second and third parts (CARTY 1991; KIRKS 1983; KLEINMAN 1990; KLEINMAN et al. 1986a; FULCHER et al. 1990). Major vascular injuries occur in about one-third of patients. Disruption of the vascular supply occurs from sudden deceleration or from the compressive force of the fixed duodenum against the spine following blunt trauma. Both ischaemic injury and direct trauma contribute to bleeding. Bleeding into the submucosa or subserosa may lead to complete or partial obstruction of the lumen. Presentation is usually with abdominal pain and vomiting with signs of peritonism and obstruction. Clinical signs may be delayed for several days after trauma has occurred. Associated biliary and pancreatic injuries occur in up to 25% of patients. If a duodenal haematoma is found during the investigation of conditions such as vomiting, failure to thrive and weight loss, NAI should be considered unless there is an appropriate history of recent trauma.

The plain abdominal radiograph may show free fluid, proximal obstruction of the bowel and ischaemic change. In suspected small bowel injuries, upper gastrointestinal contrast studies will yield the most information. In the acute phase an intramural mass with thickening of the proximal folds giving a "coiled spring" appearance is seen. In the resolving phase localised masses in the duodenal wall together with prominent thickened mucosal folds indicate previous haemorrhage (BRATU et al. 1970; KLEINMAN et al. 1986a) (Fig. 10.25). Ultrasound may directly visualise the haematoma or may demonstrate indirect signs such as proximal duodenal dilatation. A haematoma may act as a lead point causing intussusception. If possible, duodenal haematomas are managed conservatively.

Perforation of the bowel may complicate direct trauma (KLEINMAN 1990). This is likely to occur at the second and third parts of the duodenum in the retroperitoneum, or at points of mesenteric fixation at or just distal to the ligament of Treitz and the ileocaecal junction. Clinical presentation may be delayed. A delay of more than 24h in the diagnosis and repair of a duodenal laceration increases the mortality from 5% to 60% (RAPTOPOULOUS 1994). Perforation is readily diagnosed on the plain radiograph if there is sufficient free air, in which case no further imaging is needed. If the child is fit an erect chest or lateral decubitus radiograph should be obtained, which can detect as little as one or 2 ml of free air, but in a shocked child either a supine or a horizontal beam lateral radiograph may be needed. The plain film may also reveal features of bowel obstruction or an indistinct psoas shadow. Cross-sectional imaging will readily identify free fluid and dilated bowel.

A summary of the CT findings in bowel trauma are given in Table 10.8. Two pathognomonic but infrequent findings of bowel rupture on CT are extraluminal air and extravasation of oral contrast media. CT is extremely sensitive in the detection of a pneumoperitoneum provided images are reviewed

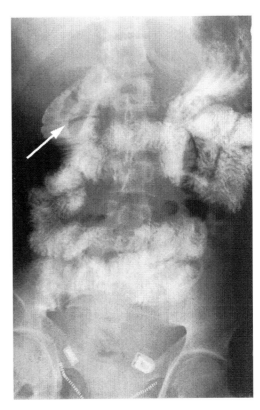

Fig. 10.25. Upper GI contrast study in a patient who sustained blunt upper abdominal trauma demonstrating two low-density filling defects in the second part of the duodenum associated with prominent thickened folds (*arrow*). The appearances are consistent with resolving duodenal haematoma

Table 10.8. CT findings in bowel injury

Pneumoperitoneum
Haemoperitoneum and free intraperitoneal fluid
Bowel wall thickening
Duodenal haematoma
Mesenteric haematoma
Bowel wall enhancement (hypoperfusion complex/shock bowel)
Extravasation of oral contrast

on wide window settings, which are most sensitive in detecting small amounts of extraluminal air. Three series found extraluminal air at CT in one-third of patients and contrast extravasation in up to one-quarter of patients (HARA et al. 1989; MIRVIS et al. 1992; RIZZO et al. 1992; SIVIT et al. 1994). The most frequent sign of bowel rupture is moderate to large amounts of unexplained peritoneal fluid. The attenuation of the fluid varies with the haematocrit and the length of time from injury. In the presence of blunt abdominal trauma, free intraperitoneal fluid is assumed to represent haemoperitoneum. The fluid may track inferiorly along the right paracolic gutter and simulate appendicitis, leading to diagnostic confusion and delays. If there is no obvious source of bleeding from the solid organs, this heightens the suspicion of bowel trauma. A specific and sensitive sign of blunt trauma is abnormally intense bowel wall enhancement as part of the hypoperfusion complex and shock bowel syndrome (TAYLOR et al. 1987; HARA et al. 1989; SIVIT et al. 1992, 1994). It results from poorly compensated hypovolaemic shock. The CT appearances may cause diagnostic confusion with bowel rupture but must be distinguished as shock bowel requires attention to haemodynamic stability and not surgery. The bowel is dilated and fluid filled with thickened walls which show intense contrast enhancement. The kidneys and major abdominal vessels also show intense enhancement and the aorta and inferior vena cava are reduced in calibre. There may be free intraperitoneal fluid. Compensatory vasoconstriction occurs, which may be so severe that the other solid organs show reduced enhancement.

Mesenteric injuries can range from trauma to small peripheral branches, resulting in local haematoma formation to complete avulsion of the superior mesenteric vessels that gives rise to mesenteric ischaemia and large collections of peritoneal blood (RIZZO et al. 1989). Later complications include the development of ischaemic strictures of the bowel (SHAH et al. 1997). CT findings of acute mesenteric injury are streaky infiltration of the mesentery, haemoperitoneum, bowel wall thickening and ill-defined mesenteric soft tissue masses representing haematoma.

10.6.2
Gastric Injuries

Gastric injury in abuse occurs in less than 1% of cases (BRUNSTING 1987). Gastric injury is rarely isolated and additional injury to the spleen, left kidney or adjacent ribs usually occurs. Gastric rupture may result, and in young children and infants the injury is usually in the greater curvature. It typically follows a meal when the stomach is full and distended. Gastric rupture is a rare consequence of failure to pass a nasogastric tube in the presence of a distended stomach which occurs secondary to duodenal obstruction or to paralysis in acute atony in neglected children. If these starved children then eat a large amount of food they become severely ill with abdominal disten-

sion, pain and vomiting. Gastric perforation and rupture is a serious event and may result in septic shock and death (KIRKS 1983; KLEINMAN 1990). Radiographically, in 60% of cases massive pneumoperitoneum is evident. Further imaging is not indicated; immediate surgery is required.

10.6.3
Colonic Injuries

The colon is relatively shielded from direct injury by the bony pelvis or because of its peripheral location within the abdomen. If colonic injuries occur, they are similar to those in the remainder of the bowel and range from focal mural contusion to perforation and laceration. The transverse colon, like the jejunum, traverses the spine and is subject to the same compressive forces. Direct stabbing with sharp implements or forced ingestion of foreign bodies may cause colonic perforation. Anal and rectal injuries may be seen in association with sexual abuse and present as perineal and pelvic abscesses, faecal peritonitis and rectal tears from forceful penetration.

10.7
Thoracic Injury

Complications of direct thoracic compression are given in Table 10.9. Although the frequency of rib fractures in NAI is high, direct contusional injury of the lungs and pleura is comparatively rare. Injuries can occur in the absence of external signs of bruising or rib fractures. The chest radiograph is usually the first investigation to be performed, often as resuscitation is taking place. Rib fractures are not always

Table 10.9. Complications of direct thoracic compression

Pulmonary contusion
Intrapulmonary haematoma
Pneumothorax
Ruptured diaphragm
Haemorrhagic effusion
Flail chest
Chylothorax
Associated intra-abdominal injuries
Associated cardiac injuries:
    Contusion, haemopericardium
    Pneumopericardium
    Myocardial ischaemia and infarction
    Ventricular septal defects
    Ventricular aneurysm

demonstrated on the initial radiograph. In all cases of suspected abuse a repeat chest radiograph should be performed 7–10 days later when fractures become easier to see during the healing phase. Bilateral fractures in 3 or more adjacent ribs or combined rib and sternal fractures produce instability leading to a flail chest. Paradoxical motion of a flail segment during respiration can impair respiratory motion and cause atelectasis. Occasionally this is complicated by herniation of lung through a defect in the chest wall produced by the flail segment. The chest radiograph also reveals lung contusion, pleural effusions and pneumonia from secondary infection or aspiration (Fig. 10.26). Other injuries difficult to detect by clinical examination such as mediastinal and pericardial haemorrhage, diaphragmatic rupture and bronchial, oesophageal and pulmonary laceration may be detected on the chest radiograph. Ideally a rapid exposure and high kilovoltage technique (120–140 kV) gives the best definition of all structures on the chest film with limited motion artefact. This is often difficult to achieve with many portable units.

Pulmonary contusion due to blunt trauma is one of the most common primary lung injuries in accidental injury secondary to blunt trauma. The radiographic changes of lung contusion may be delayed by up to 6 h (GOODMAN and PUTMAN 1981). Contusions usually occur adjacent to solid structures. A pneumothorax may result from direct compressive trauma with rupture of alveoli or a bronchus or more rarely from pulmonary laceration. Complications of laceration and contusion include bronchopleural fistula and persistent air leak, infection and abscess formation and expansion and compression of the adjacent lung by mass effect.

Haemothorax and serous effusions cannot be differentiated on radiographs although in the presence of rib fractures a presumptive diagnosis of blood can be made. At the bedside US may differentiate the two; haemothorax is of higher echogenicity than serous effusion. Injuries may preclude adequate US assessment and much of the chest is inaccessible to US. CT provides greater information and gives a better overview of thoracic and mediastinal structures. Contrast-enhanced CT can be used to assess vascular integrity. CT is much more sensitive in identifying parenchymal lung injuries and extent of disease than the plain radiograph (WAGNER et al. 1988; MIRVIS et al. 1987; SIVIT et al. 1989b) (Fig. 10.27). Both US and CT can be used to guide aspiration and/or drainage of pleural collections.

Intrathoracic injury is often accompanied by blunt abdominal trauma. The heart is relatively

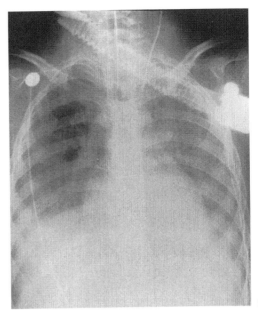

a

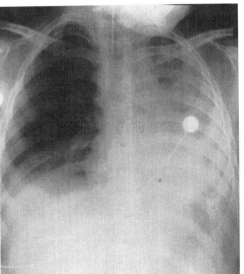

b

Fig. 10.26 a,b. Two chest radiographs of abused severely ill children demonstrating bilateral pulmonary contusion and lung consolidation/atelectasis; b also demonstrates a large left pleural effusion

protected by the thoracic cage and surrounding lungs. Rarely, with severe trauma cardiac contusional injury with haemopericardium, pneumopericardium, ventricular septal defect and ventricular aneurysm can occur (KLEINMAN 1990). Mural haemorrhages may ultimately lead to myocardial ischaemia with infarction. The presence of anterior rib fractures and sternal fractures should alert the physician to the possibility of myocardial injury.

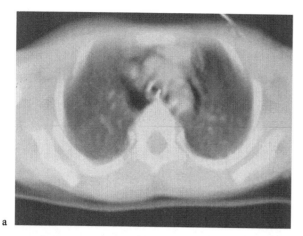

a

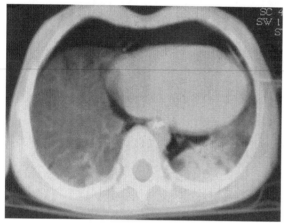

b

Fig. 10.27 a,b. Axial CT of the thorax on lung window settings in an abused patient with bilateral pneumothoraces secondary to severe chest trauma. There is associated pneumomediastinum and free retroperitoneal air tracks into the upper abdomen

Diaphragmatic Injury. Possible diaphragmatic injury should be considered with any injury of the thorax below the fourth intercostal space. In the presence of penetrating trauma the diagnosis is usually made during surgery. The diagnosis of diaphragmatic rupture is difficult especially in the presence of other injuries and few physical signs. If the initial chest radiograph shows obscuration of either hemidiaphragm following blunt trauma, rupture must be considered. Differentiation must be made from a collapsed left lower lobe with elevation of the diaphragm and stomach bubble. The chest radiograph is the initial most helpful investigation in evaluating the integrity of the hemidiaphragm after trauma. However, studies have shown that between 20% and 50% of patients with hemidiaphragm laceration will have a normal chest radiograph.

GELMAN et al. (1991) found the chest radiograph to be diagnostic or suggestive of left-sided hemidiaphragm injury in 60% of their patients. Most studies show the left side to be affected more commonly than the right (GELMAN et al. 1991; MORGAN et al. 1986). Non-specific radiological findings which are suggestive but not diagnostic are:

1. Apparent elevation of the hemidiaphragm
2. Obliteration or distortion of the contour of the hemidiaphragm
3. Displacement of the mediastinum to the contralateral side

Demonstration of gas-containing viscera in the lower thorax indicates hemidiaphragm rupture with visceral herniation.

Upper gastrointestinal contrast studies and fluoroscopy are the most sensitive investigations in assessing for diaphragmatic injury. Fluoroscopy demonstrates diaphragm movement. The position of the tip of the nasogastric tube may itself be diagnostic as it enters the thorax. Water-soluble contrast passed via the nasogastric tube is screened to see in which direction it travels. US can be performed at the bedside and can generally demonstrate an intact diaphragm provided there is good visualisation. If the child is undergoing CT for other injuries then CT is used in preference to additional fluoroscopy but if the diagnosis is uncertain, fluoroscopy must also be performed.

More recently MRI has proved useful (MIRVIS et al. 1988) but it is not suitable for unstable patients. MRI is also compromised by respiratory and cardiac motion near the diaphragm. However, it permits direct acquisition of sagittal and coronal images which give adequate demonstration of the viscera adjacent to the hemidiaphragms. MRI is used in stable patients in whom other imaging techniques are equivocal. Caution must be exerted in intubated patients because the positive pressure ventilation may delay herniation of abdominal contents into the thorax. The radiological diagnosis is delayed until on extubation respiratory embarrassment results as herniation occurs.

10.8
Injuries to the Neck, Larynx and Airway

Clinically visible oropharyngeal injuries are common in abused children. The children so injured are

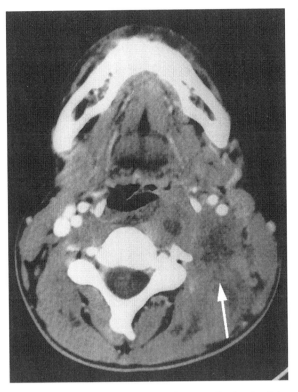

Fig. 10.28. Contrast-enhanced axial CT at the level of the pharynx in a young child with a large parapharyngeal abscess (*arrow*). (Courtesy of Doz. Dr. M. Riccabona and Professor Dr. R. Fotter, Department of Paediatric Radiology, LKH University Hospital Graz)

usually less than 1 year of age. Forceful insertion of either a blunt object such as a spoon, or penetrating objects or infliction of orosexual abuse may result in pharyngeal perforation. Any cause of retropharyngeal penetration, whether accidental or non-accidental, may result in retropharyngeal abscess or mediastinitis. Clinically, there may be a torn frenulum, inability to swallow or swelling of the soft tissues. Further complications include haemorrhage, interstitial emphysema and mediastinal pseudocyst formation.

A frontal chest radiograph may show widening of the superior mediastinum. A lateral cervical spine or a radiograph taken to show the lateral soft tissues of the neck may show impacted foreign bodies. The prevertebral soft tissues are thickened and they may contain gas or a fluid level. Oral contrast studies may show extraluminal leak of contrast. CT is not commonly performed but it will accurately demonstrate the extent of the abscess and may locate a foreign body (Fig. 10.28).

Asphyxiation. Asphyxiation frequently presents as a near-miss cot death or as sudden infant death syndrome (SIDS). Often clinical signs of battering are absent and there is no skeletal injury. Sometimes bruising is evident over the face and upper chest. There are no specific radiological signs. A chest radiograph may show evidence of aspiration. Recurrent and/or prolonged episodes may result in hypoxic ischaemic brain injury. The CT features of hypoxic ischaemic encephalopathy have been discussed in Sect. 10.3.4. In the emergency room situation, the primary duty of a doctor is to consider NAI as a cause of a child's injury in the appropriate circumstances and to ensure the safety and welfare of the child. These are certain circumstances in which a differential diagnosis must be considered. This is not discussed in this chapter as it is well discussed in standard texts. This consideration takes place once the child is in hospital. An incorrect diagnosis of NAI is a tragedy for the child and family and all reasonable causation of symptoms must be explored and excluded before the diagnosis of NAI is made. Failure to recognise signs of abuse and to act appropriately leaves a child's life at risk.

10.9
Summary

The advantages and disadvantages of the imaging techniques used in investigating NAI have been discussed with emphasis on investigations that are appropriate in the emergency situation.

Injuries inflicted in child abuse may affect any part of the body. Some of the injuries are characteristic of, or specific to, abuse. However, in many cases there is no distinction between these and accidental or innocent trauma. This emphasises the importance of the clinical history and examination and of having a high clinical index of suspicion. Good communication between the radiologist and the paediatricians is vital.

Radiological imaging serves to document the injuries and to detect occult injuries not yet clinically evident. Prior to imaging the child must be both haemodynamically and neurologically stable. In suspect cases, or if injuries are demonstrated, the radiographs should be reviewed by dedicated paediatric radiologists who have experience in dealing with abuse. There should be no hesitation in gaining a second opinion in doubtful cases. Of prime importance is the welfare of the child.

References

Ablin DS, Reinhart MA (1992) Oesophageal perforation by a tooth in child abuse. Paediatr Radiol 22:339–341

Akbarnia B, Torg JS, Kirkpatrick J, et al. (1974) Manifestations of the battered child syndrome. J Bone Joint Surg Am 56:1159–1166

Alexander R, Sato Y (1990) Incidence of impact trauma with cranial injuries ascribed to shaking. Am J Dis Child 144:724–726

Alyono D, Perry JF (1981) Value of quantitative cell count and amylase activity of peritoneal lavage fluid. J Trauma 21:345–348

Alyono D, Morrow CE, Perry JF Jr (1982) Reappraisal of diagnostic peritoneal lavage criteria for operation in penetrating and blunt trauma. Surgery 92:751–757

American Academy of Paediatrics. Committee on Child Abuse and Neglect (1993) Shaken baby syndrome; inflicted cerebral trauma. Paediatrics 92:872–875

Ammann AM, Brewer WH, Maull KI, et al. (1983) Traumatic rupture of the diaphragm: realtime sonographic diagnosis. AJR 140:915–916

Anderson WA (1982) The significance of femoral fractures in children. Ann Emerg Med 11:174

Aoki N, Masuzawa H (1984) Infantile acute subdural haematoma. Clinical analysis of 26 cases. J Neurosurg 61:273–280

Balfanz JR, Nesbit ME Jr, Jarvis C, et al. (1976) Overwhelming sepsis following splenectomy for trauma. J Paediatr 88:458–460

Ball WS (1989) Non accidental craniocerebral trauma (child abuse): evaluation with MR imaging. Radiology 173:609–610

Balthazar EJ (1989) CT diagnosis and staging of acute pancreatitis. Radiol Clin North Am 27:19–37

Balthazar EJ, Robinson DL, Megibow AJ, et al. (1990) Acute pancreatitis: value of CT in establishing prognosis. Radiology 174:331–336

Balthazar EJ, Freeny PC, Van Sonnenberg E (1994) Imaging and intervention in acute pancreatitis. Radiology 193:297–306

Beals RK, Tufts E (1983) Fractured femur in infancy: the role of child abuse. J Paediatr Orthop 3:583

Benstead JG (1983) Shaking as a culpable cause of subdural haemorrhage in infants. Med Sci Law 23:242–244

Benya EC, Bulas DI, Eichelberger MR, et al. (1995) Splenic injury from blunt abdominal trauma in children: follow-up evaluation with CT. Paediatr Radiol 95:685–688

Billimire ME, Myers PA (1985) Serious head injury in infants: accident or abuse? Paediatrics 75:340–342

Bird CR, MacMahan JR, Gilles FH, et al. (1987) Strangulation in child abuse. CT diagnosis. Radiology 163:373–375

Bratu M, Dower JC, Siegal B, et al. (1970) Jejunal haematoma, child abuse and Felson's sign. Conn Med 31:261–264

Brick SH, Taylor GA, Potter BM, et al. (1987) Hepatic and splenic injury in children: Role of CT in the decision for laparotomy. Radiology 165:643–646

Brown JK, Minns RA (1993) Non accidental head injury with particular reference to whiplash shaking and medicolegal aspects. Dev Child Neurol 35:849–869

Bruce DA, Zimmerman RA (1989) Shaken impact syndrome. Paediatr Ann 18:482–494

Bruce DA, Alari A, Bilaniuk L, et al. (1981) Diffuse cerebral swelling following head injuries in children: the syndrome of "malignant cerebral oedema". J Neurosurg 54:170–178

Brunsting L, Morton J (1987) Gastric rupture from blunt abdominal trauma. J Trauma 27:887

Burks DW, Mirvis SE, Shanmuganathan K (1992) Acute adrenal injury after blunt abdominal trauma: CT findings. AJR 162:661–663

Caffey J (1946) Multiple fractures in the long bones of infants suffering from chronic subdural haematoma. AJR 56:163–173

Caffey J (1972) On the theory and practice of shaking infants. Am J Dis Child 124:161–169

Caffey J (1974) The whiplash shaken baby syndrome: manual shaking by the extremities with whiplash induced intracranial and intraocular bleedings linked with residual permanent brain damage and mental retardation. Paediatrics 54:396–403

Carter JE, McCormick AQ (1983) Whiplash shaking syndrome: retinal haemorrhages and computed axial tomography of the brain. Child Abuse Negl 7:279–286

Carty H (1989) Skeletal manifestations of child abuse. Bone 6:3–7

Carty H (1991) The non skeletal injuries of child abuse. Part 2. The body. 1991 Year book of paediatric radiology, vol 3

Carty H (1993a) Fractures caused by child abuse. J Bone Joint Surg [Br] 75:849–857

Carty H (1993b) Case report: child abuse – necklace calcification – a sign of strangulation. BJR 66:1186–1188

Carty H (1995) Radiological features of child abuse. Curr Paediatr 5:230–235

Carty H, Ratcliffe J (1995) The shaken infant syndrome. BMJ 310:344

Chadwick DL, Chin S, Salerno C, et al. (1991) Deaths from falls in children. How far is fatal? J Trauma 31:1353–1355

Chapman S (1990) Radiological aspects of non accidental injury. J R Soc Med 83:67–71

Coant PN, Komberg AE, Brody AS, et al. (1992) Markers of occult liver injury in cases of physical abuse in children. Paediatrics 89:274–278

Cohen RA, Kaufman RA, Myers PA, et al. (1986) Cranial CT in the abused child with head inury AJR 146:97

Coleman BG, Arger PH, Rosenberg HK, et al. (1983) Grayscale sonographic assessment of pancreatitis in children. Radiology 146:145–150

Conway JJ, Collium M, Tanz RR, et al. (1993) The role of scintigraphy in detecting child abuse. Semin Nucl Med 23:321–333

Cooper A, Floyd T, Barlow B, et al. (1988) Major blunt abdominal trauma due to child abuse. J Trauma 28:1483–1487

Cox TD, Kuhn JP (1996) CT scan of bowel trauma in the pediatric patient. Radiol Clin North Am 34:807–818

Davis JW, Hoyt DB (1990) Complications in evaluating abdominal trauma: DPL versus computerised axial tomography. J Trauma 30:1506–1509

Dodds WJ, Taylor AJ, Erickson SC, et al. (1990) Traumatic fracture of the pancreas: CT characteristics. J Comput Assist Tomogr 14:375–378

Donovan PH, Sanders RC, Siegelman SS (1982) Collections of fluid after pancreatitis: evaluation by computed tomography and ultrasonography. Radiol Clin North Am 20:653–665

Duhaime AC, Gennarelli TA, Thibault LE, et al. (1987) The shaken baby syndrome: a clinical, pathological and biomechanical study. J Neurosurg 66:409–415

Duhaime AC, Alario AJ, Lewander WJ, et al. (1992) Head injury in very young children: mechanisms, injury types and ophthalmic findings in 100 hospitalised patients younger than two years of age. Paediatrics 90:179–185

Dykes L (1986) The whiplash shaken infant syndrome. What has been learned? Child Abuse Neglect 10:211–221

Edwards DK (1987) The battered child: Your day in court. In: Gosnik BB (ed) Syllabus of 12th annual San Diego Post-graduate Radiology Course. University of California, San Diego, pp 47–49

Eisenbrey A (1979) Retinal haemorrhage in the battered child. Childs Brain 5:40–44

Ellison PH, Tsai FY, Largen JA (1978) CT in child abuse and cerebral contusion. Paediatrics 62:151–154

Engrav LH, Benjamen CI, Strate RG (1975) Diagnostic perito-neal lavage in blunt abdominal trauma. J Trauma 15:845–859

Epstein JA, Epstein BS, Small M (1961) Subepicranial hy-droma. J Paediatr 4:562–566

Fagelman D, Hertz MA, Ross AS (1985) Delayed development of splenic subscapular haematoma: CT evaluation. J Comput Assist Tomogr 9:815–816

Federle M, Goldberg H, Kaiser J (1981) Evaluation of abdomi-nal trauma by computed tomography. Radiology 138:637–644

Feldman KW, Brewer DK (1984) Child abuse, cardio-pulmonary resuscitation and rib fractures. Paediatrics 73:339

Filiatrault D, Garel L (1995) Paediatric blunt abdominal trauma – to sound or not to sound? Paediatr Radiol 25:329–331

Fortune JB, Brahme J, Mulligan M, et al. (1985) Emergency intravenous pyelography in the trauma patient: a reexami-nation of the indications. Arch Surg 120:1056–1059

Friede RL, Schachnmayr W (1978) The origin of subdural neomembranes. Am J Pathol 92:69–84

Fulcher AS, Das Narla L, Brewer WH (1990) Gastric haematoma and pneumatosis in child abuse. Case report. AJR 155:1283–1284

Gelman R, Mirvis SE, Gens DR (1991) Diaphragmatic rupture due to blunt trauma: sensitivity of plain chest radiographs. AJR 156:51–57

Gentry LR, Godersky JC, Thompson B, et al. (1988) Pro-spective comparative study of intermediate field MR and CT in the evaluation of closed head trauma. AJNR 9:91–100

Gill W, Champion H, Long WB, et al. (1975) Abdominal lavage in blunt trauma. Br J Surg 62:121–124

Ginaldi BM, Nesbit M, Jarvis C (1976) Overwhelming sepsis following splenectomy for trauma. J Pediatr 88:458

Goldman SM, Sandler CM, Corriere JN Jr, et al. (1997) Blunt urethral trauma: a unified anatomical mechanical classifi-cation. J Urol 157:85–89

Goodman LR, Putman CE (1981) The SICU chest radiograph after massive blunt trauma. Radiol Clin North Am 19:111–123

Graif M, Stahl-Kent V, Ben-Ami T, et al. (1988) Sonographic detection of occult bone fractures. Pediatr Radiol 18:383–385

Guice K, Oddhem K, Eida B, et al. (1983) Haematuria after blunt abdominal trauma. When is pyelography useful? J Trauma 23:305–311

Guthkelch AN (1971) Subdural haematoma and its relation-ship to whiplash injuries. BMJ 2:430–431

Hadley MN, Sonntag VKH, Rekate HL, et al. (1989) The infant whiplash shake injury: a clinical and pathological study. Neurosurg 24:536–540

Hagirvara A, Yukioka T, Satou M, et al. (1995) Early diagnosis of small intestine rupture from blunt trauma using com-puted tomography: significance of the streaky density within the mesentery. J Trauma 38:630–633

Han JS, Kaufman B, Alfidi RJ, et al. (1984) Head trauma evalu-ation by magnetic resonance and computed tomography. Radiology 150:71–77

Han KB, Towbin RB, De Courten-Myers G, et al. (1989) Rever-sal sign on CT: effect of anoxic/ischaemic injury in chil-dren. AJNR 10:1191–1198

Hara H, Babyn PS, Bourgeois D (1989) Significance of bowel wall enhancement on CT following blunt abdominal trauma in childhood. J Comput Assist Tomogr 13:430–432

Harwood-Nash DC, Hendrick EB, Hudson AR (1971) The sig-nificance of skull fractures in children. A study of 1187 patients. Radiology 101:151

Heiberg E, Wolverson MK, Hurd RN, et al. (1980) CT recogni-tion of traumatic rupture of the diaphragm. AJR 134:369–372

Herman TE, Siegal MJ (1991) CT of the pancreas in children. AJR 157:375–379

Hesselink JR, Dowd CF, Healy ME, et al. (1988) MR imaging of brain contusions; a comparative study with CT. AJNR 9:269–278

Hilton SVW (1994) Differentiating the accidentally injured from the physically abused child; extremity trauma. In: Hilton SVW, Edwards DK (eds) Practical paediatric radiol-ogy, 2nd edn. Saunders, Philadelphia, pp 389–436

Howard MA, Bell BA, Uttley D (1993) The pathophysiology of infant subdural haematomas. Br J Neurosurg 7:355–365

Ingraham FD, Matson DD (1944) Subdural haematoma in in-fancy. J Paediatr 24:1

Jamieson DH, Babyn PS, Pearl R (1996) Imaging gastrointesti-nal perforation in paediatric blunt abdominal trauma. Paediatr Radiol 26:188–194

Jaspan T, Narborough G, Punt JAG, et al. (1992) Cerebral contusional tears as a marker of child abuse – detection by cranial sonography. Paediatr Radiol 22:237

Jeffrey RB Jr (1989) Sonography in acute pancreatitis. Radiol Clin North Am 27:5–17

Jeffrey RB, Laing FC, Federle MP, et al. (1981) Computed to-mography of splenic trauma. Radiology 141:729–732

Jeffrey RB, Federle MP, Grass RA (1983) Computed tomogra-phy of pancreatic trauma. Radiology 147:491–494

Jeffrey RB, Laing FC, Wing VW (1986) Ultrasound in acute pancreatic trauma. Gastrointest Radiol 11:44–46

Kane NM, Francis IR, Burney RE, et al. (1991) Traumatic pneumoperitoneum: implications of CT diagnosis. Invest Radiol 26:574–578

Kelly AB, Zimmerman RD, Snow RB, et al. (1988) Head trauma: comparison of MR and CT – experience in 100 patients. AJNR 9:699–708

Kempe CH, Silverman FN, Steele BF, et al. (1962) The battered child syndrome. JAMA 181:17–24

King J, Didendorf D, Apthorp J, et al. (1988) Analysis of 429 fractures in 189 battered children. J Paediatr Orthop 8:585–589

King LR, Siegel MJ, Balge DM (1995) Acute pancreatitis in children: CT findings of intra- and extrapancreatic fluid collections. Radiology 195:196–200

Kirks DR (1983) Radiological evaluation of visceral injuries in the battered child syndrome. Paediatr Ann 12:888

Klein S, Johs S, Fujitani R, et al. (1988) Haematuria following blunt abdominal trauma. The utility of intravenous pyel-ography. Arch Surg 123:1173–1177

Kleinman PK (1987a) Skeletal trauma: general considerations. In: Kleinman PK (ed) Diagnostic imaging in child abuse. Williams and Wilkins, Baltimore

Kleinman PK (1987b) Bony thoracic trauma. In: Kleinman PK (ed) Diagnostic imaging in child abuse. Williams and Wilkins, Baltimore

Kleinman PK (1990) Diagnostic imaging in child abuse. AJR 155:703

Kleinman PK (1996) Follow up skeletal survey in suspected child abuse. AJR 167:893–896

Kleinman PK, Marks SC (1988) Factors affecting visualisation of posterior rib fractures in abused infants. AJR 150:635–638

Kleinman PK, Marks SC (1996) A regional approach to the classic metaphyseal lesion in abused infants: the proximal tibia. AJR 166:421–426

Kleinman PK, Brill PW, Winchester P (1986a) Resolving duodenal-jejunal haematoma in abused children. Radiology 160:747–750

Kleinman PK, Marks SC, Blackbourne B (1986b) The metaphyseal lesion in abused infants: a radiologic-histopathological study. Am J Roentgenol 146:895–905

Kleinman PK, Marks SC, Spevak MR, et al. (1991a) Extension of growth plate cartilage into the metaphysis: a sign of healing fracture in abused infants. Am J Roentgenol 156:775–779

Kleinman PK, Belanger PL, Karellas A, et al. (1991b) Normal metaphyseal radiologic variants not to be confused with findings of infant abuse. Am J Roentgenol 156:781–783

Kleinman PK, Spevak MR, Hansen M (1992) Mediastinal pseudocyst caused by pharyngeal perforation during child abuse. Case report. AJR 158:1111–1113

Kluger Y, Paul DB, Raves JJ, et al. (1994) Delayed rupture of the spleen: myths, facts and their importance: case reports and literature review. J Trauma 36:568–571

Kogutt MS, Suischuck LE, Fagan CJ (1974) Patterns of injury and significance of uncommon fractures in the battered child syndrome. Am J Roentgenol 121:143–149

Kravitz H, Driessen G, Gomberg R, et al. (1969) Accidental falls from elevated surfaces in infants from birth to one year of age. Paediatrics 44:869–876

Krugman RD (1985) Fatal child abuse: analysis of 24 cases. Paediatrician 12:68

Kunin JR, Korobkin M, Ellis JH, et al. (1993) Duodenal injuries caused by blunt trauma: value of CT in differentiating perforation from haematoma. AJR 160:1221–1223

Lam AH, Cruz GB (1991) Ultrasound evaluation of subdural haematoma. Australas Radiol 35:330

Lane MJ, Mindelzun RE, Sandhu JS, et al. (1994) CT diagnosis of blunt pancreatic trauma: importance of detecting fluid between the pancreas and splenic vein. AJR 163:833–835

Levin HS, Amparo E, Eisenberg HM, et al. (1987) MRI and CT in relation to the neurobehavioural sequelae of mild to moderate head injury. J Neurosurg 66:706–713

Levitt MA, Criss E, Kobernik M (1985) Should emergency IVP be used more selectively in blunt trauma? Ann Emerg Med 14:959–965

Lloyd DA, Carty H, Patterson M, et al. (1997) Predictive value of skull radiography for intracranial injury in children with blunt head injury. Lancet 349:821–824

Loder RT, Bookout C (1991) Fracture patterns in battered children. J Orthop Traum 5:428–433

Ludwig S, Warman M (1984) Shaken baby syndrome. A review of twenty cases. Ann Emerg Med 13:104

Magid N, Glass T (1990) A "hole in the rib" as a sign of child abuse. Paediatr Radiol 20:334–336

McDowell HP, Fielding DW (1984) Traumatic perforation of the hypopharnyx – an unusual form of abuse. Arch Dis Child 59:888–889

McLellan BA, Hanna SS, Montoya DR, et al. (1985) Analysis of peritoneal lavage parameters in blunt abdominal trauma. J Trauma 25:393–399

Merchant WC, Gibbons MD, Gonzalez ET Jr (1984) Trauma to the bladder neck, trigone and vagina in children. J Urol 131:747–750

Merten DF, Radkowski MA, Leonidas JC (1983) The abused child: a radiological reappraisal. Radiology 146:377

Meyer DM, Thal ER, Weigett JA, et al. (1989) Evaluation of CT an DPL in blunt abdominal trauma. J Trauma 29:1168–1172

Mirvis SE, Tobin KD, Kostrubiak I, et al. (1987) Thoracic CT in detecting occult disease in critically ill patients. AJR 148:685–689

Mirvis SE, Keramati B, Buckman R, et al. (1988) MR imaging of traumatic diaphragmatic rupture. J Comput Assist Tomogr 12:147–149

Mirvis SE, Gens DR, Shanmuganathan K (1992) Rupture of the bowel after blunt trauma: Diagnosis with CT. AJR 159:1217–1221

Morgan AS, Flancbaum L, Esposito T, et al. (1986) Blunt injury to the diaphragm: an analysis of 44 patients. J Trauma 26:565–568

Morse MA, Garcia VF (1994) Selective non operative management of paediatric blunt splenic trauma: risk for missed associated injuries. J Paediatr Surg 29:23–27

Musemeche CA, Barthel M, Cosentino C, et al. (1991) Paediatric falls from heights. J Trauma 31:1347

Newton RW (1989) Intracranial haemorrhage and non accidental injury. Arch Dis Child 64:188–190

Nicolaisen GS, McAninch JW, Marshall GA, et al. (1985) Renal trauma: reevaluation of the indications for radiographic assessment. J Urol 133:183–187

Nimkin K, Teeger S, Wallach MT (1994) Adrenal haemorrhage in abused children: Imaging and post mortem findings. AJR 162:661–663

Nimkin K, Spevak M, Kleinman PK (1997) Fractures of the hands and feet in child abuse: Imaging and pathological features. Radiology 203:233–236

Noe HN, Jerkins GR (1992) Genitourinary Trauma. In: Kelalis PP, King LR, Belman AB (eds) Clinical paediatric urology, 3rd edn. Saunders, Philadelphia, pp 1353–1378

Northup WF, Simmons RL (1972) Pancreatic trauma: a review. Surgery 71:27–43

O'Connor JF, Cohen J (1987) Diagnostic imaging of child abuse. Williams and Wilkins, Baltimore

Oldham KT, Guice KS, Kaufman RA, et al. (1984) Blunt hepatic injury and elevated hepatic enzymes: a clinical correlation in children. J Paediatr Surg 19:457–461

Ommaya AK, Faas F, Yamell P (1968) Whiplash injury and brain damage. An experimental study. JAMA 204:75–79

Osborn AG, Anderson RE, Wing SD (1980) The false falx sign. Radiology 134:421–425

Ozonoff MB (1985) Emergency radiology in childhood. Emery Med Clin North Am 3:563–584

Ozonoff MB (1992) Pediatric orthopedic radiology, 2nd edn. Saunders, Philadelphia, pp 673–679

Pang D, Wilberger J (1982) Spinal cord injuries without radiographic abnormalities in children. J Neurosurg 57:114

Pappas D, Mirvis SE, Crepps JT (1987) Splenic trauma: false negative CT diagnosis in cases of delayed rupture. AJR 149:727–728

Parvin S, Smith DE, Asher WM, et al. (1975) Effectiveness of peritoneal lavage in blunt abdominal trauma. Ann Surg 181:255–261

Patrick LE, Ball TI, Atkinson GO, et al. (1992) Paediatric blunt abdominal trauma: Periportal tracking at CT. Radiology 183:689

Rance CH, Bear JW (1980) CT in the management of paediatric abdominal trauma. Aust N Z J Surg 50:506–512

Rao KG, Woodlief RM (1980) Grey scale ultrasonic demonstration of ruptured right hemidiaphragm. Br J Radiol 53:812–814

Raptopoulous V (1994) Abdominal trauma: emphasis on CT. Radiol Clin North Am 32:969–984

Reiber GD (1993) Fatal falls in childhood. How far must children fall to sustain fatal head injury? Report of cases and review of the literature. Am J For Med Pathol 14:201

Rizzo MJ, Federle MP, Griffiths BG (1989) Bowel and mesenteric injury following blunt trauma: diagnosis with CT. Radiology 173:143–148

Rizzo MJ, Federle MP, Griffiths BG (1992) Bowel and mesenteric injury following blunt trauma: diagnosis with CT. AJR 159:1217–1221

Rodriguez-Morales G, Rodriguez A, Shatney CH (1986) Acute rupture of the diaphragm in blunt trauma patients: analysis of 60 patients. J Trauma 26:438–444

Rosenthal L, Hill RO, Chuang S (1976) Observation on the use of ^{99m}Tc-phosphate imaging in peripheral bone trauma. Radiology 119:637–641

Rouse TM, Eichelberger MR (1992) Trends in paediatric trauma management. Paediatric surgery. Surg Clin North Am 72:1347–1364

Ruess L, Sivit CJ, Eichelberger MR, et al. (1995) Blunt hepatic and splenic trauma in children; correlation of a CT severity scale with clinical outcome. Paediatr Radiol 25:321–325

Salisbury FT, Alford BA (1982) Intracranial bleeding from child abuse. The value of skull radiographs. Paediatr Radiol 12:175–178

Sahuquillo-Barris J, Lamarca-Ciuro J, Vilata-Castan J, et al. (1988) Acute subdural haematoma and diffuse axonal injury after severe head trauma. J Neurosurg 68:894–900

Sandler CM, Phillips JM, Harris JD, et al. (1981) Radiology of the bladder and urethra in blunt pelvic trauma. Radiol Clin North Am 19:195–211

Sato Y, Yuh WTC, Smith WL, et al. (1989) Head injury in child abuse. Evaluation with MR imaging. Radiology 173:653

Shah P, Applegate KE, Buonomo C (1997) Stricture of the duodenum and jejunum in an abused child. Paediatr Radiol 27:281–283

Sherck JD, Oakes DD (1990) Intestinal injuries missed by computed tomography following blunt trauma: evaluation with CT. J Trauma 30:1–7

Siegel MJ, Martin KW, Worthington JC (1987) Normal and abnormal pancreas in children: US studies. Radiology 165:15–18

Silverman FN (1972) Unrecognised trauma in infants, the battered child syndrome and the syndrome of Ambroise Tardieu. Rigler Lecture. Radiology 104:337–353

Silverman PM, Baker ME, Maboney BS (1985) Atelectasis and subpulmonic fluid: CT pitfall in distinguishing pleural from peritoneal fluid. J Comput Assist Tomogr 9:763

Sivit CJ, Eichelberger MR (1995) CT diagnosis of pancreatic injury in children: significance of fluid separating the splenic vein and pancreas. AJR 165:921–924

Sivit CJ, Kaufman RA (1995) Commentary: sonography in the evaluation of children following blunt abdominal trauma: is it to be or not to be? Paediatr Radiol 25:326–328

Sivit CJ, Taylor L, Eichelberger M (1989a) Visceral injury in battered children: a changing perspective. Radiology 173:659–651

Sivit CJ, Taylor GA, Eichelberger MR (1989b) Chest injury in children with blunt abdominal trauma: evaluation with CT. Radiology 171:815–818

Sivit CJ, Taylor GA, Bulas DI, et al. (1991) Blunt trauma in children: significance of peritoneal fluid. Radiology 178:185–188

Sivit CJ, Eichelberger M, Taylor L (1992a) Blunt pancreatic trauma in children: CT diagnosis. Am J Radiol 158:1097–1100

Sivit CJ, Ingram JD, Taylor GA, et al. (1992b) Post traumatic adrenal haemorrhage in children. CT findings in 34 patients. AJR 158:1299–1302

Sivit CJ, Taylor GA, Bulas DI, et al. (1992c) Post traumatic shock in children: CT findings associated with haemodynamic instability. Radiology 182:723–726

Sivit CJ, Taylor GA, Eichelberger MR, et al. (1993) Significance of periportal low attenuation zones following blunt trauma in children. Paediatr Radiol 23:388

Sivit CJ, Eichelberger MR, Taylor GA (1994) CT in children with rupture of the bowel caused by blunt trauma: diagnostic efficacy and comparison with hypoperfusion complex. AJR 163:1195–1198

Slovis TL, Berdon WE, Haller JO, et al. (1975) Pancreatitis in the battered child syndrome. Report of two cases with skeletal involvement. AJR 125:456–461

Smeets AJ, Robben SGF, Meradji M (1990) Sonographically detected costochondral dislocation in an abused child. Pediatr Radiol 20:566–567

Snow RB, Zimmerman RD, Gandy SE, et al. (1986) Comparison of MRI and CT in the evaluation of head injury. Neurosurgery 18:45–52

Spevak MR, Kleinman PK, Belanger PL, et al. (1990) Does cardiopulmonary resuscitation cause rib fractures in infants? Post mortem radiologic-pathologic study (abstract). Radiology 177:162

Stalker HP, Kaufman RA, Towbin RB (1986) Patterns of liver injury in childhood: CT analysis. AJR 147:1199

Stanton AN (1979) Retinal haemorrhages in infancy. Br Med J 1:616

Stein JP, Freeman JA, Kaji DM, et al. (1994) Blunt renal trauma in the paediatric population: indications for radiographic evaluation. Urology 44:406–410

St. James-Roberts I (1991) Persistent infant crying. Arch Dis Child 66:653

Strouse PJ, Owings CL (1995) Fractures of the first rib in child abuse. Radiology 197:763–765

Sty JR, Starshak RJ (1983) The role of bone scintigraphy in the evaluation of the suspected abused child. Radiology 146:369–375

Taylor G, Fallat M, Eichelberger M (1987) Hypovolaemic shock in children: abdominal CT manifestations. Radiology 164:479

Taylor GA, Kaufman RA, Sivit CJ (1994) Active haemorrhage in children after thoracoabdominal trauma: clinical and CT features. AJR 162:401

Thomas NH, Robinson L, Evans A (1995) The floppy infant: a new manifestation of non accidental injury. Paediatr Neurosurg 23:188–191

Thomas SA, Rosenfield NS, Leventhal JM, et al. (1991) Long bone fractures in young children: distinguishing accidental injuries from child abuse. Paediatrics 88:471

Thornbury JR, Campbell JA, Masters SJ, et al. (1983) Skull fracture and low risk of intracranial sequelae in minor head trauma. AJR 143:661

Touloukian RJ (1968) Abdominal visceral injuries in battered children. Paediatrics 42:642

Tsai FY, Zee CS, Apthorp JB, et al. (1980) Computed tomography in child abuse head trauma. J Comput Assist Tomogr 4:277–286

Turnock RR, Sprigg A, Lloyd DA (1993) CT in the management of blunt abdominal trauma in children. Aust N Z J Surg 50:506–512

Wagner BB, Crawford WO, Schimpf PP (1988) Classification of parenchymal injuries of the lung. Radiology 167:77–82

Wilberger JE, Deeb Z, Rothfus W (1987) Magnetic resonance imaging in cases of severe head injury. Neurosurgery 20: 571–576

Williams DI (1975) Rupture of the female urethra in childhood. Eur Urol 1:129

Wing VW, Federle MP, Morris JA, et al. (1985) Tue clinical impact of CT for blunt abdominal trauma. AJR 145:1191–1194

Worlock P, Stower M, Barbor P (1986) Patterns of fractures in accidental and non accidental injury children: a comparative study. BMJ 293:100

Zimmerman RA, Bilaniuk LT, Bruce D (1978a) Interhemispheric acute subdural haematoma: a CT manifestation of child abuse by shaking. Neuroradiology 16: 39–40

Zimmerman RA, Bilaniuk LT, Gennarelli T, et al. (1978b) Cranial CT in the diagnosis and management of acute head trauma. AJR 131:27–34

Zimmerman RA, Bilaniuk LT, Bruce D (1979) Computed tomography of craniocerebral injury in the abused child. Radiology 130:687–690

Zimmerman RA, Bilaniuk LT, Hackney DB, et al. (1986) Head injury: early results of comparing CT and high field MR. AJR 147:1215–1222

Zimmerman RD, Russell EJ, Yurberg E, et al. (1982) Falx and interhemispheric fissure on axial CT: recognition and differentiation of interhemispheric subarachnoid and subdural haemorrhage. AJNR 3:635–642

11 Soft Tissue Lesions and the Acutely Swollen Limb

S.J. King

CONTENTS

11.1
Introduction

This chapter reviews the radiology of soft tissue pathology that may present acutely in children. It does not include soft tissue abnormality secondary to occult bone disease such as stress fracture or tumour or uncomplicated joint-based pathology such as ganglion or meniscal cyst where the diagnosis is clinically obvious.

11.2
Clinical Presentation

When a child develops a soft tissue lesion or swollen limb, the family may seek medical help in the emergency department. This is often because abnormalities such as these generate high levels of anxiety. Pain is a variable presentation. The lesions are often iden-

tified following minor trauma. The parents are concerned that the lesion is malignant. Fortunately a soft tissue mass and a swollen limb are relatively rare conditions and do not form a large part of the workload of paediatric radiology departments. Often the diagnosis is immediately clinically evident and imaging is only indicated to identify potential complications or to plan surgery.

It is important to stress that the correct diagnosis can often be deduced from the clinical history in these children. This information guides the radiologist to choose the best imaging techniques and ensures that each child undergoes appropriate studies. When the diagnosis is not evident, the child will be referred for imaging in an attempt to make a diagnosis.

11.3
Imaging Techniques

Plain radiographs are essential for evaluating soft tissue abnormalities in children and are the initial radiological investigation. Views in the anteroposterior and lateral projection are required. The exposure factors should allow demonstration of soft tissue as well as bone. Normally the tissue planes are sharply defined with clear margins between the muscle and subcutaneous fat. There are many soft tissue problems that can be diagnosed from radiographs. These include the radiopaque foreign body, and a vascular malformation containing phleboliths (Buetow et al. 1990; Morris and Adams 1995). Radiographs are also invaluable to look at secondary bone changes, for example, modelling abnormality, periosteal reaction or local invasion.

When a soft tissue lesion is suspected after clinical examination, plain radiographs are followed by ultrasound scanning. The development of high frequency (7.5–13 MHz) linear array transducers has led to better visualisation of soft tissue structures. Dynamic ultrasound scanning may be very helpful to show movement of a mass with muscle contraction,

S.J. King, MBChB, MRCP, FRCR, Consultant Paediatric Radiologist, Royal Liverpool Children's NHS Trust, Alder Hey Children's Hospital, Eaton Road, Liverpool L12 2AP, UK

or in cases of suspected muscle rupture to demonstrate disordered muscle contraction. Doppler ultrasound with pulsed, colour and power Doppler may also be helpful (LATIFI and SIEGEL 1994) in making a diagnosis by the demonstration of the vascular nature or otherwise of a lump. Increasingly magnetic resonance imaging (MRI) follows ultrasound examination in the imaging programme. This gives superb soft tissue contrast and the anatomical definition that may be necessary for planning a biopsy or surgery. However, MRI does have its problems. Children may require sedation or general anaesthesia in order to perform an MR study. Patient sedation is almost never required for an ultrasound examination. In many patients MRI will not differentiate benign from malignant lesions (KRANSDORF 1995a) due to lack of specificity of an abnormal signal. Some abnormalities that are readily seen on plain radiographs may not be apparent on MR scans. Examples include phleboliths in a vascular malformation, foreign bodies or soft tissue calcifications. Therefore MR scans should only be reported in conjunction with the child's radiographs to avoid mistakes in interpretation. MR sequences should include T1- and T2-weighted images together with a fat suppression sequence. Axial planes are essential, supplemented by sagittal and coronal as appropriate. Gadolinium enhancement is indicated in suspected inflammatory or neoplastic lesions.

Computed tomography (CT) can be very useful in certain circumstances, for example when looking for changes in a bone adjacent to a soft tissue mass or the patterns of calcification present in soft tissues.

Both ultrasound and MRI are helpful investigations for evaluating the acutely swollen limb. Ultrasound is indicated to diagnose a suspected vascular anomaly or pelvic mass. It is of limited use when surveying a whole limb for abnormality or looking at deep extension of a lesion. Scintigraphy can be very useful in selected children and is the technique of choice for diagnosing suspected reflex sympathetic dystrophy.

11.4
Soft Tissue Lesions

11.4.1
Mimics

When a child attends the hospital with a lump it is important to establish whether or not there is an abnormality. Muscle asymmetry may be present in normal children and mimic disease. These children are not unwell but they may attend the emergency department because of parental anxiety. They complain of a painless soft tissue mass. There may or may not be a history of sporting activity or training. On examination, there is asymmetry in one muscle or group of muscles compared with the opposite side. This is frequently around the shoulder but can occur in other muscle groups. Radiological investigations are appropriate in this situation and the initial examination is usually with ultrasound. This reveals no definite mass and the ultrasound characteristics of the soft tissues are normal. Children may require further imaging with MRI if there is still doubt about the diagnosis. Scans demonstrate normal signal characteristics from the muscle groups in question. Biopsy is not necessary in the majority of children with muscle pseudotumours (Fig. 11.1).

A clinician may refer a child for an ultrasound scan if there is doubt whether or not a mass is present. Ultrasound is a very useful technique to diagnose a soft tissue abnormality or confirm normality. A normal ultrasound examination is very reassuring for both the referring clinician and the family.

Uncommonly a normal accessory muscle can simulate a soft tissue mass. The most frequent of these is an accessory soleus muscle. It is situated on the anterior surface of the soleus muscle or on the soleal line of the tibia and fibula (YU and RESNICK 1994). The ultrasound and MRI characteristics are the same as skeletal muscle.

Children and adolescents present in the emergency department from time to time with a lump on the chest wall. Typically, the lump is painless and there is no history of injury. The mass is situated at the costal margin and is unilateral. Chest radiography reveals a bifid anterior rib, which is a congenital variant of normal. No further imaging is required.

In the adolescent age group, a lump may be seen on one side of the anterior chest wall at a costochondral or sternocostal junction and is due to hypertrophy of the cartilage. Typically the lump is painless and there is no history of injury. Radiographs are normal. Ultrasound defines the abnormality, revealing prominence of a costochondral or sternocostal junction. This produces the "lump" and no other masses are identified. Usually the ultrasound scan is sufficient to make the diagnosis and reassure the child and parents. If further imaging is required, CT or MRI can be performed. CT is preferred when bony detail is needed.

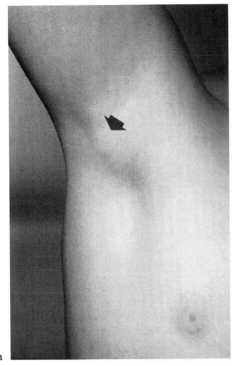

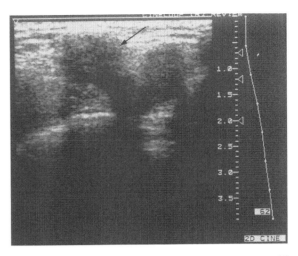

Fig. 11.2. Prominent sternocostal junction. A 15-year-old boy noticed a lump on his chest wall and came to the Emergency Department. The ultrasound scan demonstrates prominence of a sternocostal junction of a lower rib on the left side (*arrow*)

11.4.2
Trauma

A soft tissue haematoma may result from acute or remote trauma. When the history and the clinical findings are compatible there is no diagnostic difficulty. When there is no remembered injury or only trivial injury there may be a problem with diagnosis. Children who injure themselves in circumstances that they do not wish parents to know about may conceal the history or play down the level of trauma, thus causing diagnostic confusion. The features of soft tissue haematomas are well described on ultrasound (DONALDSON 1989; WICKS et al. 1978). In common with other haematomas, the appearance of an intramuscular haematoma on ultrasound examination varies depending on the stage of healing (WICKS et al. 1978). Fresh clot is usually highly echogenic. The echogenicity decreases and disappears within the first 4 days. Following this the haematoma appears cystic and develops internal echoes as the clot organises. By 4–6 weeks it reverts to a cystic appearance (DONALDSON 1989; KAPLAN et al. 1990). Repetitive injury may cause mixed patterns. Haematoma may present in previously normal tissue or when a pre-existing lesion is damaged (Fig. 11.3).

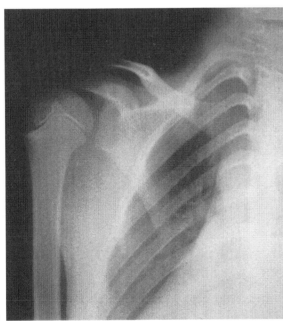

Fig. 11.1 a,b. Muscle asymmetry. a Photograph of a 12-year-old boy who complained of a painless soft tissue mass in the right axilla (*arrow*). b There is fullness of soft tissues of the axilla. Ultrasound and MR scans showed normal muscles

The cause of focal painless enlargement of the costal margin in adolescents is unknown. It may be related to local hyperaemia, caused by an episode of injury forgotten by the patient (Fig. 11.2).

Increasingly clinicians see children who have sustained sports injuries in emergency departments. Although fewer children take part in competitive sport nowadays, those who participate in sports do

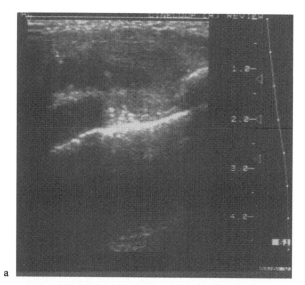

a

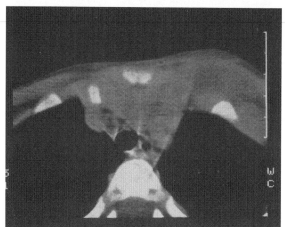

b

FIG. 11.3 a,b. Haematoma. **a** A 10-year-old boy presented with a lump over the left clavicle following trauma. The ultrasound scan shows a mixed echogenicity mass containing some cystic spaces in the soft tissues overlying the clavicle. **b** A CT scan in the same boy shows the mass to be partly of low density, consistent with fluid, and partly of soft tissue density

so intensively (CARTY 1994). Children present with both acute and chronic injuries. There is not usually any problem making the diagnosis in the acute situation. However, a child may ignore the acute lump and present when the mass has become hard. The lesion may then resemble a sarcoma on physical examination.

The appearances of an intramuscular haematoma on ultrasound examination have been described earlier. Dynamic ultrasound scanning may be useful to look at muscle contraction around the lump.

MRI may provide more information about the lesion. It is better at defining the relationship between the haematoma and surrounding muscle groups and

assessing associated muscle atrophy or fibrosis. This may be particularly useful when there is no history of injury. The signal characteristics of intramuscular haematomas are well described and variable depending on the age of the lesion (DE SMET 1993). Subacute haematomas may display high signal intensity on both T1- and T2-weighted images due to blood containing methaemoglobin (PAKTER et al. 1987) (Fig. 11.4). A chronic haematoma will have mixed signal with areas of fluid signal and areas of residual methaemoglobin (DE SMET 1993).

A partial or complete muscle tear may present some time following the injury. A muscle mass which is present may be associated with atrophy of part or all of the affected muscle. This can be seen well on MR scans, as can any compensatory hypertrophy of surrounding muscle groups. When the muscle injury is old, MRI of the torn muscle shows normal signal intensity on T1-weighted images and increased signal intensity on T2-weighted images consistent with haemosiderin deposition (DE SMET 1993). Repetitive injury may cause mixed features of acute and chronic injury on both MRI and ultrasound.

Ultrasound is excellent for monitoring healing of a muscle tear. Healing may take months or longer, particularly if the child continues to exercise the muscle (Fig. 11.5).

11.4.3
Inflammatory Lesions

Acute soft tissue abscess or inflammatory lymph nodes will rarely require any imaging. These lesions will mostly be diagnosed and managed clinically. If imaging is required, inflammatory nodes or nodal masses appear discrete on ultrasound imaging. The nodes are often of varying size. The normal node may have a central echogenic linear shadow. Increased vascularity is often shown on Doppler studies. Necrosis within a node is identified as an area of hypoechogenicity. The margins are often irregular. Malignant nodal masses differ from benign in that the nodes tend to coalesce and cease to be discrete. Calcification within a node may indicate TB or malignancy. The clinical history and other haematological tests will differentiate the two.

Diagnostic difficulty may arise with less clinically obvious inflammatory lesions including erythema nodosum, granuloma annulare, acute myositis ossificans and foreign body granuloma.

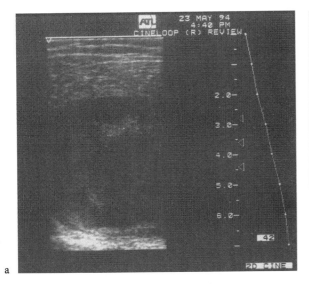

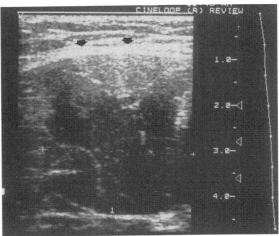

Fig. 11.5. Muscle tear. Ultrasound scan of the quadriceps muscle in a 15-year-old boy obtained with muscle contraction 1 month following an acute injury. There is a mass outlined by the calipers within the quadriceps muscle. It contains cystic and solid elements and is bulging anteriorly, although the muscle capsule is intact (*arrows*)

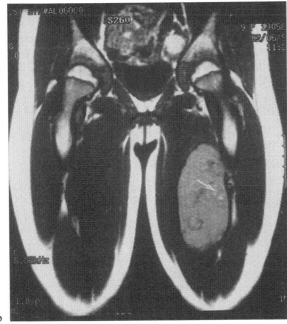

Fig. 11.4 a,b. Subacute muscle haematoma. a A 9-year-old girl presented with a firm lump in the left thigh. Ultrasound shows a predominantly cystic mass in the vastus medialis muscle. Some internal soft tissue echoes are also present. b Coronal T1-weighted MR scan demonstrates the extent of the muscle haematoma. There is mostly intermediate signal intensity in the lesion, indicating presence of methaemaglobin or proteinaceous debris. There are small areas of high signal suggesting acute bleed (*arrow*). There is no surrounding muscle atrophy

11.4.3.1
Erythema Nodosum

Erythema nodosum may present acutely. Imaging with ultrasound is not diagnostic and other clinical features should enable the clinician to make the correct diagnosis. If ultrasound is performed, the lumps appear well defined and are heterogeneous and hypoechoic (NESSI et al. 1990).

11.4.3.2
Granuloma Annulare

Occasionally children present with firm, small nodular subcutaneous swellings. These are usually painless, may be solitary or multiple and the child is otherwise healthy. The nodules are usually less than 2 cm in diameter. This condition is termed granuloma annulare. It occurs in the lower limb (ARGENT et al. 1994). The differential diagnosis of lumps on the shin in children always includes a resolving haematoma from a kick. The nodules can be difficult to define on any form of imaging technique and imaging with ultrasound and MRI is not diagnostic. The lumps have soft tissue characteristics on both ultrasound and MRI with variable infiltration into surrounding fat (Fig. 11.6). The lumps have decreased signal intensity on all MR pulse sequences. Cutaneous lesions may coexist (ARGENT et al. 1994). Biopsy can be performed if there is doubt about the diagnosis. The histological findings are reported to be indistinguishable from rheumatoid nodules. Children who have granuloma annulare do not have any manifestations of connective tissue disease and

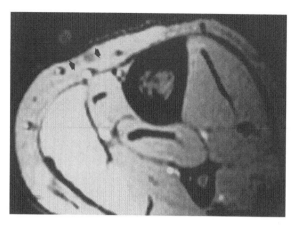

Fig. 11.6. Granuloma annulare. A 13-year-old girl presented to an Emergency Department with a 2-year history of firm nodules on the left shin. T2-weighted transverse image of the left shin. There are two soft tissue signal lesions <1 cm diameter showing poorly defined margins with subcutaneous fat (*arrows*). *, skin marker

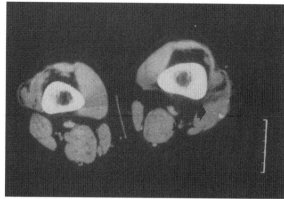

Fig. 11.7. Myositis ossificans. A 12-year-old boy presented with a hard, painful mass in the lower thigh, of 48 h duration. He gave a vague history of previous injury. The CT scan shows a poorly defined soft tissue mass with calcification (*arrow*)

the prognosis is excellent, the condition being self-limiting.

11.4.3.3
Soft Tissue Infection

Local soft tissue infection presenting as a soft tissue mass is usually diagnosed clinically and requires no imaging. Ultrasound imaging is requested when the diagnosis is uncertain or to look for necrosis or abscess formation in a lymph node mass. Deep or occult infection may present with limb swelling and is covered later in this chapter.

11.4.3.4
Myositis Ossificans

Myositis ossificans is a rare soft tissue mass of skeletal muscle. In the literature it has been referred to by a variety of synonyms, including pseudomalignant osseous tumour of soft tissue, extra-osseous localised non-neoplastic bone formation, myositis ossificans circumscripta, pseudomalignant myositis and heterotopic ossification (JELINEK and KRANSDORF 1995). Some patients with myositis ossificans give a history of trauma though the latter is not necessarily present. Myositis ossificans is a benign condition that presents as a solitary mass with progressive histological and radiological fea-

tures. These depend on the stage of evolution of the lesion when it is examined (JOHNSON 1948; KRANSDORF et al. 1991; BOOTHROYD and CARTY 1995). There are early, intermediate and late (fully mature) phases. Histology of early and intermediate lesions shows formation of peripheral lamellar bone. The mature lesion consists mainly of lamellar bone (JOHNSON 1948; KRANSDORF et al. 1991). Radiologically the soft tissue mass of myositis ossificans develops calcification then ossification. Finally the mature lesion is a well-defined bony mass with central lucency (JELINEK and KRANSDORF 1995; BOOTHROYD and CARTY 1995). Plain radiographs, ultrasound and CT are helpful especially when they demonstrate maturation of the lesion. Atypical features such as failure to ossify suggest a different diagnosis (NUOVO et al. 1992).

Plain radiographs may be normal early in the disease (BOOTHROYD and CARTY 1995). Later mineralisation is seen, which may be peripheral and appear ossified (KRANSDORF et al. 1991). Classically the mature lesion has a central lucency surrounded by a rim of bone (GOLDMAN 1976). In the early stages ultrasound scans show a low-echogenicity soft tissue mass that may be irregular and is separate from bone (KIRKPATRICK et al. 1987). Later, as calcification develops, this mass may appear irregular or orientated along the line of muscle fibre (KRAMER et al. 1979; PECK and METREWELI 1988). Calcification is appreciated best on CT scans (Fig. 11.7). MRI has recently proved helpful in diagnosing myositis ossificans. The mass has similar signal characteristics to other soft tissue tumours. However, in the early and intermediate phases of myositis ossificans MR scans demonstrate marked oedema surrounding the lesion. This sign is unusual in a primary soft tissue tumour unless there has been biopsy or haemorrhage (JELINEK and KRANSDORF 1995).

11.4.3.5
Inflammatory Pseudotumour

Inflammatory pseudotumour is a rare cause of a soft tissue mass in a limb. It is a benign condition that was previously known as plasma cell granuloma. It occurs most commonly in the lung of children or young adults (BAHADORI and LIEBOW 1973; MONZON et al. 1982) but has been described in the iliopsoas muscle (SHEDDON and NARLA 1991) and in the calf (BROWN and SHAW 1995). When it is situated peripherally it may simulate a malignancy both clinically and radiologically. Histology of the lesion shows localised proliferation of inflammatory cells including plasma cells, lymphocytes and eosinophils together with spindle cells and myofibroblasts of mesenchymal origin (BROWN and SHAW 1995; DAY et al. 1986; WU et al. 1973).

A child with an inflammatory pseudotumour may give a history of previous infection or trauma or may have been well previously. Fever and weight loss appear to be associated clinical features of the illness (BROWN and SHAW 1995; WU et al. 1973).

There are no diagnostic features on radiological investigations. Ultrasound appearances are variable. CT scans show a discreet homogeneous solid mass without calcification. It is not locally invasive. The MRI features of this condition have not been described.

The very rare diagnosis of inflammatory pseudotumour may be suggested in a child who presents with fever, weight loss and a localised mass (BROWN and SHAW 1995) but the diagnosis ultimately is made by biopsy.

11.4.3.6
Cat-scratch Disease

Cat-scratch disease is a common cause of lymph gland enlargement in children but is probably under-reported. The disease is thought to be caused by inoculation with gram-negative bacteria from a cat. The axillary lymph nodes are most frequently affected. The majority of patients with cat-scratch dis-

ease are under 18 years of age and almost all have a positive skin test. The condition is benign and self-limiting. Lymph node suppuration occurs in only a minority of children (CARITHERS 1985). Imaging is seldom required. Ultrasound will define local lymph node enlargement. The MRI features have been described as those of enlarged lymph nodes with central necrosis and surrounding soft tissue inflammation (SUNDARAM and SHARAFUDDIN 1995).

11.4.3.7
Foreign Body Granuloma

Soft tissue foreign bodies are a common problem in children attending the emergency department. Many soft tissue foreign bodies such as glass or metal are radiopaque and are readily diagnosed on radiographs. Wood and graphite may not be seen on radiographs. Glass density will depend on whether it is seen "en face" or end on. In the latter situation, there is increased density due to increased attenuation of the x-ray beam as it traverses the increased depth of the foreign body.

When performing radiographs for a suspected foreign body, two views at 90° with the puncture site marked by an external radiopaque pointer are required. All dressings should be removed wherever possible before performing the radiographs. Bone detail is not necessary but all soft tissue should be visible and radiographic exposure factors should be chosen to achieve this. Digital radiographs using edge-enhanced images are ideal. Unsharpness of the image due to patient movement must be avoided. Dedicated film/screen systems are required for soft tissue foreign body radiography and screens should be cleaned regularly to eliminate artefacts.

Ultrasound is the technique of choice for detecting objects which are not radiopaque and clinicians can use it to guide them when removing the foreign body (SHIELS et al. 1990; GOODING et al. 1987). MRI is not indicated in the acute situation, where there is not usually any difficulty making the diagnosis with radiographs and, if necessary, ultrasound. The child may, however, present to the emergency department with a soft tissue mass some time following puncture of the skin by a foreign body, possibly after a delay of weeks or months. The child with this problem does not usually present as an emergency but may do so if a mass is discovered following minor trauma. The history may be several weeks or months previously

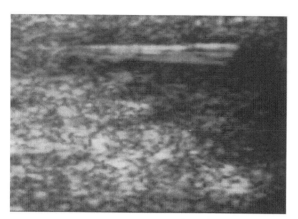

Fig. 11.8. Foreign body. A 5-year-old girl presented to the Emergency Department with a painful soft tissue mass in the left calf. She gave a history of having been pricked by a cactus spine in Spain several months previously. Ultrasound scan shows a subcutaneous linear foreign body surrounded by low-reflectivity inflammatory tissue. A cactus spine was removed surgically

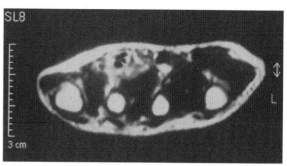

Fig. 11.9. Foreign body. A boy of 12 years presented acutely with a poorly defined swelling in the palm of the hand which was painful. A soft tissue sarcoma was suspected clinically. T2-weighted MR scan shows a thickened flexor tendon sheath and surrounding irregular oedema. There is subtle intermediate signal centrally (*arrow*). At operation, a rose thorn was removed from this area

and the clinician will not see a puncture wound and the child has forgotten the injury.

Non-radiopaque organic material which becomes embedded in soft tissue may produce soft tissue or bone changes visible on ultrasound scans and radiographs respectively. Radiographs may demonstrate a periosteal reaction of bone adjacent to the foreign body which can sometimes be confused with osteomyelitis or a bone tumour (GERLE 1971; MAYLAHN 1952). A soft tissue inflammatory reaction to a foreign body is ideally visualised by ultrasound using high-frequency linear array transducers (5–13 MHz). The foreign body appears as an echogenic focus and is surrounded by a halo of low-echogenicity inflammatory tissue. This may be poorly demarcated from surrounding tissues (SHIELS et al. 1990) (Fig. 11.8).

Magnetic resonance imaging for foreign bodies should not be done without prior ultrasound and can be reserved for a very small number of children when ultrasound examination is unhelpful. Occasionally MRI is useful if the soft tissue mass simulates a neoplasm on clinical examination or to plan surgical removal of the offending material (Fig. 11.9).

Foreign body granulomas are typically of similar signal intensity to muscle on T1-weighted images and have variable hyperintensity to muscle on T2-weighted images. The foreign body itself appears hypointense on T1- and T2-weighted images compared with muscle. However, the foreign body is not always identified on MR scans and in these children imaging does not distinguish the soft tissue lesion from a neoplasm.

11.4.3.8
Subcutaneous Fat Necrosis

Subcutaneous fat necrosis may occur in infants as a result of ischaemia to the tissues. It is associated with perinatal asphyxia or difficult labour or delivery. Subcutaneous lesions appear at about 1 month of age. They are located at the site of the trauma or ischaemia and may be seen on the limbs, although the face, buttocks and posterior trunk are more usual sites. The nodules are firm and can be either free or fixed to deep structures. They may calcify and resolve over a period of weeks or months (MALLORY 1991). Histology of the lesions reveals crystallised fat. On radiographs subcutaneous calcification is often visible. This decreases as the lesion resolves (SHACKLEFORD et al. 1975; HIGGINS et al. 1993) (Fig. 11.10).

Fat necrosis may also occur in older children following trauma. It is a common cause of a palpable soft tissue mass in children (TSAI et al. 1997). Frequently the child does not remember the episode of trauma. The most common site is the anterior tibia. MRI may be helpful. Scans show characteristic features in fat necrosis. There is no discrete mass visible and variable linear low signal intensity on T1-weighted and T2-weighted sequences and high signal intensity on T2-weighted sequences is confined to the subcutaneous tissue (TSAI et al. 1997). These

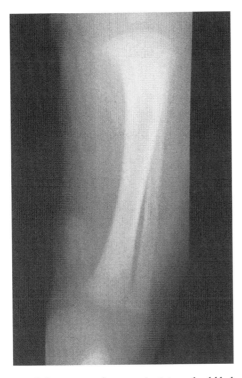

Fig. 11.10. Subcutaneous fat necrosis. A 4-week-old baby presented to the Emergency Department with a painless lump above the ankle. The birth had been normal but the baby had been treated in the Neonatal Unit for 48h for presumed sepsis. The plain frontal radiograph demonstrates localised calcification in the subcutaneous tissue of the left leg. The lesion was presumed to represent subcutaneous fat necrosis. Biopsy was not performed

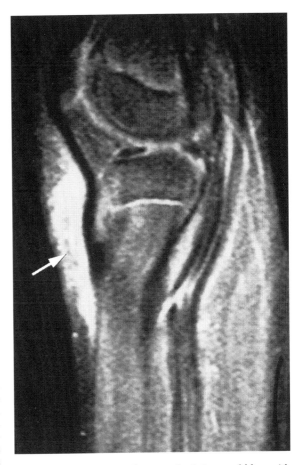

Fig. 11.11. Subcutaneous fat necrosis. A 7-year-old boy with Down's syndrome presented to the Emergency Department with a soft tissue mass and thickening over the anterior tibia. A T2-weighted MR scan demonstrates high signal intensity in the subcutaneous tissue containing linear areas of low signal intensity (arrow)

findings can render biopsy unnecessary and allow conservative management (Fig. 11.11).

Calcified soft tissue masses may occur following extravasation of intravenous infusion. The location of the mass and the previous history serve to make the diagnosis.

11.4.4
Vascular Lesions

11.4.4.1
Haemangioma

Vascular anomalies may be classified into haemangiomas, which are biologically active, or vascular malformations, which are biologically inert (MULLIKEN and GLOWACKI 1982). Haemangiomas are true endothelial tumours which have phases of rapid proliferation and slow involution. When a lesion grows, histology reveals endothelial cell division and cell multiplication (MULLIKEN and GLOWACKI 1982). All lesions contain elements of non-vascular tissue including fat, smooth muscle fibrous tissue myxoid stroma, haemosiderin, thrombus and bone (BUETOW et al. 1990).

Haemangioma is the most common soft tissue tumour in infants and children (COHEN et al. 1988). Localised haemangiomas may be subcutaneous, intramuscular or intrasynovial. Less frequently tumours are generalised. Haemangiomas are rarely present at birth. Most appear in the first weeks of life. The lesion is present on the head or neck in 60% of children with this condition. The trunk and then the extremities are the next most frequent sites. Lesions are multiple in 20% of children (LOW 1994). Typically a haemangioma grows rapidly at 3–6 months of age, is relatively stable between 6 and 18 months and

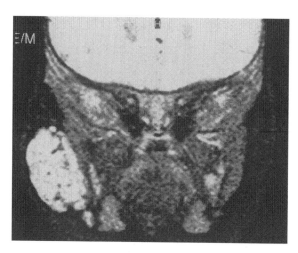

Fig. 11.12. Haemangioma. A 5-month baby girl presented with a mass over the right cheek for 1 week. The T2-weighted fat-suppressed MR scan shows a lobulated hyperintense mass infiltrating the masseter muscle and parotid gland. Signal voids represent vascular channels

then involutes slowly. Involution may take years but the majority resolve completely by the end of the first decade of life.

Plain radiographs may demonstrate a soft tissue mass. Effects on bone are rare. An example is orbital enlargement secondary to growth of an orbital haemangioma.

Ultrasound including pulsed and colour Doppler can show variable appearances. Vascular channels may be demonstrated but ultrasound may not differentiate haemangioma from a vascular malformation or even from a malignant tumour (LATIFI and SIEGEL 1994). Further information can be obtained from MRI. In the proliferative phase scans of the lesion show well-defined lobules of intermediate signal intensity on T1-weighted images and high signal intensity on T2-weighted images. During the phase of involution, fat signal is more obvious as fibro-fatty tissue increases in the lesion. An intramuscular haemangioma has a characteristic appearance on MRI. A lesion contains areas of signal void that have the configuration of vascular channels, together with a stroma of fat and fibrous tissue (Fig. 11.12).

Biopsy can be avoided when these typical findings are seen (BUETOW et al. 1990). Angiography may help surgical planning but is not usually necessary for making a diagnosis of haemangioma. The angiographic appearances are of well-defined intense lobular-parenchymal staining with peripheral and draining vessels (LOW 1994). MR scanning is preferred to angiography or CT to define the limits

of a lesion (RAUCH et al. 1984; BURROWS et al. 1983).

11.4.4.2
Vascular Malformations

Vascular malformations are present at birth though they may not be clinically evident. The lesion grows steadily with the growth of the child but may present acutely with apparent rapid growth following trauma, haematoma or puberty (LOW 1994). Usually serial clinical examinations will distinguish between vascular malformation and haemangioma. Vascular malformations do not involute. However, it may be difficult for the clinician to differentiate a vascular malformation from an haemangioma in a baby when the growth pattern of the lesion has not become apparent.

Vascular malformations comprise structurally abnormal capillaries, veins and/or arteries. These lesions do not grow or regress but enlarge in proportion with normal growth of the child (LOW 1994). Histology of a vascular malformation demonstrates flat endothelium with normal slow turnover of cells and normal numbers of mast cells.

The radiology of a vascular malformation usually helps distinguish it from a haemangioma. Plain radiographs may demonstrate skeletal overgrowth, for example, hypertrophy of a limb. A high-flow vascular malformation may cause local bony destruction or bone marrow involvement (LOW 1994). Phleboliths may be visible, indicating a venous component to the malformation (MORRIS and ADAMS 1995; LOW 1994).

Children with venous or arteriovenous malformations may present acutely with severe pain in the lesion secondary to acute thrombosis, often following direct though minor trauma.

Ultrasound is often unhelpful, failing to differentiate a vascular malformation from a haemangioma as discussed previously. Angiography is indicated prior to therapeutic embolisation and demonstrates abnormal dilated vessels without a parenchyma. Arteriovenous shunting is demonstrated if present.

MRI and MR angiography have reduced the need for direct angiography. The extent of the malformation is demonstrated and distinction between high- and low-flow lesions is possible (Fig. 11.13).

Scintigraphy is not used routinely to investigate a vascular malformation. However, technetium-99m-labelled red blood cells are taken up diffusely by a vascular malformation and homogeneously by a

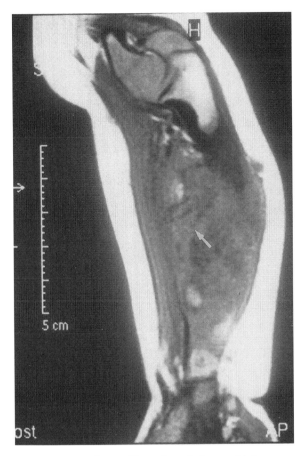

Fig. 11.13. Vascular malformation. A 2-year-old boy presented with acute swelling of the left forearm. A T1-weighted MR scan shows a large lesion in the forearm isointense to skeletal muscle containing areas of high signal intensity fat and subtle signal voids corresponding to phleboliths (*arrow*)

haemangioma. Abnormal vessels may be demonstrated in a vascular malformation (BARTON et al. 1992). Technetium-99m red blood cell scanning may be useful to screen the whole body for vascular abnormalities although it will not provide exact anatomical information.

11.4.4.3
Aneurysm

An aneurysm may present as an acute soft tissue mass in a child (BOOTHROYD and CARTY 1995). This may be a true or false aneurysm. True aneurysms follow blunt trauma to an artery. A history of injury may or may not be given. The child may have forgotten the episode of trauma (BOOTHROYD and CARTY 1995). False aneurysms are seen following direct penetrating injury to the arterial wall (BOOTHROYD and CARTY 1995; FITZGERALD et al. 1986; REY et al.

1987). A mycotic false aneurysm uncommonly follows local infection or septicaemia (WILLEMSEN et al. 1997) (Fig. 11.14).

Ultrasound scanning including pulsed and colour Doppler is the ideal way of imaging a suspected aneurysm and can distinguish between true and false aneurysms (KELLER and SIMON 1988). Vascular surgeons usually require further imaging with direct or MR angiography before operating on an aneurysm.

11.4.4.4
Lymphangioma

A child with a lymphangioma rarely presents as an emergency but may do so as a result of complications. Typically these result from sudden enlargement of the mass due to haemorrhage, or more rarely infection. Dependent on the location of the lesion, the child may present with a mass of sudden onset, pain and pressure symptoms including stridor. The parents may or may not be aware of the existence of a soft tissue mass. Lymphangiomas typically occur in infants, with 60% presenting in the first 5 years of life. Most occur in the head, neck or axilla and 10% extend into the thorax (LEVINE 1989). An uncomplicated lymphangioma does not usually cause any clinical symptoms. Haemorrhage into a lymphangioma in the neck or thorax may compromise the airway and an infant may present as an emergency with respiratory distress.

Lymphangiomas are lesions that result from sequestered lymphatic tissue that fails to communicate with the lymphatic system (LEVINE 1989). The histological appearance is mixed with variable amounts of adipose tissue, muscle and lymphoid tissue (BORECKY et al. 1995). The appearance of mixed lymphangio-haemangiomatous lesions varies, dependent on the composition and the contribution of the haemangiomatous component. A typical uncomplicated lymphangioma on ultrasound is transonic, and usually multiloculated. If there is haemorrhage into the lesion the fluid becomes echogenic. When there is a component of solid tissue, this is echogenic. On MRI, an uncomplicated lesion has a low signal on T1-weighted images and a high signal on T2-weighted images. Fresh haemorrhage shows as high signal on T1-weighted scans. Mixed lesions with solid and cystic components show heterogeneity of the signal.

Ultrasound is diagnostic in head and neck lymphangiomas but does not fully demonstrate retropharyngeal, axillary and mediastinal extension

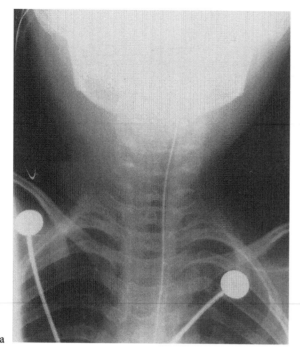

a

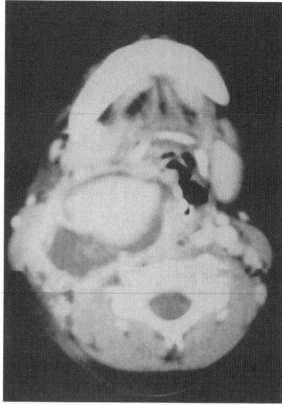

b

Fig. 11.14 a,b. External carotid artery false aneurysm. **a** A 3-year-old girl presented to the Emergency Department with an acute tender neck mass on the right. She had coughed up a little blood and was pyrexial. A plain AP radiograph of the neck demonstrates the presence of a soft tissue mass on the right side and deviation of the trachea to the left. **b** CT scan following intravenous injection of contrast medium shows a large area of low density with marked central enhancement in the right side of the neck with positive mass effect. Note the normal neck vessels on the left. Angiography demonstrated a false aneurysm of the origin of the right external carotid artery. Cause unknown

(BORECKY et al. 1995; GLASIER et al. 1987). MRI is ideal for demonstrating extension of the mass that is not clinically obvious or demonstrated on ultrasound and is indicated to map it fully. Helpful sequences include T1 following administration of intravenous gadolinium, T2 and STIR (Fig. 11.15).

The surgical treatment of lymphangiomas can be difficult and percutaneous injection of a sclerosing agent such as zein alcohol (Ethibloc) is a therapeutic option (BORECKY et al. 1995) being increasingly adopted for the lesions. Treatment of lymphangiomas is controversial. Many, especially in the mediastinum, regress spontaneously.

11.4.5
Lipomatous Tumours

Superficial fatty lumps rarely cause clinical confusion as they are usually soft well-defined masses. A

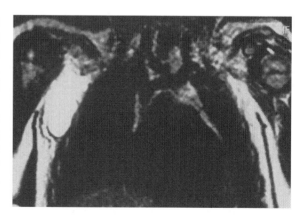

FIG. 11.15. Lymphangioma. A 13-month-old girl presented with a soft right axillary mass. Coronal fat-suppressed T1-weighted MR scan shows a loculated cystic mass in the right axilla which does not extend into the thorax

child may present acutely if the mass detected is firm or hard or if the mass appears suddenly. This is a rare though recognised presentation and causes considerable clinical confusion. An intramuscular lipoma may feel hard with muscle contraction (BJERREGAARD et al. 1989) and cause concern.

Lipomatous tumours are seen frequently in children (KRANSDORF 1995b). A variety of fatty tumours are seen in children which can be classified as simple lipomas, infiltrating lipomas, lipomatosis and lipoblastomas. Simple lipomas are well-defined subcutaneous lesions. Infiltrating lipomas infiltrate skeletal muscle and lipomatosis is where there is diffuse infiltration of fat in a region of the body. This last condition may cause significant deformity and disability and can cause local bony overgrowth. Histological examination of a simple lipoma, infiltrating lipoma and lipomatosis demonstrates mature fat cells. Lipoblastomatous lesions contain a range of fat cells from immature lipoblasts to mature lipocytes (HA et al. 1994). A lipoblastoma is a well-defined mass (Fig. 11.16). Lipoblastomatosis is unencapsulated and diffuse and invades locally into adjacent tissues.

Most childhood lipomatous lesions occur in the posterior thigh (FLETCHER and MARTIN-BATES 1988). Radiological investigations usually suggest the diagnosis. If large enough, the lesion is of fat density on plain x-rays. Ultrasound shows a mass that is hyperechoic to skeletal muscle and fat density is demonstrated on CT scans. Characteristic fat signal is seen on MRI. MRI is very helpful in children with infiltrating lipomatous conditions, to define the extent of the lesion. In addition, signal heterogeneity on MRI may be a sign of malignancy in a lipomatous tumour (SUNDARAM and SHARAFUDDIN 1995). Imaging is indicated in simple lipomas only when there is uncertainty about the nature of a mass.

11.4.6
Dermoid/Epidermoid Tumours

Dermoid and epidermoid tumours are developmental masses formed from heterotopic skin elements. They are hamartomatous lesions (LIST 1941). Most dermoid tumours do not present as an emergency, but this entity should be included in the differential diagnosis of any soft tissue mass, particularly if it lies in the midline.

Emergency presentation may be because of sudden enlargement due to infection of the lesion or more rarely because of CNS infection. Dermoid and

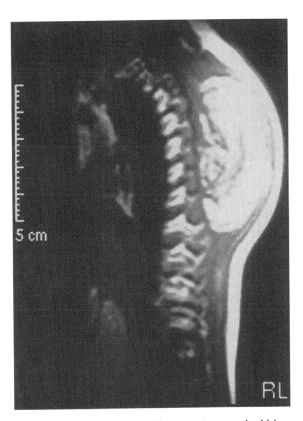

Fig. 11.16. Intramuscular lipoblastoma. A 5-month-old boy was referred by his G.P. He had a large, firm, painless mass over his back. A T1-weighted MR scan shows an encapsulated fatty mass in the muscles of the posterior thoracic wall. Biopsy showed the lesion to be a lipoblastoma

epidermoid tumours occur most frequently in the head. They are usually noted at birth or in the first few months of life. Lesions are most common at the eyebrow and anterior fontanelle (STANNARD and CURRARINO 1990). They occur in the subgaleal or subperiosteal space separate from the skin. At the vertex of the skull they may cause pressure erosion of bone but are rarely associated with a sinus tract and deep extension (STANNARD and CURRARINO 1990). Occipital and fronto-nasal lesions extend deeply and frequently communicate with the central nervous system (STANNARD and CURRARINO 1990). The differential diagnosis of these is a frontal encephalocoele, or a lesion of histiocytosis. The latter may present as a fluctuant mass anywhere on the skull vault and can grow rapidly. The mass often becomes apparent after minor trauma.

The diagnosis can usually be made from the clinical history and examination together with plain radiographs and ultrasound scan. Further imaging is probably not indicated in lesions over the skull vertex (STANNARD and CURRARINO 1990; PETER et al. 1991). However, for lesions at other sites, MRI is required to look for both a sinus track communicating intracranially and the brain structure (Fig. 11.17).

Though not due to a dermoid tumour, similar sinus tracks may be present in association with spinal column neurocutaneous markers, such as a haemangioma over the base of the spine, a hairy tuft or a sacral sinus. There is a significant risk of meningitis with these lesions. In babies under 6 months of age ultrasound is very helpful to look for a sinus track. Over 6 months, MRI is indicated to establish the presence of such a sinus track. The risk of meningitis increases if these lesions are infected.

Plain radiographs show a lucent defect in the skull with flattening of the outer table of the skull on tangential views. Ultrasound is very useful to confirm the cystic nature of the lesion and its location external to the outer table of the skull (STANNARD and CURRARINO 1990). In young babies with an open anterior fontanelle, ultrasound may also demonstrate intracranial extension and further imaging is not necessary.

11.4.7
Fibromatosis

11.4.7.1
Fibromatosis Colli

Fibromatosis colli is a benign condition of neonates and infants that is usually self-limiting. It is also known as sternomastoid tumour. In this condition a fibrotic mass forms in the belly of the sternomastoid muscle and results in torticollis. The diagnosis is usually made clinically but ultrasound will show the lesion well. The ultrasound appearances are diagnostic and other imaging or biopsy is not indicated (GLASIER et al. 1987). If a biopsy is performed the histology shows proliferated fibroblasts and residual muscle fibres (PATRICK et al. 1986). Ultrasound scans show an ovoid or round mass in the sternomastoid muscle that appears iso-, hyper- or hypoechoic to the muscle (CRAWFORD et al. 1988). (Fig. 11.18).

11.4.7.2
Fibromatosis

Children with fibromatosis have areas of proliferation of fibrous tissue in the body. Histologically there are interlacing bundles of plump spindle cells with

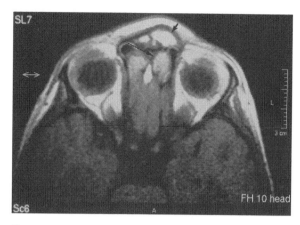

Fig. 11.17. Fronto-nasal dermoid. A 4-year-old girl presented to the Emergency Department with a soft tissue mass above the bridge of the nose. It had been present for 2 weeks. A T1-weighted MR scan shows a mixed signal lesion exterior to the skull vault (*short arrow*). A dermal sinus tract communicates deeply (*long arrow*)

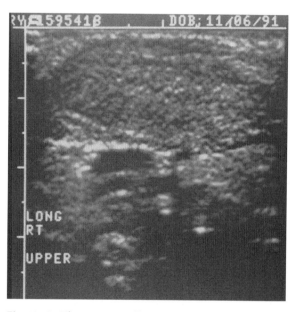

Fig. 11.18. Fibromatosis colli. A 2-week-old infant born by breech delivery had a firm mass in the right side of the neck. The ultrasound scan shows a characteristic ovoid mass slightly hyperechoic to muscle in the belly of the sternocleidomastoid muscle

variable mitotic activity (ENZINGER and WEISS 1995). Lesions are locally aggressive and may recur following resection. The fibromatoses have been classified into superficial or deep (ENZINGER and WEISS 1995). Children and adolescents most frequently have deep lesions also known as "musculo-aponeurotic fibromatoses". These may be intra- or extra-abdominal (VINNICOMBE and HALL 1994). In the young, extra-abdominal fibromatosis occurs most often in the chest wall, shoulder, back and knee. The condition grows slowly over weeks or months (VINNICOMBE and HALL 1994) and is unlikely to present as an acute mass. The CT and MRI appearances are well described and masses may be difficult to distinguish from malignant lesions on imaging studies (MOSKOVIC et al. 1992; VAN SLYKE et al. 1995).

11.4.8
Malignant Lesions

When a child develops a soft tissue mass acutely the concern is that there is a malignancy present. The majority of lesions are due to benign processes as discussed previously. Rapid growth of a lesion suggests a malignancy but biopsy is necessary to make a definite diagnosis and exclude a malignant process.

The role of imaging in a suspected lesion is to identify the borders of the lesion, to plan an appropriate biopsy approach that does not compromise subsequent limb salvage surgery and to identify metastatic spread. Initial imaging should include ultrasound with colour Doppler studies and a chest x-ray. Full staging will require nuclear medicine studies, MRI and chest CT. Dependent on the clinical examination and initial assessment, these may be done after biopsy, although MRI is usually best done before intervention.

11.4.8.1
Congenital fibrosarcoma

The most common malignant lesion in children under 1 year is congenital fibrosarcoma (KRANSDORF 1995a; VINNICOMBE and HALL 1994). In the literature this has been confused with congenital fibromatosis. Congenital fibrosarcoma is a rapidly growing tumour which may present on the trunk or in a limb. It has a high local recurrence rate and axial tumours have higher rates of metastasis and mortality than peripheral lesions (VINNICOMBE and HALL 1994). Tumour margins and extent are generally demonstrated better on MRI than CT, but bone changes are seen better on CT.

11.4.8.2
Rhabdomyosarcoma

Rhabdomyosarcoma represents 10%–15% of all solid tumours of children (ENZINGER and WEISS

Table 11.1. Proposed classification for childhood rhabdomyosarcoma and related sarcomas (from NEWTON et al. 1995)

I Superior prognosis
a) Botryoid RMS
b) Spindle cell RMS
II Intermediate prognosis
a) Embryonal RMS
III Poor prognosis
a) Alveolar RMS
b) Undifferentiated sarcoma
IV Subtypes whose prognosis is not presently evaluable
a) RMS with rhabdoid features

RMS, Rhabdomyosarcoma.

1988). Recently, a classification of rhabdomyosarcoma and related sarcomas has been developed which is based on prognosis (Table 11.1). It is hoped that a unifying classification will permit comparison among and between multi-institutional studies of children with rhabdomyosarcoma (NEWTON et al. 1995). Rhabdomyosarcomas can occur in the limbs as well as the head and neck, genitourinary tract and retroperitoneum. The clinical presentation is variable but is usually a rapidly enlarging mass on the forearm, hand or foot, which is usually non-painful. Other sites are paratesticular, the pelvic floor and chest and abdominal walls (SEBAG and DUBOIS 1994). Rhabdomyosarcomas frequently metastasise to lung, lymph nodes, mediastinum, brain, liver, and bone and local recurrence following treatment is common (HANNA and FLETCHER 1995).

Imaging is performed for diagnosis, to guide biopsy, to stage disease and to monitor the response to therapy. Ultrasound, CT and MRI all have a role. Generally there are no specific features to aid diagnosis of the tumour on imaging studies unless the mass has infiltrated the surrounding tissues or metastases are present. Open or percutaneous biopsy is required to make a diagnosis (Fig. 11.19).

11.5
The Acutely Swollen Limb

A child with an acutely swollen limb who has not sustained obvious trauma presents a diagnostic challenge. This is an uncommon clinical problem but one which usually requires the services of the radiology department.

The most common cause of limb swelling is local inflammatory change. This is most frequently due to infection.

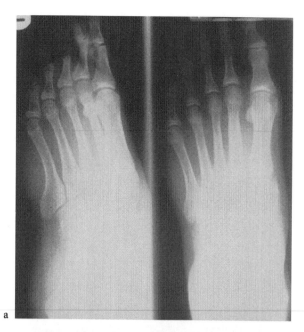

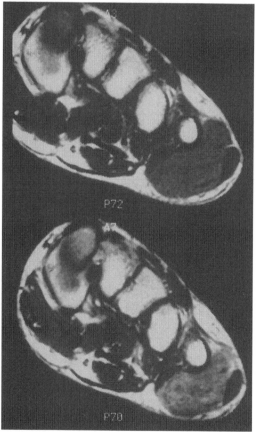

Fig. 11.19 a,b. Rhabdomyosarcoma. **a** A 15-year-old girl had a painful soft tissue mass on the lateral border of her left foot. A plain radiograph shows soft tissue swelling. The bones appear normal. **b** A T1-weighted MR scan shows a well-defined soft tissue mass with a mixed enhancement pattern following intravenous injection of gadolinium (*lower image*)

11.5.1
Soft Tissue Infection

Acute cellulitis is an infection of the subcutaneous fat which affects the superficial fascial planes. Necrotising fasciitis affects the deeper fascial planes and is much more serious. Both conditions will be apparent on plain radiographs and ultrasound scans as soft tissue thickening. However, MRI, with its inherent superior soft tissue contrast, is the best imaging technique to show which soft tissues are involved. MRI demonstrates inflammatory changes in tissues, low signal intensity on T1-weighted images and high signal intensity on T2-weighted images that appears striated (BELTRAN et al. 1987). Enhancement of tissue is seen following intravenous injection of gadolinium (Fig. 11.20).

An abscess can be differentiated from cellulitis on MRI. In the former condition, there is a well-demarcated fluid collection surrounded by a pseudocapsule and enhancement of the rim of the abscess following intravenous administration of gadolinium (BELTRAN et al. 1987).

Osteomyelitis may co-exist with soft tissue abscesses and acute limb swelling may be associated with occult bone infection, especially in the very young. Acute limb swelling may be the presenting clinical feature of occult abdominal sepsis, particularly iliopsoas abscess in neonates and infants under 1 year of age (KEARNEY and CARTY 1997). These children may have redness or induration of the skin over the groin and signs of psoas irritation may be present. Imaging studies need to be directed at the psoas muscle and spine and not simply the groin or affected leg (Fig. 11.21).

11.5.2
Inflammatory Myopathies

Inflammatory myopathies frequently present with acute limb swelling, commonly diffuse calf or thigh swelling. Proliferative myositis is characterised by infiltration of muscles by basophilic giant cells and proliferative fibroblasts. It may not be painful (JELINEK and KRANSDORF 1995). MR scanning is the preferred imaging method for demonstrating muscle abnormalities. The changes seen of diffuse subcutaneous, intramuscular and myofascial oedema and inflammation are non-specific for any myopathy (Fig. 11.22). Pyogenic bacterial myositis is uncommon in children. It is seen particularly in immun-

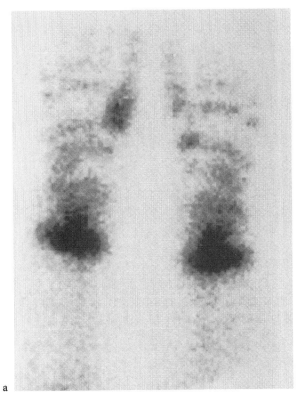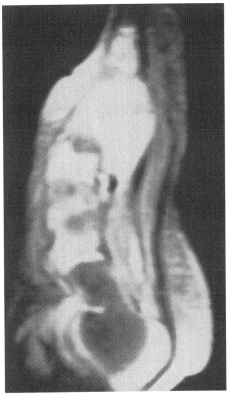

a   b

Fig. 11.20 a,b. Cellulitis and osteomyelitis. **a** A 2½-year-old girl presented to the Emergency Department with acute swelling of the right foot and lower leg. A technetium-99m labelled bone scan demonstrates uptake of isotope along the first metatarsal bone. **b** A sagittal MR scan with fat suppression and T2 weighting following injection of gadolinium shows marked enhancement of the soft tissues medial to the first metatarsal bone and in the sole of the foot. Other images showed evidence of osteomyelitis in the first metatarsal bone

ocompromised patients including those with AIDS (FLECKENSTEIN et al. 1991).

11.5.3
Vascular Abnormalities

11.5.3.1
Lymphoedema

Primary lymphoedema may present with acute limb swelling in childhood (WRIGHT and CARTY 1994). The arm or leg can be affected. The main differential diagnosis is acute deep vein thrombosis.

Primary lymphoedema more frequently affects the legs than the arms. Infrequently, the face and genitalia may be involved. The onset of the condition is at birth or in the teens around puberty. Clinical presentation occurs acutely when there is decompensation of lymphatic drainage, and often follows minor trauma. The diagnosis is usually made clinically. Typically there is pitting oedema of the affected limb. Once limb swelling secondary to a systemic cause has been ruled out, radiological investigation should commence with ultrasound, including Doppler scanning, to exclude vascular causes (WRIGHT and CARTY 1994). These include deep vein thrombosis and vascular malformations. Pelvic ultrasound is also required to exclude secondary obstructive lymphoedema.

Plain radiographs, ultrasound, CT and MRI demonstrate non-specific soft tissue oedema. Scintigraphy can be used both to image the lymphatic system and to obtain information about function and drainage. Various radiopharmaceuticals have been used, including technetium-99m labelled antimony sulphide colloid (WRIGHT and CARTY 1994). However, lymphoscintigraphy does not demonstrate fine anatomical detail. Direct lymphography provides this information and demonstrates lymphatic channels, lymph nodes and the thoracic duct, but is rarely indicated today, unless some form of operative intervention is contemplated.

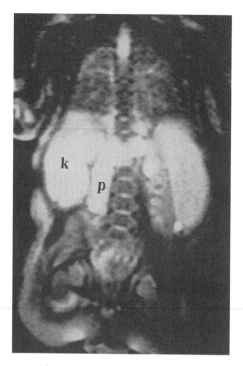

Fig. 11.21. Infective discitis and psoas abscess. A 5-week-old baby was a hospital in-patient undergoing investigations for renal abnormalities. He had unexplained pyrexia. Fat-suppressed T1-weighted coronal MR scan shows the hydronephrotic right kidney is displaced laterally by a fluid collection in the psoas muscle. (The left kidney is also hydronephrotic.) Fluid extends anterior to the spine. *K*, Right kidney; *P*, right psoas muscle

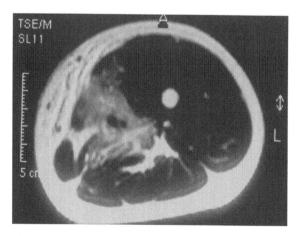

Fig. 11.22. Myositis. A 13-year-old boy presented with painful swelling of the left leg. A T2-weighted MR scan shows oedema of the muscle in the medial and posterior compartments of the thigh. Subcutaneous tissues are thickened and contain linear areas of low signal intensity

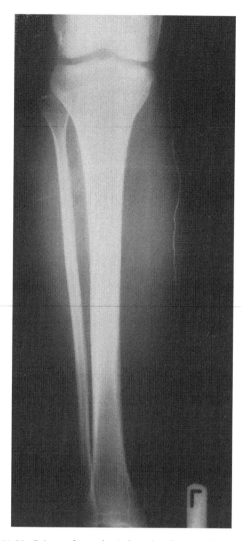

Fig. 11.23. Primary hypoplastic lymphoedema. A 15-year-old girl with acute painful swelling of the left leg. Direct lymphangiogram shows a solitary hypoplastic lymphatic vessel in the lower leg

In primary lymphoedema, lymphography may demonstrate lymphatic hypoplasia where there are small nodes in reduced numbers. There also may be reduced numbers of lymphatic channels. Alternatively the pattern may be lymphatic hyperplasia, where there are increased numbers of dilated, ectatic lymph vessels (SEBAG and DUBOIS 1994).

Children who present acutely with limb swelling usually have primary hypoplastic lymphoedema. They have hypoplasia of the proximal lymphatics, distal distension and nodal fibrosis. The condition affects boys and girls equally and presents with unilateral painful limb swelling (WRIGHT and CARTY 1994) (Fig. 11.23).

11.5.3.2
Deep Vein Thrombosis

Deep venous thrombosis (DVT) is uncommon in children, even when there are risk factors present (ROHRER et al. 1996). However, the diagnosis should be considered in any child with unilateral leg swelling or pain as it does occur in paediatric practise.

Ultrasound with Doppler studies is the appropriate imaging technique to make or exclude the diagnosis of DVT in children. The findings are the same as those in adult patients. In the larger femoral vessels the thrombus may be directly visualised. Absence of the normal venous channel will occur when the vessel is filled with clot. Colour flow Doppler shows absence of flow in complete thrombus, or turbulent flow around a thrombus. If the diagnosis is made with ultrasound, there is no need for contrast venography. This is still indicated in the acutely swollen limb with normal ultrasound. Pulmonary embolus secondary to a DVT is also rare in children.

11.5.3.3
Vascular Malformation

Mixed vascular lesions may cause acute unilateral limb swelling following trauma or thrombosis in a venous malformation. Rapid growth usually follows haemorrhage or thrombosis following trauma to the lesion (Low 1994). Ultrasound and MRI studies are required in the first instance before direct angiography is considered.

11.5.4
Reflex Sympathetic Dystrophy

Reflex sympathetic dystrophy (the preferred name) is also known as Sudek's atrophy or shoulder-hand syndrome. It occurs in children as well as in adults, and is especially seen in teenage girls following minor trauma. The aetiology of reflex sympathetic dystrophy is uncertain. It is usually preceded by injury, although a variety of causes have been reported. No cause is identified in up to one-third of patients (MERRICK 1998). Symptoms include prolonged pain that is disproportionate to the initial injury. Initially there is hyperaemia in the affected limb. This either resolves or progresses to a later atrophic stage where there is continuing pain and the limb is cold, atrophic and cyanosed. In addition there may be joint stiffness and limb swelling.

Plain radiographs are normal in the initial phase but show osteopenia and soft tissue swelling in the chronic phase. Scintigraphy using a three-phase technetium-99m bone scan can provide the diagnosis. In the early stage of the condition there is increased blood flow and diffuse soft tissue uptake in the blood flow and blood pool images. This is followed by a diffuse increase in all the bones of the affected limb in the third phase (skeletal images). These changes improve as the condition resolves or become less evident if the chronic phase ensues (MERRICK 1998) (Fig. 11.24).

Bone scan changes may be atypical in children, particularly in the early phase of the syndrome, and decreased radioisotope uptake in the affected area may be seen (LEMAHIEU et al. 1988). Bone scanning has been reported to be only 60% sensitive and inconsistent for detecting early disease (KOZIN et al. 1981; INTENZO et al. 1989).

MRI has been proposed as a useful technique for demonstrating soft tissue changes in the early phase (SCHWEITZER et al. 1995). Skin subcutaneous thickening or muscle oedema or both may be seen, together with increased signal in these tissues on T2-weighted images. Subtle soft tissue enhancement

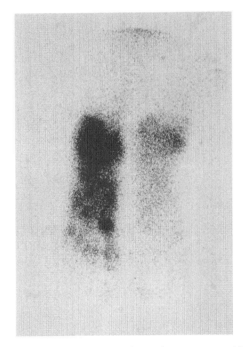

Fig. 11.24. Reflex sympathetic dystrophy. A 12-year-old boy developed painful swelling of his left leg 3 months after sustaining fractures of his metatarsal bones. The skeletal phase of the technetium-99m bone scan demonstrates diffuse increase in tracer uptake in all the bones of the left foot

follows intravenous administration of gadolinium contrast medium in the early phase of reflex sympathetic dystrophy (SCHWEITZER et al. 1995). Muscle atrophy may be seen in patients with late phase disease.

11.5.5
Miscellaneous

Complications of joint-based disease may present as a swollen limb, (the lower limbs are more often affected). For example, rupture of a popliteal cyst can cause sudden onset of pain and swelling in the calf. Popliteal cysts in young children are idiopathic but in older children the incidence of juvenile chronic arthritis increases. The presence of a popliteal cyst may or may not be known about. The symptoms of cyst rupture may be confused with vascular disease, especially DVT. Ultrasound imaging usually distinguishes DVT and a ruptured popliteal cyst. MRI is indicated to show both the extent of the burst cyst and the internal anatomy of the knee joint (Fig. 11.25).

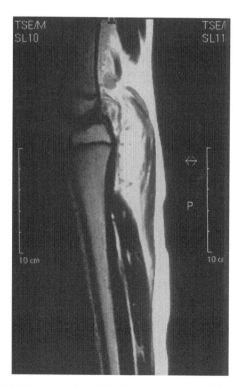

Fig. 11.25. Ruptured popliteal cyst. A 13-year-old boy with juvenile chronic arthritis presented as an emergency with pain and swelling in the calf. A T2-weighted sagittal MR scan shows fluid tracking into the posterior calf from the knee

References

Argent JD, Fairhurst JJ, Clarke NMP (1994) Subcutaneous granuloma annulare: four cases and review of the literature. Pediatr Radiol 24:527–592

Bahadori M, Liebow AA (1973) Plasma cell granuloma of the lung. Cancer 31:191–208

Barton DJ, Miller JH, Allwright SJ, et al. (1992) Distinguishing soft-tissue hemangiomas from vascular malformations using technetium-labelled red blood cell scintigraphy. Plast Reconstr Surg 89:46–55

Beltran J, Noto AM, McGhee RB, et al. (1987) Infections of the musculoskeletal system: high-field-strength MR imaging. Radiology 164:449–454

Bjerregaard P, Hagen K, Dangaard J, Koped H (1989) Intramuscular and intermuscular lipoma of the lower limb. J Bone Joint Surg [Br] 71:812–815

Boothroyd AE, Carty H (1995) The painless soft tissue mass in childhood – tumour or not? Postgrad Med J 71:10–16

Borecky N, Gudinchet F, Laurini R, et al. (1995) Imaging of cervico-thoracic lymphangiomas in children. Pediatr Radiol 25:127–130

Brown G, Shaw D (1995) Inflammatory pseudotumours in children. CT and ultrasound appearances with histopathological correlation. Clin Radiol 50:782–786

Buetow PC, Kransdorf MJ, Moser RP, et al. (1990) Radiologic appearance of intramuscular haemangioma with emphasis on MR imaging. AJR 154:563–567

Burrows PE, Mulliken JB, Fellows KE, Strand RD (1983) Childhood haemangiomas and vascular malformations. AJR 141:483–488

Carithers HA (1985) Cat-scratch disease: an overview based on a study of 1200 patients. Am J Dis Child 139:1124–1133

Carty HML (1994) Sports injuries in children – a radiological viewpoint. Arch Dis Child 70:457–460

Cohen EK, Kressel HY, Perosio T, et al. (1988) MR imaging of soft tissue haemangiomas: correlation with pathologic findings. AJR 150:1079–1081

Crawford SC, Harnsberger HR, Johnson L, et al. (1988) Fibromatosis colli of infancy: CT and sonographic findings. AJR 151:1183–1184

Day DL, Sane S, Dehner LP (1986) Inflammatory pseudotumour of the mesentery and small intestine. Pediatr Radiol 16:210–215

De Smet AA (1993) Magnetic resonance findings in skeletal muscle tears. Skeletal Radiol 22:479–484

Donaldson JS (1989) Pediatric musculoskeletal US. In: Poznanski AK, Kirkpatrick JA (eds) A categorical course in pediatric radiology. Radiological Society of North America, Illinois, pp 77–88

Enzinger FM, Weiss SW (1988) Rhabdomyosarcoma. In: Enzinger FM, Weiss SW (eds) Soft tissue tumors. Mosby, St. Louis, pp 448–488

Enzinger FM, Weiss SW (1995) In: Enzinger FM, Weiss SW (eds) Soft tissue tumours, 3rd edn Mosby, St. Louis, pp 165–268

Fitzgerald EJ, Bowsher WG, Ruttley MST (1986) False aneurysm of the femoral artery: computed tomographic and ultrasound appearances. Clin Radiol 37:585–588

Fleckenstein JL, Burns DK, Murphy FK, et al. (1991) Differential diagnosis of bacterial myositis in AIDS: Evaluation with MR imaging. Radiology 179:653–658

Fletcher CDM, Martin-Bates E (1988) Intramuscular and intermuscular lipoma: neglected diagnoses. Histopathology 12:275–287

Gerle RD (1971) Thorn-induced pseudo-tumours of bone. Br J Radiol 44:642–645

Glasier CM, Seibert JJ, Williamson SL, et al. (1987) High resolution ultrasound characterization of soft tissue masses in children. Pediatr Radiol 17:233–237

Goldman AB (1976) Myositis ossificans circumscripta: a benign lesion with a malignant differential diagnosis. AJR 126:32–40

Gooding GAW, Hardman T, Sumers M, et al. (1987) Sonography of the hand and foot in foreign body detection. J Ultrasound Med 6:441–447

Ha TV, Kleinman PK, Fraire A, et al. (1994) MR imaging of benign fatty tumours in children. Skeletal Radiol 23:361–367

Hanna SL, Fletcher BD (1995) MR imaging of soft tissue tumors. In: Weatherall PT (ed) Musculoskeletal soft-tissue imaging. Magnetic Resonance Imaging Clinics of North America. Saunders, Philadelphia, 3:629–650

Higgins JNP, Haddock JAA, Shaw DG (1993) Case report: soft tissue and perivisceral calcification occurring in an infant; a case of brown fat necrosis. Br J Radiol 66:366–368

Intenzo C, Kim S, Millin J, et al. (1989) Scintigraphic patterns of the reflex sympathetic dystrophy of the lower extremities. Clin Nucl Med 14:657–661

Jelinek J, Kransdorf MJ (1995) MR imaging of soft-tissue masses: mass-like lesions that simulate neoplasms. In: Weatherall PT (ed) Musculoskeletal soft-tissue imaging. Magnetic Resonance Imaging Clinics of North America. Saunders, Philadelphia, 3:727–741

Johnson LC (1948) Histogenesis of myositis ossificans. Am J Pathol 24:681–682

Kaplan PA, Matamoros A, Anderson JC (1990) Sonography of the musculoskeletal system. AJR 155:237–245

Kearney SE, Carty H (1997) Pelvic musculoskeletal infection in infants – diagnostic difficulties and radiological features. Clin Radiol 52:782–786

Keller PM, Simon MS (1988) Post traumatic false aneurysm simulating a soft tissue tumor. Orthopaedics 2:641–643

Kirkpatrick JS, Koman LA, Rovere GD (1987) The role of ultrasound in the early diagnosis of myositis ossificans. Am J Sports Med 15:179–181

Kozin F, Soin JS, Ryan LM, et al. (1981) Bone scintigraphy in the reflex sympathetic dystrophy syndrome. Radiology 138:437–443

Kramer FL, Kurtz AB, Rubin C, Goldberg BB (1979) Ultrasound appearance of myositis ossificans. Skeletal Radiol 4:19–20

Kransdorf MJ (1995a) Malignant soft-tissue tumors in a large referral population: distribution of diagnoses by age, sex, and location. AJR 164:129–134

Kransdorf MJ (1995b) Benign soft tissue tumors in a large referral populaiton. Distribution of specific diagnoses by age, sex and location. AJR 164:395–402

Kransdorf MJ, Meiss JM, Jelinek JS (1991) Myositis ossificans: MR appearance with radiologic-pathologic correlation. AJR 157:1243–1248

Latifi HR, Siegel MJ (1994) Colour Doppler flow imaging of pediatric soft tissue masses. J Ultrasound Med 13:165–169

Lemahieu RA, Van Laere C, Verbruggen LA (1988) Reflex sympathetic dystrophy: an under reported syndrome in children? Eur J Pediatr 147:47–50

Levine C (1989) Primary disorders of the lymphatic vessels – a unified concept. J Pediatr Surg 24:233–240

List CF (1941) Intraspinal epidermoids, dermoids and dermal sinuses. Surg Gynecol Obstet 73:525–538

Low DW (1994) Haemangiomas and vascular malformations. Semin Pediatr Surg 3:40–61

Mallory SB (1991) Neonatal skin disorders. Pediatr Clin North Am 38:745–761

Maylahn DJ (1952) Thorn-induced "tumors" of bone. J Bone Joint Surg [Am] 34:386–389

Merrick MV (1998) Essentials of nuclear medicine. Springer, London Berlin Heidelkerg New York, pp 49–50

Monzon CM, Gilchrist GS, Burgher EO, et al. (1982) Plasma cell granuloma of the lung in children. Pediatrics 70:268–274

Morris SJ, Adams H (1995) Paediatric intramuscular haemangiomata – don't overlook the phlebolith. Br J Radiol 63:208–211

Moskovic E, Serpell JW, Parsons C, et al. (1992) Benign mimics of soft tissue sarcomas. Clin Radiol 46:248–252

Mulliken JB, Glowacki J (1982) Haemangiomas and vascular malformations in infants and children. A classification based on endothelial characteristics. Plast Reconstr Surg 69:412–420

Nessi R, Betti R, Bencini PL, et al. (1990) Ultrasonography of nodular and infiltrative lesions of the skin and subcutaneous tissues. J Clin Ultrasound 18:103–109

Newton WA, Gehan EA, Webber BL, et al. (1995) Classification of the rhabdomyosarcomas and related sarcomas. Cancer 76:1073–1085

Nuovo MA, Norman A, Chumas J, Ackerman LV (1992) Myositis ossificans with atypical clinical, radiographic or pathologic findings: a review of 23 cases. Skeletal Radiol 21:87–92

Pakter RL, Fishman EK, Zerhouni EA (1987) Calf – computed tomography and magnetic resonance. Skeletal Radiol 16:393

Patrick LE, O'Shea P, Simoneaux SF, et al. (1996) Fibromatoses of childhood: the spectrum of radiographic findings. Am J Roentgenol 166:163–169

Peck RJ, Metreweli C (1988) Early myositis ossificans: a new echographic sign. Clin Radiol 39:586–588

Peter JC, Sinclair Smith C, de Villiers JC (1991) Midline dermal sinuses and cysts and their relationship to the central nervous system. Eur J Pediatr Surg 1:73–79

Rauch RF, Silverman PM, Korobkin M, et al. (1984) Coputed tomography of benign angiomatous lesions of the extremities. J Comput Assist Tomogr 8:1143–1146

Rey C, Marache P, Watel A, et al. (1987) Iatrogenic aneurysm in a brachial artery in an infant. Eur J Pediatr 146:438–439

Rohrer MJ, Cutler BS, MacDougall E, et al. (1996) A prospective study and the incidence of deep venous thrombosis in hospitalised children. J Vasc Surg 24:46–49

Schweitzer ME, Mandel S, Schwartzman RJ, et al. (1995) Reflex sympathetic dystrophy revisited: MR imaging findings before and after infusion of contrast material. Radiology 195:211–214

Sebag G, Dubois J (1994) The soft tissues. In: Carty H, Brunelle F, Shaw D, Kendall B (eds) Imaging children. Churchill Livingstone, Edinburgh, pp 1303–1368

Shackleford GD, Barton LL, McAlister WH (1975) Calcified subcutaneous fat necrosis in infancy. J Can Assoc Radiol 26:203–207

Sheddon AL, Narla LD (1991) Plasma cell granuloma presenting as an iliopsoas mass – mimicking a rhabdomyosarcoma. Pediatr Radiol 21:444

Shiels WE, Babcock DS, Wilson JL, Burch RA (1990) Localization of and guided removal of soft tissue foreign bodies with sonography. AJR 155:1277–1281

Stannard MW, Currarino G (1990) Subgaleal dermoid cyst of the anterior fontanelle; diagnosis with sonography. AJNR 11:349–352

Sundaram M, Sharafuddin MJA (1995) MR imaging of benign soft-tissue masses. In: Weatherall PT (ed) Mulsuloskeletal soft-tissue imaging. Magnetic Resonance Imaging Clinics of North America. Saunders, Philadelphia, 3:609–627

Tsai TS, Evans HA, Donnelly LF, et al. (1997) Fat necrosis after trauma: a benign cause of palpable lumps in children. AJR 169:1623–1626

Van Slyke MA, Moser RP, Madewell JE (1995) MR imaging of periarticular soft tissue lesions. In: Weatherall PT (ed) Musculoskeletal soft tissue imaging. Magnetic Resonance Clinics of North America. Saunders, Philadelphia, 3:651–667.

Vinnicombe SJ, Hall CM (1994) Infantile fibrosarcoma: radiologic and clinical features. Skeletal Radiol 23:337

Wicks JD, Silver TM, Bree RL (1978) Gray scale features of haematomas have an ultrasonic spectrum. AJR 131:977–980

Willemsen P, De Roover D, Kockx M, et al. (1997) Mycotic common carotid artery anerysm in an immunosuppressed pediatric patient: case report. J Vasc Surg 25:784–785

Wright NB, Carty HML (1994) The swollen leg and primary lymphoedema. Arch Dis Child 71:44–49

Wu JP, Yunis EJ, Fetterman G, et al. (1973) Inflammatory pseudotumours of the abdomen; plasma cell granulomas. J Clin Pathol 26:943–948

Yu JS, Resnick D (1994) MR imaging of the accessory soleus muscle: appearance in six patients and review of the literature. Skeletal Radiol 23:525–528

Subject Index

List of Contributors

Lawrence J. Abernethy, MB, ChB, FRCR
Consultant Paedriatric Radiologist
Royal Liverpool Children's NHS Trust
Alder Hey Children's Hospital
Eaton Road
Liverpool L12 2AP
UK

Richard E. Appleton, MB, BS, FRCPCH
Consultant Paediatric Neurologist
Royal Liverpool Children's NHS Trust
Alder Hey Children's Hospital
Eaton Road
Liverpool L12 2AP
UK

Helen Carty, MB, FRCR, FRCPI, FRCP, FFRCSI
Professor of Paediatric Radiology
Royal Liverpool Children's NHS Trust
Alder Hey Children's Hospital
Eaton Road
Liverpool L12 2AP
UK

Andrew W. Duncan, MD, FRCR, FRCPh, DMRD
Consultant Paediatric Radiologist
Clinical Senior Lecturer in Paediatric Radiology
University of Bristol
Department of Radiology
Bristol Royal Hospital for Sick Children
St. Michael's Hill
Bristol BS2 8BJ
UK

David Grier, MB, FRCR, Psch
Consultant Radiologist
Bristol Royal Hospital for Sick Children
St. Michael's Hill
Bristol BS2 8BJ
UK

Katharine E. Halliday, MB, FRCR
Queen's Medical Centre
Nottingham NG7 2UH
UK

Anne S. Hollman, MB, ChB, MRCP, FRCR
Consultant Paediatric Radiologist
Department of Paediatric Radiology
Royal Hospital for Sick Children
Yorkhill
Glasgow G3 8SJ
UK

Susan J. King, MBChB, MRCP, FRCR
Consultant Paediatric Radiologist
Royal Liverpool Children's NHS Trust
Alder Hey Children's Hospital
Eaton Road
Liverpool L12 2AP
UK

Sumaira Macdonald, MB, BCh, FRCR
Consultant Paediatric Radiologist
Royal Hospital for Sick Children
Yorkhill
Glasgow G3 8SJ
UK

Clive W. Majury, FRCR, FFRRCSI
Consultant Radiologist
Ulster Hospital
Upper Newtownards Road
Dundonald
Belfast BT16 0RH
United Kingdom

William Ramsden, BM, FRCR
Consultant Paediatric Radiologist
St. James's University Hospital
Beckett Street
Leeds LS9 7TF
UK

Dr. Padma Rao, BSc Hons, MB BS, MRCP, FRCR
Lecturer in Paediatric Radiology
Royal Liverpool Children's NHS Trust
Alder Hey Children's Hospital
Eaton Road
Liverpool L12 2AP
UK

John M. Somers, MB, BS, FRCR
Consultant Paediatric Radiologist
Queen's Medical Centre
Nottingham NG7 2UH
UK

Louise E. Sweeney, MB, FRCR
Consultant Radiologist
X-Ray Department
Royal Belfast Hospital for Sick Children
180 Falls Road
Belfast BT12 6BE
United Kingdom

Neville B. Wright, MB, DMRD, FRCR
Consultant Paediatric Radiologist
Manchester Children's Hospitals NHS Trust
Royal Manchester Children's Hospital
Hospital Road
Pendlebury
Manchester M27 4HA
UK

R.E. Richard Wright, FRCR, FFRRCSI
Consultant Radiologist
Ulster Hospital
Upper Newtownards Road
Dundonald
Belfast BT16 ORH
United Kingdom

MEDICAL RADIOLOGY
Diagnostic Imaging and Radiation Oncology

Titles in the series already published

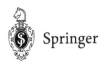 Springer

MEDICAL RADIOLOGY
Diagnostic Imaging and Radiation Oncology

Titles in the series already published

RADIATION ONCOLOGY

Lung Cancer
Edited by C. W. Scarantino

Innovations in Radiation Oncology
Edited by H. R. Withers
and L. J. Peters

**Radiation Therapy of Head
and Neck Cancer**
Edited by G. E. Laramore

Gastrointestinal Cancer – Radiation Therapy
Edited by R. R. Dobelbower, Jr.

**Radiation Exposure and
Occupational Risks**
Edited by E. Scherer, C. Streffer,
and K.-R. Trott

**Radiation Therapy of Benign
Diseases - A Clinical Guide**
S.E. Order and S.S. Donaldson

**Interventional Radiation Therapy
Techniques - Brachytherapy**
Edited by R. Sauer

Radiopathology of Organs and Tissues
Edited by E. Scherer,
C. Streffer, and K.-R. Trott

**Concomitant Continuous Infusion
Chemotherapy and Radiation**
Edited by M. Rotman
and C. J. Rosenthal

**Intraoperative Radiotherapy –
Clinical Experiences and Results**
Edited by F. A. Calvo,
M. Santos, and L. W. Brady

**Radiotherapy of Intraocular
and Orbital Tumors**
Edited by W. E. Alberti
and R. H. Sagerman

**Interstitial and Intracavitary
Thermoradiotherapy**
Edited by M. H. Seegenschmiedt
and R. Sauer

**Non-Disseminated Breast Cancer
Controversial Issues
in Management**
Edited by G. H. Fletcher
and S. H. Levitt

**Current Topics in Clinical Radiobiology
of Tumors**
Edited by H.-P. Beck-Bornholdt

**Practical Approaches to Cancer Invasion
and Metastases**
A Compendium of Radiation
Oncologists' Responses to 40 Histories
Edited by A. R. Kagan with the
Assistance of R. J. Steckel

Radiation Therapy in Pediatric Oncology
Edited by J. R. Cassady

Radiation Therapy Physics
Edited by A. R. Smith

Late Sequelae in Oncology
Edited by J. Dunst and R. Sauer

Mediastinal Tumors. Update 1995
Edited by D.E. Wood
and C.R. Thomas, Jr.

**Thermoradiotherapy
and Thermochemotherapy**

Volume 1:
Biology, Physiology, and Physics

Volume 2:
Clinical Applications
Edited by M. H. Seegenschmiedt,
P. Fessenden, and C. C. Vernon

Carcinoma of the Prostate
Innovations in Management
Edited by Z. Petrovich,
L. Baert, and L.W. Brady

**Radiation Oncology
of Gynecological Cancers**
Edited by H. W. Vahrson

Carcinoma of the Bladder
Innovations in Management
Edited by Z. Petrovich,
L. Baert, and L. W. Brady

**Blood Perfusion and Microenvironment
of Human Tumors**
Implications for Clinical
Radiooncology
Edited by M. Molls and P. Vaupel

**Radiation Therapy of Benign Diseases.
A Clinical Guide**
2nd Revised Edition
S. E. Order and S. S. Donaldson

**Carcinoma of the Kidney and Testis,
and Rare Urologic Malignancies**
Innovations in Management
Edited by Z. Petrovich,
L. Baert, and L. W. Brady

**Progress and Perspectives
in the Treatment of Lung Cancer**
Edited by P. Van Houtte, J. Klastersky,
and P. Rocmans

**Combined Modality Therapy of
Central Nervous System Tumors**
Edited by Z. Petrovich, L. W. Brady,
M. L. Apuzzo, and M. Bamberg

Age-Related Macular Degeneration
Current Treatment Concepts
Edited by W. A. Alberti, G. Richards,
and R. H. Sagerman

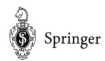 Springer

10415271R0

Made in the USA
Lexington, KY
23 July 2011